Total Parenteral Nutrition

Total Parenteral Nutrition

Second Edition

Edited by

Josef E. Fischer, M.D.

Christian R. Holmes Professor and
Chairman of Surgery, University of
Cincinnati College of Medicine;
Surgeon-in-Chief, University Hospital,
Cincinnati

Little, Brown and Company
Boston/Toronto/London

Library of Congress Catalog Card No. 91-62295

ISBN 0-316-28379-7
Printed in the United States of America
MV-NY

To Karen, Erich, and Alexandra

Contents

II. Specific Aspects

III. Supplemental Techniques

Preface

Much time has elapsed since publication of the first edition of *Total Parenteral Nutrition*. Since that time, the field of total parenteral nutrition (TPN) has matured in a number of ways. It is fair to say that there is no longer the unabashed enthusiasm that greeted the advent of TPN as an almost miraculous therapy. Shortcomings and complications have become appreciated, and we have a much better idea of which patients are appropriate for nutritional support and which (and it turns out to be a far greater number than originally thought) are not. We are aware of our limitations, of what we can and cannot do. A whole new series of solutions and approaches has been advocated, some of which have efficacy and some of which do not. Especially during the past eight years, the gut has been rediscovered; it is fair to say that there is much greater emphasis on the use of the gut, when possible, and there is greater effort to use the gut than had heretofore been appreciated.

Most exciting, however, is the ushering in of the principles of nutritional pharmacology. We are at the threshold of this era in nutritional support. Nutritional pharmacology, a phrase coined by Dr. J. Wesley Alexander, is the utilization of normal nutritional components in either supranormal amounts or in specified, directed amounts in order to achieve pharmacologic rather than nutritional effects. Although still in its infancy, examples of such nutritional pharmacologic approaches abound in this volume.

As with the previous edition, this volume captures parenteral nutrition, a rapidly evolving field still in its youth, at a specific point in time. When a third edition is published, it is certan that there will have been a tremendous evolution in what we understand and what we can do for our patients.

J.E.F.

Contributing Authors

J. Wesley Alexander, M.D., Sc.D.
Professor of Surgery, and Director of
Transplantation Division, University of
Cincinnati College of Medicine, Cincinnati

Adrian Barbul, M.D.
Associate Professor of Surgery, Johns
Hopkins University School of Medicine;
Assistant Surgeon-in-Chief, Sinai Hospital
of Baltimore, Baltimore

Daniel W. Benson, M.D.
Resident, Department of Surgery,
University of Cincinnati Medical Center,
Cincinnati

Robert H. Bower, M.D.
Associate Professor of Surgery, University
of Cincinnati College of Medicine; Director
of Nutrition Support Service, University
Hospital, Cincinnati

Murray F. Brennan, M.D.
Attending Physician, Department of
Surgery, Memorial Sloan-Kettering Cancer
Center, New York

Gordon P. Buzby, M.D.
Associate Professor of Surgery, University
of Pennsylvania School of Medicine;
Attending Physician, Hospital of the
University of Pennsylvania, Philadelphia

Frank B. Cerra, M.D.
Professor of Surgery, University of
Minnesota Medical School—Minneapolis;
Director of Surgical Critical Care and
Nutrition Support Service, University of
Minnesota Hospital and Clinic, Minneapolis

Nicolas V. Christou, M.D., Ph.D.
Associate Professor of Surgery, McGill
University Faculty of Medicine; Attending
Surgeon and Director of Surgical Intensive
Care Unit, Department of Surgery, Royal
Victoria Hospital, Montreal

John M. Daly, M.D.
Jonathan E. Rhoads Professor of Surgery,
University of Pennsylvania School of
Medicine; Chief, Division of Surgical
Oncology, Hospital of the University of
Pennsylvania, Philadelphia

Crystal L. Davis, R.N., B.S.N.
Nurse Clinician, Nutrition Support Service,
University of Cincinnati Medical Center,
Cincinnati

Josef E. Fischer, M.D.
Christian R. Holmes Professor and
Chairman of Surgery, University of
Cincinnati College of Medicine;
Surgeon-in-Chief, University Hospital,
Cincinnati

James F. Flowers, M.D.
Chief Surgical Resident, Virginia Mason
Medical Center, Seattle

Herbert R. Freund, M.D.
Professor of Surgery, Hebrew
University-Hadassah Medical School; Chief
of Surgery, Hadassah University
Hospital-Mount Scopus, Jerusalem

Michele M. Gottschlich, Ph.D.
Adjunct Assistant Professor of Health and
Nutrition Sciences, University of Cincinnati
College of Medicine; Director of Nutrition
Services, Shriners Burns Hospital,
Cincinnati

JoAnn Gough, C.R.N.I.
Clinical Director of I.V. Therapy, Virginia
Mason Medical Center, Seattle

Per-Olof Hasselgren, M.D.
Associate Professor of Surgery, University
of Cincinnati College of Medicine,
Cincinnati

Graham L. Hill, M.D.
Professor and Chairman of Surgery,
Auckland Hospital, Auckland, New
Zealand

Darryl T. Hiyama, M.D.
Assistant Clinical Professor of Surgery,
University of California, Los Angeles,
UCLA School of Medicine, Los Angeles;
Attending Surgeon, Olive View Medical
Center, Sylmar, California

Danny O. Jacobs, M.D., M.P.H.
Assistant Professor of Surgery, Harvard
Medical School; Associate Surgeon, Brigham
and Women's Hospital, Boston

Khursheed N. Jeejeebhoy, Ph.D.
Professor of Medicine, University of
Toronto Faculty of Medicine; Attending
Gastroenterologist, St. Michael's Hospital,
Toronto

John M. Kinney, M.D.
Visiting Professor and Physician,
Rockefeller University; Attending Physician,
Departments of Medicine and Surgery,
St. Luke's-Roosevelt Hospital, New York

Jarol B. Knowles, M.D.
Assistant Professor of Medicine, McGill
University Faculty of Medicine; Attending
Physician, Division of Gastroenterology,
Royal Victoria Hospital, Montreal

Scott A. Kripke, M.D.
Research Fellow, Harrison Department
of Surgical Research, University of

Pennsylvania School of Medicine,
Philadelphia

Richard J. LaFrance, Pharm. D.
Pharmacy Manager, New England Critical
Care, Seattle

Shujun Li, M.D.
Associate Professor of Surgery, Beijing
Medical University, Beijing; Clinical Fellow,
Nutritional Support, University of
Cincinnati Medical Center, Cincinnati

Daniel K. Lowe, M.D.
Associate Professor of Surgery, Yale
University School of Medicine, New Haven

James D. Luketich, M.D.
Attending Physician, Hospital of the
University of Pennsylvania, Philadelphia

Clyde I. Miyagawa, Pharm. D.
Clinical Pharmacy Specialist, University
Hospital, Cincinnati

Randall S. Moore, M.D.
Assistant Professor of Gastroenterology and
Hepatology, University of Minnesota
Medical School—Minneapolis; Medical
Director of Comprehensive Home
Alimentation Management Program and
Director, Nutrition Section, University of
Minnesota Hospital and Clinic, Minneapolis

James L. Mullen, M.D.
Associate Professor of Surgery, University
of Pennsylvania School of Medicine;
Director, Nutrition Support, Hospital of the
University of Pennsylvania, Philadelphia

Marsha E. Orr, R.N., M.S.
Associate Director, Nutrition Support,
University of Cincinnati Medical Center,
Cincinnati

Michael D. Peck, M.D., Sc.D.
Assistant Professor of Surgery, University
of Miami School of Medicine; Assistant
Director, University of Miami-Jackson
Memorial Burn Center, Jackson Memorial
Hospital, Miami

John L. Rombeau, M.D.
Associate Professor of Surgery, University
of Pennsylvania School of Medicine;
Attending Surgeon, Hospital of the
University of Pennsylvania, Philadelphia

John A. Ryan, Jr., M.D.
Clinical Associate Professor of Surgery,
University of Washington School of
Medicine; Head of General Surgery,
Virginia Mason Medical Center, Seattle

Harry C. Sax, M.D.
Assistant Professor of Surgery, University
of Rochester School of Medicine and
Dentistry; Attending Surgeon and Medical
Director, Adult Nutritional Support Service,
The Strong Memorial Hospital, Rochester

Lisa M. Sclafani, M.D.
Instructor of Surgery, Cornell University
Medical College; Assistant Attending
Surgeon, Departments of Surgery and
Nutrition, Memorial Sloan-Kettering Cancer
Center, New York

Harry M. Shizgal, M.D.
Professor of Surgery, McGill University
Faculty of Medicine; Senior Surgeon, Royal
Victoria Hospital, Montreal

J.M. Tellado, M.D.
Attending Surgeon, Cirugia General III,
Hospital General Gregorian Maronon,
Madrid, Spain

Michael H. Torosian, M.D.
Assistant Professor of Surgery, University
of Pennsylvania School of Medicine;
Attending Surgeon, Hospital of the
University of Pennsylvania, Philadelphia

Daniel von Allmen, M.D.
Resident in Surgery, University of
Cincinnati Medical Center, Cincinnati

Glenn D. Warden, M.D.
Professor of Surgery, University of
Cincinnati College of Medicine; Chief of
Staff, Shriners Burns Hospital, Cincinnati

Brad W. Warner, M.D.
Fellow, Pediatric Surgery, University of
Cincinnati College of Medicine; Fellow,
Pediatric Surgery, Children's Hospital
Medical Center, Cincinnati

Douglas W. Wilmore, M.D.
Frank Sawyer Professor of Surgery, Harvard
Medical School; Medical Director of
Nutrition Support Service, Brigham and
Women's Hospital, Boston

I

General Principles

Indications

Harry C. Sax
Per-Olof Hasselgren

HISTORICAL PERSPECTIVES

The history of parenteral nutrition dates to early attempts to infuse various substrates into the veins. Shortly after William Harvey described blood circulation in 1628, Christopher Wren gave intravenous injections of morphine to a dog and oleic acid to a horse, using hollowed goose quills as needles. Attempts at the infusion of various nutrients continued intermittently, usually employing alcohol or milk. The systemic effects were at times disastrous. With the development of protein hydrolysates in the 1930s, peripheral intravenous infusions of amino acids were utilized in the therapy of patients who could not tolerate enteral feedings [16]. However, the near iso-osmolality required of peripheral infusions made provision of adequate non-protein calories by glucose alone impossible. Although the development of lipid infusions improved the situation, it was not until 1952 that Aubaniac's description of subclavian vein cannulation [5] opened the door for hy-

pertonic infusions of glucose, amino acids, and fats into the central circulation. Stanley Dudrick, working in the laboratory of Jonathan Rhoads, was able to demonstrate normal growth and development of beagle puppies, supported solely by intravenous nutrients [14, 15]. A report of growth, positive nitrogen balance, and normal development of a baby girl with intestinal atresia was published by the same group in 1968 [47]. The early 1970s brought rapid growth to this new therapeutic modality with refinements in delivery systems and techniques. As parenteral nutritional support of increasingly ill patients was undertaken, new disease-specific formulations were introduced to address the pathophysiologic changes associated with renal, cardiac, and hepatic failure. The 1980s not only brought new technologies to the field, making provision of total parenteral nutrition (TPN) safe and easy, but also demanded demonstration of therapeutic efficacy to this expensive modality. One must therefore be cognizant of those disease states

Table 1-1. Indications for Total Parenteral Nutrition

Primary therapy
  Efficacy shown
    Short-gut syndrome
    Enterocutaneous fistula
    Renal failure due to acute tubular necrosis
    Hepatic failure (acute decompensation in the face of cirrhosis)
    Burns (when combined with aggressive enteral support)
  Efficacy not shown
    Inflammatory bowel disease
    Anorexia nervosa

Supportive therapy
  Efficacy shown
    Acute radiation enteritis
    Chemotherapy enteritis
    Perioperative support of the clearly malnourished patient
  Efficacy not shown
    Chronic pancreatitis
    Perioperative support in "cardiac cachexia"
    Chronic protein loss from wounds or disease in excess of enteral repletion
    Prolonged respiratory support with ileus

Areas under investigation
  Cancer support
  Sepsis and trauma
  General perioperative support

where TPN is clearly beneficial and, should one choose, be able to defend its use in less clear-cut but still indicated situations. This chapter attempts to define indications, pointing out pitfalls where appropriate, and discusses marginal indications. The indications for TPN are summarized in Table 1-1.

PRIMARY THERAPY: EFFICACY SHOWN

Short-Gut Syndrome

Perhaps the leading use of TPN in the pediatric population is the support of infants with inadequate absorptive surface, due to either congenital defect or loss from necrotizing enterocolitis. In the adult population, short-gut syndrome is usually due to midgut volvulus, multiple resections for Crohn's disease, or mesenteric vascular catastrophe. In many cases TPN is a useful adjunct in supporting the patient while awaiting hypertrophy of the remaining bowel to the point that enteral feeding is tolerated. Patients with as little as 30.5 cm (12 in.) of jejunum, with an intact ileocecal valve and pylorus, have eventually been able to support themselves enterally. A combination of parenteral and enteral support in the interim may be beneficial. The pediatric population presents a somewhat more difficult problem, as long-term TPN is associated with a high rate of significant hepatic dysfunction, leading, in some cases, to acute and chronic liver disease including fulminant hepatic failure and death [34, 41]. This has led some pediatric surgeons to suggest that, if presented with an infant with less than 5 cm of bowel and no ileocecal valve, no attempt at salvage should be made. Our own view is that the hepatic failure in infants and children is probably preventable and that these children should be salvaged.

The patient with short-gut syndrome has deficiencies in absorption of fat-soluble vitamins and vitamin B_{12}, and should be supplemented accordingly. Massive diarrhea may lead to large losses of zinc and magnesium. If prolonged parenteral support is anticipated, cholecystectomy should be performed at the time of initial laparotomy. The incidence of cholelithiasis approaches 100% in patients with short-gut syndrome who receive TPN at home.

Enterocutaneous Fistula

The overall mortality associated with enterocutaneous fistulas has not dramatically decreased since the advent of TPN [20, 43]. However, parenteral nutrition plays an important role in the increased rate of spontaneous closure by breaking the cycle of ongoing protein loss in the succus entericus followed by attempts to increase enteral intake with resultant increased losses. Extensive work by Fischer and others has shown that with TPN the majority of fistulas will close on their own if they do not have the following characteristics: (1) malignancy, (2) adjacent abscess, (3) end fistula, (4) bowel discontinuity, and (5) distal stricture. It should be noted that even if the fistula cannot be closed by TPN alone, the patients tend to be in better condition to tolerate operative therapy after a course of TPN [36].

Renal Failure

The patient with renal failure presents an additional challenge in nutrition due to an ongoing catabolic state. There are wide variations in fluids and electrolytes, and the accumulation of metabolic breakdown products with resultant uremia leads to acidosis. Oral intake is often poor due to anorexia or vomiting from uremia. Major operative intervention or infection is common in patients with renal failure. Although dialysis is effective in correcting fluid and electrolyte imbalance and uremia, additional protein is lost in the dialysate, leading to further catabolism. In the past, dietary manipulations involved protein restriction in an attempt to decrease urea production. However, with the advent of TPN, the provision of "high-quality" protein in the form of essential amino acids became possible. The first randomized prospective trial of this solution in patients who had acute renal failure associated with surgical disease was carried out by Abel and colleagues at the Massachusetts General Hospital [1]. The infusion of hypertonic dextrose and essential amino acids led to a quicker recovery from postoperative acute renal failure than did equicaloric infusion of hypertonic dextrose alone. Overall hospital mortality was not improved; however, in patients with serious complications, such as sepsis, there was improved survival. While subsequent trials have not shown a clear survival advantage to the use of TPN in acute renal failure, nitrogen balance can certainly be improved in these severely catabolic patients [17, 18]. It should be obvious that reversal of the inciting factor (e.g., hypotension or sepsis) is of paramount importance. TPN solutions for renal failure are usually of a higher dextrose concentration in deference to volume con-

straints, and glucose control may be a problem. If the patients are receiving concomitant dialysis, there appears to be no advantage to the use of only essential amino acids, and a balanced amino acid solution is appropriate.

Hepatic Failure

The liver plays a key role in overall organism metabolism. Specifically, its involvement in gluconeogenesis and protein synthesis requires a constant flux of basic nutrients. The amino acids present a continuum in their clearance characteristics. The branched-chain amino acids (BCAAs) leucine, isoleucine, and valine require almost no hepatic function for metabolism, while the aromatic and sulfur-containing amino acids (e.g., phenylalanine and methionine) are cleared only by the liver [19]. It would follow, therefore, that hepatic impairment is characterized by alterations in the ratio between the BCAAs and the aromatic and sulfur-containing amino acids [35].

During hepatic failure, alterations in the blood-brain barrier lead to increased intracerebral concentrations of tryptophan and aromatic amino acids. It is hypothesized that these changes cause neurotransmitter alterations with the development of encephalopathy. Plasma BCAA levels are depressed, as they are catabolized by skeletal muscle peripherally as an energy source [28, 33, 38].

Early proposals for the treatment of hepatic failure centered on protein restriction and purgatives such as lactulose and neomycin. These methods failed to address the basic requirement for substrate to allow liver repair and regeneration. In the mid-1970s, a disease-specific amino acid formulation for hepatic failure was proposed. Its aim was to alter the abnormal peripheral concentrations by increasing levels of the BCAAs and decreasing the aromatic and sulfur-containing amino acids. Clinical studies of the efficacy of these new solutions were plagued by small numbers of patients and lack of homogeneity of the patient population [30, 38, 46]. The patients who would appear to benefit most from specialized solutions are those with acute encephalopathy superimposed on chronic liver disease. The largest study was the U.S. Multicenter Trial with 80 patients. Hypertonic glucose with F080 (the precursor of Hepatamine) was compared with hypertonic glucose and neomycin. Nitrogen equilibrium or positive nitrogen balance was achieved in these protein-intolerant patients. A higher percentage of the patients woke up sooner with F080 and there was a trend toward lower in-hospital mortality, but statistical significance was not reached [9]. Using fat as the nonprotein substrate showed no advantage [30].

It would seem logical that the BCAA-enriched formulations may be of some benefit in the protein-intolerant patient with encephalopathy if one uses wake-up time as the key parameter. The oral formulations (HepaticAid II) have benefited outpatients with chronic liver disease. Disease-specific TPN does not appear to be of clear benefit in fulminant hepatic failure (although a few anecdotal studies claim efficacy) or after hepatic insult such as resection for malignant disease. It is appropriate to support these patients parenterally with standard formulations, reserving hepatic formulations for encephalopathy.

Burns

It has become increasingly clear that the gut plays a major hormonal and bacteriologic role during sepsis. Early, aggressive utilization of the gut decreases the hypermetabolism associated with burns and may improve survival in burn patients [39], and maintenance of gut mucosal integrity is a cornerstone in the prevention of bacterial translocation with subsequent sepsis. Although most septic patients have impaired gastric emptying, the utilization of transpyloric small-bore feeding tubes or jejunostomies will allow at least partial support of the patient via an enteral route. A combined parenteral and enteral approach may also be of benefit, especially in the burn patient, if the gut alone cannot support caloric needs. These are truly hypermetabolic patients, and malnutrition is central to the development of fatal sepsis. The infectious

complications associated with central lines in thermally injured patients may be minimized by utilizing lines for multiple purposes and by rotating line sites every 3 days.

PRIMARY THERAPY: EFFICACY NOT SHOWN

Inflammatory Bowel Disease

The patient with Crohn's disease or ulcerative colitis may require TPN either as primary therapy or as an adjunct to surgical intervention. The patient with Crohn's disease is more likely to have a fistula or short gut. Because the small bowel is primarily involved, a decreased absorptive surface with resultant malnutrition compounds the problem.

Acute exacerbations of symptomatology are relieved by periods of bowel rest with TPN support. The patient with Crohn's disease and short gut after resection may require home TPN while the remainder of his or her bowel hypertrophies to the point that it can provide adequate absorption. Because Crohn's disease frequently affects young females, pregnancy may mandate parenteral nutrition to meet increased calorie and nitrogen requirements. Although fistulas associated with Crohn's disease close with TPN, they tend to reopen. TPN is a useful adjunct to surgical therapy in this situation.

Ulcerative colitis solely involves the colon and rarely responds (over the long term) to TPN. Whereas surgery is to be avoided in the patient with Crohn's disease, surgery is curative in the patient with ulcerative colitis. The current therapy of choice is total colectomy with ileoanal pull-through (Soave procedure). Because this requires stripping of the rectum, a quiescent mucosa is mandatory. TPN has been utilized in the perioperative preparation of patients with ulcerative colitis, as a period of bowel rest appears to aid in "cooling down" the mucosa.

Anorexia Nervosa

Although the treatment of these patients with an inherently normal gastrointestinal tract is primarily psychiatric, malnutrition is clearly rampant. With the advent of soft-bore nasoenteral tubes, the gut is the preferred route to replenishment. In the patient who absolutely refuses therapy that involves the sensations associated with eating, TPN is a useful bridge when combined with effective psychotherapy [21]. [Editor's Note: It may be that parenteral nutrition may be helpful in accepting psychotherapy. The wastage of protein in starvation may affect the brain, and these patients may not be able to deal with psychotherapy until nutritionally repleted.]

SUPPORTIVE THERAPY: EFFICACY SHOWN

Acute Radiation Enteritis and Chemotherapy Enteritis

Numerous clinical studies have been carried out utilizing TPN as an adjunct to chemotherapy, radiation therapy, or surgery [29]. As is common in this type of study, numbers are small and it is easy to commit a type II error. An exception was the study of Müller et al. in which patients undergoing esophagogastrectomy seemed to benefit from perioperative TPN, although the benefits were not confined to an identifiable malnourished group [32]. Taking these studies as a group, there appears to be a reduction in perioperative mortality with a brief (7-day) period of preoperative TPN in clearly malnourished patients with serum albumin levels less than 3.0 g/dl, greater than 4.5-kg (10-lb.) weight loss, and lack of recall anergy [12]. Chemotherapy trials have mixed results, although there are more infectious complications in those patients receiving TPN. There appears to be neither an advantage nor a disadvantage to the use of TPN in all patients receiving radiation therapy; TPN is beneficial in the subgroup with radiation enteritis as shown by Copeland et al. [13]. By the same token, the gut is one of the organ systems most affected by chemotherapy due to its high metabolic rate. TPN is a useful adjunct during periods when the gut cannot support the cancer pa-

tient. Further work is emerging from the laboratory of Souba at the University of Florida which demonstrates gut mucosal protection by the amino acid glutamine during methotrexate therapy. In these groups of patients, TPN is an indicated adjunct, although use of the gut remains preferable, even in small amounts.

Perioperative Support of the Clearly Malnourished Patient

Growing evidence supports the advantages of enteral feeding in the patient with a functioning gastrointestinal tract [3, 31, 44]. It is perfectly appropriate to initiate TPN in the severely malnourished patient with, for example, esophageal carcinoma, and then achieve enteral access at the time of laparotomy and transition to enteral support in the postoperative period.

SUPPORTIVE THERAPY: EFFICACY NOT SHOWN

Chronic Pancreatitis

At least two studies have shown no advantage of TPN early in the course of acute pancreatitis. In both studies, a higher rate of catheter line infection and prolonged hospital stay were observed in patients receiving TPN [23, 42]. TPN is appropriate in the patient with a postpancreatitis phlegmon or pseudocyst, if necessary, while awaiting its maturation or spontaneous resolution [40]. We have also used home TPN in patients with chronic pancreatitis and severe parenchymal involvement not associated with correctable surgical lesions. One must also consider the enteral route in these patients, especially if access to the jejunum is achieved during surgery and an elemental or other chemically defined diet is utilized. TPN is appropriate in the fulminantly ill patient with acute pancreatitis or abscess.

Cardiac Cachexia

Although one does not associate atherosclerotic cardiovascular disease with malnutrition, a subgroup of patients with chronic congestive heart failure is clearly at nutritional risk. The so-called "cardiac cachexia" revolves around a chronic low-flow state. The general unpalatability of a cardiac diet, anorexia, and malabsorption lead to protein-calorie malnutrition. The hypoalbuminemic state is exacerbated by the peripheral edema already present [27]. Experimental work in dogs has demonstrated this to be a vicious cycle, with malnutrition directly affecting left ventricular function and increasing intestinal edema, making malabsorption more prominent [2].

Clearly, not all patients with cardiac disease will require TPN. However, the subgroup of patients with long-standing cardiac failure, especially on a valvular basis, may well benefit from perioperative support. [*Editor's Note:* The recovery of cardiac muscle and function is disappointingly slow. Nutritional support may be required for a prolonged period of time and, at that, recovery may be limited.]

Chronic Protein Loss

Patients with large open wounds or protein wasting states may not be able to maintain themselves by the enteral route alone. TPN is appropriate in this setting. Nitrogen balance studies are helpful in guiding support levels.

Respiratory Failure with Ileus

Many debilitated patients require respiratory support in conjunction with the treatment of pneumonia or sepsis. It is of vital importance to maintain their nutritional status, as catabolism of the respiratory muscles will take place in starvation. Gastric atony is common, and usually some form of small-bore tube can be introduced into the duodenum for enteral support. In the patient who cannot tolerate enteral nutrition, TPN is a vital adjunct in eventual weaning from the ventilator. Although one should remain cognizant of the previous concerns with carbon dioxide overproduction, these problems can be minimized with careful monitoring to prevent

overfeeding. The maintenance and repletion of muscle stores are paramount.

AREAS UNDER INVESTIGATION

Cancer Support

Perhaps no area of nutritional support sparks more controversy than the use of parenteral support in the cancer patient. Tumors are nutritional sinks, and the goal of support is to supplement the host without accelerating growth of the tumor. A great deal of confusion arises within the literature in that different tumors have different responses to substrates. The methylcholanthrene sarcoma in the guinea pig appears to prefer glutamine [11]. Growth of other tumors can be slowed in relation to the host by high levels of insulin, presumably robbing the tumor of glucose [11]. The rates of response to nutritional supplementation after starvation are variable. Grube et al. have elegantly shown an early peak in DNA synthesis in tumor cells of a rat mammary carcinoma 4 hours after the institution of TPN; tissues in the remainder of the organism showed an increased synthetic rate only hours later. This "therapeutic window" may have clinical significance when considering chemotherapeutic intervention, although this remains unproved [22, 24, 25].

A final aspect of the oncology patient is the so-called "anorexia of cancer." This multifactorial response involves mechanical and neurohormonal changes leading to alterations in oral intake and cachexia in excess of what one would expect from tumor burden alone. While some have advocated home TPN in these patients, we do not endorse this policy as it adds expense, prolongs the suffering, and, overall, fails to benefit the patient. Central catheters in the cancer patient may be appropriate for the administration of parenteral analgesics or hydration.

Trauma and Sepsis

The septic and posttraumatic states are characterized by a net afflux of amino acids from skeletal muscle to the liver. This peripheral breakdown is presumably of teleologic advantage to provide substrates for hepatic protein synthesis for host defense and repair [26]. Studies of the amino acid patterns in sepsis resemble those of hepatic failure, with additional prominence of sulfur-containing amino acids, not unreasonable in view of the prevalence of hepatic functional impairment in sepsis. It would seem logical, therefore, that a BCAA enriched-solution could be of advantage in the septic patient. Several studies have shown a trend toward improved hepatic protein synthesis with a 45% BCAA solution [6, 10, 35]; however, the advantage over conventional (22% BCAA) TPN is minimal unless the patient is clearly septic, and the cost differential great.

In the parenteral support of the septic patient, one must prevent provision of excessive calories and the subsequent overproduction of carbon dioxide and respiratory insufficiency [4]. [Editor's Note: This complication has been emphasized far beyond its occurrence or clinical utility. No one seems to have read the original manuscript in which depleted septic patients were suddenly given more than twice their caloric needs. In practice, while one should be aware of the possibility of this complication, and measuring VCO_2 is useful, it is very unusual to be unable to wean a patient from the ventilator because of excessive carbon dioxide production.] One approach is to use a 15% dextrose–based TPN solution with additional nonprotein calories provided by lipids. Although the question of immunomodulation by specific fatty acids remains to be clarified, we have found this combination to be effective, especially in the glucose-intolerant patient.

General Perioperative Support

Once again, it is difficult to find "pure" studies of significant size to draw conclusions regarding perioperative support in the non-cancer patient. This group would include patients malnourished on the basis of esophageal stricture or dysmotility, ulcer disease, pancreatitis, ulcerative colitis, or Crohn's disease. In a prospective, observational study of all patients admitted to the Philadelphia Veterans' Administration Medical Center, Buzby et al. followed 368 patients and divided them according to malignant, nonmalignant, gastrointestinal, and thoracic procedures. Overall complication rates ranged from 30 to 38%. Those patients undergoing thoracotomy for nonmalignant disease had few complications and were excluded from further study [8]. Criteria for malnutrition were then identified based on albumin, transferrin, and ideal body weight, and an at-risk group isolated. Analysis of preliminary results from this study suggests that perioperative nutrition for 7 to 10 days preoperatively results in a decreased incidence of operative complications, while in those who are only moderately or mildly malnourished the increased incidence of non–catheter-related infections outweighed the benefit of perioperative nutrition [7].

The duration of preoperative nutritional support is also controversial. Starker et al. have proposed that early diuresis of extracellular fluid in response to TPN augurs a favorable prognosis. A concomitant rise in serum albumin level reflects this diuresis and not hepatic protein synthesis. More appropriate measures of response to nutritional support would include the short-turnover proteins transferrin and retinol-binding prealbumin [45].

Preoperative TPN may well play a role in the reduction of perioperative complications in a carefully selected group of severely malnourished patients.

CONCLUSION

Since its inception, TPN has become ubiquitous and life-saving in medical care. Its benefits have been clearly established in the short-gut syndrome, as an adjunct in the patient with enterocutaneous fistula, and as supportive therapy in patients with renal or hepatic failure or sepsis. The role of TPN in perioperative therapy, especially the malnourished and the cancer patient, is yet to be defined and provides an area of intensive and exciting research.

REFERENCES

1. Abel, R. M., Beck, C. M., Jr., Abbott, W. M., Ryan, J. A., Barnett, G. O., and Fischer, J. E. Improved survival from acute renal failure after treatment with intravenous essential L-amino acids and glucose: Results of a prospective, double-blind study. *N. Engl. J. Med.* 288:695, 1973.
2. Abel, R. M., Grimes, J. B., Alonso, D., Alonso, M., and Gay, W. A., Jr. Adverse hemodynamic and ultrastructural changes in dog hearts subjected to protein-calorie malnutrition, *Am. Heart J.* 97:733, 1979.
3. Andrassy, R. J., DuBois, T., Page, C. P., Patterson, R. S., and Paredes, A. Early postoperative nutritional enhancement utilizing enteral branched-chain amino acids by way of a needle catheter jejunostomy. *Am. J. Surg.* 150:730, 1985.
4. Askanazi, J., Elwyn, D. H., Silverberg, P. A., Rosenbaum, S. H., and Kinney, J. M. Respiratory distress secondary to a high carbohydrate load: A case report. *Surgery* 88:596, 1980.
5. Aubaniac, R. L'injection intraveineuse sousclaviculaire. Avantage et technique. *Presse Med.* 60:1456, 1952.
6. Bower, R. H., Muggia-Sullam, M., Vallgren, S., et al. Branched chain amino acid-enriched solutions in the septic patient: A randomized, prospective trial. *Ann. Surg.* 203:13, 1986.
7. Buzby, G. P. Case for preoperative nutritional support. Presented at the American College of Surgeons 1988 Clinical Congress Postgraduate Course "Pre- and Postoperative Care: Metabolism and Nutrition," Chicago, IL, October 25–28, 1988.
8. Buzby, G. P., Williford, W. O., Peterson, O. L., et al. A randomized clinical trial of total parenteral nutrition in malnourished surgical patients: The rationale and impact of previous clinical trials and pilot study on protocol design. *Am. J. Clin. Nutr.* 47:357, 1988.
9. Cerra, F. B., Cheung, N. K., Fischer, J. E., et al. Disease-specific amino acid infusion (F080) in hepatic encephalopathy: A prospective, randomized, double-blind, controlled trial. *J. Parenter. Enter. Nutr.* 9:288, 1985.
10. Cerra, F. B., Mazuki, J., Teasley, K., et al. Nitrogen retention in critically ill patients is proportional to the branched chain amino acid load. *Crit. Care Med.* 11:775, 1983.
11. Chance, W. T., Cao, L., Kim, M. W., Nelson, J. L., and Fischer, J. E. Reduction of tumor growth following treatment with a glutamine antimetabolite. *Life Sci.* 42:87, 1988.
12. Chwals, W. J., and Blackburn, G. L. Perioperative nutritional support in the cancer patient. *Surg. Clin. North Am.* 66:1137, 1986.
13. Copeland, E. M., Souchon, E. A., MacFayden, B. V., Jr., Rapp, M. A., and Dudrick, S. J. Intravenous hyperalimentation as an adjunct to radiation therapy. *Cancer* 39:609, 1977.
14. Dudrick, S. J. The genesis of intravenous hyperalimentation. *J. Parenter. Enter. Nutr.* 1:23, 1977.
15. Dudrick, S. J., Wilmore, D. W., Vars, H. M., and Rhoads, J. E. Long-term total parenteral nutrition with growth, development, and positive nitrogen balance. *Surgery* 64:134, 1968.
16. Elman, R., and Weiner, D. O. Intravenous alimentation with special reference to protein (amino acid) metabolism. *J.A.M.A.* 122:796, 1939.
17. Feinstein, E. I., Blumenkrantz, M. J., Healy, M., et al. Clinical and metabolic responses to parenteral nutritional in acute renal failure: A controlled double-blind study. *Medicine* 60:124, 1981.
18. Feinstein, E. I., Kopple, J., Silberman, H., and Massry, S. G. Total parenteral nutrition with high or low nitrogen intakes in patients with acute renal failure. *Kidney Int.* 26(Suppl. 16):S319, 1983.
19. Felig, P. H. Amino acid metabolism in man. *Annu. Rev. Biochem.* 44:933, 1975.
20. Fischer, J. E. The management of gastrointestinal cutaneous fistulae. *Contemp. Surg.* 29:104, 1986.
21. Forster, J. The use of total parenteral nutrition in the treatment of anorexia nervosa. In J. L. Rombeau and M. D. Caldwell (eds.), *Parenteral Nutrition.* Philadelphia: W. B. Saunders, 1986. Pp. 520–523.
22. Gamelli, R. L., and Foster, R. S. Effects of protein calorie malnutrition and refeeding of fluorouracil toxicity. *Arch. Surg.* 118:1192, 1983.
23. Goodgame, J. T., and Fischer, J. E. Parenteral nutrition in the treatment of acute pancreatitis: Effect on complications and mortality. *Am. Surg.* 186:651, 1977.
24. Grube, B. J., and Gamelli, R. L. Nutritional modulation of tumor growth. *J. Surg. Res.* 45:120, 1988.
25. Grube, B. J., Gamelli, R. K., and Foster, R. S., Jr. Refeeding differentially affects tumor and host cell proliferation. *J. Surg. Res.* 39:535, 1985.
26. Hasselgren, P. O., Pedersen, P., Sax, H. C., Warner, B. W., and Fischer, J. E. Current concepts of protein turnover and amino acid transport in liver and skeletal muscle during sepsis. *Arch. Surg.* 123:992, 1988.
27. Heymsfield, S. B., Smith, J., Read, S., and Whitworth, H. B., Jr. Nutritional support in cardiac failure. *Surg. Clin. North Am.* 61:635, 1981.

28. Hiyama, D. T., and Fischer, J. E. Nutritional hepatic failure: Current thought in practice. *Nutr. Clin. Pract.* 3:96, 1988.
29. Klein, S., Simes, J., and Blackburn, G. L. Total parenteral nutrition and cancer clinical trials. *Cancer* 58:1378, 1986.
30. Michel, H., Pomier-Layrargues, G., Duhamel, O., Lacombe, B., Cuilleret, G., and Bellet, H. Intravenous infusion of ordinary and modified amino acid solutions in the management of hepatic encephalopathy (controlled study, 30 patients). (Abstract) *Gastroenterology* 79:1038, 1980.
31. Mochizuki, H., Trocki, O., Dominioni, L., Brackett, K. A., Joffe, S. N., and Alexander, J. W. Mechanism of prevention of postburn hypermetabolism and catabolism by early enteral feeding. *Ann. Surg.* 200:297, 1984.
32. Müller, J. M., Keller, H. W., Brenner, U., Walter, M., and Holzmüller, W. Indications and effects of preoperative parenteral nutrition. *World J. Surg.* 10:53, 1986.
33. Nespoli, A., Bevilacqua, G., Staudacher, C., Rossi, N., Salerno, F., and Castelli, M. R. Pathogenesis of hepatic encephalopathy and hyperdynamic syndrome in cirrhosis: Role of false neurotransmitters. *Arch. Surg.* 116:1129, 1981.
34. Peden, V. H., Witzleben, C. L., and Skelton, M. A. Total parenteral nutrition. *J. Pediatr.* 78:180, 1971.
35. Pelosi, G., Proietti, R., Magglini, S. I., Santori, R., Giammaria, A., and Manni, C. Anticatabolic properties of branched chain amino acids in trauma. *Resuscitation* 10:153, 1983.
36. Rose, D., Yarborough, M. F., Canizaro, P. C., and Lowry, S. F. One hundred and fourteen fistulas of the gastrointestinal tract treated with total parenteral nutrition. *Surg. Gynecol. Obstet.* 163:345, 1986.
37. Rosen H. M., Yoshimura, N., Hodgman, J. M., and Fischer, J. E. Plasma amino acid patterns in hepatic encephalopathy of differing etiology. *Gastroenterology* 72:483, 1977.
38. Rossi-Fanelli, F., Riggio, O., Cangiano, C., et al. Branched chain amino acids vs lactulose in the treatment of hepatic coma: A controlled study. *Dig. Dis. Sci.* 27:929, 1982.
39. Saito, H., Trocki, O., Alexander, J. W., Kopcha, R., Heyd, T., and Joffe, S. N. The effect of route of nutrient administration on the nutritional state, catabolic hormone secretion, and gut mucosal integrity after burn injury. *J. Parenter. Enter. Nutr.* 11:1, 1987.
40. Sax, H. C. Nutritional support in pancreatitis. In C. L. Lang (ed.), *Nutritional Support in Critical Care.* Rockville, MD: Aspen, 1987. Pp. 265–273.
41. Sax, H. C., and Bower, R. H. Hepatic complications of total parenteral nutrition. *J. Parenter. Enter. Nutr.* 12:615, 1988.
42. Sax, H. C., Warner, B. W., Talamini, M. A., et al. Early total parenteral nutrition in acute pancreatitis: Lack of beneficial effects. *Am. J. Surg.* 153:117, 1987.
43. Soeters, P. B., Ebeid, A. M., and Fischer, J. E. Review of 404 patients with gastrointestinal fistula. Impact of parenteral nutrition. *Ann. Surg.* 190:189, 1979.
44. Souba, W. W., Smith, R. J., and Wilmore, D. W. Glutamine metabolism by the intestinal tract. *J. Parenter. Enter. Nutr.* 9:608, 1985.
45. Starker, P. M., LaSala, P. A., Askanazi, J., Todd, G., Hensle, T. W., and Kinney, J. M. The influence of preoperative total parenteral nutrition upon morbidity and mortality. *Surg. Gynecol. Obstet.* 162:569, 1986.
46. Strauss, E., Santos, W. R., DaSilva, E. C., Lacet, C. M., Capacci, M. L. L., and Bernardini, A. P. A randomized controlled clinical trial for the evaluation of the efficacy of an enriched branched-chain amino acid solution compared to neomycin in hepatic encephalopathy. (Abstract) *Hepatology* 3:862, 1983.
47. Wilmore, D. W., and Dudrick, S. J. Growth and development of an infant receiving all nutrients exclusively by vein. *J.A.M.A.* 203:860, 1968.

Solutions Available

Michael H. Torosian
John M. Daly

The development and initial clinical application of parenteral nutrition, as currently practiced in the United States, were performed by Rhoads, Dudrick, Wilmore, and associates at the University of Pennsylvania [10, 11]. In order to achieve the goal of improving nutritional status, parenteral nutrient solutions must be formulated to satisfy not only daily maintenance requirements, but also additional demands of nutritional repletion, normal growth and development, and disease and stress states including malignancy, severe burn injury, trauma, and other critical illnesses.

Parenteral nutrient solutions have been developed to provide adequate calories and protein to achieve a positive energy-nitrogen balance and to promote host tissue synthesis. The energy sources most commonly employed in parenteral solutions include dextrose and lipid emulsions; crystalline amino acid solutions usually provide the nitrogen source. In some instances, individual formulations have been developed and are re-served for patients with specific disease states. Electrolytes, vitamins, and minerals are included in the composition or supplied as additives to parenteral solutions. This chapter reviews the currently available parenteral nutrient solutions and the advantages and disadvantages of these formulations.

ENERGY SOURCES

Glucose

Glucose provides the source of carbohydrate calories in parenteral nutrient solutions that are currently available. The advantages of using glucose in parenteral solutions are that it is a physiologic substrate, easily purified for intravenous administration, and inexpensive, and can be prepared in high concentrations for central intravenous infusion [24, 37]. Although glucose may be administered as the sole caloric source, glucose is generally administered in combination with lipids to meet daily caloric requirements.

Caloric requirements of individuals may be estimated by calculating basal energy expenditure (BEE) using the Harris-Benedict formula and adding various factors to account for injury in disease states [16]. The Harris-Benedict formulas for estimating BEE for males and females, respectively, are:

BEE (kcal) = 66.5 + 13.7 × weight (kg)
              + 5 × height (cm) − 6.8 × age (yr)
BEE (kcal) = 65.5 + 9.6 × weight (kg)
              + 1.7 × height (cm) − 4.7 × age (yr)

Alternatively, actual resting energy expenditure in patients may be measured at the bedside by indirect calorimetry [26, 30]. Indirect calorimetry measurement prevents errors inherent in estimating energy expenditure by predetermined formulas. The rate of glucose metabolism in patients varies from 0.4–1.4 g/kg/hr; an average adult under normal conditions metabolizes glucose at a rate of 0.5 g/kg/hr [9].

Glucose is commercially available as dextrose monohydrate. In this form, each gram of glucose monohydrate provides 3.4 kcal. Because of this low caloric density, hypertonic solutions have been formulated to contain adequate calories in limited volumes of fluid. The majority of standard parenteral nutrient solutions contain dextrose concentrations between 25 to 35%; the osmolarity of these solutions ranges from 1200 to 1700 mOsm/liter. The hypertonicity of these solutions requires administration by the central venous system. The maximum glucose concentration generally tolerated by peripheral venous infusion is 10%. The commercially available glucose preparations with caloric content and osmolarity are outlined in Table 2-1.

When supplied with lipids as the energy source, a minimum of 100 to 150 g of glucose should be administered daily. This amount of glucose is required for the "nitrogen-sparing" effect of carbohydrate to inhibit gluconeogenesis [36]. Furthermore, to achieve optimal nitrogen balance, glucose should be infused simultaneously with the parenteral nitrogen source [32, 36].

Table 2-1. Dextrose Solutions

Dextrose Concentration (%)	Caloric Density (kcal/liter)	Osmolarity (mOsm/liter)
5	170	252
10	340	505
20	680	1010
30	1020	1515
40	1360	2020
50	1700	2525
60	2040	3030
70	2380	3535

Lipid

Fat emulsions are used in parenteral nutrition to prevent fatty acid deficiency and as a caloric source. To prevent fatty acid deficiency, 4 to 10% of the daily caloric intake should consist of fat emulsion [12]. All lipid solutions contain the essential fatty acid linoleic acid. Fatty acid deficiency can be avoided by providing two to three bottles of 500 ml of 10% lipid weekly to adults who are receiving total parenteral nutrition.

Lipid emulsions offer several advantages for use as a caloric source. First, lipid emulsions have a high caloric density at 9 kcal/g. A 500-ml bottle of 10% or 20% fat emulsion provides 555 (1.1 kcal/ml) or 1000 kcal (2.0 kcal/ml), respectively. Second, these solutions are prepared isotonically by the addition of glycerin which makes peripheral intravenous infusion feasible [19]. Third, lipid is an ideal caloric source for patients who are relatively glucose intolerant (e.g., diabetic, septic, or cancer patients). [Editor's Note: It is now generally agreed that administered lipid emulsions are cleared in septic patients. What is controversial is whether the fat is totally utilized and at what point in the course of sepsis efficient fat utilization decreases (see Chap. 22).]

With adequate provision of nitrogen, the combination of lipid and carbohydrate as an energy source has similar effects on nitrogen balance and weight gain compared with ad-

Table 2-2. Lipid Emulsions

	Intralipid (Kabi Vitrum)	Liposyn II (Abbott)	Soyacal (Alpha Therapeutic)
Triglyceride source	Soybean	Safflower & soybean	Soybean
Fatty acid content (%)			
Linoleic	50.0–54.0	65.8	49.0–60.0
Oleic	26.0	17.7	21.0–26.0
Palmitic	9.0–10.0	8.8	9.0–13.0
Linolenic	8.0– 9.0	4.2	6.0– 9.0
Stearic	0	3.4	3.0– 5.0
Egg yolk phospholipids (%)	1.2	1.2	1.2
Glycerin (%)	2.25	2.5	2.21
Caloric density (kcal/ml)			
10% Emulsion	1.1	1.1	1.1
20% Emulsion	2.0	2.0	2.0
Osmolarity (mOsm/liter)			
10% Emulsion	280	320	280
20% Emulsion	330	340	315

ministration of carbohydrate alone [38]. The addition of lipid to the parenteral nutrient regimen has additional advantages of reducing the incidence of hepatic dysfunction and decreasing carbon dioxide generation [45]. The latter phenomenon is of particular importance in patients with marginal respiratory reserve. Although greater quantities of parenteral lipid have been administered, it is generally recommended that a maximum of 60% of total nonprotein calories be provided as lipid. Lipid quantities in excess of this amount may exceed the patient's metabolic capacity for effective clearance and oxidation of fat [18, 46].

The clearance and oxidation kinetics of parenteral lipid depend to a great extent on the clinical condition of the patient. At low concentrations of triglycerides, plasma clearance rate is dependent on triglyceride concentration [18, 19]. Above a critical triglyceride concentration at which lipoprotein lipase binding sites are saturated, a maximum clearance capacity that is independent of triglyceride concentration is reached. This maximum clearance capacity varies depending on the clinical state of the patient. Maximum clearance capacity is increased following starvation or

trauma and in states of severe catabolism. By increasing starvation from 19 to 39 hours, triglyceride clearance in patients increased from 1.9 to 5.7 g/kg/day to 4.43 to 8.23 g/kg/day. When the 39-hour fast was combined with a surgical procedure, the triglyceride clearance rate rose to 5.06 to 30.39 g/kg/day [18].

Lipid emulsions of soybean oil and/or safflower oil are used in the commercially available nutrient solutions (Table 2-2). Compared with soybean oil, safflower oil contains a greater percentage of linoleic acid and much less linolenic acid [5, 47]. Since linolenic acid can be formed after providing the essential linoleic acid, this difference in composition may not be clinically significant. Both purified plant oils are emulsified with glycerin added to render the emulsion isosmotic. Egg phospholipids are added to stabilize the emulsion and to regulate the size of the fat particles. When prepared in this manner, the fat droplets are similar in size to chylomicrons which are naturally formed after absorption of dietary lipid from the small intestine [19, 23].

In the past, fat emulsions have not been admixed with other components of the parenteral nutrient solution because of reported physical and chemical instability. Fat emulsions were typically "piggybacked" to a carbohydrate and amino acid solution and were infused into a distal intravenous-tubing injection site. However, refinements in technique have allowed admixture of lipid, carbohydrate, and protein in a common bag. These combined nutrient systems are termed complete nutritive mixtures ("three-in-one") or total nutrient admixtures [13, 33]. Physicochemical stability of all components of this system, including vitamins and trace elements, has been documented by numerous studies [35]. Initial development and clinical utilization of these combined formula mixtures were conducted in Europe and Canada; these admixture solutions are now also available in the United States [3, 33, 34].

Toxicity associated with parenteral lipid administration is minimal. The most common adverse effects include fever, chills, shivering, chest and/or back pain, and vomiting [20, 47]. Uncommon reactions that have been reported include abnormalities in blood coagulation, transient elevations of transaminase and alkaline phosphatase levels, and anemia [28, 47]. The previously documented pulmonary embolic complications associated with intravenous lipid are no longer observed as the initial cottonseed emulsions have been replaced by soybean and safflower emulsions [44].

Despite the low incidence of complications, a test dose is recommended when one initiates parenteral lipid emulsion. In adults and children, 10% fat emulsion should be infused at a rate of 1 ml/min and 0.1 ml/min, respectively, for the first 15 to 30 minutes. The initial infusion of 20% fat emulsion should be one-half this rate. If no reactions are observed during this initial infusion period, full infusion is begun.

Fructose

Fructose is a naturally occurring monosaccharide that offers an alternative to dextrose as a source of carbohydrate calories. Fructose has been used in 5% and 10% solutions combined with glucose and xylitol in Europe, but its use has not gained popularity in the United States [39]. Fructose offers several advantages to dextrose. First, fructose does not require insulin for initial uptake and phosphorylation [16, 43]. However, since most adult tissues cannot utilize fructose directly but require its conversion to glucose in the liver, this theoretic advantage is limited. [*Editor's Note:* Since fructose utilization principally utilizes the hexose monophosphate shunt, the advantage over glucose is hardly even theoretical.] Second, hyperglycemia and glycosuria occur less with fructose than with corresponding amounts of glucose [16].

Fructose is also associated with several disadvantages. First, rapid infusion of fructose has been associated with lactic acidosis, hypophosphatemia, elevated serum bilirubin and uric acid levels, and depletion of hepatic adenine nucleotides [4, 43]. Second, fructose is contraindicated in patients with fructose intolerance [41]. Third, most laboratories do not measure fructose, although measurement techniques could be introduced. Finally, use of fructose as the sole energy source is limited by the total dose and rate of infusion that can be tolerated [39].

Invert Sugar

Invert sugar consists of equal parts of dextrose and fructose. The caloric density of invert sugar is approximately 4 kcal/g. Both 5% and 10% solutions of invert sugar are commercially available. Clinical experience using invert sugar as a caloric source, however, is limited.

Maltose

Maltose is a disaccharide that consists of two linked glucose monomers. Maltose is theoretically attractive as a caloric source since the caloric density is twice that of an isotonic dextrose solution. However, previous studies have demonstrated urinary losses of over 25% of the administered maltose dose with an infusion rate of 0.25 g/kg/hr [15]. Thus, actual utilizable calories delivered to the individual are limited.

Sorbitol and Xylitol

Sorbitol and xylitol are alcohol sugars. Like fructose, both sorbitol and xylitol are only partially insulin independent [25]. However, sorbitol, which is dehydrogenated to fructose and xylitol, cannot be used directly by peripheral tissues [1, 25]. Both require conversion to glucose in the liver. In addition, sorbitol and xylitol are associated with numerous severe toxic effects, including lactic acidosis, hepatic failure, hyperuricemia, and depletion of liver adenosine triphosphate and inorganic phosphate [1].

Glycerol

Glycerol is a naturally occurring sugar alcohol with a caloric density of 4.32 kcal/g [7]. As a sole energy source, a 3% glycerol solution is now available combined with 3% amino acids. Nutritional maintenance in a protein-sparing regimen is possible with this glycerol-based solution [40]. The use of glycerol as an exclusive energy source is relatively recent and requires further clinical investigation.

Ethanol

Ethanol has a caloric density of 7.1 kcal/g [22]. However, the use of ethanol as a caloric source is not recommended because of its toxicity. Ethanol is toxic to muscle, brain, liver, and other host tissues [42]. Ethanol is also associated with hypoglycemia (by inhibiting gluconeogenesis), impairs leukocyte migration and phagocytosis, and can irritate pulmonary alveoli [29]. [*Editor's Note:* Ethanol was utilized in the early days of parenteral nutrition and, it is believed, caused several cases of pancreatitis.] Five and 10% solutions of ethanol are commercially available.

PROTEIN SOURCES

Standard Parenteral Nutrition

Nutritional maintenance and repletion require provision of both adequate calories and nitrogen. Original protein sources in parenteral solutions consisted of hydrolysates of naturally occurring proteins (e.g., fibrin and casein). Parenteral administration of protein hydrolysates is associated with several disadvantages, including inefficient utilization of dipeptides and tripeptides with large urinary nitrogen losses and a high incidence of hyperammonemia [8]. In addition, the composition of the hydrolysate is dependent on the protein source and not related to the nitrogen requirements of the patient. Chemically defined solutions of crystalline amino acids have now replaced protein hydrolysates as the source of nitrogen in parenteral nutrient solutions. [*Editor's Note:* Hydrolysates did contain glutamine, now looked on as advantageous.]

Crystalline amino acids consist of L-amino acid solutions free of ammonia and the metabolically inefficient dipeptides and tripeptides. Concentrated amino acids have been formulated to provide a physiologic ratio of essential and nonessential amino acids for optimal protein synthesis. Commercially available solutions consist of 40 to 50% essential amino acids and 50 to 60% nonessential amino acids.

Commercially available amino acid solutions are available in a range of concentrations from 3 to 11.4%. The composition of available 8.5% amino acid solutions is shown in Table 2-3. The individual amino acid composition of specific formulations is constant regardless of final amino acid concentration. Although slight differences between different products exist in the amounts of essential and nonessential amino acids, the clinical significance of these differences has not been demonstrated. Premixed maintenance electrolytes are available in some amino acid solutions.

Specific Clinical Situations

Protein-Sparing Effect
Protein-sparing therapy utilizes the body's own fat stores as the major energy source. Three to 5.5% amino acid solutions are admixed with or without 5% dextrose to pro-

Table 2-3. 8.5% Amino Acid Solutions

	FreAmine II (McGaw)	Aminosyn (Abbott)	Travasol (Travenol)	Novamine (Cutter)
Essential amino acids (mg/100 ml)				
L-Leucine	770	810	526	590
L-Isoleucine	590	620	406	420
L-Valine	560	680	590	550
L-Phenylalanine	480	380	526	590
L-Tryptophan	130	150	152	140
L-Methionine	450	340	492	420
L-Threonine	340	460	356	420
L-Lysine	620	624	492	673
Nonessential amino acids (mg/100 ml)				
L-Alanine	600	1100	1760	1200
L-Arginine	810	850	880	840
L-Histidine	240	260	372	500
L-Proline	950	750	356	500
L-Serine	500	370	356	500
L-Tyrosine	—	44	34	340
L-Glutamic acid	—	—	—	20
L-Aspartic acid	—	—	—	420
Glycine	1190	1100	1760	250
Cysteine	20	—	—	590
				40
Total nitrogen (g/100 ml)	1.3	1.3	1.4	1.35
Osmolarity (mOsm/liter)	810	850	860	750

vide nitrogenous substrates for protein synthesis. Maintenance electrolytes are required for protein-sparing therapy. This parenteral regimen is only indicated in selected patients with abundant fat stores and without significant protein depletion, and in those without severe metabolic stress. Its efficacy has not been demonstrated.

Trauma and Severe Catabolic Stress

Trauma and severe catabolic stress are associated with large urinary nitrogen losses and plasma aminograms characterized by low branched-chain amino acids (BCAAs)— leucine, isoleucine, and valine [2]. To replete the BCAA supply and normalize the plasma aminogram, BCAA-enriched formulas have been advocated. FreAmine HBC (high branched-chain) consists of 6.9% amino acids with increased concentration of BCAA and

has been formulated for hypercatabolic patients (Table 2-4). Dextrose needs to be added to FreAmine HBC prior to administration. The use of this parenteral therapy in severely catabolic patients has demonstrated a small positive effect in terms of whole-body nitrogen balance in comparison with a standard amino acid formulation.

Hepatic Disease

Acute deterioration in patients with chronic liver disease (particularly cirrhosis) has been associated with increased serum levels of aromatic amino acids and decreased levels of BCAA [14]. To correct these amino acid imbalances and reverse the associated encephalopathy, Hepatamine 8% has been formulated with increased BCAA and decreased aromatic amino acids—phenylalanine, tryptophan, threonine, and methionine (see Table 2-4). Hepatamine requires mixture with dextrose (50–70%) prior to administration. Despite several years of clinical study with this product, the efficacy of Hepatamine in treating patients with hepatic encephalopathy remains controversial. [*Editor's Note:* Several recent reviews concluded that an amino acid solution deficient in aromatic amino acids and enriched with BCAA is efficacious in the treatment of hepatic encephalopathy.]

Renal Failure

To prevent the development of hyperuremia in patients with acute renal failure, amino acid mixtures with high levels of essential amino acids have been formulated. The compositions of three commercially available products are shown in Table 2-5. All solutions require admixture with glucose as a caloric source for nutritional repletion. Despite the theoretical advantages offered by solutions high in essential amino acids, the clini-

Table 2-4. Branched-Chain Amino Acid–Enriched Solutions

	FreAmine HBC 6.9% (McGaw)	Hepatamine 8% (McGaw)
Essential amino acids (mg/100 ml)		
L-Isoleucine	760	900
L-Leucine	1370	1100
L-Valine	880	840
L-Lysine	410	610
L-Methionine	250	100
L-Phenylalanine	320	100
L-Threonine	200	450
L-Tryptophan	90	66
Nonessential amino acids (mg/100 ml)		
L-Alanine	400	770
L-Arginine	580	600
L-Histidine	160	240
L-Proline	630	800
L-Serine	330	800
Glycine	330	900
L-Cysteine	20	20
L-Amino acids (g/100 ml)	6.9	8.0
Osmolarity (mOsm/liter)	625	785

Table 2-5. Essential Amino Acid–Enriched Solutions

	Nephramine 5.4% (McGaw)	Renamin (Travenol)	Aminosyn 5.2% (Abbott)
Essential amino acids (mg/100 ml)			
L-Leucine	880	600	726
L-Isoleucine	560	500	462
L-Phenylalanine	880	490	726
L-Methionine	880	500	726
L-Threonine	400	380	330
L-Valine	640	820	528
L-Lysine	640	450	535
L-Tryptophan	200	160	165
Nonessential amino acids (mg/100 ml)			
L-Arginine	—	630	600
L-Histidine	250	420	429
L-Cysteine	20	—	—
L-Alanine	—	560	—
L-Proline	—	350	—
L-Serine	—	300	—
L-Tyrosine	—	40	—
Glycine	—	300	—
Total nitrogen (g/100 ml)	0.65	1.0	0.79
Osmolarity (mOsm/liter)	440	600	475

cal efficacy of these products in patients with renal failure has not been conclusively demonstrated [6]. Early studies comparing these essential amino acid mixtures and glucose with glucose alone demonstrated improvement in mortality with the former solution in patients with acute renal failure. However, more recent studies comparing glucose admixed with either essential amino acids alone or a balanced amino acid formulation have failed to demonstrate clear benefit. Thus, an alternative approach for patients with acute renal failure is to administer standard parenteral nutrient regimens and to aggressively dialyze the patient.

Fluid and Electrolytes

Adequate fluid and electrolytes must be provided to patients receiving parenteral nutrition. Fluid and electrolyte requirements must be individualized depending on preexisting abnormalities, ongoing losses, and considerations imposed by clinical problems (e.g., cardiac, renal, and pulmonary disease). Both intracellular and extracellular electrolytes must be administered in the parenteral nutrient regimen. Intracellular electrolytes, specifically potassium, phosphate, and magnesium, are necessary for optimal anabolism and are rapidly incorporated into cells after adequate parenteral nutrition is initiated. Sodium, potassium, chloride, acetate, phosphate, magnesium, and calcium may be added directly to parenteral nutrient solutions.

Bicarbonate is incompatible with acidic parenteral nutrient solutions and cannot be added directly. However, acetate and lactate, precursors of bicarbonate, are chemically compatible as admixtures to parenteral nutrient solutions. Multiple electrolyte solutions have been developed to simplify solution admixture in patients receiving standard parenteral nutrient formulations. Some amino acid solutions are commercially available with maintenance electrolytes already added. In certain circumstances, however, premixed electrolyte combinations are not clinically appropriate and electrolytes must be added in-

dividually. Careful assessment of fluid and electrolyte balance is required throughout the entire period of parenteral nutrient administration.

Vitamins

Vitamins are required for optimal nutritional repletion, to maintain cellular integrity, and to sustain subcellular metabolism. In 1978, guidelines for parenteral vitamin administration for adult and pediatric patients were established by the Nutrition Advisory Group of the Department of Foods and Nutrition of the American Medical Association [31]. Based on these recommendations, a parenteral multivitamin (MVI-12) preparation has been formulated. Ten milliliters of this preparation added daily to the parenteral nutrient solution meets the guidelines for adults established by the American Medical Association. The composition of commercially available vitamin mixtures is shown in Table 2-6.

Vitamin K is not a component of any of the vitamin mixtures formulated for adults. Maintenance requirements can be satisfied by adding vitamin K in the parenteral nutrient solution. For treatment of vitamin K deficiency, it is generally recommended that daily intramuscular injections be administered [31].

Certain diseases or treatments may induce other specific vitamin-deficient states. In these situations, specific vitamin supplementation is accomplished by using single-entity preparations. Single-entity products are commercially available for vitamins K, A, D, E, B_1 (thiamine), B_2 (riboflavin), B_3 (niacin), B_6 (pyridoxine), B_{12} (cyanocobalamin), C, and folic acid [27].

Trace Elements

Guidelines for the parenteral administration of zinc, copper, manganese, and chromium have been established [17]. Although the precise requirements of these trace elements are difficult to determine and may vary depending on the clinical situation, these micronutrients should be part of a complete paren-

Table 2-6.   Multivitamin Preparations

	MVI-12 (Armour)	MCV 9 + 3 (Lymphomed)	Multivitamin Additive (Abbott)	Berocca Parenteral Nutrition (Roche)
A (IU)	3300	3300	3300	3300
D (IU)	200	200	200	200
Thiamine (B_1) (mg)	3.0	3.0	3.35	3.0
Riboflavin (B_2) (mg)	3.6	3.6	4.93	3.6
Niacin (B_3) (mg)	40	40	40	40
Pantothenic acid (B_5) (mg)	15	15	15	15
Pyridoxine (B_6) (mg)	4.0	4.0	4.86	4.0
B_{12} (mg)	5.0	5.0	5.0	5.0
Ascorbic acid (C) (mg)	100	100	100	100
E (IU)	10	10	10	10
Folic acid (mg)	400	400	400	400
Biotin (mg)	6.0	6.0	6.0	6.0

teral nutrient system. States of trace element deficiency have developed in the past when these micronutrients were omitted from parenteral solutions. Single- and multiple-entity trace element solutions are commercially available (Table 2-7) [17, 21].

Iodide, selenium, and molybdenum are additional trace elements with requirements that have not been well established. These trace elements should be added to solutions for patients receiving prolonged parenteral nutrition and perhaps in other selected instances. Single-entity products are available for each of these trace elements.

FUTURE RESEARCH

Total parenteral nutrition requires the provision of adequate calories, protein, fluid, electrolytes, vitamins, and trace elements. Current clinical investigation is focused on two divergent concepts. First, total nutrient admixture systems combine all parenteral nutrients in a common administration unit. These systems offer the advantage of convenience of administration for patients receiving standard parenteral nutrition and the potential for reducing iatrogenic infectious complications. In contrast, the development of inno-

Table 2-7.   Multiple Trace Element Preparations

	Multiple Trace Element Additives (Abbott)	Multiple Trace Metal Additives (IMS)	Multiple Trace Element Solution (American Quinine)	Multe-Pak-4 & Multe-Pak-5* (Solo Pak)	MTE-4 & MTE-5* (Lymphomed)
Zinc sulfate (mg)	4.0	4.0	1.0 or 5.0	1.0 or 5.0	1.0
Copper sulfate (mg)	1.0	1.0	0.4 or 1.0	0.4 or 5.0	0.4
Manganese sulfate (mg)	0.8	0.5	0.1 or 0.5	0.1 or 0.5	0.1
Chromium chloride (mg)	10.0	10.0	4.0 or 10.0	4.0 or 10.0	4.0

*Multe-Pak-5 and MTE-5 also contain 20.0 μg of selenium.

vative modular formulas for patients with specific disease states is being actively pursued. Both concepts in parenteral nutrient therapy have definite roles in the future and require further clinical investigation.

REFERENCES

1. Ahnefeld, F. W., Bassler, K. H., and Bauer, B. L. Suitability of nonglucose carbohydrates for parenteral nutrition. *Eur. J. Intens. Care Med.* 1:105, 1975.
2. Askanazi, J., Carpenter, Y. A., and Michelson, C. B. Muscle and plasma amino acids following injury: Influence of intercurrent infection. *Ann. Surg.* 792:78, 1980.
3. Barat, A. C., Harrie, K., Jacob, M., Diamantidis, T. G., and McIntosh, N. C. Effect of amino acid solutions on total nutrient admixture stability. *J. Parenter. Enter. Nutr.* 11:384, 1987.
4. Bergstrom, J., Hultman, E., and Roch-Norlund, A. E. Lactic acid accumulation in connection with fructose infusion. *Acta Med. Scand.* 184:359, 1968.
5. Bivins, B. A., Rapp, R. P., Record, K., Meng, H. C., and Griffen, W. O., Jr. Parenteral safflower oil emulsion (Liposyn 10%): Safety and effectiveness in treating or preventing essential fatty acid deficiency in surgical patients. *Ann. Surg.* 191:307, 1980.
6. Blackburn, G. L., Etter, G., and Mackenzie, T. Criteria for choosing amino acid therapy in acute renal failure. *Am. J. Clin. Nutr.* 31:1841, 1978.
7. Brennan, M. F., Fitzpatrick, G. F., Cohen, K. H., and Moore, F. D. Glycerol: Major contributor to the short-term protein-sparing effect of fat emulsions in normal man. *Ann. Surg.* 182:386, 1975.
8. Christensen, H. N., Lynch, E. L., and Power, J. H. The conjugated, nonprotein amino acids of plasma. III: Peptidemia and hyperpeptiduria as a result of the intravenous administration of partially hydrolyzed casein (Amigen). *J. Biol. Chem.* 166:649, 1946.
9. Dudrick, S. J., MacFayden, B. V., Jr., Van Buren, C. T., Ruberg, R. L., and Maynard, A. T. Parenteral hyperalimentation: Metabolic problems and solutions. *Ann. Surg.* 176:259, 1972.
10. Dudrick, S. J., and Rhoads, J. E. New horizons for intravenous feeding. *J.A.M.A.* 215:939, 1971.
11. Dudrick, S. J., Wilmore, D. W., and Vars, H. M. Long-term total parenteral nutrition with growth in puppies and positive nitrogen balance in patients. *Surg. Forum* 18:356, 1967.
12. Elwyn, D. H. Nutritional requirements of

adult surgical patients. *Crit. Care Med.* 8:9, 1980.
13. Epps, D. R., Knutsen, C. V., and Kaminski, M. V. Clinical results with total nutrient admixture for intravenous infusion. *Clin. Pharm.* 2:268, 1983.
14. Fischer, J. E., and Bower, R. H. Nutritional support in liver disease. *Surg. Clin. North Am.* 61:653, 1981.
15. Forster, H., and Hoos, I. The suitability of maltose for parenteral nutrition. *Eur. J. Intensive Care Med.* 1:141, 1975.
16. Friedman, G. J. Diet in the treatment of diabetes mellitus. In R. S. Goodhart and M. E. Shils (eds.), *Modern Nutrition in Health and Disease.* Philadelphia: Lea & Febiger, 1980.
17. Guidelines for essential trace element preparations for parenteral use. *J.A.M.A.* 241:2051, 1979.
18. Hallberg, D. Studies on the elimination of exogenous lipids from the blood stream: The effect of fasting and surgical trauma in man on the elimination rate of a fat emulsion injection intravenously. *Acta Physiol. Scand.* 65:153, 1965.
19. Hallberg, D. Therapy with fat emulsion. *Acta Anaesthesiol. Scand. Suppl.* 55:131, 1974.
20. Hallberg, D., Holm, I., Obel, A. L., Schuberth, O., and Wretlind, A. Fat emulsions for complete intravenous nutrition. *Postgrad. Med. J.* 43:307, 1967.
21. Hauer, E. C., and Kaminski, M. V., Jr. Trace metal profile of parenteral nutrition solutions. *Am. J. Clin. Nutr.* 31:264, 1978.
22. Heuckenkamp, P. U., Sprandel, U., and Liebhardt, E. W. Studies concerning ethanol as a nutrient for intravenous alimentation in man. *Nutr. Metab.* 21 (Suppl. 1):121, 1977.
23. Jeejeebhoy, K. N. Total parenteral nutrition. *Ann. Rev. Coll. Phys. Surg. Can.* 9:287, 1976.
24. Lee, H. A. Intravenous nutrition. *Br. J. Hosp. Med.* 2:719, 1974.
25. Lee, H. A., and Wretlind, A. Non-protein energy sources in parenteral nutrition. *Acta Chir. Scand. Suppl.* 466:6, 1976.
26. Long, C. L., Schaffel, N., and Geiger, J. W. Metabolic response to injury and illness: Estimation of energy and protein needs from indirect calorimetry and nitrogen balance. *J. Parenter. Enter. Nutr.* 3:452, 1979.
27. Lowry, S. F., Goodgame, J. T., Maher, M. M., and Brennan, M. F. Parenteral vitamin requirements during intravenous feeding. *Am. J. Clin. Nutr.* 31:2149, 1978.
28. McNiff, B. L. Clinical use of 10% soybean oil emulsion. *Am. J. Hosp. Pharm.* 34:1080, 1977.
29. Meng, H. C. Parenteral nutrition: Principles, nutrient requirements, and techniques. *Geriatrics* 30:97, 1975.
30. Mirtallo, J. M., Fabri, P. J., and Radcliffe, K.

Evaluation of nitrogen utilization in patients receiving total parenteral nutrition. *J. Parenter. Enter. Nutr.* 7:136, 1983.

31. Multivitamin preparations for parenteral use: A statement by the Nutrition Advisory group. *J. Parenter. Enter. Nutr.* 3:258, 1979.

32. Nube, M., Bos, L. P., and Winkelman, A. Simultaneous and consecutive administration of nutrients in parenteral nutrition. *Am. J. Clin. Nutr.* 32:1505, 1979.

33. Pamperl, H., and Kleinberger, G. Morphologic changes of Intralipid 20% liposomes in all-in-one solutions during prolonged storage. *Infusionstherapie* 9:86, 1982.

34. Pamperl, H., and Kleinberger, G. Stability of intravenous fat emulsions. *Arch. Surg.* 117:859, 1982.

35. Shenkin, A., Fraser, W. D., McLelland, A. J. D., Fell, G. S., and Gordon, O. J. Maintenance of vitamin and trace element status in intravenous nutrition using a complete nutritive mixture. *J. Parenter. Enter. Nutr.* 11:238, 1987.

36. Shenkin, A., and Wretlind, A. Complete intravenous nutrition including amino acids, glucose and lipids. In J. R. Richards and J. M. Kinney (eds.), *Nutritional Aspects of Care in the Critically Ill.* Edinburgh: Churchill-Livingstone, 1977.

37. Shils, M. E. Guidelines for total parenteral nutrition. *J.A.M.A.* 220:1721, 1972.

38. Shizgal, H. M., and Forse, R. A. Protein and caloric requirements with total parenteral nutrition. *Ann. Surg.* 192:562, 1980.

39. Singh, V. N. Non-glucose carbohydrate as an alternate energy source (Abstract). Presented at the 7th Clinical Congress, American Society of Parenteral and Enteral Nutrition, Washington, D.C., January 17, 1983.

40. Tao, R. C. Glycerol: Its metabolism and use as an intravenous energy source. *J. Parenter. Enter. Nutr.* 7:479, 1983.

41. Trissel, L. A. (Ed.). *Handbook of Injectable Drugs* (2nd ed.). Bethesda, MD: American Society of Hospital Pharmacists, 1980.

42. Vanamee, P. Parenteral nutrition. In Nutrition Reviews' *Present Knowledge in Nutrition.* New York: Nutrition Foundation, 1976.

43. Wilmore, D. W. (ed.). *The Metabolic Management of the Critically Ill.* New York: Plenum, 1977.

44. Wilmore, D. W., Moyland, J. A. Helmkamp, G. M., and Pruitt, B. A., Jr. Clinical evaluation of a 10% intravenous fat emulsion for parenteral nutrition in thermally injured patients. *Ann. Surg.* 178:503, 1973.

45. Wolfe, B. M., and Chock, E. Energy sources, stores, and hormonal controls. *Surg. Clin. North Am.* 61:509, 1981.

46. Wolfe, B. M., and Ney, D. M. Lipid metabolism in parenteral nutrition. In J. L. Rombeau and M. D. Caldwell (eds.), *Parenteral Nutrition.* Philadelphia: W. B. Saunders, 1986.

47. Wretlind, A. Current status of Intralipid and other fat emulsions. In H. C. Meng and D. W. Wilmore (eds.), *Fat Emulsions in Parenteral Nutrition.* Chicago: American Medical Association, 1976.

Catheter-Related Complications of Total Parenteral Nutrition

James F. Flowers
John A. Ryan, Jr.
Jo Ann Gough

In the 1950s and 1960s the major obstacle to providing complete intravenous nutrition, adequate to sustain positive nitrogen balance and sufficient to achieve growth, was the lack of a satisfactory delivery system for hyperosmolar solutions. These solutions, highly concentrated to avoid excessive volume, were sclerosing when given through short catheters in peripheral veins; longer plastic catheters, threaded through antecubital veins and terminating in the superior vena cava, were notorious for early thrombophlebitis and were, therefore, not suitable for long-term use. Clearly, another approach was needed.

In 1968 Dudrick et al. [15] solved the problem by adapting subclavian vein catheterization for the infusion of hypertonic solutions of glucose and amino acids. Subclavian vein catheterization was first used for rapid access to the central venous system in the treatment of battle injuries [2] and was later used to measure central venous pressure [68]. Using this approach for the administration of hyperalimentation, Dudrick et al. proved that long-term total parenteral nutrition (TPN) could be safe and effective.

The basic principles of the technique Dudrick et al. described have changed little in the two decades since its introduction and widespread acceptance. The tip of the catheter resides in the superior vena cava so that solutions with a concentration of 1500 mOsm/liter (five times the osmolarity of plasma) can be infused at a rate of 2 to 3 ml/min while being diluted by a blood flow of 2 to 5 liter/min (a dilution factor of at least a thousand). The venipuncture itself is in a large vein, decreasing the likelihood of thrombophlebitis. Although there have been minor modifications in the materials and methods of administering intravenous nutrition, this original piece of work still stands as a landmark in modern medicine.

A large body of data on the incidence, prevention, recognition, and treatment of various catheter-related complications has accumulated. These data will continue to accumulate as long as new patient populations are defined, new catheters are invented, new insertion techniques are employed, new diagnostic modalities are refined, and new treatment options evolve. However, strict adherence to basic surgical principles, awareness of the array of potential clinical problems, enforcement of an institutional protocol, and scientific review of the published experience of others remain the keys to maintaining an acceptably low complication rate in the administration of TPN.

CATHETER SELECTION

The ideal catheter for TPN should be easy to insert and maintain in a central vein; should be atraumatic and nonreactive to the skin, soft tissues, and venous endothelium; and should be nonthrombogenic and resistant to bacterial colonization. In general, the smallest catheter adequate for delivery is best.

In the past, stiff, relatively thrombogenic materials such as polyvinyl chloride and polyethylene were used because their insertion was simple and easy. More recently, softer, more flexible, less thrombogenic catheters, such as those made of polyurethane and especially those made of silicone elastomer, have become available. These catheters, which can be inserted more safely with the Seldinger technique described below, are increasing in popularity and should lead to fewer complications.

Silicone elastomer catheters are available in a wide variety of lengths and calibers. The simplest are the short catheters (15–25 cm) for direct percutaneous access to central veins, designed for use in the hospital. Other catheters are designed for long-term use out of the hospital. They may be placed through a subcutaneous tunnel where they are stabilized by a polyester cuff.

Silicone elastomer catheters have also been designed for entry into the central venous system via the peripheral veins of the antecubital fossa, thus eliminating the risks of insertion directly into the great veins. Despite occasional problems with superficial thrombophlebitis or misdirection, these catheters have been useful in selected cases for intermediate-term use in both inpatients and outpatients.

Catheters are also available with pressure-sensitive two-way valves at the distal ports. This design feature helps prevent air embolism and minimizes reflux of blood into the catheter tip between uses, reducing the required frequency of flushing with heparinized saline solution.

Multilumen catheters have gained popularity because they provide additional access for venous blood sampling, venous pressure monitoring, and administration of medications and blood products. However, their concomitant use for TPN has been associated with a dramatic increase in catheter-related sepsis [49, 67, 70]. Every reasonable attempt should be made to avoid using multilumen catheters for TPN, and the indications for their exceptional use should be reexamined on a regular basis.

CATHETER INSERTION

Anatomy of Central Veins

The superior vena cava is the largest of all veins, but its location deep in the chest behind the sternum makes it inaccessible except through the arm or the neck (Fig. 3-1). It will accept a catheter that has been passed through the subclavian or internal jugular vein.

The subclavian vein lies within the costoclavicular-scalene triangle, which is bordered by the clavicle anteriorly, the anterior scalene muscle posteriorly, and the flat surface of the first rib inferiorly (Fig. 3-2). The subclavian vein courses over the dome of the pleural space and is covered by the medial 5 cm of the clavicle. It arises as the axillary vein laterally and becomes the subclavian vein as it crosses over the first rib. The confluence of the subclavian and internal jugular veins forms the innominate vein, which is short and nearly vertical on the right side and longer and more nearly horizontal on the left side. These, in turn, form the superior vena cava. The subclavian artery and brachial

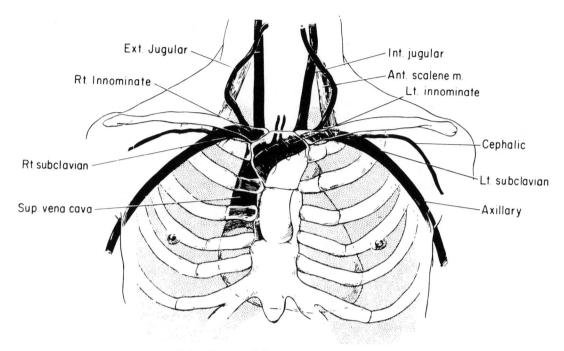

Figure 3-1. Venous anatomy of the thoracic inlet.

plexus lie dorsal to the anterior scalene muscle (see Fig. 3-2).

The internal jugular vein lies behind the sternocleidomastoid muscle in the carotid sheath, usually anterior and lateral to the carotid artery and the vagus nerve (Fig. 3-3). The junction of the subclavian vein and the internal jugular vein lies just beneath the sternoclavicular joint on each side. The thoracic duct on the left and the right lymphatic duct empty into the venous system at these junctions.

Etiology and Incidence of Insertion Complications

The danger in percutaneous insertion of needles and catheters into the subclavian or internal jugular veins lies in the possibility of inadvertent puncture or laceration of the important structures in proximity to these veins. Table 3-1 lists many of the potential complications of central venous catheterization. Table 3-2 lists the specific complications of insertion that occurred in one series [55]. Figure 3-4 depicts some of these graphically. Direct complications of the insertion itself are usually manifest immediately or in the first few days. Others such as venous thrombosis, catheter thrombosis, and catheter-related sepsis develop later and are classified separately.

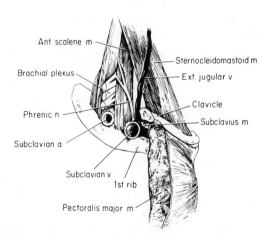

Figure 3-2. Costoclavicular-scalene triangle.

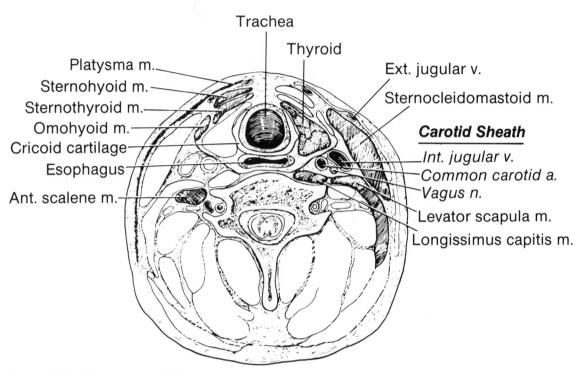

Figure 3-3. Cross section of the neck at the cricoid cartilage.

The incidence of complications related to catheter insertion has been reported to be 2 to 7% in several large series [34, 47, 55, 56, 59]. However, the definition of an insertion complication is not uniform in the literature, making comparisons difficult. In the largest series reported to date [70], only 21 (1.3%) of 1647 patients had major complications of insertion that required invasive treatment or resulted in death (0.1%), although the overall complication rate, including minor complications, was 5.7%. In general, pneumothorax and great vessel injury are the most commonly reported complications.

Prevention of Insertion Complications: Preparation and Technique

Percutaneous venipuncture of the central veins for TPN should not be treated as an emergency but rather as a sterile, precise surgical procedure with ample preparation. The patient should have an orientation visit from the TPN nurse, during which the patient learns what to expect and has an opportunity to ask questions. Although procedures may be routine for the physicians and nurses, they may cause anxiety in patients. The nurse should teach the Valsalva maneuver, which increases the pressure in the veins of the thoracic inlet. Practicing this in advance and during the procedure gives the patient a feeling of helping rather than helplessness. Familiarity with the Trendelenburg position and the Valsalva maneuver, expectation of the postinsertion chest x-ray, and knowledge of proper care of the insertion site and tubing gain the patient's cooperation and minimize anxiety. The nurse should also check in advance that the bed is suitable for Trendelenburg positioning and that adequate lighting is available.

The role of the nurse during the procedure includes attention to asepsis, positioning the patient, and providing proper equip-

Table 3-1. Complications of Central Venous Catheterization

Pleural space
  Pneumothorax
  Hemothorax
  Hydrothorax
Arterial injury
  Hematoma
  False aneurysm
  Fistula
  Stenosis
Venous injury
  Hematoma
  Thrombosis
  Hepatic vein occlusion
  Venobronchial fistula
Cardiac injury
  Myocardial perforation (hydropericardium,
    tamponade)
  Coronary sinus occlusion
  Cardiac arrhythmias, including heart block
Mediastinum
  Hemomediastinum
  Hydromediastinum
Tracheal injury
Nerve injury
  Brachial plexus
  Phrenic nerve
  Vagus nerve
  Recurrent laryngeal nerve
Lymphatic injury
  Chylothorax
  Lymph fistula
Embolic events
  Air embolism
  Catheter embolism
  Pulmonary thromboembolism
Catheter-related sepsis
Septic thrombosis
Misdirection (neck, contralateral arm, azygos
    vein, etc.)
  Thrombophlebitis

Table 3-2. Complications of Catheter Insertion (355 Catheters in 200 Consecutive Patients)

Complication	No.
Pneumothorax	6
Thrombophlebitis	3
Carotid artery laceration	1
Mediastinal hematoma	1
Hydrothorax	1
Brachial plexus injury	2
Total	14

Data from Ryan, J. A., Jr., Abel, R. M., Abbott, W. M., et al. Catheter complications in total parenteral nutrition: A prospective study of 200 consecutive patients. *N. Engl. J. Med.* 290:757, 1974.

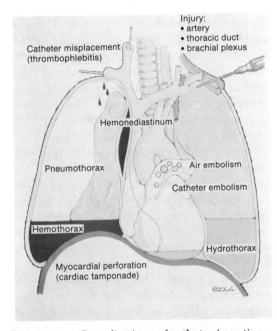

Figure 3-4. Complications of catheter insertion.

ment. Being available to comfort the patient throughout the procedure by providing physical contact and reassurance is invaluable.

The patient should be brought into a state of normal blood volume by transfusions or intravenous fluid therapy before venipuncture is attempted. Occasionally, it is necessary to suspend anticoagulation therapy or to infuse specific blood components to correct coagulopathies. The patient should be premedicated with short-acting benzodiazepines or narcotics in order to minimize discomfort and help ensure calmness and cooperation. The patient who is psychologically prepared as well as adequately premedicated is less likely to move at an inopportune time during insertion.

A mobile cart maintained by the TPN team should be provided with all necessary items (e.g., catheters, instruments, dressings, gowns, gloves, masks, intravenous adminis- tration sets, and so on). Once the patient is positioned, the operative field is cleansed with a 10% acetone and 70% isopropyl alco- hol solution, and povidone-iodine antiseptic solution is then applied and allowed to air- dry. The physician wears sterile gown and gloves, and all personnel, including the pa- tient, wear masks. Sterile drapes are placed to provide a wide field in which to work.

Infraclavicular Subclavian Vein

The infraclavicular approach to the subcla- vian vein for access to the central circulation has several advantages. The cutaneous entry site of the catheter in the pectoral skin below the clavicle has proved to be an excellent place to keep clean and maintain a sterile dressing because it is flat, is relatively immo- bile, and does not collect perspiration or other secretions. The patient's arm and neck are free for normal motion, enhancing long- term comfort and convenience. These advan- tages make this the preferred route for TPN in adults.

Three preliminary measures for position- ing patients for percutaneous access to the subclavian vein are in common use: (1) The Trendelenburg position and Valsalva maneu- ver are employed to increase venous pres- sure, decreasing the chance of air embolism and possibly distending the vein to facilitate its puncture. (2) A rolled sheet or towel is placed beneath the vertebral column between the scapulae, increasing the separation be- tween the subclavian vein and the apex of the lung by allowing the shoulders to fall back and permitting the medial aspect of the clavicles to rise. (3) The patient's head is turned away from the insertion site, improv- ing visualization of the musculoskeletal land- marks and straightening the course of the vein. [Editor's Note: It has never been my practice to have the patient turn his or her head—the catheter is not as easy to place. This has been confirmed (see below) by non- invasive studies.]

More recently, studies correlating gross an- atomic dissection with MRIs have challenged each of these guidelines [33]. Although the

Trendelenburg position remains useful for enlarging the veins of the neck, fibrous at- tachments surrounding the subclavian vein may actually prevent any significant disten- tion with this maneuver. Shoulder retraction, although facilitating a horizontal approach, may actually compress the subclavian vein in its anteroposterior dimension between the clavicle and the first rib, making the veni- puncture or threading of the catheter more difficult. Turning the head to the contralat- eral side tends to increase the angle formed at the confluence of the subclavian and internal jugular veins, making passage of the guide- wire into the neck more likely. These obser- vations suggest that a neutral position may be more favorable for successful catheteriza- tion. Nevertheless, any measures to elevate a low venous pressure, whether by fluid re- suscitation, Trendelenburg positioning, or the Valsalva maneuver, are certainly indi- cated to decrease the chance of air embolism.

The preferred approach is via the left sub- clavian vein, because, as seen in Figure 3-1, its continuation as the left innominate vein makes a more gentle arch into the superior vena cava than does the corresponding path on the right side. This makes misdirection less likely and outweighs the slightly in- creased risk of lymphatic injury on the left side.

Figure 3-5 demonstrates the important landmarks for subclavian vein catheteriza- tion. The landmarks are the sternal notch in the midline and a point on the underside of the clavicle at the junction of its medial third and lateral two-thirds [36, 37]. These two points help identify the course of the axillary vein as it crosses the first rib and continues as the subclavian vein. In selecting the actual entry site on the skin, however, one should plan to avoid the dense costoclavicular liga- ments in the tight angle between the medial third of the clavicle and the first rib. Entering this area not only makes passage of a soft, flexible catheter difficult and contributes to kinking of both the guidewire and the cathe- ter, but also may eventually cause catheter- fragment embolism due to chronic pinching action and friction on the catheter [1]. The

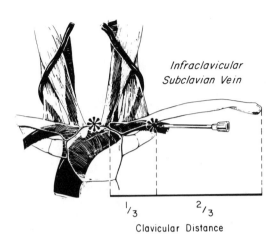

Infraclavicular Subclavian Vein

$^1/_3$ $^2/_3$

Clavicular Distance

Figure 3-5. Infraclavicular approach to sub-clavian vein catheterization.

key to avoidance of this problem is in entering both the skin and the vein more laterally, taking into account the length of the needle and aiming for the vein just as it begins to cross the first rib. Two to 4 cm below the junction of the middle and lateral thirds of the clavicle should be an ideal entry point in most adult patients. A skin wheal is raised in this area with 1 ml of 1% lidocaine, and additional local anesthetic is delivered to the periosteum beneath the clavicle with a small-bore needle. A longer, larger-bore needle, usually 16 or 18 gauge, is provided for the actual venipuncture and will accommodate a flexible spring guidewire with an open J tip.

With the index finger of one hand in the sternal notch and the thumb along the clavicle, the landmarks are established. The needle is inserted horizontally with the bevel up, passing through the skin, subcutaneous tissue, and pectoralis major muscle, just beneath the clavicle, aiming toward the sternal notch. A small-barrel syringe is selected so it can be easily depressed into a horizontal position parallel to the chest wall as the needle approaches the vein. Pain may be elicited when the needle pierces the fascia of the subclavius muscle or touches the periosteum of the clavicle, but it is important to hold this horizontal position throughout the venipuncture to avoid entering the pleural space. As the patient performs a Valsalva maneuver,

the physician advances the needle while gently aspirating the syringe. If no blood returns, the needle is withdrawn slowly while gentle aspiration continues. If venous blood is not found, the needle is withdrawn entirely, and another attempt is made. If arterial bleeding ensues, direct pressure is applied. If air is aspirated, the needle is removed, the patient is observed for signs of pneumothorax, and a chest x-ray is obtained.

If several attempts are unsuccessful, the opposite side is used. Once the vein is entered and blood aspirated, three maneuvers help to position the needle so the guidewire will thread easily into the superior vena cava: (1) The syringe is elevated cephalad so the tip of the needle in the subclavian vein will be pointed down the course of the innominate vein. (2) The needle itself is rotated 90 degrees so the bevel is pointed downstream. (3) The patient turns his or her head toward the side of the insertion site to create an acute angle between the jugular vein and the subclavian vein, making passage of the guidewire toward the heart and away from the neck more likely.

At this point, the hub of the needle is immobilized and the syringe is disconnected while the patient again performs a Valsalva maneuver. While blood flows freely from the open needle, the flexible-tip guidewire is threaded into the vein for a distance of approximately 15 to 20 cm. The needle is then removed, leaving the tip of the guidewire in the superior vena cava. The catheter is trimmed, if necessary, to the proper length, and its tip is inserted over the guidewire up to the level of the skin. The end of the guidewire must protrude through the hub of the catheter. The two are then advanced as a unit through the soft tissues into the vein all the way to the catheter hub, and the guidewire is then removed. Alternatively, an introducer-dilator apparatus may first be passed into position over the guidewire, after which the guidewire and dilator are removed, the catheter inserted, and the introducer split apart with extraction. In either case, aspiration with a syringe is used at each step to ensure adequate blood return. Only very gentle force should be necessary, and any undue resistance should warn of potential misdirection. Fluoroscopic guidance may be necessary in some cases to safely achieve final positioning. This Seldinger technique represents a significant technical improvement, reducing trauma by permitting the use of smaller needles and preventing catheter embolism by eliminating the need for a catheter-inside-the-needle system. The larger introducer systems, however, do pose a threat if they are not handled with respect during insertion. Moving the guidewire back and forth slightly at frequent intervals during the insertion helps to maintain the intraluminal position and ensure safe passage of the introducer.

Once in place, the catheter is secured to the skin with a monofilament suture passed through the dermis and tied to the hub or its flanges. The area is cleansed of any blood, and povidone-iodine ointment is placed at the entry site. The catheter hub is attached to a short length of sterile extension tubing included beneath the sterile dressing. Standard intravenous tubing and a fresh bottle of isotonic solution are then connected, and patency of the entire system is checked by lowering the bottle below the level of the heart while backflow of blood into the intravenous tubing is observed. This is the final check to make sure the catheter tip lies within the vascular space. This solution is used initially until the chest x-ray confirms that the tip of the catheter is properly positioned in the superior vena cava.

Internal Jugular Vein

The internal jugular vein may be preferred for catheterization in four subsets of patients. In the emphysematous patient on positive pressure ventilation, the increased risk of a tension pneumothorax may be significantly reduced by an approach to the central circulation through the neck rather than the chest. In the patient with a coagulopathy or thrombocytopenia, a carotid artery injury may be more easily controlled with direct pressure in the neck than a similar injury to the subclavian artery. In patients whose venous anat-

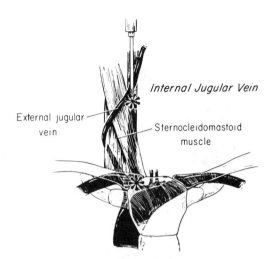

Figure 3-6. Anterior approach to internal jugular vein catheterization.

omy or thrombotic occlusion makes it difficult to pass a guidewire into the superior vena cava from the subclavian approach, the internal jugular vein may provide a useful alternative. Finally, in any patient in whom permanent vascular access for hemodialysis is planned in the upper extremities, it may be wise to avoid the subclavian veins for hyperalimentation, because any thrombotic complications here may eventually compromise graft or fistula outflow.

The right internal jugular vein is preferred because it provides the most direct route to the superior vena cava, minimizing the chance of misdirection. Figure 3-6 illustrates the landmarks in the anterior approach to this vein. In the Trendelenburg position, the patient extends his or her neck and turns the head slightly to the opposite side. The needle is inserted at the anterior border of the sternocleidomastoid muscle just below the superficial course of the external jugular vein. The needle is inserted parallel and just lateral to the carotid artery, which is palpated throughout the procedure with the fingertips of the left hand. The angle of approach should be 30 to 45 degrees above the horizontal, aiming for a point just deep to the sternal head of the clavicle. The V-shaped indentation formed by the sternal and clavicular insertions of the sternocleidomastoid muscle may be palpated as an additional landmark immediately lateral to the anticipated point of vein entry. Other approaches to this vein have been described, but we believe this is the simplest and most direct method with the lowest chance of injury to surrounding structures. Once the syringe aspirates blood from the internal jugular vein, the guidewire is threaded through the needle into the innominate vein and superior vena cava. Catheter insertion follows as described for subclavian vein catheterization.

Supraclavicular Subclavian Vein

The supraclavicular approach to the subclavian vein has been favored by some [71]. It offers no advantages in comfort or daily care, however, and may place the apices of the lung at significant risk if there is any difficulty in locating the vein. For these reasons, we have not found this approach to be a useful alternative.

Antecubital Vein

This technique employs a long-arm silicone elastomer catheter that is inserted through the antecubital fossa via the basilic or cephalic vein into the superior vena cava. This approach avoids the insertion complications of subclavian or internal jugular venipuncture [28]. Patients must have easily visible or palpable veins, however, and threading the catheter into the superior vena cava may be technically difficult. Superficial thrombophlebitis occasionally develops, necessitating early removal of the catheter. Nevertheless, experience has shown that, when successful, this technique yields excellent results [21, 52]. In some hospitals, intravenous therapy team nurses are inserting these catheters at the bedside or even on an outpatient basis.

Recognition and Treatment of Insertion Complications

A chest x-ray should be taken and read promptly after every catheter insertion. This should identify misdirection, pneumothorax, hemothorax, or other early complications. A subsequent chest x-ray should also be obtained whenever there is any question of catheter malfunction or any clinical deterioration that may be attributable to an insertion-related complication.

Misdirection

The catheter tip may be found on completion chest x-ray to be in the neck, contralateral arm, or azygos vein. This should be managed by repositioning the catheter under sterile conditions with a guidewire and fluoroscopy. Hypertonic solutions are not well tolerated in veins more peripheral than the innominate veins or superior vena cava. Ideally, the tip of the catheter should be at the junction of the superior vena cava and the right atrium. This point is approximately 20 to 25 cm from the left internal jugular or left subclavian approach or 15 to 20 cm from the right side in an average adult.

Pneumothorax

When a patient develops dyspnea, chest pain, cyanosis, or shock following placement of a subclavian or internal jugular catheter, tension pneumothorax should be suspected. Physical examination may reveal decreased breath sounds and hyperresonance on the affected side with tracheal deviation to the contralateral side and jugular venous distention. Although a chest x-ray confirms the diagnosis, treatment should be carried out on clinical grounds alone in the face of cardiopulmonary instability. A large-bore needle or chest tube should be placed through the second intercostal space in the midclavicular line. Clinical improvement should be prompt if the diagnosis is correct. If chest x-ray indicates that the catheter is still in the vascular space and placement of the needle or chest tube solves the clinical problem, then there is no reason to remove the catheter. Smaller pneumothoraces without tension may be evacuated or managed expectantly. [*Editor's Note:* Tension pneumothorax is unusual, but pneumothorax may occur in up to 6% of insertions. Pain behind the clavicle after an insertion is almost always an indication of pneumothorax.]

Arterial Injury

Pulsatile blood return or expanding hematoma at the time of attempted venipuncture usually indicates arterial injury. Prompt removal of the needle and application of direct pressure are usually sufficient to stop the bleeding, although injuries to the subclavian artery may not be easily controlled in patients with an underlying coagulopathy. A chest x-ray may reveal a subpleural hematoma or hemothorax. Proximal dissection of a hematoma into the mediastinum may make the diagnosis more difficult. A large-bore chest tube should be placed posteriorly on the affected side in unstable patients to help clarify the diagnosis and remove any blood or air. Neck exploration or thoracotomy is rarely necessary for evacuation of the hematoma and direct control of the bleeding. Chronic stenosis, arteriovenous fistula, and pseudoaneurysm formation are potential late sequelae.

Catheter Embolism

Catheter embolism is fortunately a less common event now that the catheter-inside-the-needle systems have been almost completely abandoned. This complication usually represents an error in technique due to shearing off of the catheter tip by the sharp bevel of the needle when the catheter is withdrawn during placement. The catheter fragment may lodge anywhere from the insertion site to the pulmonary artery and can cause thrombosis, sepsis, or arrhythmia. Paradoxic catheter emboli have been reported [44]. The treatment is retrieval with an angiographic guidewire snare technique performed under fluoroscopic guidance [6].

Placement of catheters over a guidewire or through a soft introducer has virtually eliminated this problem. There is one exception, however. Subclavian vein catheterization through the extreme medial aspect of this vein has been associated with catheter embolism occurring as a late complication [1]. This complication is attributed to the chronic pinching action on the catheter as it passes between the clavicle and the first rib. In some cases, difficulties with catheter patency or

recognition of the "pinch-off sign" on chest x-ray at the point of catheter compression may warn of impending catheter transection. This is an indication for catheter removal and replacement through a more lateral entry site.

Arrhythmias

Supraventricular or ventricular arrhythmias are occasionally encountered as a result of irritation of the endocardium by a guidewire. Various forms of heart block—even complete heart block in a patient with preexisting left bundle branch block—may occur. Promptly repositioning the wire in the superior vena cava usually solves the problem, but medical therapy, pacemaker intervention, or even cardioversion may be required. The catheter itself can cause these same arrhythmias, but selecting the correct catheter length combined with fluoroscopic positioning should prevent this complication.

Lymphatic Injury

Lymphatic injury usually involves the thoracic duct on approaches from the left side and is recognized by clear lymph drainage from the insertion site. This is managed by catheter removal and the application of direct pressure. Chronic sequelae are rare, although chylothorax has been reported [65].

Nerve Injury

As seen in Figure 3-2, the subclavian artery and brachial plexus are deep and posterior to the subclavian vein, being separated from it by the width of the intervening anterior scalene muscle. Knowledge of these anatomic relationships and maintenance of a strictly horizontal approach to the subclavian vein in a supine patient should prevent a brachial plexus injury. Prompt removal of the needle or catheter is indicated if a nerve injury is suspected. Fortunately, permanent neurologic damage is rare.

Myocardial Perforation

This surgical emergency may develop acutely or insidiously. It is a result of positioning the catheter beyond the cavoatrial junction. Constant motion of the catheter with the cardiac cycle may cause abrupt or gradual erosion through the myocardium and into the pericardial space, particularly with the stiffer catheter materials. As the pericardium begins to fill with hypertonic solution, effusion and eventual tamponade may develop [4, 64]. In a complex deteriorating clinical situation, this complication may be difficult to recognize unless a high index of suspicion concerning central venous catheters is maintained. The diagnosis may be suggested or confirmed by chest x-ray or echocardiography, but an attempt at aspiration through the distal port of the catheter should be made prior to its removal or repositioning. This may be a life-saving measure, providing prompt diagnosis and treatment while avoiding an emergency pericardiocentesis. Silicone elastomer catheters should be much less prone to this complication than catheters of stiffer materials.

Caval Perforation

Just as with myocardial perforation, this complication may develop insidiously, and a high index of suspicion is required. A stiff catheter tenting the wall of the superior vena cava or a widening mediastinum on chest x-ray, coupled with the inability to aspirate blood from the catheter, is virtually diagnostic. Catheter removal is usually sufficient, but prevention and early diagnosis are essential. Hydromediastinum and hemomediastinum have been reported as lethal complications [10, 32, 43]. Pericardial tamponade may also occur if the caval perforation is within the pericardial reflection.

Air Embolism

Air embolism is an unusual but dramatic and potentially fatal complication. Air embolism may occur in unguarded moments during the process of insertion when the syringe is removed in order to thread the catheter or guidewire. It may also occur if the intravenous tubing becomes inadvertently detached from the intravenous catheter, or after the intravenous catheter has been pulled out and before the tract can seal. Hypovolemia, upright posture, and deep, spontaneous inspi-

rations are predisposing factors due to creation of an unfavorable pressure gradient. Air embolism can be prevented if the patient performs a Valsalva maneuver while in the Trendelenburg position as the catheter is being inserted or when the tubing is being changed; if the patient is instructed to place his or her finger over the hub of the catheter (breaking sterile technique) in an emergency such as an accidental tubing disconnection; and if, whenever the catheter is removed, antibiotic ointment and occlusive dressing are placed over the insertion site for 24 hours. Catheters with two-way valves at each port are designed to reduce the possibility of air embolism during tubing changes and other manipulations, but the usual precautions should still be followed.

The symptoms of air embolism are dyspnea, chest pain, and depressed mental status. The physical findings vary from tachypnea, tachycardia, cyanosis, and elevated central venous pressure, to shock and cardiac arrest. The characteristic mill-wheel churning murmur heard over the precordium is caused by frothing of air at the pulmonic valve. Bubbles may be seen on chest x-ray or echocardiogram. The differential diagnosis is that of any cardiopulmonary collapse, but any patient found in this condition with an open central venous catheter is highly suspect for an air embolus. Treatment includes covering the catheter immediately and placing the patient head down while in the left lateral decubitus position [16, 46]. The principle is to put the right side up so that the air will be trapped in the right atrial appendage or right ventricular apex. Death is caused by obstruction of the pulmonary outflow tract or paradoxic embolization to the coronary or cerebral circulation through a patent foramen ovale. Attempts may be made to aspirate the air with a central venous catheter passed into the right heart. However, if cardiac arrest unresponsive to conventional cardiopulmonary resuscitation (CPR) occurs, then emergency left thoracotomy at the bedside is indicated, with aspiration of the right ventricle and direct cardiac massage [58]. Two hundred milliliters of air in the right heart can be fatal, and only seconds are required for this volume to pass through an open catheter [19]. This emphasizes the importance of preventing even brief periods of exposure of the open system to atmospheric pressure.

VENOUS THROMBOSIS

Etiology and Incidence

The initial assumption that great vein thrombosis would not occur secondary to TPN has clearly been disproved. Venous thrombosis in this setting should not be surprising, considering how many patients receiving TPN satisfy Virchow's triad of conditions predisposing to thrombus formation: venous stasis, hypercoagulable state, and local trauma. Patients requiring TPN are often volume-depleted or subject to low-flow states. Their blood may be hypercoagulable due to sepsis, major surgical trauma, or malignancy. The catheters inevitably create local trauma at the puncture site and irritation of the intima.

Added to this triad is the constant presence of an intravascular foreign body. A fibrin sheath forms on all types of indwelling catheters, and it has been suggested that this may be the first step in thrombus formation [29, 50]. This sheath originates at the intimal injury, either where the catheter enters the vessel or where the catheter tip touches the intima. By 1 to 7 days, the entire catheter is surrounded by an unorganized, unendothelialized fibrin sleeve that is apparent on venography even in the absence of any clinical signs of thrombosis.

Clinically significant major venous thrombosis has been reported in up to 5% of patients in recent large series [47, 59, 70]. Clinically silent thrombi were found at autopsy in an additional 4% of patients in one study [55].

Prevention

Two preventative measures have been recommended. Silicone elastomer and polyurethane catheters have been reported to cause a lower incidence of fibrin sheath formation than either polyethylene or polyvinyl chloride catheters [63, 66], although the exact correlation of this finding with clinical great vein thrombosis is not yet clear. Silicone elastomer is even softer and less thrombogenic than polyurethane and would, therefore, seem to be the ideal material for the prevention of great vein thrombosis. The addition of heparin to the infusion solution to prevent great vein thrombosis has also been suggested [9, 17, 31]. One to 3000 U/liter of TPN solution is recommended to prevent local thrombosis without causing systemic anticoagulation. Others have challenged the efficacy of this regimen [40], but we have routinely used it unless there is a specific contraindication.

Recognition

Recognition of great vein thrombosis is impeded by the variability of its presentation. Thrombosis may be asymptomatic and only discovered when the physician is unable to insert a new catheter, or it may be an incidental finding at autopsy. Pain and swelling of the arm and neck suggest the diagnosis, which may be confirmed by venography or ultrasound-Doppler duplex scanning. Occasionally, signs and symptoms of pulmonary embolism may be the first clue to thrombosis. Certainly, an intravenous catheter should be considered the possible source of an otherwise unexplained pulmonary embolus if upper-extremity or superior vena cava thrombosis can be documented radiographically. Fortunately, pulmonary emboli from TPN catheters must be rare, as no cases were documented in three recent series [47, 59, 70].

Treatment

The conventional treatment of major venous thrombosis is removal of the catheter and 6 to 12 weeks of systemic anticoagulation. This should be accompanied by a search for any specific etiologic factors such as large catheter size, thrombogenic material, the presence of infection, or malposition of the tip, which may have contributed to thrombus formation and which may be corrected or avoided if another catheter must be placed. Thrombolytic therapy is now being more frequently employed to restore venous patency, especially when the situation is clinically urgent [14, 38, 54, 60, 61]. The advent of tissue plasminogen activator (TPA) for use in this setting should represent a significant improvement in safety and effectiveness [62].

Special Case: Septic Thrombosis

Suppurative or septic thrombophlebitis of the great veins is fortunately rare, since it has devastating clinical significance. The most common presentation is unrelenting septicemia of unknown etiology, with or without signs of venous occlusion. Venography and blood cultures confirm the diagnosis.

Treatment with high-dose, long-term antibiotics and systemic anticoagulation has only resulted in occasional success [48]. The addition of thrombolytic therapy may improve medical management, but this has not been thoroughly evaluated.

Direct surgical attack on the veins of the thorax is a major undertaking. Excision of the superior vena cava for septic thrombosis has not been reported. However, there have been isolated reports documenting successful drainage or excision of infected veins at the level of the thoracic inlet in conjunction with extraction of purulent thrombus from the more central veins using a Fogarty catheter [26, 53, 69]. This approach is obviously hazardous but may be necessary if the combination of antibiotics, anticoagulation, and thrombolysis is not effective.

CATHETER THROMBOSIS

Thrombotic occlusion of the catheter represents only a small fraction of mechanical difficulties in most large series. Presumably, stasis in the catheter or reflux of blood at the distal tip is primarily responsible for this problem. Intrinsic surface properties of some catheter materials may predispose to platelet

aggregation, and a period of subclinical non-occlusive thrombosis may occur [63, 66].

Prophylactic heparin has been recommended for prevention of catheter thrombosis [9], as well as prevention of venous thrombosis [17, 31] and catheter-related sepsis [3]. Based on these studies, we recommend heparin as long as it is not clinically contraindicated.

Thrombolytic therapy has proved to be extremely useful in restoring patency to thrombosed catheters [22, 23, 30]. Our protocol consists of instilling urokinase into the catheter followed by attempted aspiration 10 minutes later. An aliquot of a 5000 U/ml solution equal in volume to the luminal volume of the catheter is used for each injection. This procedure may be repeated, if necessary, so long as systemic thrombolysis is not induced. We have found this method to be very effective in avoiding the need for catheter replacement with the attendant risks of reinsertion.

CATHETER-RELATED SEPSIS

One of the most frequent and potentially serious complications in patients receiving TPN is septicemia related to the catheter. Patients are treated with TPN because of severe and complex medical and surgical illnesses. The typical patient is recovering from an operation; has multiple tubes and drains; and may have pneumonia, urinary tract infection, wound infection, intra-abdominal abscesses, or fistulaes. In such a patient, the etiology of a septic episode is not always clear. When the possibility of catheter-related sepsis is added, the picture becomes even more difficult to sort out.

Definition

Catheter-related sepsis in a patient receiving TPN is defined clinically as an episode of sepsis for which no anatomic septic focus can be identified and which resolves on removal of the hyperalimentation catheter. Laboratory confirmation may be provided by recovery of the same organism from the catheter tip and a peripheral blood culture. In the absence of this confirmation, the clinical definition remains sufficient for patient management.

Etiology

The weight of evidence strongly suggests that most cases of catheter-related sepsis in the patient receiving TPN are secondary to ingrowth of skin organisms along the outside of the catheter or breaks in a closed system, allowing organisms to gain access to the inside of the catheter.

This conclusion is the result of systematic study of all potential sources of catheter-related sepsis. The role of contamination in the solution was examined and found to be an extremely rare cause of catheter-related sepsis. This is due not only to stringent preparation techniques, but also to the fact that TPN solutions are surprisingly poor growth media [22, 55, 56]. Hematogenous seeding of intravenous catheters must also be uncommon, because the incidence of catheter sepsis (3–11%) is so much lower than that of concurrent anatomic infections (38–84%) and because the organisms responsible for catheter-related sepsis are rarely the same as those in other infections [12, 13, 47, 55, 56, 59, 70].

Organisms normally found on the skin of hospitalized patients and on the hands of hospital personnel are the most commonly cultured organisms in cases of catheter-related sepsis. Most large series list the following organisms as the leading sources of catheter-related sepsis: *Staphylococcus aureus, Staphylococcus epidermidis, Streptococcus viridans*, and *Candida albicans* [47, 55, 56, 59]. Much less commonly seen are the common gram-negative rod pathogens, such as *Klebsiella, Pseudomonas, Serratia*, and *Escherichia coli*, although the incidence of gram-negative pathogens in one series [70] was 23% of all cases of catheter-related sepsis, considerably higher than in other reports.

The hypothesis that skin flora are primarily responsible for catheter-related sepsis is also supported by abundant epidemiologic evidence. Institutions that have established and enforced protocols dealing with strict aseptic technique in catheter insertion and nursing care have witnessed a striking decrease in the incidence of catheter-associated sepsis [20, 55, 56].

Catheter-related sepsis has a strong correlation with positive findings on cultures from the skin entry site [5, 59]. If the skin entry point for a catheter becomes infected, then the catheter should be removed. Convincing evidence for this policy is provided by the finding that skin cultures are positive in over 50% of patients with proven catheter-related sepsis, but less than 10% are positive in those whose catheters were removed for suspected catheter sepsis and subsequently proven free of infection [59]. The number of attempted catheterizations also has a direct relationship to the incidence of catheter-related sepsis [59]. Skin injury by multiple needle punctures enhances low-grade skin infection that can lead to an infected catheter.

At least two studies have identified the use of multilumen venous catheters (triple lumen catheters, pulmonary artery catheters) for TPN with a threefold increase in the incidence of catheter-related sepsis [49, 70]. This is presumably due to the expanded opportunity to break and enter the closed system on a more frequent basis. [*Editor's Note:* It is not so much the breaking into a closed system, but that the patients with triple lumen catheters have no other venous access, thereby increasing manipulations.] The analysis is complicated, however, by the fact that patients selected for triple lumen and pulmonary artery catheters tend to be more critically ill and, hence, more susceptible to infection. Further study is needed to determine what effect placing a second catheter solely for TPN would have on overall patient morbidity. Nevertheless, the conclusion that increasing exposure of the TPN system to a contaminated environment invites infectious complications is inescapable.

Incidence

Data collected at the Centers for Disease Control (CDC) from 31 hospitals administering

Table 3-3. **Incidence of Catheter Sepsis Related to Total Parenteral Nutrition**

Study	Medical Center	Year	Patients	Incidence of Catheter Sepsis (% of Patients) All Pathogens	Fungi	Mortality (%)
Ryan et al. [55]	Massachusetts General	1974	200	11	4	1
Sanders and Sheldon [56]	San Francisco General	1976	172	4.7	1.7	0
Padberg et al. [47]	New England Deaconess	1981	104	4.8	0	0
Jones et al. [34]	St. Barnabas, New Jersey	1984	307	4.5	1.5	0
Sitzmann et al. [59]	Johns Hopkins	1985	200	7.5	0.5	NS[a]
Wolfe et al. [70]	University of California, Davis	1986	1647	6.5[b]	1.6	0.6

[a]NS = Not stated.
[b]When multilumen catheters were excluded in this series, the rate of catheter sepsis was approximately 3%.

TPN to a total of 2078 patients under a formal protocol revealed an overall incidence of catheter-related sepsis of 7% [24]. Table 3-3 summarizes the incidence of catheter sepsis (4.5–11%) related to TPN in several large institutional series spanning 13 years since that benchmark survey from the CDC was reported in 1973.

Prevention

When Dudrick et al. first introduced TPN in 1968 [15], they established two principles for catheter care: (1) aseptic technique in the insertion and maintenance of the catheter, and (2) restricted use of the catheter for nutrient solutions only. These two principles still hold true today as the most important guidelines for minimizing catheter-related sepsis.

Importance of Protocol
Strict adherence to a protocol specifying aseptic technique for handling the catheter and restricting its use is the cornerstone of prevention. An institution offering TPN should establish and enforce an institution-wide standard of care, and the backbone of this standard should be the intravenous therapy nurse or TPN special nurse. This nurse should be well trained in aseptic technique, should have special training in TPN, should

be a skilled teacher and communicator, and should be firm enough to ensure that the nursing and medical staffs adhere to the protocol. A multidisciplinary TPN committee composed of physicians, nurses, pharmacists, and dietitians should be created and meet regularly to review the implementation of this protocol. Several studies have clearly documented the dramatic effect that a team approach to TPN can have on reducing complications [8, 18, 27, 39, 45, 55].

Catheter Care
All central line catheter care, including dressing and tubing changes, should be performed by the intravenous therapy team. Having a small number of nurses caring for the catheters helps in achieving standard, routine care of these lines and facilitates communication if any problems should arise. All administration sets should be changed with the dressings every 48 hours. The area should be cleansed with 10% acetone and 70% isopropyl alcohol solution, followed by a povidone-iodine solution. An antiseptic ointment should be applied to the puncture and suture sites following catheter placement. A transparent dressing is preferred. During this procedure, the nurse should wear a clean gown, mask, and sterile gloves. If possible, the patient should also wear a mask.

Prophylactic Heparin

Heparin in doses of 1 to 3 U/ml added to the TPN solution has been reported to reduce the incidence of catheter-related sepsis by preventing fibrin sheath formation [3]. This effect is attributed to the elimination of a potential nidus for colonization of bacteria on the catheter surface. The correlation of catheter thrombogenicity with positive findings on catheter-tip cultures [63] and the dramatic effect that thrombolytic therapy has had as an adjunct in the treatment of catheter-related sepsis in situ [23, 57] would seem to strengthen the argument that nonocclusive catheter thrombosis has at least a permissive role in the pathogenesis of catheter-related sepsis. Others [35] have not been able to demonstrate a reduction in catheter-related sepsis with the use of prophylactic heparin, perhaps due to the recent trend toward the use of less thrombogenic catheter materials. Nevertheless, we continue to use heparin in TPN solutions in the absence of any contraindications.

Routine Change of Catheter

No proof of an increased incidence of catheter-related sepsis with longevity of an individual hyperalimentation catheter exists [55]. Catheters should be left in place as long as they are functioning properly and are not infected. Unnecessary changes of catheters generate additional risks of an insertion complication and contribute to further endothelial damage and skin trauma.

Summary of Preventative Measures

The following list of guidelines may be helpful in reducing or minimizing catheter-related sepsis in the administration of TPN:

1. Institutional protocol with regular review by TPN committee
2. "Watchdog" TPN nurse
3. Aseptic technique in insertion and in routine management
4. Catheter use for nutrients only
5. No multilumen catheters
6. Sterile solutions with laminar flow technique in preparation
7. Intravenous tubing and dressing changes every 48 hours
8. No prophylactic antibiotics or antibiotic flushes
9. No routine changes of catheters without a specific indication
10. Removal of catheters for infection at skin sites
11. Use of soft, nonthrombogenic catheters, preferably silicone elastomer
12. Insertion technique of minimal trauma (Seldinger)
13. Addition of heparin (1 to 3 U/ml) to TPN solution

[*Editor's Note:* In addition, our own practice is to culture the skin surrounding the catheter in quantitative fashion. If cultures reveal a concentration of organisms greater than 10^3 organisms/cm^2 consideration should be given to removing the catheter.]

Recognition of Catheter-Related Sepsis

Clinical Findings

Recognition of catheter-related sepsis can be difficult, especially in the context of a critically ill patient with multiple potential foci of infection. When the patient receiving TPN develops a new fever, hyperglycemia, glycosuria, or other signs of sepsis, a full evaluation is initiated, including blood cultures and inspection of the catheter entry site. If a tissue infection such as pneumonia, urinary tract infection, or abdominal abscess is diagnosed, it is treated with antibiotics or surgical drainage. If no tissue diagnosis is made, then the catheter is suspected. However, several studies have documented that the incidence of suspected catheter-related sepsis is at least three times greater than that of proved catheter sepsis [47, 51, 55, 59]. Because of this consistent finding, we do not immediately remove a catheter unless the patient is florid, with shaking chills, septic shock, or recent positive findings on blood cultures for skin flora or fungal organisms. Local infection of the catheter entry site would be another indication for immediate catheter removal and abandonment of this insertion site. If none of these findings is present, however, we may leave the catheter in place despite the fever, or exchange it over a guidewire and culture the tip while continuing the search for another source of infection. [*Editor's Note:* In our experience, if the quantitative skin culture around the catheter shows less than 10^3 organisms/cm^2, removing the catheter almost never cures the sepsis, unless yeast is the offending organism, in which case the site of entry is almost never the skin.]

Microbiologic Evidence

Cultures of a catheter tip removed for suspected sepsis or of blood drawn through the catheter prior to its removal may help to identify catheter colonization. At least two methods have been proposed to distinguish colonization or contamination from true infection [11, 42]. However, a blood culture of the same organism from a remote site is needed to secure the diagnosis of true catheter-related sepsis on laboratory evidence alone.

The probability of catheter colonization or sepsis has been reported to be high when cultures of the skin around the catheter entry site are positive [5, 59]. Based on this finding, it has been recommended that insertion sites be cultured routinely in critically ill patients, moving to a new area for venous access when results are positive, even in the absence of any systemic signs of catheter-related sepsis. However, this approach must be balanced against the difficulty in interpreting skin culture results and the risks of insertion complications at the new site.

Special Case: Candida Septicemia

Table 3-3 lists the incidence of fungal catheter-related sepsis in several large series of patients receiving TPN. Although the incidence of this complication seems to be declining, a basic understanding of the pathophysiology of *Candida* infection is important in caring for patients receiving TPN. *Candida* is a normal saprophyte in the gastrointestinal tract, vagina, and respiratory tract. It colo-

nizes bladder catheters, drains, intravenous catheters, and open wounds. *Candida* infection, as opposed to *Candida* colonization, usually appears in a compromised host. A typical victim would be a malnourished patient receiving antibiotics, steroids, chemotherapy, radiation therapy, or other forms of treatment that alter normal flora or impair the host immune response. The diagnosis of *Candida* septicemia is usually made by positive results on blood cultures. However, widespread colonization and a septic presentation may be an adequate indication for catheter removal or exchange even in the absence of documented fungemia.

Treatment of Catheter-Related Sepsis

Catheter Removal

The basic treatment of catheter-related sepsis remains the removal of the catheter. We maintain the patient on isotonic glucose solutions through a peripheral vein for 24 hours in order to allow the suspected bacteremia to clear. If new central venous access is necessary, a separate skin site is selected. Unless there is an obvious ongoing anatomic source of fever, we do not start antibiotics following removal of the catheter, but we do perform surveillance blood cultures following its removal to ensure clearance of the bacteremia. Usually the fever disappears promptly if it is caused by an infected catheter, and by the time results of cultures of the catheter tip and blood are available, the patient has recovered from the septic episode. An exception would be a case of clearly documented fungal catheter-related sepsis when fungemia is apt to persist. In this setting, systemic antifungal therapy should continue until blood culture results are consistently negative.

Guidewire Exchange

In order to avoid unnecessary venipunctures, we and others [7, 41, 51, 59, 70] have gained experience with catheter exchange over a guidewire for patients with fever in whom we do not strongly suspect catheter-related sepsis. Strict aseptic technique is used, and blood samples for culture are drawn through the catheter as well as from a remote site. The skin around the catheter should be reexamined for signs of infection. If the site is grossly purulent, then the site must be abandoned. In the absence of this finding, a guidewire is passed through the catheter, the catheter is withdrawn completely, and the tip is cultured according to described methods. A new catheter is then inserted over the guidewire, and its position is confirmed on chest x-ray.

If the blood drawn from the original catheter shows positive results on culture, or the cultured material of the catheter tip yields significant growth, then at least catheter colonization is likely. The new catheter must be removed in this situation, and the site abandoned, even if the patient's fever has abated in the interim. A positive blood culture of the same organism from a peripheral site is diagnostic of catheter-related sepsis in this setting. If the catheter tip and catheter-obtained blood cultures are negative, then the new catheter may be left in place despite the fever.

Treatment In Situ

In situ treatment of catheter-related sepsis with a combination of systemic antibiotics and local thrombolytic agents has been reported with a significant improvement in successful salvage rates [23, 57]. Culture-proved cases of both gram-positive and gram-negative organisms were included in these reports, as well as one case of fungal sepsis. The hypothesis is that the formation of a fibrin sheath or thrombus, even if nonocclusive and subclinical, may either predispose the catheter to infection or prevent antibiotics and host defenses from clearing the infection. This is certainly a promising treatment strategy for clinically stable outpatients with tunneled and cuffed, long-term permanent catheters, and may also shed some light on the pathogenesis of catheter-related sepsis. Simple catheter removal, however, remains the treatment of choice for inpatients with temporary percutaneous catheters or for any unstable patient.

Long-Term Surveillance

Once a patient has had documented catheter-related sepsis, close observation, including repeat blood cultures, is necessary. If the fever fails to abate, or if positive blood cultures persist after the catheter has been removed, then antibiotics should be initiated or continued, and search for another focus of infection should be aggressively resumed. The possibility of an occult septic thrombosis should also be considered in this situation.

Patients with fungal catheter-related sepsis are especially prone to ongoing systemic involvement. Special attempts at limiting *Candida* colonization should be made. For example, patients with gastrointestinal tract dysfunction and stool cultures that are positive for *Candida* should be given prophylactic oral antifungal therapy to clear the bowel of superinfection. A second line of defense involves supporting the reticuloendothelial system and other immune defense mechanisms by discontinuing any unnecessary antibiotics, reducing glucocorticoids as much as possible, and suspending other forms of chemotherapy as the situation permits. Disseminated candidiasis can occur long after an isolated, positive blood culture, and may be insidious in its onset. Surveillance blood cultures and regular funduscopic examinations are essential in this patient population. If tissue invasion persists or recurs, additional systemic antifungal treatment is indicated.

REFERENCES
1. Aitken, D. R., and Minton, J. P. The "pinch-off sign": A warning of impending problems with permanent subclavian catheters. *Am. J. Surg.* 148:633, 1984.
2. Aubaniac, R. L'injection intraveineuse sous-claviculaire: Avantages et technique. *Presse Med.* 60:1456, 1952.
3. Bailey, M. J. Reduction of catheter-associated sepsis in parenteral nutrition using low-dose intravenous heparin. *Br. Med. J.* 1:1671, 1979.
4. Bertrand, Y. M., Reynaert, M. S., De Meulder, A., Louon, A., and Bauer, G. Reversible cardiac tamponade during prolonged parenteral feeding. *Intensive Care Med.* 9:95, 1983.
5. Bjornson, H. S., Colley, R., Bower, R. H., Duty, V. P., Schwartz-Fulton, J. T., and Fischer, J. E. Association between microorganism

growth at the catheter insertion site and colonization of the catheter in patients receiving total parenteral nutrition. *Surgery* 92:720, 1982.

6. Block, P. C. Transvenous retrieval of foreign bodies in the cardiac circulation. *J.A.M.A.* 224:241, 1973.

7. Bozzetti, F., Terno, G., Bonfanti, G., et al. Prevention and treatment of central venous catheter sepsis by exchange via a guidewire: A prospective controlled trial. *Ann. Surg.* 198:48, 1983.

8. Bozzetti, F., Terno, G., Camerini, E., Baticci, F., Scarpa, D., and Pupa, A. Pathogenesis and predictability of central venous catheter sepsis. *Surgery* 91:383, 1982.

9. Brismar, B., Hardstedt, C., Jacobson, S., Kager, L., and Malmborg, A. S. Reduction of catheter-associated thrombosis in parenteral nutrition by intravenous heparin therapy. *Arch. Surg.* 117:1196, 1982.

10. Chute, E., and Cerra, F. Late development of hydrothorax and hydromediastinum in patients with central venous catheters. *Crit. Care Med.* 10:868, 1982.

11. Cleri, D. J., Corrado, M. L., and Seligman, S. J. Quantitative culture of intravenous catheters and other intravascular inserts. *J. Infect. Dis.* 141:781, 1980.

12. Copeland, E. M., MacFayden, B. V., McGown, C., and Dudrick, S. J. The use of hyperalimentation in patients with potential sepsis. *Surg. Gynecol. Obstet.* 138:377, 1974.

13. Dillon, J. D., Schaffner, W., Van Way, C. W., and Meng, H. C. Septicemia and total parenteral nutrition: Distinguishing catheter-related from other septic episodes. *J.A.M.A.* 223:1341, 1973.

14. Druy, E. M., Trout, H. H., III, Giordano, J. M., and Hix, W. R. Lytic therapy in the treatment of axillary and subclavian vein thrombosis. *J. Vasc. Surg.* 2:821, 1985.

15. Dudrick, S. J., Wilmore, D. W., Vars, H. M., and Rhoads, J. E. Long-term total parenteral nutrition with growth, development, and positive nitrogen balance. *Surgery* 64:134, 1968.

16. Durant, T. M., Long, J., and Oppenheimer, M. J. Pulmonary (venous) air embolism. *Am. Heart J.* 33:269, 1947.

17. Fabri, P. J., Mirtallo, J. M., Ruberg, R. L., et al. Incidence and prevention of thrombosis of the subclavian vein during total parenteral nutrition. *Surg. Gynecol. Obstet.* 155:238, 1982.

18. Faubion, W. C., Wesley, J. R., Khalidi, N., and Silva, J. Total parenteral nutrition catheter sepsis: Impact of the team approach. *J. Parenter. Enter. Nutr.* 10:642, 1986.

19. Flanagan, J. P., Gradisar, I. A., Gross, R. J., and Kelly, T. R. Air embolus: A lethal complication of subclavian venipuncture. *N. Eng. J. Med.* 281:488, 1969.

20. Freeman, J. B., Lemire, A., and MacLean, L. D. Intravenous alimentation and septicemia. *Surg. Gynecol. Obstet.* 135:708, 1972.

21. Geiss, A. C., Flanagan, S. J., and Grossman, A. Evaluation of 75 patients with the long arm silastic catheter. *J. Parenter. Enter. Nutr.* 3:462, 1979.

22. Gilligan, J. E., Phillips, P. J., Wong, C. H., and Kimber, R. J. Streptokinase and blocked central venous catheter. *Lancet* 2:1189, 1979.

23. Glynn, M. F. X., Langer, B., and Jeejeebhoy, K. N. Therapy for thrombotic occlusion of long-term intravenous alimentation catheters. *J. Parenter. Enter. Nutr.* 4:387, 1980.

24. Goldmann, D. A., and Maki, D. G. Infection control in total parenteral nutrition. *J.A.M.A.* 223:1360, 1973.

25. Goldmann, D. A., Martin, W. T., and Worthington, J. W. Growth of bacteria and fungi in total parenteral nutrition solutions. *Am. J. Surg.* 126:314, 1973.

26. Hoffman, M. J., and Greenfield, L. J. Central venous septic thrombosis managed by superior vena cava Greenfield filter and venous thrombectomy: A case report. *J. Vasc. Surg.* 4:606, 1986.

27. Hoshal, V. Intravenous catheters and infection. *Surg. Clin. North Am.* 52:1407, 1972.

28. Hoshal, V. L., Jr. Total intravenous nutrition with peripherally inserted silicone elastomer central venous catheters. *Arch. Surg.* 110:644, 1975.

29. Hoshal, V. L., Jr., Ause, R. G., and Hoskins, P. A. Fibrin sleeve formation on indwelling subclavian central venous catheters. *Arch. Surg.* 102:253, 1971.

30. Hurtubise, M. R., Bottino, J. C., Lawson, M., and McGredie, K. B. Restoring patency of occluded central venous catheters. *Arch. Surg.* 115:212, 1980.

31. Imperial, J., Bistrian, B. R., Bothe, A., Jr., Bern, M., and Blackburn, G. L. Limitation of central vein thrombosis in total parental nutrition by continuous infusion of low-dose heparin. *J. Am. Coll. Nutr.* 2:63, 1983.

32. Jebson, P. J., and Rempe, L. E. Perforation of intrathoracic great veins by parenteral nutrition catheters. *J. Parenter. Enter. Nutr.* 6:528, 1982.

33. Jesseph, J. M., Conces, D. J., Jr., and Augustyn, G. T. Patient positioning for subclavian vein catheterization. *Arch. Surg.* 122:1207, 1987.

34. Jones, K. W., Seltzer, M. H., Slocum, B. A., Cataldi-Betcher, E. L., Goldberger, D. J., and Wright, F. R. Parenteral nutrition complications in a voluntary hospital. *J. Parenter. Enter. Nutr.* 8:385, 1984.

35. Kudsk, K. A., Powell, C., Mirtallo, J. M., Fabri, P. J., and Ruberg, R. L. Heparin does not

reduce catheter sepsis during total parenteral nutrition. *J. Parenter. Enter. Nutr.* 9:348, 1985.

36. Land, R. E. Anatomic relationships of the right subclavian vein: A radiologic study of pertinence to percutaneous subclavian venous catheterization. *Arch. Surg.* 102:178, 1971.

37. Land, R. E. The relationship of the left subclavian vein to the clavicle: Practical considerations pertinent to the percutaneous catheterization of the subclavian vein. *J. Thorac. Cardiovasc. Surg.* 63:546, 1972.

38. Landercasper, J., Gall, W., Fischer, M., et al. Thrombolytic therapy of axillary-subclavian venous thrombosis. *Arch. Surg.* 122:1072, 1987.

39. Lyman, B., Pendleton, S. H., and Pemberton, L. B. The role of the nutritional support team in preventing and identifying complications of parenteral and enteral nutrition. *Q.R.B.* 13:232, 1987.

40. Macoviak, J. A., Melnik, G., McLean, G., et al. The effect of low-dose heparin on the prevention of venous thrombosis in patients receiving short-term parenteral nutrition. *Curr. Surg.* 41:98, 1984.

41. Maher, M. M., Henderson, D. K., and Brennan, M. F. Central venous catheter exchange in cancer patients during total parenteral nutrition. *J.N.I.T.A.* 5:54, 1982.

42. Maki, D., Weise, C., and Sarafin, H. W. A semiquantitative culture method for identifying intravenous-catheter-related infection. *N. Engl. J. Med.* 296:1305, 1977.

43. McDonnell, P. J., Qualman, S. J., and Hutchins, G. M. Bilateral hydrothorax as a life-threatening complication of central venous hyperalimentation. *Surg. Gynecol. Obstet.* 158:577, 1984.

44. Nash, G., and Moylan, J. S. Paradoxical catheter embolism. *Arch. Surg.* 102:213, 1971.

45. Nelson, D. B., Kien, C. L., Mohr, B., Frank, S., and Davis, S. D. Dressing changes by specialized personnel reduce infection rates in patients receiving central venous parenteral nutrition. *J. Parenter. Enter. Nutr.* 10:220, 1986.

46. Oppenheimer, M. J., Durant, T. M., and Lynch, P. Body position in relation to venous air embolism and the associated cardiovascular-respiratory changes. *Am. J. Med. Sci.* 225:362, 1953.

47. Padberg, F. T., Jr., Ruggiero, J., Blackburn, G. L., and Bistrian, B. R. Central venous catheterization for parenteral nutrition. *Ann. Surg.* 193:264, 1981.

48. Paige, C., Pinson, C. W., Antonovic, R., and Strausbaugh, L. J. Catheter-related thrombophlebitis of the superior vena cava caused by *Candida glabrata. West. J. Med.* 147:333, 1987.

49. Pemberton, L. B., Lyman, B., Lander, V., and Covinsky, J. Sepsis from triple-versus single-lumen catheters during total parenteral nutrition in surgical or critically ill patients. *Arch. Surg.* 121:591, 1986.

50. Peters, W. R., Bush, W. H., McIntyre, R. D., and Hill, L. D. The development of fibrin sheath on indwelling venous catheters. *Surg. Gynecol. Obstet.* 137:43, 1973.

51. Pettigrew, R. A., Lano, S. D. R., Haydock, D. A., Parry, B. R., Bremner, D. A., and Hill, G. L. Catheter-related sepsis in patients on intravenous nutrition: A prospective study of quantitative catheter cultures and guidewire changes for suspected sepsis. *Br. J. Surg.* 72:52, 1985.

52. Priac, G. W., and Vanway, C. W. The long arm Silastic catheter: A critical look at complications. *J. Parenter. Enter. Nutr.* 2:124, 1978.

53. Pruitt, B. A., Stein, J. M., Foley, F. D., Moncrief, J. A., and O'Neill, J. A. Intravenous therapy in burn patients: Suppurative thrombophlebitis and other life-threatening complications. *Arch. Surg.* 100:399, 1970.

54. Rubenstein, M., and Creger, W. P. Successful streptokinase therapy for catheter-induced subclavian vein thrombosis. *Arch. Intern. Med.* 140:1370, 1980.

55. Ryan, J. A., Jr., Abel, R. M., Abbott, W. M., et al. Catheter complications in total parenteral nutrition: A prospective study of 200 consecutive patients. *N. Engl. J. Med.* 290:757, 1974.

56. Sanders, R. A., and Sheldon, G. F. Septic complications of total parenteral nutrition: A five year experience. *Am. J. Surg.* 132:214, 1976.

57. Schuman, E. S., Winters, V., Gross, G. F., and Hayes, J. F. Management of Hickman catheter sepsis. *Am. J. Surg.* 149:627, 1985.

58. Shires, T., and O'Banoin, J. Successful treatment of massive air embolism producing cardiac arrest. *J.A.M.A.* 167:1483, 1958.

59. Sitzmann, J. V., Townsend, T. R., Siler, M. C., and Bartlett, J. G. Septic and technical complications of central venous catheterization: A prospective study of 200 consecutive patients. *Ann. Surg.* 202:766, 1985.

60. Smith, N. L., Ravo, B., Soroff, H. S., and Khan, S. A. Successful fibrinolytic therapy for superior vena cava thrombosis secondary to long-term total parenteral nutrition. *J. Parenter. Enter. Nutr.* 9:55, 1985.

61. Steed, D. L., Teodori, M. F., Peitzman, A. B., McAuley, C. E., Kapoor, W. N., and Webster, M. W. Streptokinase in the treatment of subclavian vein thrombosis. *J. Vasc. Surg.* 4:28, 1986.

62. Stewart, A., and Mayne, E. E. Rapid resolution of subclavian vein thrombosis by tissue plasminogen activator. (Letter) *Lancet* 1:890, 1988.

63. Stillman, R. M., Soliman, F., Garcia, L., and

Sawyer, P. N. Etiology of catheter-associated sepsis: Correlation with thrombogenicity. *Arch. Surg.* 112:1497, 1977.

64. Suddleson, E. A. Cardiac tamponade: A complication of central venous hyperalimentation. *J. Parenter. Enter. Nutr.* 10:528, 1986.

65. Thurer, R. J. Chylothorax: A complication of subclavian vein catheterization and parenteral hyperalimentation. *J. Thorac. Cardiovasc. Surg.* 71:465, 1976.

66. Welch, G. W., McKell, D. W., Silverstein, P., and Walker, H. L. The role of catheter composition in the development of thrombophlebitis. *Surg. Gynecol. Obstet.* 138:421, 1974.

67. Williams, W. W. Infection control during parenteral nutrition therapy. *J. Parenter. Enter. Nutr.* 9:735, 1985.

68. Wilson, J. N., Grow, J. B., Demong, C. V., Prevedel, A. E., and Owens, J. C. Central venous pressure in optimal blood volume maintenance. *Arch. Surg.* 85:563, 1962.

69. Winn, R. E., Tuttle, K. L., and Gilbert, D. N. Surgical approach to extensive thrombophlebitis of the central veins of the chest. *J. Thorac. Cardiovasc. Surg.* 81:564, 1981.

70. Wolfe, B. M., Ryder, M. A., Nishikawa, R. A., Halsted, C. H., and Schmidt, B. F. Complications of parenteral nutrition. *Am. J. Surg.* 152:93, 1986.

71. Yoffa, D. Supraclavicular subclavian vena puncture and catheterization. *Lancet* 2:614, 1965.

Metabolic Complications

Daniel von Allmen
Josef E. Fischer

Over the past two decades, as the use of parenteral nutrition has increased in frequency and duration, a great variety of metabolic disorders have been reported. Despite increased knowledge of and improvements in the composition of parenteral nutrition solutions, metabolic complications occur in 5 to 10% of adult patients [49]. Inability to tolerate a nutrient load, deficiencies of essential components, and toxic reactions to specific components have all been described. It is important, therefore, that the clinician administering total parenteral nutrition (TPN) be aware of these metabolic disorders and recognize their signs and symptoms in order to make appropriate adjustments in therapy.

COMPLICATIONS RELATED TO FLUID AND ELECTROLYTES

Administration of fluid to a patient receiving parenteral nutrition requires the same basic considerations applied to any patient. Abnormal fluid losses due to diarrhea and fistula and drain output require appropriate replacement, while underlying medical problems such as cardiac disease and renal failure predispose to fluid overload. Fluid overload, a more common complication, is often related to administration of a predetermined number of calories in a typical 1 kcal/ml solution without regard for the volume infused. Treatment consists of decreasing the rate of fluid administration and optimizing cardiac and renal function. Caloric intake can be effectively maintained either by increasing the concentration of glucose calories supplied or by adding fat, especially as the 20% emulsion, as a caloric source. Supplying 30% or more of the nonprotein caloric requirement as a 10% or 20% lipid emulsion can effectively decrease complications related to fluid overload and excess glucose administration [33, 37]. In a prospective randomized crossover trial, postoperative cancer patients received isocaloric formulations with approximately one-third of the calories supplied as fat in either 10% or

20% emulsions. The group administered 20% emulsions received significantly less fluid and developed significantly fewer signs of fluid overload than did the group receiving 10% lipid emulsion.

Abnormalities of sodium are commonly linked to fluid administration. Hypernatremia results from restricted fluid intake in a patient unable to respond appropriately to the hyperosmolarity by increased oral intake of free water. Hyponatremia, on the other hand, commonly results from free-water overload rather than a sodium deficit.

Alkalosis and increased insulin levels due to administration of solutions containing high concentrations of glucose can cause a redistribution of potassium into cells, resulting in lower serum potassium levels. Redistribution along with gastrointestinal losses from diarrhea or renal losses associated with diuretic therapy can contribute to a significant hypokalemia. Treatment requires frequent monitoring of serum potassium levels and adjusting administration as indicated. Conversely, acidosis, renal impairment, and excess potassium administration can lead to hyperkalemia, requiring appropriate reductions in the potassium dose.

Abnormalities of chloride metabolism were common with the first-generation crystalline amino acid solutions. These formulas contained amino acids including lysine as chloride salts, which, when fully metabolized, was equivalent to infusing hydrochloric acid, resulting in hyperchloremic metabolic acidosis [26]. In subsequent formulations, acetate has been substituted as an anion, and chloride is maintained in a 1:1 ratio with sodium. In a report by Caldwell et al. [10], no cases of hyperchloremic acidosis were found in 92 patients receiving an acetate-balanced formulation. Hypochloremic metabolic alkalosis remains a risk in patients undergoing sustained gastric decompression.

Serum calcium levels are usually maintained at the expense of bone demineralization in the face of decreased dietary intake. Significant hypocalcemia can develop in patients with severe pancreatitis. Administration of large amounts of phosphate salts can also contribute to a lowering of serum calcium levels. In contrast, administration of intravenous phosphate and acetate-balanced solutions has been shown to decrease hypercalciuria and may be beneficial in maintaining calcium stores in patients receiving long-term TPN [7, 52]. Appropriate calcium replacement is required to prevent bone demineralization in adults and growth retardation in children and to support anabolic metabolism. In malnourished patients, serum calcium levels may be low due to decreased levels of albumin, to which half of calcium is bound, while levels of ionized calcium remain normal. Hypercalcemia results from excessive administration and can lead to pancreatitis [29].

Magnesium is an important cofactor in several enzymes responsible for anabolism. Inadequate magnesium replacement aggravated by abnormally high magnesium losses, as seen in gastrointestinal disorders, can lead to the clinical syndrome of hypomagnesemia. It is manifested by apathy, weakness, seizures, arrhythmias, hallucinations, ileus, and hyperreflexia. Symptoms occur when serum levels drop below 1.0 mEq/liter. In addition, renal potassium and phosphate losses are increased by hypomagnesemia [25, 43], which can contribute to the development of hypokalemia and hypophosphatemia. Weakness of the respiratory muscles associated with hypomagnesemia may exacerbate respiratory insufficiency [15]. Symptoms resolve rapidly with magnesium replacement.

Hypophosphatemia is commonly found during the initial phases of nutritional support in previously debilitated, malnourished patients. Dietary restriction alone is unlikely to produce hypophosphatemia, but with refeeding there is a redistribution of phosphate into muscle, which can become symptomatic. Increased renal excretion of phosphate occurs with alkalosis, hypokalemia, hypomagnesemia, steroid and diuretic treatment, and diabetes mellitus.

Signs and symptoms of hypophosphatemia include tremor, paresthesias, ataxia, decreased platelet and erythrocyte survival, impaired leukocyte function, and weakness. As with hypomagnesemia, hypophosphatemia has been linked to respiratory failure [36] and difficulty in weaning patients from assisted ventilation [1]. Symptoms of this disorder may occur within several days of initiating nutritional support and can be prevented by including 10 to 15 mmol of phosphate per liter of solution.

COMPLICATIONS RELATED TO CARBOHYDRATE METABOLISM

Patients with normal insulin response can be expected to tolerate a glucose infusion of 0.5 g/kg/hr [39], and up to 1.2 g/kg/hr has been administered without complication [16]. However, some studies indicate that with a glucose infusion of more than 5 mg/kg/min (0.3 g/kg/hr), direct oxidation of glucose and physiologically significant increases in protein synthesis cannot be expected [9]. Conditions of stress, such as sepsis or surgery, result in decreased glucose tolerance and hyperglycemia in as many as 25% of patients on TPN. Infusion of large amounts of glucose can also unmask latent diabetes, making hyperglycemia one of the most common metabolic complications encountered with parenteral nutrition. Treatment of the problem relies on increasing the percentage of calories provided as fat, beginning highly concentrated glucose infusions slowly, and adding insulin to the solution when necessary.

Hyperosmolar hyperglycemic nonketotic coma is a serious complication related to carbohydrate metabolism, which is rarely encountered, but worthy of mention. Continued infusion of hypertonic glucose solutions in the face of increasing hyperglycemia results in glycosuria and an osmotic diuresis. As hyperosmolality, hypovolemia, and intracellular dehydration progress, a metabolic acidosis develops in the absence of serum or urine ketone bodies. The patient progresses along a clinical course of stupor, coma, and death. McCurdy [32] reported a 40% mortality from this uncommon complication.

Treatment requires rehydration with hypotonic fluid and administration of insulin after stopping the hypertonic glucose infusion. Careful monitoring of serum electrolytes is essential during rehydration. The syndrome is easily prevented by frequent monitoring of serum and urine glucose levels, particularly when parenteral nutrition is first instituted, and by providing a significant proportion of total calories as fat [34].

Hypoglycemia can be seen after sudden withdrawal of a prolonged infusion of a highly concentrated glucose solution. This phenomenon is uncommon in adults, but is seen frequently in children. Symptoms include diaphoresis, confusion, and agitation. Treatment consists of reinstituting an infusion of 10% glucose and frequent measurement of serum glucose levels.

A further consideration when infusing formulations containing high glucose concentration is the potential effect of carbohydrate metabolism on respiration. Metabolism of carbohydrates results in increased production of carbon dioxide that must be compensated by increased minute ventilation. Theoretically, this could precipitate respiratory failure in patients with preexisting respiratory disease or interfere with weaning from mechanical ventilation. Askanazi et al. [3] and others [2, 12, 14] demonstrated hypercarbia with glucose infusion. The circumstances of the study reported by Askanazi et al. are rarely mentioned and are probably responsible for the effect seen. The patients were depleted and largely septic; the glucose load was increased precipitously to 2.25 times their requirement. This rarely happens in most normal clinical situations. Thus, the excessive publicity given this study is misplaced. Moreover, the clinical significance of these findings is not clear, since others have found that only with carbohydrate overfeeding and net lipogenesis does the respiratory quotient exceed 1.0 to a sufficient degree that increased carbon dioxide production becomes clinically important [46, 50]. This potential hazard can be avoided as long as the patient's calorie requirement is not greatly exceeded.

COMPLICATIONS RELATED TO LIPID METABOLISM

In 1971, Collins et al. [11] reported on two adults receiving TPN who had abnormal fatty acid profiles. One patient developed an accompanying rash and anemia that rapidly corrected after administration of an intravenous fat emulsion containing linoleic and linolenic acids. Essential fatty acid deficiency in patients receiving parenteral nutrition is now a well-recognized clinical syndrome. It develops when no exogenous dietary fatty acids are available and endogenous fat stores are not accessible due to the inhibitory effect of increased insulin levels on lipolysis during administration of TPN. Essential fatty acid deficiency is characterized by a diffuse scaly dermatitis that begins on the face, extremities, and skin folds and then becomes generalized. Alopecia, thrombocytopenia, anemia, and poor wound healing can occur with the skin rash within 1 to 2 months of beginning fat-free nutritional support. The changes in serum fatty acids appear within 2 weeks of fat-free parenteral nutrition.

Biochemically, the syndrome is characterized by alterations in the serum fatty acid profile. Normally, linoleic acid, an essential fatty acid, is elongated and desaturated to arachidonic acid, a tetraene. In the absence of linoleic acid, oleic acid is metabolized to eicosatrienoic acid, a triene. A triene-tetraene ratio greater than 0.4 is indicative of essential fatty acid deficiency.

Linolenic acid deficiency was found to cause neurologic symptoms including tremor, paresthesias, and visual changes in a child receiving parenteral nutrition rich in linoleic acid [19]. The symptoms resolved with linolenic acid supplementation. Thus, it appears that both linoleic and linolenic acid are essential components of TPN.

Administration of lipid emulsions has been associated with impairment of a number of different organ systems including pulmonary, renal, hepatic, and pancreatic. In addition, disorders of blood coagulation, hemolytic anemia, and compromise of the immune system have all been reported. These effects are all thought to be due to high serum levels of triglycerides and that with careful administration of lipids and monitoring of serum triglyceride and cholesterol levels, complications can be avoided. There is no evidence to suggest that lipids affect pancreatitis in the absence of an underlying lipid metabolism disorder, but fatal cases of recrudescence of pancreatitis following the administration of 20% lipid emulsions have been reported.

Allergic reactions consisting of sweating, flushing, headache, and dizziness have also been reported during infusion of lipid emulsions.

TRACE METAL ABNORMALITIES

Zinc is an important constituent of many enzymes, and is required for the synthesis of DNA and RNA. When a patient is zinc deficient, clinical signs and symptoms of impaired taste and smell, mental disturbances, growth retardation, impaired leukocyte function, and perioral exfoliative dermatitis develop [22]. Darkening of skinfolds also occurs. Zinc deficiency is also associated with impaired wound healing. Animal [40] and human [45] studies have demonstrated marked improvement in wound healing with zinc supplementation in zinc-depleted patients. Wolman et al. [51] demonstrated a correlation between zinc administration and positive nitrogen balance in zinc-depleted patients receiving parenteral nutrition. Since many patients placed on TPN are at high risk for preexisting zinc depletion, it is important to provide adequate zinc supplementation during therapy.

Copper is also an essential cofactor for a number of enzyme systems. Deficiency leads to primarily hematologic disorders including anemia, leukopenia, and neutropenia in adults. In children, copper deficiency also causes osteoporosis, possibly through abnormalities of collagen and ascorbic acid metabolism.

Normal dietary requirements of copper are 1.3 to 1.6 mg/day, of which 10 to 30% is absorbed through the proximal intestine. Normal copper balance is maintained by infusion of 0.3 mg/day of copper in adults. There is an enterohepatic circulation for copper that may be disrupted by severe diarrhea or proximal stomas, and copper requirements are increased in these cases. In general, copper deficiency is seen only in patients receiving long-term TPN. Liver disease, on the other hand, can lead to accumulation of copper and toxic effects in the kidney and liver.

Chromium is essential to the function of glucose tolerance factor, which acts peripherally to potentiate the effects of insulin. Deficiency leads to impaired carbohydrate metabolism and a clinical picture consistent with insulin-resistant diabetes mellitus [20]. Symptoms of peripheral neuropathy, ataxia, and encephalopathy have also been reported [17, 23]. Findings consistent with chromium deficiency occur as early as 5 months after initiation of chromium-deficient TPN.

Selenium is a catalyst for the enzyme glutathione peroxidase, which is an important antioxidant pathway. Deficiency of selenium may make the patient susceptible to toxic effects of peroxides, especially when accompanied by a deficiency of vitamin E, with which it shares many properties [30]. Low selenium levels lead to a myopathy causing severe muscle pain and impaired cardiac function.

HYPERAMMONEMIA

An elevated blood ammonia level is a common finding in infants and children receiving parenteral nutrition. Because high protein intake may lead to elevated ammonia levels [21], the amount of protein intake for infants should be restricted to 2.5 g/kg/day to avoid this complication. Hyperammonemia has also been attributed, in part, to infusion of hydrolysate amino acid solutions that contain 10 to 30 mg/dl of preformed ammonia. However, the significance of preformed ammonia is unclear, since increased ammonia levels have also been noted in patients receiving crystalline amino acid formulations that contain no ammonia. Arginine is important in the urea cycle, and a deficiency of this amino

acid may contribute to the development of hyperammonemia. Current commercial formulations available for children contain higher concentrations of arginine than did previous solutions.

The effect of various solutions on ammonia levels in children was examined by Seashore et al. [41]. In that study, ammonia levels were followed in 45 infants and children on TPN. A 73% incidence of hyperammonemia was found, with a higher incidence and severity in premature infants (< 2500 g). There was no significant difference in ammonia levels between infants receiving protein hydrolysates and those treated with crystalline amino acid–based formulas. Symptoms of lethargy leading to frank coma developed in four infants, but resolved after discontinuing TPN. In one child, high serum ammonia levels resolved after switching to a formulation high in arginine. Six of seven infants maintained on the high arginine TPN also had one or more elevated ammonia levels recorded. Thus, hyperammonemia may occur despite reductions in protein intake and modification of the TPN formula. Increased ammonia levels are usually not associated with clinical signs and symptoms, making diagnosis dependent on routine monitoring of serum ammonia levels.

HEPATIC AND BILIARY COMPLICATIONS

Hepatic complications are one of the most common metabolic abnormalities associated with parenteral alimentation. The findings associated with hepatic abnormalities encompass a diverse array of biochemical and morphologic findings related to the duration and composition of the nutritional support as well as the age of the patient. Distinct patterns emerge when considering hepatic complications in adults and children. Adults usually have relatively benign biochemical and morphologic changes, while TPN-associated hepatic abnormalities in infants and neonates can be progressive and even fatal.

Adults

In adults the most common laboratory finding is that of elevated transaminase levels that usually peak 10 to 15 days after instituting TPN and resolve slowly without change in therapy. Peak SGOT and SGPT are typically three to seven times the normal values. Elevation of alkaline phosphatase has been reported to peak both earlier and later in the treatment course than the transaminases. Bilirubin elevations occur late, if at all, in adults and are usually due to sepsis, as hyperbilirubinemia is rarely, if ever, due to TPN. The pathophysiology of these changes is not clear. Rapid infusion of high dextrose formulas has been implicated as one contributing factor. Klein and Nealon [24] noted that prior to 1980, large amounts of high dextrose solutions were infused and there was a high incidence of liver function test (LFT) abnormalities. In subsequent years, glucose infusions have been decreased and fat substituted as a calorie source. During this time, the incidence and degree of LFT abnormalities have decreased [4]. Meguid et al. [34] demonstrated in a prospective randomized controlled study that patients receiving solutions containing one-third of calories as fat had fewer and less dramatic elevations of transaminase levels than did patients treated with high concentrations of glucose.

Morphologically, the most common abnormality seen in the adult liver is steatosis. Fatty infiltration beginning in the periportal areas is seen within 5 days of initiating therapy and resolves rapidly after discontinuation of TPN. The lipid accumulation is mostly in the form of triglycerides, and its appearance coincides temporally with the development of abnormal LFT results, although no cause-and-effect relationship has been established. As with the hepatic enzymes, infusion of high glucose loads is associated with the development of steatosis [28]. While many mechanisms have been proposed, the exact pathophysiology of the TPN-associated morphologic changes remains unclear. Glucose overload with accumulation of acetyl CoA leading to increased fatty acid synthesis, decreased fatty acid oxidation due to L-carnitine deficiency, and decreased lipoprotein synthesis due to protein malnutrition or essential fatty acid deficiency have all been proposed as possible mechanisms. Results of recent animal studies suggested that the changes in hepatic metabolism leading to steatosis may be mediated by alterations in the portal glucagon-insulin ratio [27].

Cholestasis and gallbladder disease are potential complications of long-term parenteral nutrition. Messing et al. [35] demonstrated sludge formation in the gallbladder in 50% of patients after 4 to 6 weeks of therapy. Gallstone formation was demonstrated in 6 of 14 patients who developed gallbladder sludge. Warner and coworkers [44] obtained hepatobiliary scans in patients receiving parenteral nutrition, and found the scans unreliable as indicating cholecystitis. Liver bioposy specimens obtained in patients receiving long-term TPN have shown signs of bile stasis with periportal inflammation in some cases, but progressive fibrosis is very rare. Biochemical and morphologic evidence of bile stasis and biliary sludging resolve with resumption of enteral feeding [13].

Infants

In infants the predominant finding associated with parenteral nutrition is cholestasis. Beale et al. [6] studied 62 premature infants with isolated respiratory disease who received TPN, and documented cholestasis in 23%. The incidence increased with the duration of therapy and was inversely correlated to the patient's gestational age and weight. Elevated direct bilirubin levels are the most accurate measure of TPN-associated cholestasis, but elevations are seen late in the progression of disease. Measurements of transaminases, alkaline phosphatase, and total bilirubin have not been found to be clinically useful in making the diagnosis [47].

Morphologic changes in infants consist primarily of hepatocyte and canalicular cholestasis and periportal inflammation. Discontinuation of TPN leaves mild residual periportal fibrosis. Continuing TPN in the face of cholestasis can lead to micronodular cirrhosis [13], liver failure, and death.

As in adults, the exact pathogenesis of these changes remains unclear. Immaturity of liver function, especially of bile salt metabolism [5], toxicity from high calorie fat and carbohydrate infusion [28], amino acids [8], gastrointestinal surgery [38], sepsis [48], and intestinal bacteria overgrowth [18] have all been implicated in hepatobiliary dysfunction. Further studies are necessary to completely elucidate the mechanisms involved.

Thus, liver function abnormalities are a common finding in both infants and adults receiving TPN. However, it is important to note that patients who are candidates for TPN are usually at high risk for developing other unrelated complications resulting in changes in hepatic function. All potential causes of hepatobiliary dysfunction, especially sepsis, should be investigated before ascribing liver function abnormalities to TPN.

METABOLIC BONE DISEASE

Metabolic bone disease is a rare and poorly understood complication of long-term parenteral nutrition. The syndrome typically presents with lower-extremity and back pain or pathologic fractures. A radiologic workup and laboratory studies including urine and serum calcium levels, phosphate levels, and serum vitamin D levels may or may not be diagnostic. In addition, bone biopsy may be necessary to complete the workup. Findings of elevated urine calcium and low vitamin D_3 levels have been reported. However, normal findings on workup do not rule out the possibility of metabolic bone disease. Seligman et al. [42] reported a case of a woman receiving TPN for 26 months who presented with pathologic rib fractures due to metabolic bone disease in the face of a normal radiologic and laboratory findings. In that patient, bone mineral mass progressively decreased over the ensuing 22 months, and evidence of osteomalacia was found on examination of a bone biopsy specimen. A sophisticated metabolic workup did not suggest a correlation

with the patient's preexistent small bowel disease or medical therapy.

The pathogenesis of this lesion is obscure, but has been related to abnormal metabolism of vitamin D, aluminum, calcium, protein, and glucose [31]. Withdrawal of vitamin D_3 or cessation of TPN leads to resolution of the symptoms. It is unlikely that vitamin D toxicity due to excess intake is responsible, since serum levels are not elevated. Similarly, biochemical evidence of phosphate deficiency or phosphate-induced secondary hyperparathyroidism has not been found to explain the osteomalacia.

The syndrome usually subsides after discontinuation of TPN or withholding of vitamin D. Bone remineralization occurs slowly after resolution of symptoms and may take months or years to complete.

REFERENCES

1. Agusti, A. G. N., Torres, A., Estopa, R., and Agustiuidal, A. Hypophosphatemia as a cause of failed weaning: The importance of metabolic factors. *Crit. Care Med.* 12:142, 1984.
2. Amene, P. C., Sladen, R. N., Feeley, T. W., and Fisher, R. Hypercapnia during total parenteral nutrition with hypertonic glucose. *Crit. Care Med.* 15:171, 1987.
3. Askanazi, J., Rosenbaum, S. H., Hyman, A. L., et al. Respiratory changes induced by large glucose loads of total parenteral nutrition. *J.A.M.A.* 243:1444, 1980.
4. Baker, A. L., and Rosenberg, E. H. Hepatic complications of total parenteral nutrition. *Am. J. Med.* 82:489, 1989.
5. Balistreri, W. F. Neonatal cholestasis. *J. Pediatr.* 106:171, 1985.
6. Beale, E. F., Nelson, R. M., Bucciarelli, R. C., Donnelly, W. H., and Eitzman, D. V. Intrahepatic cholestasis associated with parenteral nutrition in premature infants. *Pediatrics* 64:342, 1979.
7. Berkelhammer, C. H., Wood, R. J., and Sitrin, M. D. Acetate and hypercalciuria during total parenteral nutrition. *Am. J. Clin. Nutr.* 48:1482, 1988.
8. Black, D. D., Suttle, E. A., Whittington, P. F., Whittington, G. L., and Korones, S. D. The effect of short-term total parenteral nutrition on hepatic function in the neonate: A prospective randomized function demonstrating alteration of hepatic canalicular function. *J. Pediatr.* 99:445, 1981.

9. Burke, J. F., Wolfe, R. R., Mullany, C. J., Mathews, D. E., and Bier, D. M. Glucose requirements following burn injury: Parameters of optimal glucose infusion and possible hepatic and respiratory abnormalities following excessive glucose intake. *Ann. Surg.* 190:274, 1979.

10. Caldwell, M. D., O'Neill, J. A., Meng, H. C., and Stahlman, M. H. Evaluation of a new amino acid source for use in parenteral nutrition. *Ann. Surg.* 185:153, 1977.

11. Collins, F. D., Sinclair, A. J., Royle, J. P., Coats, D. A., Meynard, A. T., and Leonard, R. F. Plasma lipids in human linoleic acid deficiency. *Nutr. Metab.* 13:150, 1971.

12. Covelli, H. D., Black, J. W., Olsen, M. W., and Beckman, J. F. Respiratory failure precipitated by high carbohydrate loads. *Ann. Intern. Med.* 95:579, 1981.

13. Dahms, B. B., and Halpin, T. C. Serial liver biopsies in parenteral nutrition-associated cholestasis of early infancy. *Gastroenterology* 81:136, 1981.

14. Dark, D. S., Pingleton, S. K., and Kerby, G. R. Hypercapnia during weaning: A complication of nutritional support. *Chest* 88:141, 1985.

15. Dhingra, S., Solven, F., Wilson, A., and McCarthy, D. S. Hypomagnesemia and respiratory muscle power. *Am. Rev. Respir. Dis.* 129:497, 1984.

16. Dudrick, S. J., Wilmore, D. W., Vars, H. M., and Rhoads, J. E. Can intravenous feeding as the sole means of nutrition support growth in the child and restore weight loss in an adult? An affirmative answer. *Ann. Surg.* 169:974, 1969.

17. Freund H., Atamian, S., and Fischer, J. E. Chromium deficiency during total parenteral nutrition. *J.A.M.A.* 241:496, 1981.

18. Freund, H. R., Muggia-Sullam, M., LaFrance, R., Enrione, E. B., Popp, M. B., and Bjornson, H. S. A possible beneficial effect of metronidazole in reducing TPN-associated liver function derangements. *J. Surg. Res.* 38:356, 1985.

19. Holuran, R. T., Johnson, S. B., and Hatch, T. F. A case of human linolenic acid deficiency involving neurologic abnormalities. *Am. J. Clin. Nutr.* 35:617, 1982.

20. Jeejeebhoy, K. N., Chu, R. C., Marliss, E. B., Greenberg, G. R., and Bruce-Robertson, S. Chromium deficiency, glucose intolerance, and neuropathy reversed by chromium supplementation, in a patient receiving long-term parenteral nutrition. *Am. J. Clin. Nutr.* 30:531, 1977.

21. Johnson, J. D., Albritton, W. L., and Sunshine, P. Hyperammonemia accompanying parenteral nutrition in newborn infants. *J. Pediatr.* 81:154, 1972.

22. Kay, R. G., Tasman-Jones, C., Pybus, J., Whitling, R., and Black, H. A syndrome of acute zinc deficiency during total parenteral nutrition. *Ann. Surg.* 183:331, 1976.

23. Kein, C. L., Veillon, C., Patterson, K. Y., and Farrel, P. M. Mild peripheral neuropathy but biochemical chromium sufficiency during 16 months of "chromium-free" total parenteral nutrition. *J. Parenter. Enter. Nutr.* 10:662, 1986.

24. Klein, S., and Nealon, W. H. Hepatobiliary abnormalities associated with total parenteral nutrition. *Semin. Liver Dis.* 8:237, 1988.

25. Knochel, J. P. The pathophysiology and clinical characteristics of severe hypophosphatemia. *Arch. Intern. Med.* 137:203, 1977.

26. Kushner, R. F. Total parenteral nutrition-associated metabolic acidosis. *J. Parenter. Enter. Nutr.* 10:306, 1986.

27. Li, S., Nussbaum, M. S., McFadden, D. W., Gapen, C. L., Dayal, R., and Fischer, J. E. Addition of glucagon to total parenteral nutrition (TPN) prevents hepatic steatosis in rats. *Surgery* 104:350, 1988.

28. Lowry, S. F., and Brennan, M. F. Abnormal liver function during parenteral nutrition: Relation to infusion excess. *J. Surg. Res.* 26:300, 1979.

29. Maurou, R. R. Acute pancreatitis secondary to iatrogenic hypercalcemia: Implications of hyperalimentation. *Arch. Surg.* 108:213, 1974.

30. McClain, C. J. Trace metal abnormalities in adults during hyperalimentation. *J. Parenter. Enter. Nutr.* 8:722, 1984.

31. McCullough, M. L., and Hsu, N. Metabolic bone disease in home parenteral nutrition. *J. Am. Diet. Assoc.* 87:915, 1987.

32. McCurdy, D. K. Hyperosmolar hyperglycemic nonketotic diabetic coma. *Med. Clin. North Am.* 54:683, 1970.

33. Meguid, M. M., Akahoshi, M., Debonis, D., Hayashi, R. J., and Hammond, W. G. Use of 20% fat emulsion in total parenteral nutrition. *Crit. Care Med.* 14:29, 1986.

34. Meguid, M. M., Akahoshi, M., Jeffers, F., Hayashi, R. J., and Hammond, W. G. Amelioration of metabolic complications of conventional total parenteral nutrition. A prospective randomized study. *Arch. Surg* 119:1294, 1984.

35. Messing, B., Bories, C., Kunstlinger, F., and Bernier, J. J. Does total parenteral nutrition induce sludge formation and lithiasis? *Gastroenterology* 84:1012, 1983.

36. Newman, J. H., Neff, T. A., and Ziporin, P. Acute respiratory failure associated with hypophosphatemia. *N. Engl. J. Med.* 296:1101, 1977.

37. Paluzzi, M., and Meguid, M. M. A prospective randomized study of the optimal source of nonprotein calories in total parenteral nutrition. *Surgery* 103:711, 1987.

38. Postuma, R., and Trevenen, C. L. Liver disease in infants receiving total parenteral nutrition. *Pediatrics* 63:110, 1979.
39. Sanderson, I., and Deitel, M. Insulin response in patients receiving concentrated infusions of glucose and casein hydrolysate for complete parenteral nutrition. *Ann. Surg.* 179:387, 1974.
40. Sanstead, H. H., Lanier, V. C., Shepard, G. H., and Gillespie, D. D. Zinc and wound healing: Effects of zinc deficiency and supplementation. *Am. J. Clin. Nutr.* 23:514, 1970.
41. Seashore, J. H., Seashore, M. R., and Riley, C. Hyperammonemia during total parenteral nutrition in children. *J. Parenter. Enter. Nutr.* 6:114, 1972.
42. Seligman, J. V., Surinder, S. B., Deitel, M., Bayley, T. A., and Khanna, R. Metabolic bone disease in a patient on long-term total parenteral nutrition: A case report with review of literature. *J. Parenter. Enter. Nutr.* 8:722, 1984.
43. Shils, M. E. Experimental human magnesium depletion. *Medicine* 48:61, 1969.
44. Warner, B. W., Hamilton, F. N., Silberstein, E. B., et al. The value of hepatobiliary scans in fasted patients receiving total parenteral nutrition. *Surgery* 102:595, 1987.
45. Weismann, K., Hjorth, N., and Fischer, A. Zinc depletion syndrome with acrodermatitis during long-term intravenous feeding. *Clin. Exp. Dermatol.* 1:237, 1976.
46. Weissman, C., and Hyman, A. L. Nutrition care of the critically ill patient with respiratory failure. *Crit. Care Clin.* 3:185, 1987.
47. Whitington, P. F. Cholestasis associated with total parenteral nutrition in infants. *Hepatology* 5:693, 1985.
48. Wolf, A., and Pohlandt, F. Bacterial infection: The main cause of acute cholestasis in newborn infants receiving short term parenteral nutrition. *J. Pediatr. Gastroenterol. Nutr.* 8:297, 1989.
49. Wolfe, B. M., Ryder, M. A., Nishikawa, R. A., Halsted, C. H., and Schmidt, B. F. Complications of parenteral nutrition. *Am. J. Surg.* 152:93, 1986.
50. Wolfe, R. R., O'Donnell, T. F., Stone, M. D., Richmond, D. A., and Burke, J. F. Investigation of factors determining the optimal glucose infusion rate in total parenteral nutrition. *Metabolism* 29:892, 1980.
51. Wolman, S. L., Anderson, G. H., Marliss, E. B., and Jeejeebhoy, K. N. Zinc in total parenteral nutrition: Requirements and metabolic effects. *Gastroenterology* 76:458, 1979.
52. Wood, R. J., Sitrin, M. D., Cusson, G. J., and Rosenberg, I. H. Reduction of total parenteral nutrition-induced urinary calcium loss by increasing the phosphorus in the total parenteral nutrition. *J. Parenter. Enter. Nutr.* 10:188, 1986.

Pharmaceutical Considerations in Total Parenteral Nutrition

Richard J. LaFrance
Clyde I. Miyagawa

Since 1968, when Dudrick [46, 47] proved the concept of parenteral nutrition practicable, many technological advances have been made. Today we enjoy the luxury of a vast array of nutritional formulation components as well as administration equipment. We have also gained extensive experience in the provision of safe and effective parenteral nutrition. This chapter reviews formulation preparation, components of parenteral nutrient formulations, specific formulations, and stability and compatibility issues associated with parenteral nutrient formulations.

PATIENT REQUIREMENTS AND PARENTERAL NUTRITION COMPONENTS

When formulating a parenteral nutrition admixture, one must provide certain basic elements to meet the patient's nutritional requirements. These essential elements include nitrogen, a caloric source (dextrose, glycerol, or fat), electrolytes, vitamins, trace elements, and water.

Nitrogen

Crystalline amino acid solutions provide the nitrogen source for parenteral nutrition. There are several manufacturers of general-purpose amino acid formulations that vary in concentrations from 3 to 15%. These products also vary in protein and nitrogen content, amino acid profiles, osmolarity, pH, and electrolyte composition. A comparison of four commercially available general-purpose amino acid solutions is presented in Table 5-1 [3].

Nonprotein Calories

Dextrose

Dextrose is the most common and least expensive caloric source used for parenteral nutrition. Intravenous solutions contain dextrose monohydrate which provides 3.4 kcal/g.

Table 5-1. General-Purpose Amino Acid Formulations

Preparation Manufacturer	Aminosyn II 10% (Abbott)	FreAmine III 10% (Kendall-McGaw)	Travasol 10% (Baxter)	Novamine 15% (Baxter)
Protein concentration (%)	10	10	10	15
Nitrogen (g/100 ml)	1.53	1.53	1.65	2.37
Essential amino acids (mg/100 ml)				
Isoleucine	660	690	600	749
Leucine	1000	910	730	1040
Lysine	1050	730	580	1180
Methionine	172	530	400	749
Phenylalanine	298	560	560	1040
Threonine	400	400	420	749
Tryptophan	200	150	180	250
Valine	500	660	580	960
Nonessential amino acids (mg/100 ml)				
Alanine	993	710	2070	2170
Arginine	1018	950	1150	1470
Histidine	300	280	480	894
Proline	722	1120	680	894
Serine	530	590	500	592
Tyrosine	270	—	40	39
Glycine	500	1400	1030	1040
Cysteine	—	<24	—	—
Glutamic acid	738	—	—	749
Aspartic acid	700	—	—	434
Electrolytes (mEq/liter)				
Calcium	—	—	—	—
Sodium	45.3	10	—	—
Potassium	—	—	—	—
Magnesium	—	—	—	—
Chloride	—	<3	40	—
Acetate	71.8	89	60–87	151
Phosphate (mmol/liter)	—	10	—	—
mOsm/liter	873	950	970–1000	1388
pH	5.0–6.5	6.5	6	5.2–6.0
Calories/liter	—	—	—	—

From *American Hospital Formulary Service: Drug Information.* Section 40:20. Caloric agents. Bethesda, MD: American Society of Hospital Pharmacists, 1990. Reprinted with permission.

Dextrose is commercially available in various concentrations ranging from 5 to 70%.

Glycerol
Glycerin (glycerol) is another commercially available caloric source. The only commercially available product that makes use of this nonprotein caloric source is ProcalAmine (Kendall-McGaw), which contains 3% amino acids and 3% glycerin (Table 5-2) and is intended for peripheral parenteral nutrition [3]. Each liter of ProcalAmine provides 29 g of protein equivalent and 130 nonprotein calories [121].

Fat
Another nonprotein caloric source used in the provision of parenteral nutrition is intravenous fat emulsion. These products are also used to correct or prevent essential fatty acid deficiency. Fat emulsions are oil-in-water emulsions and use soybean oil or a combination of soybean and safflower oils as the source of fatty acids. Commercially available products are available in 10% and 20% concentrations (Table 5-3) [3]. The 10% fat emulsion provides 1.1 kcal/ml while the 20% fat emulsion provides 2 kcal/ml. It is recommended that total calories provided by fat

Table 5-2. 3% Glycerin and 3% Amino Acid Peripheral Formulation

	ProcalAmine (Kendall-McGaw)
Protein concentration (%)	3
Nitrogen (g/100 ml)	0.46
Essential amino acids (mg/100 ml)	
Isoleucine	210
Leucine	270
Lysine	220
Methionine	160
Phenylalanine	170
Threonine	120
Tryptophan	46
Valine	200
Nonessential amino acids (mg/100 ml)	
Alanine	210
Arginine	290
Histidine	85
Proline	340
Serine	180
Tyrosine	—
Glycine	420
Cysteine	<20
Glutamic acid	—
Aspartic acid	—
Electrolytes (mEq/liter)	
Calcium	3
Sodium	35
Potassium	24
Magnesium	5
Chloride	41
Acetate	47
Phosphate (mmol/liter)	3.5
mOsm/liter	735
pH	6.8
Calories/liter	130

From *American Hospital Formulary Service: Drug Information.* Section 40:20. Caloric agents. Bethesda, MD: American Society of Hospital Pharmacists, 1990. Reprinted with permission.

should not exceed 60% of nonprotein calories [177].

Electrolytes

Most commercially available amino acid formulations are available with and without added electrolytes. When choosing an amino acid source without added electrolytes, it is important to take into account the electrolyte content of the amino acid formulation when determining electrolyte requirements for the patient. In addition, three factors must be considered when determining the electrolyte requirements for a patient receiving parenteral nutrition. First, if the patient has preexisting electrolyte deficits, they should be corrected immediately. Second, excessive fluid and electrolyte losses can lead to chronic deficits if these losses are not recognized and replaced early in the patient's course. Finally, daily electrolyte needs of the patient must be determined (Table 5-4) [126]. Using these three factors, one can determine the amounts of electrolyte additive that should be added to the parenteral nutrition admixture daily. If the patient has excessive electrolyte deficits or losses, it would be prudent to replace these losses separately from the parenteral nutrition admixture. This allows one the flexibility to change the replacement solution at any time without having to discard an expensive parenteral nutrition admixture.

At the University of Cincinnati Medical Center, we restrict the amount of allowable additives (Table 5-5). The maximum additive per liter may only be exceeded with the approval of the Nutrition Support Service. These limits were established to minimize the risk of incompatibilities and wasting of parenteral nutrition admixtures.

Trace Elements

Trace elements have important biologic function. In 1979, the American Medical Association (AMA) Department of Foods and Nutrition established guidelines for essential trace element preparations for parenteral nutrition (Table 5-6) [4]. Several commercial parenteral multiple trace element products were designed to meet these guidelines. Today, in addition to zinc, copper, chromium, and manganese, for which there are established guidelines, newer products are available with selenium, iodide, and molybdenum as well.

Another important trace element is iron. We do not routinely supplement iron. If a patient should require iron supplementation,

Table 5-3. Intravenous Fat Emulsions

	Intralipid 10% (Baxter)	Intralipid 20% (Baxter)	Liposyn II 10% (Abbott)	Liposyn II 20% (Abbott)	Nutrilipid 10% (Kendall-McGaw)	Nutrilipid 20% (Kendall-McGaw)	Soyacal 10% (Alpha Therapeutic)	Soyacal 20% (Alpha Therapeutic)
Concentration (%)	10	20	10	20	10	20	10	20
Fat content (g/100 ml)								
Safflower oil	—	—	5	10	—	—	—	—
Soybean oil	10	20	5	10	10	20	10	20
Fatty acids (%)								
Linoleic acid	50	50	65.8	65.8	49–60	49–60	49–60	49–60
Oleic acid	26	26	17.7	17.7	21–26	21–26	21–26	21–26
Palmitic acid	10	10	8.8	8.8	9–13	9–13	9–13	9–13
Stearic acid	3.5	3.5	3.4	3.4	3–5	3–5	3–5	3–5
Linolenic acid	9	9	4.2	4.2	6–9	6–9	6–9	6–9
Egg phosphatides (g/100 ml)	1.2	1.2	up to 1.2	1.2	1.2	1.2	1.2	1.2
Glycerin (g/100 ml)	2.25	2.25	2.5	2.5	2.21	2.21	2.21	2.21
mOsm/liter	260	260	276	258	280	315	280	315
pH	6.0–8.9	6.0–8.9	8	8.3	6.0–7.9	6.0–7.9	6.0–7.9	6.0–7.9
Calories/ml	1.1	2	1.1	2	1.1	2	1.1	2

From *American Hospital Formulary Service: Drug Information*. Section 40:20. Caloric agents. Bethesda, MD: American Society of Hospital Pharmacists, 1989. Reprinted with permission.

Table 5-4. Daily Electrolyte Recommendations

Electrolyte	Recommendations
Sodium	Daily needs may range from 100–150 mEq May add as sodium acetate or chloride Do not use sodium bicarbonate since it is incompatible
Chloride	Add similar quantity to total sodium content
Potassium	Daily needs may range from 80–100 mEq Anabolic patient may require 150–200 mEq daily May add as chloride, phosphate, or acetate salt
Calcium	Requirements may range from 5–15 mEq/day Most commonly used salt is gluconate
Magnesium	Requirement may range from 8–30 mEq/day Available as the sulfate salt
Phosphorus	Requirements range from 15–45 mM/day Available as potassium and sodium phosphate

From Pestana, C. *Fluid and Electrolytes in the Surgical Patient* (3rd ed.). Baltimore: Williams & Wilkins, 1985. Reprinted with permission.

it is administered apart from the parenteral nutrition admixture.

Vitamins

Vitamins, like trace elements, are important components of a parenteral nutrition formula. In 1979, the AMA Nutrition Advisory Group (NAG) [5] published recommendations for parenteral vitamin formulations (Table 5-7). Several parenteral vitamin formulations designed to meet these recommendations are commercially available.

Vitamin K (5 mg) is added to the parenteral nutrition admixture once a week, but not for patients receiving the anticoagulant warfarin. Because vitamin K is not included in adult multivitamin formulations, it is necessary to add it separately. Other vitamins may also need to be supplemented, depending on the patient's metabolic requirements.

SPECIALTY AMINO ACID FORMULATIONS

As the medical community has expanded its knowledge of the metabolic needs of specific disease states, we have seen the develop-

Table 5-5. Allowable Additive Supplementation of Electrolytes and Insulin

Additives	Available Products (Injection)	Maximum Allowable Total per Liter
Calcium	Calcium gluconate Calcium chloride	9 mEq
Magnesium	Magnesium sulfate	12 mEq
Phosphate	Sodium phosphate Potassium phosphate	21 mM
Potassium	Potassium chloride Potassium acetate	80 mEq
Sodium	Sodium chloride Sodium acetate	Patient tolerance and/or need
Chloride	Sodium chloride Calcium chloride Potassium chloride	Limited by amount of cation
Acetate	Sodium acetate Potassium acetate	Limited by amount of cation
Insulin	Regular human insulin	50 U

Table 5-6. Guidelines for Daily Parenteral Trace Elements (Adult Dose)

Zinc*	2.5–4.0 mg
Copper	0.5–1.5 mg
Chromium	10–15 μg
Manganese	0.15–0.80 mg

*Zinc—additional 2 mg for acute catabolic state; additional 12 mg/liter for small-bowel fluid loss; additional 17.1 mg/kg of stool or ileostomy output.
From the American Medical Association Department of Foods and Nutrition. Guidelines for essential trace element preparations for parenteral use: A statement by an expert panel. *J.A.M.A.* 241:2051, 1979. Reprinted with permission.

ment of disease-specific amino acid formulations. Although a detailed review of these specialty formulations is beyond the scope of this chapter, all commercially available specialty formulations are briefly described. Please refer to chapters on specific diseases for more in-depth discussion of specialty amino acid usage.

Renal Disease

There are currently four commercially available amino acid products that have been specifically formulated for patients with renal failure (Table 5-8) [3]. All four products contain high levels of essential amino acids as well as histidine, which is considered an essential amino acid in patients with renal dysfunction. One product also contains arginine and another contains nonessential amino acids in lower concentrations as compared to general-purpose amino acid formulations. Use of these specialty amino acid formulations for renal failure remains controversial [1, 20, 61, 108].

Liver Disease

Only one disease-specific amino acid formulation has been tested and approved for the treatment of liver disease (Table 5-9) [32]. Dietary studies, abnormal amino acid patterns associated with hepatic encephalopathy, and the false neurotransmitter theory led to the development of this product [56, 137]. This disease-specific amino acid formulation contains higher concentrations of branched-chain amino acids (BCAAs) and lower concentrations of aromatic amino acids and methionine than do general-purpose amino acid formulations.

Table 5-7. Recommended Multivitamin Additions

A multivitamin product that meets the American Medical Association Nutrition Advisory Group's guidelines [5] for vitamin therapy is added to the parenteral nutrition formula daily. The vitamin composition is as follows:

Ascorbic acid (C)	100 mg
Vitamin A (retinol)	1 mg
Ergocalciferol (D)	5 μg
Thiamine (B_1) (as the hydrochloride)	3 mg
Riboflavin (B_2) (as riboflavin-phosphate sodium)	3.6 mg
Pyridoxine HCl (B_6)	4 mg
Niacinamide	40 mg
Dexpanthenol (*d*-pantothenyl alcohol)	15 mg
Vitamin E (*d*-alpha-tocopheryl acetate)	10 mg
Biotin	60 μg
Folic acid	400 μg
Cyanocobalamin (B_{12})	5 mg

with propylene glycol 30%, and citric acid, sodium citrate, and sodium hydroxide for pH adjustment.

From American Medical Association Department of Foods and Nutrition. Multivitamin preparations for parenteral use: A statement by the Nutrition Advisory Group. *J. Parenter. Enter. Nutr.* 3:258, 1979. Reprinted with permission.

Table 5-8.   Specialty Amino Acid Formulations—Renal Disease

	Aminosyn RF 5.2% (Abbott)	NephrAmine 5.4% (Kendall-McGaw)	Aminess 5.2% (Baxter)	RenAmine 6.5% (Baxter)
Protein concentration (%)	5.2	5.4	5.2	6.5
Nitrogen (g/100 ml)	0.787	0.64	0.66	1
Essential amino acids (mg/100 ml)				
Isoleucine	462	560	525	500
Leucine	726	880	825	600
Lysine	535	640	600	450
Methionine	726	880	825	500
Phenylalanine	726	880	825	490
Threonine	330	400	375	380
Tryptophan	165	200	188	160
Valine	528	640	600	820
Nonessential amino acids (mg/100 ml)				
Alanine	—	—	—	560
Arginine	600	—	—	630
Histidine*	429	250	412	420
Proline	—	—	—	350
Serine	—	—	—	300
Tyrosine	—	—	—	40
Glycine	—	—	—	300
Cysteine	—	<20	—	—
Glutamic acid	—	—	—	—
Aspartic acid	—	—	—	—
Electrolytes (mEq/liter)				
Calcium	—	—	—	—
Sodium	—	5	—	—
Potassium	5.4	—	—	—
Magnesium	—	—	—	—
Chloride	—	<3	—	31
Acetate	105	44	50	60
Phosphate (mmol/liter)	—	—	—	—
mOsm/liter	475	435	416	600
pH	4.5–6	6.5	6.4	5–7
Calories/liter	—	—	—	—

*Histidine is considered an essential amino acid in patients with renal dysfunction.
From *American Hospital Formulary Service: Drug Information*. Section 40:20. Caloric agents. Bethesda, MD: American Society of Hospital Pharmacists, 1990. Reprinted with permission.

Metabolic Stress

It is well recognized that patients become hypercatabolic secondary to the metabolic state created by trauma and sepsis. Unique nutritional needs and amino acid patterns have been associated with these disease states. BCAA-enriched formulations have been developed to meet these unique nutritional needs [25, 48, 110]. Two products are BCAA-enriched formulations while the third is a BCAA additive (Table 5-10) [3].

Formulations for Infants and Young Children

Infants and young children have their own unique nutritional needs. Amino acids such as histidine, tyrosine, cysteine, and taurine, which are nonessential amino acids in adults, may be essential for infants and small children. Two formulations have been developed to meet the special needs of this patient population (Table 5-11). L-Cysteine hydrochloride (50 mg/ml) is also available from

Table 5-9. Specialty Amino Acid Formulations—Liver Disease

	Hepatamine 8% (Kendall-McGaw)
Protein concentration (%)	8
Nitrogen (g/100 ml)	1.2
Essential amino acids (mg/100 ml)	
Isoleucine	900
Leucine	1100
Lysine	610
Methionine	100
Phenylalanine	100
Threonine	450
Tryptophan	66
Valine	840
Nonessential amino acids (mg/100 ml)	
Alanine	770
Arginine	600
Histidine	240
Proline	800
Serine	500
Tyrosine	—
Glycine	900
Cysteine	<20
Glutamic acid	—
Aspartic acid	—
Electrolytes (mEq/liter)	
Calcium	—
Sodium	10
Potassium	—
Magnesium	—
Chloride	<3
Acetate	62
Phosphate (mmol/liter)	10
mOsm/liter	785
pH	6.5
Calories/liter	—

From *American Hospital Formulary Service: Drug Information*. Section 40:20. Caloric agents. Bethesda, MD: American Society of Hospital Pharmacists, 1990. Reprinted with permission.

Abbott Laboratories as an amino acid additive.

ASEPTIC MANUFACTURING PROCEDURE

The manufacturing of parenteral nutrient admixtures should only be accomplished by well-trained pharmacy technicians under the supervision of a registered pharmacist. The manufacturing procedure should be conducted within the confines of a certified laminar air-flow hood. Strict guidelines for aseptic manufacturing technique need to be followed to ensure delivery of sterile parenteral nutrient admixtures. Finally, to minimize the potential for microbial growth, the National Coordinating Committee on Large-Volume Parenterals recommends that parenteral admixtures be refrigerated immediately or utilized within 24 hours of final admixture [115].

PARENTERAL NUTRITION FORMULATION PREPARATION

The preparation of parenteral nutrition base formulations may be accomplished by two methods. The first method utilizes the gravity flow technique whereby the amino acid, dextrose, and intravenous fat emulsion flow from their source containers into the final admixture container. This method is relatively time-consuming, especially for an institution that compounds a large number of parenteral nutrient admixtures daily. Also, the degree of accuracy achieved using this method is limited.

A second method for preparation of parenteral nutrition base formulations makes use of automated, high-speed multichannel pumping devices. There are currently several commercially available units that are highly accurate and can reduce preparation time significantly. They also allow the utilization of concentrated amino acid–dextrose solutions that can be diluted to the desired final concentration with sterile water. Using larger-volume, concentrated amino acid–dextrose solutions may decrease overall inventory as well as space for storage, and thus reduce cost.

Disadvantages of the automated mixing method include the cost of the mixing device. An institution would need to be admixing a significant number of parenteral nutrient admixtures on a daily basis to justify the cost of

Table 5-10.   Specialty Amino Acid Formulations—Metabolic Stress

	Aminosyn-HBC 7% (Abbott)	FreAmine 6.9% HBC (Kendall-McGaw)	BranchAmin 4% (Baxter)
Protein concentration (%)	7	6.9	4
Nitrogen (g/100 ml)	1.12	0.97	0.443
Essential amino acids (mg/100 ml)			
Isoleucine	789	760	1380
Leucine	1576	1370	1380
Lysine	265	410	—
Methionine	206	250	—
Phenylalanine	228	320	—
Threonine	272	200	—
Tryptophan	88	90	—
Valine	789	880	1240
Nonessential amino acids (mg/100 ml)			
Alanine	660	400	—
Arginine	507	580	—
Histidine	154	160	—
Proline	448	630	—
Serine	221	330	—
Tyrosine	33	—	—
Glycine	660	330	—
Cysteine	—	<20	—
Glutamic acid	—	—	—
Aspartic acid	—	—	—
Electrolytes (mEq/liter)			
Calcium	—	—	—
Sodium	7	10	—
Potassium	—	—	—
Magnesium	—	—	—
Chloride	≤40	<3	—
Acetate	72	57	—
Phosphate (mmol/liter)	—	—	—
mOsm/liter	665	620	316
pH	4.5–6	6.5	6
Calories/liter	—	—	—

From *American Hospital Formulary Service: Drug Information.* Section 40:20. Caloric agents. Bethesda, MD: American Society of Hospital Pharmacists, 1990. Reprinted with permission.

this method. Also, extreme caution must be exercised while using this device to prevent contamination of the pump tubing. Any break in aseptic technique has the potential to contaminate multiple units of parenteral nutrient admixtures.

ADDITIVES TO PARENTERAL NUTRITION FORMULATIONS

Once again, adherence to strict aseptic manufacturing technique is crucial to the prep-aration of a sterile parenteral nutrient admixture. The addition of electrolytes, trace elements, and vitamins to the parenteral nutrition base formulation may be accomplished by two methods.

The first method, used by a majority of institutions, is the manual additive method. Using this method, each electrolyte, multivitamin, and multiple trace element formulation is drawn up into an individual syringe and added separately. This method is very time-consuming and can significantly increase the risk of microbial contamination.

Table 5-11.   Specialty Amino Acid Formulations—Infant/Young Children Formulations

	Aminosyn-PF 10% (Abbott)	TrophAmine 10% (Kendall-McGaw)
Protein concentration (%)	10	10
Nitrogen (g/100 ml)	1.52	1.55
Essential amino acids (mg/100 ml)	a	b
Isoleucine	760	820
Leucine	1200	1400
Lysine	677	820
Methionine	180	340
Phenylalanine	427	480
Threonine	512	420
Tryptophan	180	200
Valine	673	780
Nonessential amino acids (mg/100 ml)		
Alanine	698	540
Arginine	1227	1120
Histidine[c]	312	480
Proline	812	680
Serine	495	380
Tyrosine[c]	44	240
Glycine	385	360
Cysteine[c]	—	<16
Glutamic acid	820	500
Aspartic acid	527	320
Electrolytes (mEq/liter)		
Calcium	—	—
Sodium	3.4	5
Potassium	—	—
Magnesium	—	—
Chloride	—	<3
Acetate	46	97
Phosphate (mmol/liter)	—	—
mOsm/liter	834	875
pH	5.0–6.5	5–6
Calories/liter	—	—

[a]Aminosyn-PF 10% also contains taurine (70 mg/100 ml).
[b]TrophAmine 10% also contains taurine (250 mg/100 ml).
[c]Histidine, tyrosine, cysteine, and taurine are considered as essential amino acids in infants and young children.
From *American Hospital Formulary Service: Drug Information.* Section 40:20. Caloric agents. Bethesda, MD: American Society of Hospital Pharmacists, 1990. Reprinted with permission.

An automated compounding device recently became commercially available. This multichannel device is highly accurate and has the potential to save considerable time and decrease the use of syringes and needles. As far as cost and potential for microbial contamination, the disadvantages are similar to those of the automated device for base formulation preparations. Another disadvantage is the lack of large-volume additive source containers.

PARENTERAL NUTRITION FORMULARY AND GUIDELINES

Protocol

The following protocol is used by the Nutrition Support Service at the University of Cincinnati Medical Center:

Seven standard formulations are available for adult parenteral nutrition at the University of Cincinnati Hospital and the Christian R. Holmes Division. The Department of Pharmacy will only accept those parenteral nutrition orders written on the standardized forms. If a patient's condition requires a formulation other than the seven available, the "Individualized Parenteral Nutrition Formulation Form" will be utilized.

In an effort to promote cost-effective therapy as well as enhance educational experience, the nutrition support physician should be consulted prior to writing the initial order for review and provision of selected order forms.

1. Central Formulation
   a. *Indications.* The majority of patients who require parenteral nutrition can use this standard formulation.
   b. *Composition.* This formulation consists of 500 ml of an 8.5% general-purpose amino acid solution and 500 ml of 50% dextrose. Each 1000 ml of this formulation contains 42.5 g of amino acids, 250 g of dextrose, and 6.5 g of nitrogen. The caloric content of this formulation is 1020 kcal/liter (850 kcal as nonprotein calories).
      (1) Kcal/ml = 1.02
      (2) Nitrogen = 6.5 g/liter
      (3) Kcal:nitrogen ratio = 131:1
2. Modified Substrate Formulation
   a. *Indications.* This formulation contains 15% dextrose and is designed to have fat emulsion administered to substitute for the lower concentration of carbohydrate calories. This formulation is used in patients who cannot tolerate the higher glucose load or in patients who show evidence of carbohydrate overfeeding.
   b. *Composition.* This formulation consists of 500 ml of an 8.5% general-purpose amino acid solution and 500 ml of 30% dextrose. Each 1000 ml of this formulation contains 42.5 g of amino acids, 150 g of dextrose, and 6.5 g of nitrogen. The caloric content of this formulation is 680 kcal/liter (510 kcal as nonprotein calories).
      (1) Kcal/ml = 0.68
      (2) Nitrogen = 6.5 g/liter
      (3) Kcal:nitrogen ratio = 78:1
3. Cardiac Formulation
   a. *Indications.* This formulation contains a balanced amino acid protein source in hypertonic dextrose in order to give a reduced volume in patients with fluid intolerance. The similarity in nonprotein substrate composition to renal formula makes this a good transition from renal formulation to a balanced amino acid formulation.
   b. *Composition.* This formulation consists of 500 ml of a 10% general-purpose amino acid solution and 500 ml of 70% dextrose. Each 1000 ml of this formulation contains 50 g of amino acids, 350 g of dextrose and 7.65 g of nitro-

gen. The caloric content of this formulation is 1390 kcal/liter (1190 kcal as nonprotein calories).
      (1) Kcal/ml = 1.39
      (2) Nitrogen = 7.65 gm/liter
      (3) Kcal:nitrogen ratio = 156:1
4. Renal Formulation
   a. *Indications.* The amino acid source is essential L-amino acids (NephrAmine). This formulation is indicated in patients with acute tubular necrosis who can tolerate modest fluid administration and who do not have severe hyperkalemia or other electrolyte disturbances. This solution may be useful in delaying dialysis. Once the patient has been converted to chronic dialysis, parenteral nutrition should be changed to a more balanced formulation (see standard central and/or cardiac formulations).
   b. *Composition.* This formulation consists of 250 ml of a 5.4% essential amino acid solution and 500 ml of 70% dextrose. Each 750 ml of this formulation contains 12.75 g of essential amino acids, 350 g of dextrose, and 1.6 g of nitrogen. The caloric content of this formulation is 1240 kcal/750 ml (1190 kcal as nonprotein calories).
      (1) Kcal/ml = 1.65
      (2) Nitrogen = 1.6 g/750 ml
      (3) Kcal:nitrogen ratio = 744:1
5. Hepatic Formulation
   a. *Indications.* Approximately 50% of patients with chronic liver disease who present to the hospital with either grade 0 or grade 1 hepatic encephalopathy will tolerate standard central formulation at low doses, 50 to 60 g of protein equivalent per 24 hours. Patients who present with grade 2 or greater encephalopathy, or who fail the above, are candidates for hepatic formulation. The efficacy of the hepatic formulation has been demonstrated only with glucose as the source of calories. Hepatic formulation is enriched with 35% BCAA, alanine and arginine, and reduced amounts of the aromatic and sulfur-containing amino acids.
   b. *Composition.* This formulation consists of 500 ml of an 8% branched-chain–enriched amino acid solution (35% BCAA) and 500 ml of 50% dextrose. Each 1000 ml of this formulation contains 40 g of amino acids, 250 g of dextrose and 6 g of nitrogen. The caloric content of this formulation is 1010 kcal/liter (850 kcal as nonprotein calories).
      (1) Kcal/ml = 1.01
      (2) Nitrogen = 6 g/liter
      (3) Kcal:nitrogen ratio = 142:1
6. Stress Formulation
   a. *Indications.* This formulation is a 5% amino acid solution enriched with 45% BCAA high

in leucine. It contains 17.5% dextrose in response to the decreased calorie-nitrogen ratio required in the stressed patient as well as glucose intolerance frequently encountered. This is indicated in critically ill, hypermetabolic, traumatized, or septic patients in the immediate postinjury period. Lipid emulsion may be added as an additional source of calories.

b. *Composition.* This formulation consists of 750 ml of a 6.9% branched-chain–enriched amino acid solution (45% BCAA) and 250 ml of 70% dextrose. Each 1000 ml of this formulation contains 52 g of amino acids, 175 g of dextrose, and 7.3 g of nitrogen. The caloric content of this formulation is 903 kcal/liter (595 kcal as nonprotein calories).
  (1) Kcal/ml = 0.803
  (2) Nitrogen = 7.3 g/liter
  (3) Kcal:nitrogen ratio = 82:1

7. Peripheral Formulation
  a. *Indications.* This formulation contains 3.5% amino acids in 5% dextrose. To provide an adequate calorie-nitrogen ratio, lipid emulsion should be administered with peripheral formulation. This is indicated in patients who have no central venous access or in whom central venous catheterization is contraindicated. Difficulties include increased cost and difficulties with venous access due to phlebitis. May be indicated for 3 to 5 days of nutrition support in patients who one is not certain may be able to take an adequate oral intake.
  b. *Composition.* This formulation consists of 500 ml of a 7% general-purpose amino acid solution and 500 ml of 10% dextrose. Each 1000 ml of this formulation contains 35 g of amino acids, 50 g of dextrose, and 5.5 g of nitrogen. The caloric content of this formulation is 310 kcal/liter (170 kcal as nonprotein calories).
  (1) Kcal/ml = 0.31
  (2) Nitrogen = 5.5 g/liter
  (3) Kcal:nitrogen ratio = 31:1

8. Individualized Nutrition Formulation
  As stated previously, this formulation can only be utilized when the seven standardized formulations do not meet a patient's specific metabolic needs. When used, each individual ingredient must be specified on the appropriate order form. Orders for "Total Nutrient Admixtures" should be written on this form.

Points to Remember

1. Stability
  Each parenteral nutrition day begins at 2 P.M. and all bags of parenteral nutrition formulation are given a 24-hour expiration date. No bag of parenteral nutrition formulation may be infused beyond the 24-hour expiration date.

2. Incompatibilities
  a. Bicarbonate salts must not be added to parenteral nutrition formulations since they create a number of incompatibilities and are ineffective given in this manner.
  b. Medicinal agents not mentioned (such as all antibiotics, cardioactive agents, colloids, and electrolytes not specified as compatible) must not be admixed or administered with parenteral nutrition formulations due to resultant incompatibilities.
  c. Phosphate supplementation must be ordered in terms of millimoles (mM) of phosphate. Please note that phosphate is available only as the sodium or potassium salts, and that when the potassium salt is used for "added" phosphate it must not exceed the maximum allowable concentration of potassium (i.e., 80 mEq).

The Ordering Process

All parenteral nutrition orders must be written using the Physician's Order Forms UMC 375-382. Orders not on the appropriate form will not be honored by the Pharmacy.

1. Initial Orders
  The order for a new parenteral nutrition patient must be received by the Pharmacy before 2 P.M. with line placement confirmation before 3 P.M. in order to receive parenteral nutrition formulation that day. All **initial** orders must be signed by a Nutrition Support physician (in collaboration with the patient's resident physician) in order to be honored by the Pharmacy. This will ensure appropriate use of specialty solutions and avoid waste.

2. Daily Orders
  a. Subsequent daily orders must be received in the Pharmacy before 9:30 A.M. in order to be honored. For late orders, 5% dextrose in water should be administered at the previously ordered rate since the Pharmacy will not prepare parenteral nutrition formulations until the next day's orders are received. The Nutrition Support physician may approve late orders for preparation when clinically indicated.
  b. Parenteral nutrition orders must be written daily and only a 24-hour supply of formulation should be ordered. It is unacceptable to order several days' supply of formulation in advance.
  c. Order forms for the Central Formulation and the Modified Substrate Formulation are available on the patient care units. For all other order forms, the initial form will be

provided by the nutrition support physician. Thereafter, a form for the subsequent day will be delivered with the parenteral nutrition bags. This form should be stamped and put with the patient's doctor's orders to be filled out by the resident physician.

3. Standing Orders

    A Physician's Standing Order sheet stamped with the patient's identification plate should be dated, timed, signed, and placed in the patient's chart along with the initial order for TPN (Fig. 5-1).

Administration

1. Central formulations should always be infused through a **new** subclavian or internal jugular catheter that terminates in the superior vena cava or brachiocephalic vein and is confirmed by portable chest x-ray, with appropriate documentation of the position of the catheter in the patient's chart.
2. The initial and subsequent sterile dressing procedure should be performed by verified nursing personnel.
3. Insertion of this catheter should never be an emergency. Adequate time should be allowed for hydration, correction of clotting abnormalities, and stabilization of the patient prior to insertion of the catheter. (See "Procedures: Percutaneous Subclavian Vein Catheterization" in *Nutrition Support Handbook* for description of placement technique of central venous catheter.)

Infusion

1. All central formulations except for renal and cardiac formulations are generally begun at a rate of 40 ml/hr. Due to the higher dextrose concentration, renal and cardiac formulations are generally begun at a rate of 30 ml/hr.
2. The rate can be advanced 20 ml/hr/day to target calories in the absence of hyperglycemia. With renal and cardiac formulations, the rate should be advanced 10 ml/hr/day to target calories.
3. With the exception of lipid emulsion, the catheter cannot be used for any other infusion of medication, blood sampling, or CVP monitoring.

Monitoring

1. Vital signs every 6 hours
2. Urine S and A every 6 hours
3. 24-Hour intake and output
4. Weight three times per week
5. Blood work twice weekly (see Fig. 5-1)

STABILITY OF PARENTERAL NUTRITION FORMULATIONS

Parenteral nutrient admixtures, because of their complex nature, are subject to stability problems. It is not always possible to determine the stability or compatibility of the formulation being prepared from the available reference sources. Extreme caution should be used in deciding to prepare a formulation for which there are no documented data on stability or compatibility.

Current data support the stability of amino acid–dextrose base solutions plus electrolytes stored under refrigeration for up to 30 days [124]. These admixtures should be refrigerated immediately after preparation. If the admixture is not refrigerated, it should be infused within 24 hours [115].

An increasingly popular formulation for the provision of parenteral nutrition is the total nutrient admixture [6, 28, 45, 123]. This admixture combines amino acids, dextrose, electrolytes, trace elements, and vitamins with intravenous fat emulsions. Total nutrient admixtures have an entirely different set of stability problems from the amino acid–dextrose base solutions.

Acidic pH is very disruptive to fat emulsions; therefore, intravenous fat emulsions should never be combined directly with dextrose or any acidic solution. However, it is safe to admix with amino acid–dextrose solutions, since the amino acid solution's buffering capacity protects the fat emulsion from the effect of the dextrose solution. It is also acceptable to co-infuse amino acids, dextrose, and intravenous fat emulsion into the same container [172].

Not all amino acid formulations can be used in total nutrient admixtures. In addition, it is not acceptable to use commercially available intravenous fat emulsions interchangeably. Prior to admixing, one should always refer to the manufacturer's product information for compatibility data.

Additives such as divalent and trivalent cations as well as excessive amounts of some trace elements are known to be disruptive to these emulsions. One should never exceed the established limits for these cations [172].

UMC-374
Revised 5/88

University of Cincinnati Hospital
Physician's Checklist/Order Sheet

All applicable orders have been checked. A line has been placed
through orders that have been voided. ORDERS NOT CHECKED
ARE NOT TO BE FOLLOWED. Orders have been modified
according to the medical condition of the patient. These orders
have been dated, timed and signed by a physician. As an order is
filled, the individual doing so must date/time and initial in the
space provided. Further orders will be added as needed.

PAGE __1__ OF __1__

ORDER NUMBER	✓	PHYSICIAN'S STANDING ORDERS PARENTERAL NUTRITION	ORDER NOTED (DATE/TIME)	(INITIAL)
1.	✓	Infuse only through a new subclavian or internal jugular		
		or existing implanted catheter which terminates in		
		superior vena cava or brachiocephalic vein.		
2.	✓	STAT portable chest x-ray.		
3.	✓	Initial and subsequent dressing by nurse (per Nursing		
		Procedure).		
4.	✓	Infuse D_5W at 40 ml/hr until TPN is available.		
5.	✓	Administration via infusion device.		
6.	✓	Catheter may be used only for TPN except by order of		
		Nutritional Support physician.		
7.	✓	Vital signs Q 6 hours.		
8.	✓	Urine sugars Q 6 hours with Diastix.		
9.	✓	Intake and Output Q 24 hours.		
10.	✓	Weights Monday, Wednesday, and Friday.		
11.	✓	Blood Work:		
		MONDAY: Renal (4203), Bone (4041) & Hepatic (4162)		
		Profiles.		
		THURSDAY AND PRIOR TO STARTING PARENTERAL NUTRITION:		
		Renal (4203), Bone (4041) & Hepatic (4162) Profiles,		
		CBC (4032), Prothrombin Time (4204), Transferrin (4706),		
		Prealbumin (4705), Retinol Binding Protein (4707),		
		Magnesium (4229), Cholesterol & Triglyceride (4726),		
		Amino Acid Profile (4265).		
12.	✓	STAT blood glucose for 1/4% or greater glycosuria.		
13.	✓	If parenteral nutrition solution is interrupted, infuse		
		D_5W at the same rate until it is restarted.		
14.	✓	Notify Nutritional Support for catheter removal and		
		culture Mon.-Fri. 9:00 a.m.-4:00 p.m.		

Physician's signature _____

White-Chart   Yellow-Kardex

Date _____ Time _____

Developed by ___Robert H. Bower, M.D.___   Date __4/88__

Figure 5-1. Physician's standing orders.

Storage and stability data are limited and can vary from product to product. If the data cannot be found in current references or literature, it is prudent to contact the manufacturer for the latest product information.

COMPATIBILITY OF PARENTERAL NUTRITION SOLUTIONS

Parenteral nutrition solutions provide a viable alternative to the intravenous administration of medications. This can limit the number of intravenous lines in patients with limited peripheral access, and decrease the volume of fluid administered in patients whose fluid intake is being restricted. Although parenteral nutrition solutions provide a greater buffering capacity than either dextrose or saline solutions, the physical and chemical stability of drugs in parenteral nutrition solutions still poses a major problem to clinicians [33]. This concern involves the physical stability of the solution itself as well as the physicochemical stability of the additives. Variables such as base amino acid solutions, concentration of additives, solution pH, temperature, and length of storage time must be considered in determining the physicochemical stability.

Stability studies of drugs in parenteral nutrition solutions have utilized varying study conditions and have resulted in conflicting data. Earlier studies demonstrated the need for determination of chemical stability in addition to visual compatibility [9, 91, 146]. Subsequent studies utilized more specific determinants of stability such as microbiologic assays and high-pressure liquid chromatography. However, there still exists inaccurate interpretation of analytical methods [162]. In a recent review, Niemiec and Vanderveen [116] discussed the problems in methodology associated with parenteral nutrition stability studies.

Calcium and Phosphate Salts

Calcium phosphate solubility is dependent on factors such as calcium and phosphate salt concentrations [9, 49, 74, 116, 146], solution pH [116, 146], solution temperature [49, 85, 116], amino acid concentration [116, 135], calcium salt [49], duration of infusion [85, 88, 116, 146], addition of calcium before phosphate [91, 146], and magnesium availability [129, 166]. Table 5-12 summarizes some of the more valuable calcium phosphate compatibility studies performed in varying parenteral nutrition solutions.

Phosphate exists simultaneously in both the monovalent and the divalent forms. The ratio is dependent on solution pH and is described by the equation:

$$HPO_4^{-2} \underset{[OH^-]}{\overset{[H^+]}{\rightleftharpoons}} H_2PO_4^-$$

Dibasic calcium phosphate is very insoluble (30 mg/100 ml) while monobasic calcium phosphate is relatively soluble (1800 mg/100 ml). With an increase in pH, a greater amount of dibasic phosphate is available to bind with free calcium to form dibasic calcium phosphate precipitate. At low pH, monobasic phosphate predominates. The pH of parenteral nutrition solutions is determined primarily by the concentration and type of amino acids. (There are minimal effects on solution pH with varying dextrose concentrations.) Parenteral nutrition solutions containing lower concentrations of protein are more susceptible to calcium phosphate precipitation since titratable acidity decreases as a direct function of amino acid dilution [49, 116, 130]. Eggert et al. [49] constructed calcium phosphate precipitation curves that demonstrated a greater solubility of calcium and phosphate in a solution of Aminosyn 2%–dextrose 20% (pH 5.1) than in a solution of FreAmine III 2%–dextrose 20% (pH 6.4). Poole et al. [130] observed that increased concentrations of Aminosyn allowed for greater solubility of both calcium and phosphate in a parenteral nutrition model. Fitzgerald and MacKay [57] used TrophAmine as the source of amino acids, and although no statistical comparison of calcium and phosphate solubility was made, they concluded that with the use of TrophAmine-dextrose solutions

Table 5-12. Calcium Phosphate Stability

Reference	Parenteral Nutrition Solution	Assessment for Precipitate	Solution pH	Temperature (°C)	Mg	Duration (hr)	Comments
Kaminski et al. [85]	Freamine 4.25% Dextrose 25%	Visual	Not reported	Not reported	No	Not reported	15 mEq/liter of calcium glucoheptonate visually compatible with 30 mEq/liter of phosphate
Kobayashi and King [91]	Protein hydrolysate 4% Dextrose 20%	Visual	5.22–6.18	Room temperature	Yes	24	20 mEq/liter of calcium gluconate visually compatible with 20 mEq of potassium phosphate; addition of phosphate to the parenteral solution before calcium
Schuetz and King [146]	Veinamine 4% Dextrose 25%	Visual	6.2–6.6	22	Yes	24	15 mEq/liter of calcium gluconate visually compatible with 40 mEq/liter of potassium phosphate; addition of phosphate to the parenteral solution before calcium
Eggert et al. [49]	Aminosyn 2% Dextrose 20% Aminosyn 1% Dextrose 10%	Visual and spectrophotometric absorbance	5.1 5.4	[a]	No		Generation of calcium-phosphate precipitation curves for vary-

Reference	Composition	Detection method	pH	Temperature (°C)	Precipitation	Number	Purpose
	FreAmine III 4% Dextrose 25%		6.3				ing concentrations of FreAmine III and Aminosyn using potassium phosphate and calcium gluconate
	FreAmine III 2% Dextrose 20%		6.4				
	FreAmine III 1% Dextrose 10%		6.6				
	FreAmine III 1% Dextrose 10% NaOH to pH 7.0		7.0				
Poole et al. [130]	Aminosyn 0.5% with Dextrose 10%, 25%; Aminosyn 2% with Dextrose 10%, 15%, 25%; Aminosyn 4% with Dextrose 10%, 25%	Visual	Not reported	25	No	30	Generation of calcium-phosphate curves for varying concentrations of Aminosyn using calcium gluconate and sodium phosphate
Knight et al. [88]	Travasol 1% Dextrose 10%	Visual	5.3–6.1	b	No	b	Use of calcium-phosphate solubility products to predict compatibility
Fitzgerald and MacKay [57]	TrophAmine (0.8 g/dl), dextrose 10%; TrophAmine (1.5 g/dl), dextrose 10%; TrophAmine (2 g/dl), dextrose 10%	Visual microscopic	4.9–5.5	25c	No	18c	Generation of calcium-phosphate precipitation curves for varying concentrations of TrophAmine using calcium gluconate and potassium phosphate

aOne-half of samples were assessed after heating to 37°C; the other one-half of samples were left standing for 18 hr at room temperature (25°C) and then heated to 37°C.
bSamples were evaluated at room temperature (22°C) immediately after preparation or after 20 hr of refrigeration (7°C).
cSamples were evaluated after sitting at room temperature for 18 hr; samples were then placed in a water bath at 37°C for 30 min and reevaluated.

From LaFrance, R. J., Miyagawa, C. I., and Youngs, C. H. F. Pharmacotherapeutic considerations in enteral and parenteral therapy. In (C. E. Lang (ed.), Nutritional Support in Critical Care. Rockville, MD: Aspen Publishers, 1987. P. 407. Reprinted with permission.

(pH 4.9–5.5), a slightly greater concentration of phosphate can be solubilized as compared with the amino acid–dextrose solutions used by Eggert et al. [49]. Therefore, the choice of amino acid preparation as well as the concentration of amino acids may allow for more or less calcium and phosphate to be administered in parenteral nutrition solutions.

Several investigators attempted to increase the solubility of calcium and phosphate in parenteral nutrition solutions by exogenously lowering the pH of the solution [57, 130]. Utilizing the essential amino acid cysteine HCl, they were able to lower the pH of standard solutions and thereby increase calcium and phosphate solubility.

An increase in the temperature of parenteral nutrition solutions increases the dissociation of calcium. This increases the amount of calcium ion available to complex with phosphate and results in a decrease in calcium and phosphate solubility [74]. Eggert et al. [49] observed a decrease in calcium and phosphate solubility when they compared solutions immediately prepared to those placed in a water bath at 37°C for 30 minutes. The placement of the solution in a water bath of 37°C was intended to duplicate the placement of parenteral nutrition solutions in incubators of infants receiving hyperalimentation solutions. Robinson and Wright [135] also demonstrated the decreased solubility of calcium and phosphate at 37°C by the observance of a noticeable precipitate within 12 hours in a parenteral nutrition solution. Similar solutions at room temperature (26°C) and refrigeration (5°C) were visually clear at 24 hours. Although lower temperatures may potentially allow for a greater amount of calcium and phosphate to be solubilized, premature infants do not tolerate the infusion of cold fluids.

The dissociation of calcium chloride in solution is greater than that of calcium gluconate. Dissociation of either calcium salt leads to the availability of free calcium to bind with phosphate. Henry et al. [74] observed that a greater concentration of calcium in the form of the gluconate salt can be admixed in parenteral nutrition solutions with sodium phosphate than can calcium in the form of the chloride salt. The order of calcium and phosphate addition to parenteral nutrition solutions can also affect the solubility of these electrolytes [91, 116, 146]. It is recommended that phosphate be added and diluted as much as possible prior to the addition of calcium. Many studies do not evaluate the effect of magnesium on calcium phosphate solubility [49, 57, 85, 88]. However, the presence of magnesium may influence the interaction between calcium and phosphate [24, 166]. Calcium phosphate precipitation may occur immediately on admixture in parenteral nutrition solutions, or may occur gradually over 12 to 24 hours in solutions bordering on compatibility [116, 146].

In an effort to simulate the administration of lipid and a parenteral nutrition solution through a common intravenous line, Eggert et al. [49] admixed lipid emulsion (Intralipid, Cutter) with a parenteral nutrition solution composed of either FreAmine III 2% or FreAmine III 1% with dextrose 10% in a ratio of 7.5:1 (parenteral nutrition solution:lipid). There was an increase in pH of both solutions after the addition of lipid. However, the pH increased to a greater degree in the 1% solution than in the 2% solution. Eggert et al. [49] suggested that the infusion of lipid into an intravenous line containing a parenteral nutrition solution that has a calcium and phosphate content bordering on the precipitation curve for that solution be avoided in order to prevent an increase in solution pH and the resultant formation of calcium-phosphate crystals, which may be infused into the patient or obstruct the catheter. Fitzgerald and MacKay [57], using a similar model except for the substitution of TrophAmine for FreAmine III, did not observe an increase in solution pH following the addition of lipid in a 7.5:1 ratio. The combined addition of cysteine and lipid actually caused a decrease in solution pH from 5.5 to 4.9.

Data from studies evaluating the compatibility of calcium and phosphate in parenteral nutrition solutions are specific for the amino acid product and amino acid concentration used in that particular study. Furthermore, the compatibility information is also specific for temperature, storage time, and solution pH. Conflicting and inconcise information has been reported due to varying methodology (i.e., temperature, storage time, solution, pH, etc.), subjective assessment methods for precipitation, failure to include magnesium in precipitation models, and unreported accuracy and calibration for aliquot volume measurements.

The calcium and phosphate precipitation curves generated by Eggert et al. [49] provide a useful reference for the preparation of parenteral nutrition solutions in which FreAmine III and Aminosyn are utilized. Precipitation curves for FreAmine III can be applied to Travasol solutions [116]. The avoidance of solutions with borderline calcium phosphate compatibilities is recommended since variables such as temperature, time, and lipid infusion may cause delayed precipitation.

Thiamine

Thiamine is sensitive to degradation by sulfite ions in an alkaline pH [175]. At molar (4–10-fold excess) concentrations of sulfite, the cleavage of thiamine to the inactive thiazole and pyrimidine moieties occurs instantaneously at pH 6 and is complete within 48 hours at pH 5 [175]. This is of major concern since currently available crystalline amino acid products contain up to a maximum of 500 mg of sodium bisulfite (9.6 mM) per 500 ml as an antioxidant and, when combined with usual concentrations of thiamine in parenteral nutrition solutions, result in a large molar excess of sulfite and thiamine [116].

Thiamine has been shown to be stable for 24 hours in intravenous solutions that do not contain sulfite [161]. However, its stability in parenteral nutrition solutions containing bisulfite is questionable [26, 34, 145]. Scheiner et al. [145] observed the extent of degradation of 3 mg of thiamine (MVI-12, Armour Pharmaceutical Company) when added to 500 ml of undiluted FreAmine III 8.5% and 500 ml of undiluted Travasol 5.5% over 24 hours. At room temperature, only 3 to 8% and 29% of added thiamine remained in the FreAmine III

8.5% and Travasol 5.5% solutions, respectively. At 7°C, 37 and 67% of thiamine remained in the FreAmine III 8.5% and Travasol 5.5%, respectively. No effect of lighting on thiamine stability was demonstrated. It was concluded that due to the significant degradation of thiamine in bisulfite-containing solutions, these solutions are inadequate for the intravenous administration of vitamin preparations containing thiamine.

Chen et al. [34] demonstrated a 26% loss of thiamine in a parenteral nutrition solution over 8 hours at room temperature in direct sunlight. No significant losses were observed when the same solutions were placed in fluorescent light or indirect sunlight over 8 hours. However, unlike Scheiner et al. [145], Chen et al. [34] placed 50 mg of thiamine (Multivitamin concentrate, Lypho-Med Inc.) in a parenteral nutrition solution composed of 8.5% amino acid, 500 ml of 50% dextrose, and electrolytes. Bowman and Nguyen [26] observed a 40% loss of thiamine in 500 ml of undiluted Travasol 10% after 22 hours at 31°C. However, when the same amount of thiamine (50 mg from Multivitamin concentrate, Lypho-Med Inc.) was admixed with a parenteral nutrition solution composed of 500 ml of 8.5% amino acid and 500 ml of 50% dextrose, negligible losses were observed.

Table 5-13 summarizes the results and conditions of the three studies discussed. Chen et al. [34] and Bowman and Nguyen [26] observed substantially lower losses of thiamine than did Scheiner et al. [145]. This may be attributed to the differences in the sulfite-thiamine ratio. Scheiner et al. [145] tested thiamine dosages of 3 mg/500 ml of undiluted amino acid solutions with a resultant sulfite-thiamine ratio of 6.67. Chen et al. [34] and Bowman and Nguyen [26] evaluated a significantly larger dose of thiamine (50 mg) in parenteral nutrition solutions with a resultant sulfite-thiamine ratio of 1.0. The larger doses of thiamine used by Chen et al. [34] and Bowman and Nguyen [26], in face of sulfite concentrations of 0.02% in the evaluation by Scheiner et al. [145], probably resulted in the higher levels of thiamine recovered.

Although Scheiner et al. [145] used a

Table 5-13. Thiamine Stability

Reference	Solution	pH	Temperature (°C)	Storage Time (hr)	% Thiamine Remaining	% Sulfite in Solution	Thiamine Added to Solution (mg)	Sulfite-Thiamine Ratio
Scheiner et al. [145]	500 ml Freamine III 8.5%	6.5	23	24	3–8	0.02	3	6.67
	500 ml Travasol 5.5%	5.5	23	24	29		3	
	500 ml Freamine III 8.5%	6.5	7	24	37	0.02	3	6.67
	500 ml Travasol 5.5%	5.5	7	24	67		3	
Chen et al. [34]	500 ml 8.5% amino acid plus 500 ml of 50% dextrose plus electrolytes	—	23*	8	74	0.05	50	1.0
Bowman and Nguyen [26]	500 ml Travasol 10% plus 500 ml of 50% dextrose	5.6–5.9	31	22	60	0.1	50	2.0
	500 ml of 8.5% amino acid plus 500 ml of 50% dextrose	5.6–5.9	31	22	100	0.05	50	1.0

*Direct sunlight.

From LaFrance, R. J., Miyagawa, C. I., and Youngs, C. H. F. Pharmacotherapeutic considerations in enteral and parenteral therapy. In C. E. Lang (ed.), *Nutritional Support in Critical Care.* Rockville, MD: Aspen Publishers, 1987. P. 407. Reprinted with permission.

model that did not realistically simulate amino acid–dextrose mixtures, they did utilize thiamine dosages (3 mg) that conformed with AMA NAG guidelines [5]. Their results have since been confirmed [155]. Although Chen et al. [34] and Bowman and Nguyen [26] used realistic amino acid–dextrose mixtures, they utilized thiamine dosages (50 mg) that did not conform with AMA NAG guidelines [5]. Thiamine stability in parenteral nutrition solutions that simulate solutions utilized in actual clinical practice needs to be addressed to fully determine the effect of thiamine degradation by sulfite. The loss of thiamine depends on solution pH, storage time, temperature, and sulfite-thiamine ratio. Until thiamine stability in parenteral nutrition solutions is clarified, patients who are predisposed to thiamine deficiency should be monitored closely, and alternative routes of thiamine administration devised [116]. Intravenous vitamins in general should be added to the parenteral nutrition solutions immediately prior to administration, and these solutions should be infused over a period of time no longer than 24 hours.

Vitamin A

The poor availability of vitamin A from parenteral nutrition solutions has been documented in the literature [64, 67, 72, 77, 87, 104, 113, 134, 153]. Depending upon solution storage time, temperature, infusion time, and the type of administration equipment used, vitamin A losses have ranged from 40 to 89% [72, 104, 153].

Moorhatch and Chiou [113] observed a 75% decrease in unbound retinol acetate over 24 hours using polyvinylcholoride intravenous bags protected from light at room temperature. Shenai et al. [153] demonstrated a 75% loss of vitamin A over 24 hours in a neonatal parenteral nutrition infusion using glass bottles. They also attributed vitamin A losses to photodegradation or oxidation after 12 hours. Although other studies have not adequately evaluated net losses of vitamin A secondary to photodegradation, Kishi et al. [87] attributed significant losses to sunlight exposure. Gillis et al. [64] were able to document mean effluent recoveries of 31, 68, and 64% of vitamins A, D, and E, respectively, after 24 hours from a simulated parenteral nutrition solution with radioactively labeled vitamins A, D, and E. All solutions were admixed in polyvinylchloride bags and run through an infusion chamber with attached intravenous tubing, extension set, and inline filter. Maximal loss occurred in the effluent within the first 1½ hours. Howard et al. [77] found a 50% loss of vitamin A from a home parenteral nutrition solution stored for 1 week at 4°C in a polyvinylchloride bag. Riggli and Brandt [134] demonstrated a loss of 77 to 98% of vitamin A analyzed spectrofluorometrically.

The chemical properties of vitamin A suggest that the significant losses are due to absorption from the parenteral nutrition solution into the plastic matrix of polyvinylchloride bags and intravenous administration sets with a resultant physiocochemical bond [113]. Absorption appears to continue over time without saturation to binding sites, and the total extent of absorption is dependent on temperature and exposure time. Howard et al. [77] were able to extract a portion of absorbed vitamin A from polyvinylchloride bags with the use of a solvent.

Based on substantial losses of vitamin A by as much as 75%, it is recommended that (1) intramuscular or oral vitamin A is preferable in patients with severe vitamin A depletion, or (2) a threefold to fourfold increase in the dose of vitamin A be administered in parenteral nutrition solutions [116, 153]. Preliminary studies indicate that vitamin A losses may be minimized if admixed with lipid preparations. No changes in lipid stability were observed [67].

Folic Acid

Folic acid has been demonstrated to be visually compatible in parenteral nutrition solutions [91, 146]. It was originally reported that folic acid was chemically unstable when combined with other vitamins. Riboflavin, thiamine, ascorbic acid, and pyridoxine had been shown to increase the degradation of folic acid. However, these reports evaluated the stability of folic acid in oral multivitamin solutions and not in parenteral nutrition solutions [17, 149, 159]. Recently, the chemical stability of folic acid in parenteral nutrition solutions has been demonstrated [14, 34, 97].

Louie and Stennett [97] demonstrated the chemical stability of varying concentrations of folic acid (0.25 mg, 0.5 mg, 0.75 mg, 1.0 mg) in a parenteral nutrition solution composed of 500 ml of 7% crystalline amino acids, 500 ml of 50% dextrose, and 5 ml of multivitamin concentration emulsion over 48 hours. In addition, chemical stability was also demonstrated at room temperature (21°C) and refrigeration (6°C) under fluorescent and dark storage conditions. No trace minerals were added to the solutions evaluated. Barker et al. [14] observed the chemical stability of 1.0 to 1.5 mg of folic acid when added to various amino acid–dextrose parenteral nutrition formulations that included electrolytes, vitamins, and trace minerals for at least 1 week. Stability was documented at 4°C and 25°C when the various solutions were protected from light. Chen et al. [34] observed the stability of 1 mg of folic acid in a parenteral nutrition solution composed of 500 ml of 8.5% crystalline amino acids, 500 ml of 50% dextrose, electrolytes, multivitamin concentrate, and trace elements in a variety of lighting conditions (i.e., fluorescent, indirect sunlight, and direct sunlight).

Many factors are associated with the visual and chemical stability of folic acid in various solutions. The pH of the solution is important in determining the chemical stability of folic acid. It is relatively insoluble at pH values below 5.0 unless diluted in a sufficient volume [14, 116]. Most parenteral nutrition solutions, however, maintain a pH between 5 and 6, and thereby ensure folic acid stability. Heavy metal ions have been reported to decrease the stability of folic acid [93, 100]. However, the chemical and physical stability of folic acid in the presence of parenteral nutrition solutions containing trace elements has been documented [14, 34, 91, 146]. Earlier studies suggested that riboflavin in the presence of air and light may increase the

rate of oxidative cleavage of folic acid [17, 149, 159]. Louie and Stennett [97] suggested that the preparation of parenteral nutrition solutions in air-evacuated containers may protect folic acid from oxidative cleavage. No appreciable evidence of folate absorption onto the polyvinylchloride plastic of the container, administration set, or inline membrane filter has been demonstrated [14].

Phytonadione

There is very little literature documenting the stability of phytonadione in parenteral nutrition solutions. Although it has been demonstrated to be visually compatible for 24 hours in a parenteral nutrition model, skepticism concerning the stability of phytonadione in light has been voiced [9, 96, 146]. Niemiec and Vanderveen [116] stated that there is only a 10 to 15% loss of phytonadione potency over 24 hours on exposure to sunlight or fluorescent light. It is common practice in many institutions to add 10 mg of phytonadione to 1 bag or bottle of parenteral nutrition solution daily or weekly. Although there are no studies documenting the chemical stability of phytonadione in parenteral nutrition solutions, it appears that prothrombin times are maintained with no serious adverse effects.

Other B Vitamins

Cyanocobalamin has been shown to be visually compatible in parenteral nutrition solutions over 24 hours [146]. However, no chemical stability has been documented.

Chen et al. [34] evaluated the activity of riboflavin-5-phosphate as measured by microbiologic assay in a parenteral nutrition solution composed of 500 ml of 8.5% crystalline amino acids, 500 ml of 50% dextrose, electrolytes, trace elements, and other vitamins. There was a 47 and 100% loss of activity with indirect and direct sunlight, respectively, in 8 hours. Minimal losses of riboflavin were experienced under fluorescent lighting. Niacinamide was found to be stable under all lighting conditions over an 8-hour period.

Pyridoxine demonstrated an 86% loss of activity over 8 hours under direct sunlight as determined by microbiologic assay. There was minimal loss observed under fluorescent lighting and indirect sunlight.

Trace Element Preparations

Boddapati et al. [22] reported that the concentration of four trace elements (copper, zinc, manganese, and chromium) remained within 99% of the confidence levels in a parenteral nutrition solution composed of 500 ml of 8.5% amino acids, 500 ml of 50% dextrose, electrolytes, and multivitamins over 24 hours at elevated temperatures and during refrigeration. There was no difference in recovery of the various trace elements between glass and plastic intravenous containers. Inline filtration had no appreciable effect on trace element concentrations during a 3-hour infusion.

Insulin

The addition of insulin to parenteral nutrition solutions appears to result in both chemical and physical stability [9, 91]. However, many variables have been associated with a decrease in the availability of insulin from parenteral nutrition solutions secondary to adsorptive losses. Adsorption can occur to the delivery unit (glass bottle, polyvinylchloride bag), administration set, and inline filter [66, 160, 170]. Reportedly, insulin adsorption occurs fairly rapidly (15 seconds) on surface contact. This is followed by the development of an equilibrium state over a period of 1 to 5 hours and results in a relatively constant rate of insulin delivery [66, 75, 127, 128, 160, 165, 170, 173]. The extent of insulin adsorption varies from 3 to 80% [116] and is dependent on variables such as type and length of administration tubing [173], type of delivery unit [76], temperature [164], insulin concentration, concentration of amino acid [43], and duration of infusion [170].

The addition of albumin to decrease the extent of insulin adsorption has been shown to be of minimal value [160, 170]. Weber et al.

[170] observed marginal reductions with the addition of 0.375% albumin to a parenteral nutrition model. It is therefore not recommended that albumin be added to decrease adsorptive losses.

Niemiec and Vanderveen provided an extensive review of insulin availability from parenteral nutrition solutions [116]. They stated that although up to 50% adsorptive losses can occur, the admixture of insulin in parenteral nutrition solutions is clinically effective in controlling serum glucose concentrations. They recommended that if insulin is to be added to parenteral nutrition solutions, (1) 50% of the previous day's sliding-scale insulin requirements be added to the next day's parenteral nutrition solution, and (2) increments no smaller than 5 U/day be used.

Hydrochloric Acid

The administration of hydrochloric acid in the treatment of severe metabolic alkalosis should be via a catheter in a large central vein [152]. The physical and chemical stability of hydrochloric acid in a parenteral nutrition model has been demonstrated [107]. Mirtallo et al. [107] evaluated the addition of 40, 60, and 100 mEq of hydrochloric acid to a parenteral nutrition solution composed of 500 ml of 50% dextrose, 500 ml of Travasol 8.5%, and electrolytes. Over a period of 24 hours at room temperature (25°C), single-assay determination of amino acid concentrations revealed minor decreases in proline and histidine concentrations only. There was no change in the titratable acidity of the solutions at 24 hours. The authors stated that although some amino acid concentrations are decreased in the presence of hydrochloric acid, the effect on the nutritional status of the patient is minimal.

Sodium Bicarbonate

The addition of sodium bicarbonate to acidic parenteral nutrition solutions can result in effervescence and the formation of carbon dioxide with a resultant loss of the bicarbonate ion [161]. In addition, the potential for the formation of insoluble calcium and magnesium carbonate also exists [161]. With the availability of acetate and lactate salts to serve as bicarbonate precursors, it has been recommended that the addition of sodium bicarbonate to parenteral nutrition solutions be avoided [116]. However, patients with renal failure may not utilize bicarbonate precursors to the same degree that normal human subjects can [102, 133].

Henann and Jacks [73] evaluated the physical and chemical compatibility of sodium bicarbonate (50–150 mEq) in various parenteral nutrition models composed of 500 ml of dextrose 50% and 500 ml of 10% Intralipid with either 500 ml of 8.5% FreAmine III, 8.5% FreAmine III with electrolytes, 5.4% NephrAmine, or 5.2% Aminosyn RF. All admixtures were stored at room temperature (25°C), protected from light, and assessed over a period of 7 days. There were no changes in solution pH during the evaluation period regardless of the amount of sodium bicarbonate added. In those solutions that contained Intralipid, there was an increase in pH after 1 week. No solution demonstrated significant effervescence when sodium bicarbonate was added except those solutions containing 5.2% Aminosyn RF and 150 mEq of sodium bicarbonate. There were no physical incompatibilities observed, and bicarbonate loss was minimal as demonstrated by measured total carbon dioxide content (bicarbonate and carbonic acid). Henann and Jacks [73] concluded that since effervescence was minimal, and solution pH was unchanged over the study period, bicarbonate was physically and chemically compatible in their parenteral nutrition model. However, with the initial addition of sodium bicarbonate to the various solutions, the solution pH increased from a baseline pH of 6.2 to as high as 7.3 following the addition of 150 mEq of sodium bicarbonate. This increase in pH could potentially effect the physical compatibility of other electrolytes including calcium and phosphate. Therefore, caution must be used with the addition of sodium bicarbonate to parenteral nutrition solutions in which a change in solution pH may affect the compatibility of other additives.

Heparin

Heparin in concentrations of 1000 to 20,000 U/liter has been shown to be visually compatible in parenteral nutrition solutions [9, 91]. In the prevention of subclavian vein thrombosis, heparin in 1000 U/liter [27, 99] does not appear to be as efficacious as heparin in 3000 U/liter [53, 157] when admixed with standard parenteral nutrition models. No changes in coagulation tests were observed with 3000 U/liter of heparin.

Certain drugs such as vancomycin, tobramycin, gentamicin, amikacin, and dobutamine have been reported to be incompatible with heparin [147]. In a standard neonatal parenteral nutrition solution (10% Aminosyn, 5% dextrose injection, standard electrolytes, vitamins, trace elements, and heparin sodium in 1.0 U/ml), these drugs were evaluated for physical stability when admixed with the parenteral nutrition solution. Vancomycin (30 mg), tobramycin (5 mg), gentamicin (5 mg), amikacin (15 mg), and dobutamine (10 mg/kg/m) were infused at a rate set to simulate clinical conditions. No precipitation was observed with any of the drugs.

In an isolated case report, Forster [58] reported on the possible unresponsiveness to heparin as a complication of parenteral nutrition. It is speculated that decreased levels of antithrombin III were responsible for the lack of heparin activity. No clear association between parenteral nutrition and depressed antithrombin III levels was made.

Albumin

Albumin has been stated to be visually compatible in parenteral nutrition solutions over 24 hours [116]. However, Mirtallo et al. [106] demonstrated a significant increase in bacterial and fungal growth in parenteral nutrition solutions containing albumin. They recommended that if the administration of albumin is necessary, it should be given separate from the parenteral nutrition solution. Other problems associated with the concomitant administration of albumin include occlusion of inline filters with albumin concentrations greater than 25 g/per liter [116], and an increase in cost following the routine addition of albumin to parenteral nutrition solutions [109]. Mirtallo and coworkers [109] recommended the routine administration of 12.5 g of albumin per liter of parenteral nutrition solutions only when the serum albumin concentration is less than 2.5 g/100 ml. Once serum albumin concentrations exceed 2.5 g/100 ml, albumin therapy should be discontinued. The addition of albumin is not recommended for the purpose of decreasing adsorption of insulin to parenteral nutrition delivery systems [116].

Antibiotics

The direct addition of antibiotics to parenteral nutrition solutions or the coadministration of antibiotics via a secondary infusion line may be of benefit in patients with fluid restriction and limited venous access, and may result in a decrease in nursing time and the number of venipuncture sites. However, most clinicians are wary of the use of parenteral nutrition catheters for concomitant administration of parenteral nutrition solutions and antibiotics since the relative risks of catheter contamination and central vein thrombosis secondary to intermittent antibiotic administration and central line manipulation are unknown [116]. The risk of antibiotic binding to cellulose or polycarbonate inline filters is minimal and should not decrease significantly the total amount of drug administered [41, 140, 141]. However, Ennis et al. [52] recovered only 38% of a 60-mg dose of gentamicin infused through a Pall Ultipor 0.2-μm filter. This was attributed to the low specific gravity of the gentamicin-containing solution.

There have been numerous studies demonstrating the visual compatibility [9, 146] and microbiologic activity [35–37, 55, 132, 146] of various antibiotics after the addition to parenteral nutrition solutions. However, these studies differed from one another in the doses of antibiotics employed, the amino acid preparation used, and the tests used to determine microbiologic stability.

Scheutz and King [146] demonstrated the visual and microbiologic stability of ampicillin (0.5 g, 1.0 g), gentamicin (80 mg), cephalothin (2 g), and kanamycin (500 mg) in a liter of parenteral nutrition solution (4.5% crystalline amino acids, 25% dextrose, electrolytes, and multivitamins) for up to 24 hours. However, there was a minimal decrease in ampicillin activity after 12 hours. Although not evaluating for microbiologic activity, Athanikar et al. [9] observed unacceptable levels of particulate matter when ampicillin (1 g) was added to a liter of parenteral nutrition solution (4.25% crystalline amino acids and 25% dextrose). However, the following antibiotics were visually and microscopically compatible: carbenicillin (8 g), cephalothin (2 g), cefazolin (1 g), clindamycin (600 mg), erythromycin glucceptate (1 g), gentamicin (80 mg), kanamycin (500 mg), methicillin (1 g), oxacillin (500 mg), penicillin G (1 million U), and tetracycline (500 mg).

Feigin et al. [55] observed that antibiotic stability may vary depending on the source of protein used. In general, all antibiotics evaluated were more stable in the protein hydrolystate than in the crystalline amino acid mixtures. With various antibiotics in either crystalline amino acid, protein hydrolysate, or essential amino acid models (including electrolytes and vitamins), no visual evidence of incompatibility was noted in any test mixture with ampicillin, kanamycin, clindamycin, penicillin G, carbenicillin, methicillin, and cephalothin. However, based on microbiologic activity as determined by zone inhibition, ampicillin and kanamycin were observed to be the least stable in all three protein solutions. Ampicillin (1 g/liter) was unstable at 25°C in the crystalline and essential amino acid formulas after 6 to 12 hours. Kanamycin (250 mg/liter) losses were significant after 24 hours at 37°C in all three protein solutions. Clindamycin (250 mg/liter) and penicillin G (5 million U/liter) were stable in all protein solutions at all temperatures for 24 hours. Carbenicillin (1 g/liter) was stable in all solutions for 24 hours except the essential amino acid formula.

Reed et al. [132] evaluated the physical and microbiologic stability of gentamicin (50 mg/liter), tobramycin (50 mg/liter), carbenicillin (1.5 g/liter), penicillin G (0.4 million U/liter), methicillin (1.5 g/liter), clindamycin (0.1 g/liter), cephalothin (0.6 g/liter), and chloramphenicol (0.7 g/liter) in a liter of parenteral nutrition solution (3.5% protein hydrolystate, 15% dextrose, electrolytes, and multivitamins). No significant loss of microbiologic activity, as determined by minimum inhibitory concentration at room temperature or refrigeration, was observed over 24 hours. However, some loss of activity was noted at 36 hours when tobramycin was combined with cephalothin or methicillin, and methicillin combined with gentamicin. No physical incompatibilities were detected visually.

Colding and Anderson [35] observed the microbiologic stability as determined by a paper disk method of gentamicin (50 mg/liter), ampicillin (1.5 g/liter), carbenicillin (6 g/liter), and polymyxin B (50 mg/liter) in a liter of a crystalline amino acid–fructose model at 29°C over 24 hours. The concentration of gentamicin and polymyxin B was unchanged. However, the concentration of ampicillin and carbenicillin decreased by 22 and 31%, respectively, without any appreciable visual incompatibility. There was a 20 to 30% decrease in the cystine content in those solutions containing penicillin. These losses were attributed to chemical binding with penicillin breakdown products. Colding et al. [36, 37] in two subsequent studies were able to demonstrate therapeutic serum levels of gentamicin and ampicillin in newborn infants who received a continuous infusion of ampicillin and gentamicin over 24 hours following mixture in a parenteral nutrition solution.

Kamen et al. [84] evaluated the physical and chemical stability of 13 antibiotics in a parenteral nutrition solution (1.5% amino acids, 15% dextrose, vitamins, calcium, and standard electrolyte concentrations). The antibiotics were diluted with either 1 or 2 parts of parenteral nutrition solution and let sit for 6 hours at room temperature. Physical and chemical stability was demonstrated for the following antibiotics: amikacin, azlocillin, cefamandole, cephalothin, gentamicin, mezlocillin, moxalactam, nafcillin, oxacillin, penicillin, piperacillin, ticarcillin, and tobramycin.

Baptista and Lawrence [12] evaluated the physical compatibility of secondary infusions of antibiotics in a total nutrient admixture (10% amino acids, 70% dextrose, 20% lipid emulsion, electrolytes, and multivitamins). Criteria for compatibility of the lipid in the total nutrient admixture included the complete absence of (1) creaming, (2) oiling out, and (3) phase separation. Except for tetracycline, no antibiotic (ampicillin, 2g/1500 ml; cefamandole, 2 g/1500 ml; cefazolin, 1 g/1500 ml; cefoxitin, 1 g/1500 ml; cephapirin, 1 g/1500 ml; clindamycin, 600 mg/1500 ml; erythromycin lactobionate, 1 g/1500 ml; gentamicin, 80 mg/1500 ml; kanamycin, 500 mg/1500 ml; oxacillin, 1 g/1500 ml; penicillin G, 2 million U/1500 ml; ticarcillin, 3 g/1500 ml; and tobramycin, 80 mg/1500 ml) resulted in creaming, oiling out, or phase separation. The effect of tetracycline on the lipid emulsion was attributed to the highly acidic pH of the ascorbic acid in the tetracycline product. Further studies assessing the changes in particle-size distribution of the lipid emulsion over time are necessary before routine addition of antibiotics to total nutrient admixtures can be recommended. Table 5-14 summarizes the studies discussed above.

Abnormal serum liver enzyme levels and intrahepatic cholestasis are common in adults receiving parenteral nutrition solutions. Metronidazole has been shown to prevent the expected rise in enzyme levels on liver function tests associated with total parenteral nutrition [31, 50, 92]. Capron et al. [31] demonstrated minimal elevations in serum alkaline phosphatase, Y-glutamyl transferase, and alanine aminotransferase in eight patients receiving metronidazole, 500 mg twice a day, along with their parenteral nutrition solution. Subsequent reports by Elleby and Solhang [50] and by Lambert and Thomas [92] verified the results of Capron et al. [31]. The postulated mechanisms for the parenteral nutrition solution elevation of liver enzyme levels include (1) hepatotoxicity of parenteral nutrition solutions, and (2) changes in biliary bile acid composition with an increase in toxic lithocholic acid [59]. The increase in lithocholic acid production may be secondary to the overgrowth of anaerobic intestinal bacteria, which may result in the production of hepatic endotoxins as well as lithocholic acid [118, 122]. The prevention by metronidazole of hepatic abnormalities would highly implicate the role of anaerobic bacteria. A large prospective trial is needed to confirm these findings before metronidazole prophylaxis can be advocated in patients receiving parenteral nutrition solutions.

In an animal model, concomitant administration of aminoglycoside antibiotic and lysine demonstrated an additive nephrotoxic potential as evidenced by a decrease in glomerular filtration rate, cast formation, and tubular necrosis [101]. Well-designed trials in humans are necessary to characterize the possible additive risks that parenteral nutrition solutions and aminoglycoside antibiotics may have on nephrotoxicity.

The visual and chemical stability of antibiotics in parenteral nutrition solutions is dependent on many factors including (1) concentration of the antibiotic, (2) temperature, (3) length of time that the antibiotic is combined with the parenteral nutrition solution, (4) amino acid profile of the parenteral nutrition solution, (5) concomitant administration of multiple drugs, and (6) the assay method used. Until control and specificity of the above factors can be manipulated to provide consistent, well-documented, and accurate data, it would appear that the admixture of antibiotics with parenteral nutrition solutions should be limited.

Amphotericin B

Amphotericin B (100 mg/liter) has been shown to form an unacceptable amount of particulate matter on admixture with a parenteral nutrition solution composed of 500 ml of FreAmine 8.5% and 500 ml of 50% dextrose [9]. Amphotericin B, which exists as a colloid in aqueous mixture, is disrupted by the ionic nature of amino acid solutions and results in the formation of an insoluble precipitate [9]. Amphotericin B has also been shown to be unstable in solutions with pH values less than 6.0 [83].

Histamine Antagonists

Cimetidine
Cimetidine hydrochloride (300–1200 mg/liter) has been shown to be chemically and physically compatible for 24 hours in parenteral nutrition solutions containing crystalline amino acids and dextrose [13, 138, 163, 179, 180]. Tsallas and Allen [163] observed no appreciable change in pH, color or clarity, and cimetidine concentration over 24 hours at 4°C or room temperature. The stability of cimetidine in total nutrient admixtures (5% injection, 20% dextrose injection, and 3% intravenous fat emulsion) in concentrations up to 1800 mg/1500 ml has been demonstrated by Baptista et al. [13]. Cimetidine concentrations in the samples were 98.9 to 101.4% of the initial concentration at 48 hours with no appreciable change in pH. No signs of creaming, oiling out, or phase separation were observed.

The routine addition of cimetidine to parenteral nutrition solutions in the prevention of gastric stress ulceration and the treatment of metabolic alkalosis secondary to nasogastric suctioning has been reported [15, 42, 114, 139, 176]. Moore et al. [112] were able to demonstrate steady-state serum cimetidine concentrations of 0.6 to 1.0 μg/ml in four patients receiving parenteral nutrition solutions providing 900 to 1300 mg/day of cimetidine. Unfortunately, gastric pH analysis was not performed to document the efficacy of delivered cimetidine infusions via parenteral nutrition. However, the use of continuous cimetidine infusions (1200 mg/day) provided by parenteral nutrition solutions has been shown to maintain gastric pH above 4 to 7 with serum cimetidine concentrations greater than 0.5 μg/ml [120, 125]. Therefore, it appears that cimetidine added to parenteral nu-

Table 5-14. Antibiotic Stability

Antibiotic	Visual Compatibility	Microbiologic Compatibility	Duration of Evaluation (hr)	Temperature (°C)	Dose (per liter)	Comments	References
Ampicillin sodium	I	I	24	25–37	1 g		82, 133
Carbenicillin di-sodium	C	C	24	4–37	1.0–1.5 g	Decreased microbiologic activity in spite of visual compatibility at doses of 6 g/liter	73, 82, 102, 133
Cefamandole naftate	C		24	37	1–2 g	2 g in total nutrient admixture (1500 ml)	53, 157
Cefazolin sodium	C C		24	4 25	1 g 1 g	Without additives; 1 g in total nutrient admixture (1500 ml)	53, 82
Cefoxitin sodium	C			25	1 g	1 g in total nutrient admixture (1500 ml)	53
Cephalothin sodium	C	C	12–24	4–25	1–2 g	Unstable at temperatures >25°C	82, 133, 136
Cephapirin sodium	C			25	1 g	1 g in total nutrient admixture (1500 ml)	53
Chloramphenicol sodium succinate	C	C	24	4–25	700 mg		102
Clindamycin phosphate	C C	C	24	4–37 25	100–600 mg 600 mg	600 mg in total nutrient admixture (1500 ml)	53, 82, 102, 133
Erythromycin gluceptate	C		24	4	1 g	Without additives	82

Drug	C/I	Hours			Concentration	Comments	References
Erythromycin lactobionate	C			25	1 g	1 g in total nutrient admixture (1500 ml)	53
Gentamicin sulfate	C	12–24	4–29		50–80 mg		27, 53, 73, 82, 99, 102, 133
	C			25	80 mg	80 mg in total nutrient admixture (1500 ml)	
Kanamycin sulfate	C	24	22		500 mg		53, 82, 133, 136
	I	6–24		25–37	250 mg	500 mg in total nutrient admixture (1500 ml)	
Methicillin sodium	C	24	4–25		1.0–1.5 g	Unstable at temperatures >25°C	82, 102, 133
Oxacillin sodium	C	24	4		500 mg		82, 133
	C			25	1 g	Without additives; 1 g in total nutrient admixture (1500 ml)	
Penicillin G	C	24	4–37		0.4–5.0 million U		82, 102, 133
	C			25	2 million U	2 million U in total nutrient admixture (1500 ml)	53
Polymyxin B sulfate	C	24	29		40 mg		73
Tetracycline hydrochloride	C	24	4		500 mg	May chelate with divalent ions in solution	51, 82
	I			25	500 mg	500 mg in total nutrient admixture (1500 ml)	53
Ticarcillin disodium	C			25	3 g	3 g in total nutrient admixture (1500 ml)	53
Tobramycin sulfate	C	24	4–25		50–80 mg		82, 102
	C			25	80 mg	80 mg in total nutrient admixture (1500 ml)	53

C = compatible; I = incompatible.

From LaFrance, R. J., Miyagawa, C. I., and Youngs, C. H. F. Pharmacotherapeutic considerations in enteral and parenteral therapy. In C. E. Lang (ed.), *Nutritional Support in Critical Care.* Rockville, MD: Aspen Publishers, 1987. P. 407. Reprinted with permission.

trition solutions, in addition to being physically and chemically compatible, is probably effective in maintaining gastric pH above 4.

Potentially, cimetidine may be incompatible when admixed with aminophylline, various antibiotics, and hydrochloric acid. In addition, on exposure to cold temperatures, cimetidine may precipitate out of solution [112, 176]. However, rewarming will redissolve the drug without causing a loss of potency [116].

Ranitidine

Ranitidine hydrochloride has been demonstrated to be stable both visually and chemically in standard parenteral nutrition solutions. Walker and Bayliff [168], utilizing a high-performance liquid chromatography assay, observed a decrease in initial ranitidine concentrations by approximately 5% every 24 hours. The time to reach 90% of the initial concentration averaged 51 hours. The rate of degradation was independent of the initial concentration of ranitidine (100 mg, 200 mg, or 300 mg in 1200 ml of parenteral nutrition solution). Similar results were obtained by Bullock et al. [29] with concentrations of 50 to 100 μg/ml of ranitidine. No visual changes or pH changes occurred by 24 hours, and more than 90% of the initial ranitidine concentration was measured at 24 hours. In addition, ranitidine did not substantially affect concentrations of the amino acids in the parenteral nutrition solution.

However, the stability of ranitidine in a total nutrient admixture containing 5% intravenous fat emulsion is questionable. Cano et al. [30] did not observe any major pH or visual changes over 72 hours in admixtures containing 100 mg or 200 mg of ranitidine. However, approximately 10% of the initial concentration of ranitidine was lost in 12 hours. By 72 hours there was a loss of approximately 80% of ranitidine activity. Although the authors assayed the contents of only one bag of each solution for drug concentration, the data suggest that it may not be advisable to administer ranitidine in total nutrient admixtures.

Metoclopramide

Recent reports demonstrate the chemical and physical compatibility of metoclopramide in parenteral nutrition models [7, 116]. Niemiec and Vanderveen [116] stated that metoclopramide in doses of 5 mg and 20 mg is chemically stable in a parenteral nutrition solution composed of Travasol 2.75%, 25% dextrose, and electrolytes for up to 72 hours at room temperature. It is also suggested that a loading dose (10 mg IV or IM) can be administered before beginning a parenteral nutrition solution containing metoclopramide [116].

Narcotics

Based on what few data are available concerning the stability of narcotics in parenteral nutrition models, parenteral nutrition solutions may potentially provide convenient vehicles for the concomitant administration of narcotics and nutrition in patients where only a single intravenous catheter site is available.

Cutie and Waranis [38] demonstrated the visual and chemical stability of 80 mg of hydromorphone in a liter of various crystalline amino acid products for 24 hours. All solutions were mixed in glass bottles, stored at 25°C, and protected from light. Macias and coworkers [98] observed the visual and chemical stability, as determined by high-pressure liquid chromatography, of 300 mg of morphine sulfate and meperidine hydrochloride, each added separately to a parenteral nutrition model composed of 1500 ml of 8.5% amino acids, 1500 ml of 50% dextrose, electrolytes, multivitamins, and trace elements. The parenteral nutrition solutions were admixed in 3-liter polyvinylchloride bags and stored at room temperature (21.5°C) with no protection from environmental light. There was no evidence of precipitation, color change, turbidity, evolution of gas, or loss of either drug due to adsorption by the plastic container.

The concomitant administration of narcotics with parenteral nutrition solutions requires consideration of the risks of continuous narcotic infusions. In addition, total daily narcotic requirements must be stabilized in order to avoid varying the administration rate of the parenteral nutrition solution. It is suggested that daily narcotic dosage requirements be initially titrated using intermittent infusions of the narcotic. The total 24-hour dosage requirement should then be administered over 24 hours by a peripheral venous route, allowing for further dosage adjustments. Once the patient's pain is controlled with a stabilized narcotic dose, the parenteral nutrition solution can then be used as the vehicle for narcotic administration [98, 116]. Further studies are required to demonstrate the stability of other narcotics in parenteral nutrition solutions.

Animal models have demonstrated a marked depression of hepatic drug metabolism capabilities in response to the intravenous administration of amino acid–dextrose solutions as compared to enteral administration [89, 90]. Knodell et al. [89, 90] observed that a decrease in the hepatic mixed function oxidase activity was responsible for an approximately 50% decrease in pentobarbital clearance as well as a significant reduction in demethylation of meperidine in rats receiving a parenteral nutrition solution intravenously. Postulated mechanisms for the decrease in drug metabolism include sepsis, differences in gut and pancreatic hormones received by the liver, and distribution and/or disposition of the infused amino acids. These studies demonstrate that the route of alimentation delivery can influence hepatic drug metabolism in rats. If animal model data can be duplicated in humans receiving parenteral nutrition solutions, then dosage adjustments of drug regimens may be necessary.

Iron Dextran

Iron dextran is not routinely added to parenteral nutrition solutions. Stead et al. [156] stated that the routine administration of iron in parenteral nutritional solutions is not necessary since the lowered serum iron observed in malnourished patients is secondary to defects in iron mobilization rather than lowered whole-body stores. In addition, there are potential problems associated with the compatibility [158], availability [143, 174], and administration [23, 103, 171] of iron dextran with parenteral nutrition solutions. Will and Groden [174] reported that the average utilization of iron dextran in iron-deficient patients was 39% after 3 weeks. Also, hyperferremia or hypotransferrinemia secondary to iron administration may make patients more susceptible to bacterial and fungal infections [23, 103, 171].

However, the routine administration of iron in parenteral nutrition solutions [119, 178] or temporary co-infusion of iron with parenteral solutions [62, 68] has been advocated. Wan and Tsallas [169] evaluated the chemical and physical stability of iron dextran (100 mg/liter) in a Travasol-dextrose solution containing typical additives. Iron recovery, as determined by atomic absorption spectroscopy, was reported to be greater than 86% over 18 hours at room temperature. No physical incompatibilities were observed. Although the authors stated that the addition of daily recommended doses of iron dextran to parenteral nutrition solutions is chemically and physically stable, the effects of varying temperatures, pH, storage time, lighting conditions, and mixture with vitamins were not assessed.

Norton et al. [119] evaluated the iron dosage needed to restore serum iron levels in patients receiving parenteral nutrition solutions. Over a 3-week study period, patients received 0, 25, 87.5, or 175 mg of iron dextran per week via their parenteral nutrition solution. Serum iron levels increased with increasing dosages of iron. However, iron at 175 mg/week increased serum levels above the normal range in 80% of patients after 3 weeks. Hemoglobin, reticulocyte count, and total iron binding capacity did not increase, and no increased incidence of sepsis was observed. The authors recommended that the daily administration of 12.5 mg of iron dextran (87.5 mg/week) via parenteral nutrition solution not only is free of chemical and physical instability, but also will result in an increase of serum iron levels.

Sayers et al. [143] suggested that iron citrate is safe and effective when admixed with a parenteral nutrition solution. They propose that iron citrate may be superior to iron dextran based upon utilization in hemoglobin synthesis. Also, the use of iron dextran may confuse the interpretation of serum iron measurements, since the compound, which cannot be distinguished from nontransferrin iron, may circulate for days. Therefore, iron-deficient individuals may present with spuriously elevated serum iron levels.

Iron dextran is not approved for admixture with any vehicle [116]. Before the routine addition of any iron salt to parenteral nutrition solutions can be recommended, further studies must be done to evaluate the chemical stability and availability under simulated clinical conditions of use (i.e., temperature, time, pH, and vitamin admixture).

Cardiotonic Agents

Drugs such as dopamine, furosemide, isoproterenol, levarterenol, lidocaine, metaraminol, and methyldopate have been shown to be physically compatible in a parenteral nutrition model and deemed acceptable for administering with amino acid–dextrose solutions [10, 69, 116, 148]. However, since many of these agents along with other cardiovascular drugs (i.e., nitroprusside, nitroglycerin, dobutamine, etc.) require continuous titration of dosage administration to maximize hemodynamic response, it is not recommended that these agents be mixed with parenteral nutrition solutions.

However, there may be instances where the administration of cardiotonic agents as a secondary infusion into parenteral nutrition solutions may be necessary. Baptista et al. [11] evaluated the stability of dopamine, furosemide, isoproterenol, lidocaine, methyldopate, and norepinephrine in a total nutrient admixture (10% amino acids, 70% dextrose, 20% lipid emulsion, electrolytes, trace minerals, and multivitamins). Volumes were simulated for mixing of primary and secondary infusions in triplicate using 1:1 dilution

methods [2]. Dopamine, furosemide, isoproterenol, lidocaine, and norepinephrine in either 5% dextrose injection or 0.9% sodium chloride, and methyldopate in 0.9% sodium chloride did not disrupt the lipid emulsion in the total nutrient admixture, as evidenced by the lack of creaming, oiling out, and phase separation at 0, 1, and 4 hours after mixing. Methyldopate, when diluted in 5% dextrose injection, however, cracked the lipid emulsion on testing and retesting. Although visual compatibility was demonstrated, the chemical stability of cardiovascular agents in total nutrient admixtures as well as standard parenteral nutrition solutions must be evaluated before routine admixture can be recommended.

Digoxin

Digoxin has been demonstrated to be chemically stable in concentrations of 0.25 mg/99 ml in dextrose-saline intravenous fluids stored at 4°C and 23°C for 48 hours in glass [151]. Its visual and chemical stability in parenteral nutrition models has also been verified [11, 21, 54]. Baptista et al. [11] demonstrated the visual stability of digoxin (0.625 mg) in 0.9% sodium chloride and 5% dextrose when mixed as a secondary infusion with a total nutrient admixture. Blackstone et al. [21] reported on the chemical stability, as demonstrated by radioimmunoassay, of digoxin (0.25–1.0 mg/liter) in parenteral nutrition solutions for up to 96 hours in plastic intravenous bags at 4°C. Two patients maintained adequate serum digoxin levels after receiving parenteral nutrition solutions with added digoxin. Fagerman and Dean [54] described the achievement of therapeutic serum digoxin levels by adding 0.125 to 0.25 mg of digoxin to 12-hour nocturnal infusions of parenteral nutrition solutions.

Reports have demonstrated that drugs administered in very low concentrations may present problems in regard to binding to in-line filters. However, digoxin does not appear to bind significantly to cellulose or polycarbonate membrane filters [41, 140, 141] and did not appear to affect the serum digoxin concentrations obtained by Fagerman and Dean [54]. Further accumulation of data concerning chemical and visual stability must occur before the routine addition of digoxin to parenteral nutrition solutions can be recommended.

Urokinase

Thrombolytic agents have been shown to successfully restore patency to occluded central catheters [8, 65, 78]. Baumgartner et al. [16] evaluated the stability and activity of 1 ml of urokinase (2500 IU/ml) when admixed with 1 ml of a crystalline amino acid–dextrose solution. Urokinase activity was maintained as determined by spectrophotometric assay in duplicate. It was concluded that the catalytic activity of urokinase is retained after being mixed with a standard parenteral nutrition model, and that urokinase can be used to restore patency to occluded parenteral nutrition catheters.

Aminophylline

Aminophylline has been demonstrated to be stable in parenteral nutrition solutions [9, 117]. Athanikar and coworkers [9] observed no physical incompatibility by visual inspection of 50 mg of aminophylline in a liter of parenteral nutrition solution (500 ml of FreAmine 8.5% and 500 ml of 50% dextrose) over 24 hours.

Niemiec et al. [117] evaluated the stability of aminophylline in dosages of 0.25 to 1.50 mg/ml in parenteral nutrition models composed of 25% dextrose with either FreAmine III 4.25%, Aminosyn 3.5%, or Travasol 4.25%. All solutions contained typical electrolytes and vitamins, and were evaluated for physical and chemical compatibility over 24 hours at room temperature and refrigeration (4°C) under normal lighting conditions. Additional solutions containing 1% amino acids at room temperature were also evaluated. Chemical stability as demonstrated by high-pressure liquid chromatography revealed aminophylline recovery rates of 100% after 24

hours at room temperature. Refrigeration or decreased amino acid concentration did not affect aminophylline stability. The addition of alkaline medications such as aminophylline to parenteral nutrition solutions containing borderline concentrations of calcium and phosphate salts, and composed of amino acid concentrations less than 2.5%, should be avoided. The minimal buffering capacity of amino acid solutions with a concentration less than 2.5% may not tolerate the addition of aminophylline and may result in calcium-phosphate precipitation [49, 117].

Corticosteroids

Data concerning the chemical and physical stability of corticosteroids in parenteral nutrition solutions are limited to hydrocortisone sodium succinate [80, 86] and methylprednisolone sodium succinate [9].

Isaacs et al. [80] reported on the visual compatibility of hydrocortisone sodium succinate (5 mg/liter) in a 900-mOsm parenteral nutrition model without B vitamins. Hydrocortisone sodium succinate (Solu-Cortef, Upjohn) (100–500 mg) has been shown to be visually compatible in parenteral nutrition models composed of dextrose, vitamins, and either crystalline amino acids [84] or protein hydrolysates [116].

Athanikar et al. [9] demonstrated the visual compatibility of methylprednisolone sodium succinate (Solu-Medrol, Upjohn) (250 mg/liter) in a parenteral nutrition model composed of FreAmine II 4.25%, 25% dextrose, electrolytes, and vitamins for 24 hours at 4°C.

Although various corticosteroids have demonstrated visual compatibility in parenteral nutrition models, there are no data to support any chemical stability. In addition, hydrocortisone and methylprednisolone both contain phosphate buffers that preclude the mixture of their concentrated form with magnesium or calcium salts [116]. It is suggested that corticosteroids be administered as an intravenous piggyback or as a slow intravenous push rather than admixed with parenteral nutrition solutions [116].

Antineoplastics

Fluorouracil

Although fluorouracil (5-FU) (500 mg) in a liter of 5% dextrose and 0.9% sodium chloride injection is chemically stable for 72 hours, it is recommended that it be administered intravenously in undiluted form [116]. However, Lemon et al. [94], Moertel and Reitemeier [111], and Seifert et al. [150] demonstrated less myelosuppression and an enhanced therapeutic benefit with a continuous 4-day infusion of 5-FU. Levels of fluorouracil in plasma and bone have been reported to be 50 to 100 times higher following a rapid intravenous injection than after a 96-hour continuous infusion [60].

Visual compatibility of 5-FU (500 mg) in a liter of parenteral nutrition solution (4.25% amino acids and 25% dextrose) over 24 hours at 4°C has been demonstrated [60]. However, direct sunlight or intense lighting may cause partial degradation with a resultant color change to dark amber, and microprecipitation may result from exposure to low temperature [71].

Hardin and Clibon [70] observed no evidence of visual incompatibility or pH change over 48 hours following the addition of 0.1% 5-FU in a parenteral nutrition solution (4.25% amino acids, 25% dextrose, electrolytes, and vitamins) at room temperature under normal lighting. There was a 96.6 to 99.9% recovery of 5-FU at 48 hours as determined by high-pressure liquid chromatography analysis. These results were similar to those obtained in an earlier report by Hardin and Clibon [70] in which they obtained a 90 to 100% recovery over 24 hours of a 1 mg/ml concentration, and a 82 to 94% recovery of a 4 mg/ml concentration.

Cytarabine

Cytarabine has been demonstrated to be visually and chemically compatible in parenteral nutrition solutions [39, 146]. Athanikar et al. [9] found cytarabine (100 mg/liter) to be visually compatible in a parenteral nutrition model over 24 hours at 4°C with no appreciable change in pH. Quock and Sakai [131]

were able to demonstrate the chemical compatibility of cytarabine (50 μg/ml) in a pediatric parenteral nutrition solution (2.125% amino acids, 10% dextrose, electrolytes, vitamins, and trace elements) at 8°C and 25°C. Cytarabine concentration, as determined by high-pressure liquid chromatography analysis, was 93.3 to 104.4% of the initial concentration at 48 hours. There was no change in pH or color of the solutions at 96 hours.

The potential benefits of combining antineoplastic agents with parenteral nutrition solutions include preserving future veins for intravenous access and reducing the total volume of fluid administered, while simultaneously providing nutritional support and chemotherapy. Although cytarabine and 5-FU have demonstrated physical and chemical stability in parenteral nutrition models, controversy exists, especially with 5-FU, over the toxicity and effectiveness of continuous intravenous chemotherapy versus bolus administration.

Lipid Emulsion–Amino Acid–Carbohydrate Solutions (Total Nutrient Admixture)

In recent years, total nutrient admixtures have been used with increased frequency in patients requiring parenteral nutrition. However, very little information is available on the physical and chemical stability of drugs in total nutrient admixtures. Baptista and Lawrence [12] demonstrated the physical stability of ampicillin, cefamandole, cefazolin, cefoxitin, cephapirin, clindamycin, erythromycin lactobionate, ticarcillin, and tobramycin when admixed as a secondary infusion with a total nutrient admixture containing electrolytes and vitamins. Baptista et al. [11] observed the physical stability of dopamine, furosemide, isoproterenol, lidocaine, and norepinephrine in either 5% dextrose or 0.9% sodium chloride, and methyldopate in 0.9% sodium chloride when admixed as a secondary infusion with a total nutrient admixture containing electrolytes, minerals, and vitamins. Cimetidine has also been shown to be stable in a total nutrient admixture [13]. Physical stability was defined as a lack of creaming, oiling out, or phase separation.

Electrolyte concentration and pH can affect the stability of fats in total nutrient admixtures [18, 28]. Most amino acid solutions have minimal effects when added to lipid emulsions. However, fat emulsion stability can be increased or decreased depending on the pH of specific amino acids. Recently, Sayeed et al. [142] demonstrated the stability of Liposyn II with varying concentrations of amino acids and dextrose. If added to dextrose and amino acids in proper order, fat emulsions are chemically and physically stable [18, 28, 142]. However, this will vary with the type of crystalline amino acid and fat emulsion employed.

Compatibility and stability of electrolyte, vitamin, and trace elements must also be addressed to determine the maximum concentrations that are compatible in total nutrient admixtures [79, 81]. Shenkin et al. [154] observed no differences in blood concentrations of trace minerals and vitamins in patients receiving a total nutrient admixture or a separate infusion of trace minerals and vitamins. Potential problems may arise with the precipitation of calcium and phosphate salts, since fat emulsions have the ability to increase solution pH [49]. Conversely, the addition of divalent cations (calcium) can result in immediate emulsion breakdown. Trace elements have not been shown to alter stability of total nutrient admixtures. Total nutrient admixtures may also support bacterial growth to a greater degree than parenteral nutrition solutions without lipid emulsions, although some controversy exists [40, 44, 45, 63,95, 105, 144, 167].

CONCLUSIONS

The use of parenteral nutrition solutions for the administration of medications is a viable option in patients whose fluid intake is restricted or who have limited venous access. However, the addition of various medications to parenteral nutrition solutions is dependent on physical as well as chemical stability. Unfortunately, inadequate study design has limited the applicability of stability studies to clinical practice. There are many unanswered questions that require extensive well-designed evaluations. With the advent of total nutrient admixtures, the number of questions have increased substantially.

REFERENCES

1. Abel, R. M., Beck, C. H., Jr., Abbott, W. M., Ryan, J. A., Jr., Barnett, G. O., and Fischer, J. E. Improved survival from acute renal failure after treatment with intravenous essential L-amino acids. *N. Engl. J. Med.* 228:695, 1973.
2. Allen, L. V., Levinson, R. S., and Phisutsinthop, D. Compatibility of various admixtures with secondary additives at Y-injection sites of intravenous administration sets. *Am. J. Hosp. Pharm.* 34:939, 1977.
3. *American Hospital Formulary Service: Drug Information.* Section 40:20. Caloric agents. Bethesda, MD: American Society of Hospital Pharmacists, 1990.
4. American Medical Association Department of Foods and Nutrition. Guidelines for essential trace element preparations for parenteral use: A statement by an expert panel. *J.A.M.A.* 241:2051, 1979.
5. American Medical Association Department of Foods and Nutrition. Multivitamin preparations for parenteral use: A statement by the Nutrition Advisory Group. *J. Parenter. Enter. Nutr.* 3:258, 1979.
6. Ang, S. D., Canham, J. E., and Daly, J. M. Parenteral infusion with an admixture of amino acids, dextrose, and fat emulsion solution: Compatibility and clinical safety. *J. Parenter. Enter. Nutr.* 11:23, 1987.
7. Arend, K., McGraw, D., and Hagman, D. Compatibility of intravenous metoclopramide injection. Presented at the 18th clinical midyear meeting of the ASHP, Atlanta, Georgia, December 1983.
8. Arisz, L., Tugzess, A. M., Donker, A. J. M., Meijers, S., Sibinga, T. S., and Van der Hem, G. K. The use of streptokinase in obstructed arteriovenous shunts. *Postgrad. Med. J.* 49 (Suppl.):99, 1973.
9. Athanikar, N., Boyer, B., Deamer, R., et al. Visual compatibility of 30 additives with a parenteral nutrition solution. *Am. J. Hosp. Pharm.* 36:511, 1979.
10. Baptista, R. J. Medications compatible with hyperalimentation solutions. *Nutr. Supp. Serv.* 3:13, 1983.
11. Baptista, R. J., Dumas, G. J., Bistrian, B. R., Condella, F., and Blackburn, G. L. Compati-

bility of total nutrient admixtures and secondary cardiovascular medications. (Letter) *Am. J. Hosp. Pharm.* 42:777, 1985.

12. Baptista, R. J., and Lawrence, R. W. Compatibility of total nutrient admixtures and secondary antibiotic infusions. *Am. J. Hosp. Pharm.* 42:362, 1985.

13. Baptista, R. J., Palombo, J. D., Tahan, S. R., et al. Stability of cimetidine hydrochloride in a total nutrient admixture. *Am. J. Hosp. Pharm.* 42:2208, 1985.

14. Barker, A., Hebron, B. S., Beck, P. R., and Ellis, B. Folic acid and total parenteral nutrition. *J. Parenter. Enter. Nutr.* 8:3, 1984.

15. Barton, C. H., Vaziri, N. D., Ness, R. L., Saiki, J.K., and Mirahmadi, K. S. Cimetidine in the management of metabolic alkalosis induced by nasogastric drainage. *Arch. Surg.* 114:70, 1979.

16. Baumgartner, T. G., Sitren, H. S., Hall, J., and Lottenberg, R. The stability of urokinase in parenteral nutrition solutions. *Nutr. Supp. Serv.* 1:41, 1985.

17. Biamonte, A. R., and Schneller, G. H. A study of folic acid stability in solutions of the B complex vitamins. *J. Am. Pharmacol. Assoc.* (sci. ed.) 40:313, 1951.

18. Black, C. D., and Popovich, N. G. Stability of intravenous fat emulsions. *Arch. Surg.* 115:891, 1980.

19. Black, C. D., and Popovich, N. G. A study of intravenous emulsion compatibility: Effects of dextrose, amino acids, and selected electrolytes. *Drug Intell. Clin. Pharm.* 15:184, 1981.

20. Blackburn, G. L., Etter, G., and Mackenzie, T. Criteria for choosing amino acid therapy in acute renal failure. *Am. J. Clin. Nutr.* 31:1841, 1978.

21. Blackstone, M., Lee, P., and Reynolds, E. Use of digoxin in total parenteral nutrition fluids. Presented at the 15th annual midyear clinical meeting of the ASHP, San Francisco, December 7, 1980.

22. Boddapati, S., Yang, K., and Murty, R. Intravenous solution compatibility and filter-retention characteristics of trace element preparations. *Am. J. Hosp. Pharm.* 38:1731, 1981.

23. Bothe, A., Benotti, P., Bistrian, B. R., and Blackburn, G. L. Use of iron with total parenteral nutrition. (Letter) *N. Engl. J. Med.* 293:1154, 1975.

24. Boulet, M., and Marier, J. R. Precipitation of calcium phosphates from solutions at near physiological concentrations. *Arch. Biochem. Biophys.* 93:157, 1961.

25. Bower, R. H., Muggia-Sullam, M., Vallgren, S., et al. Branched chain amino acid–enriched solutions in the septic patient: A

randomized, prospective trial. *Ann. Surg.* 203:13, 1986.

26. Bowman, B. B., and Nguyen, P. Stability of thiamine in parenteral nutrition solutions. *J. Parenter. Enter. Nutr.* 7:567, 1983.

27. Bozzetti, F., Scarpa, D., Terno, G., et al. Subclavian venous thrombosis due to indwelling catheters: A prospective study on 52 patients. *J. Parenter. Enter. Nutr.* 7:560, 1983.

28. Brown, R., Quercia, R. A., and Sigman, R. Total nutrient admixture: A review. *J. Parenter. Enter. Nutr.* 10:650, 1986.

29. Bullock, L., Parks, R. B., Lampasona, V., and Mullins, R. E. Stability of ranitidine hydrochloride and amino acids in parenteral nutrient solutions. *Am. J. Hosp. Pharm.* 42:2683, 1985.

30. Cano, S. M., Montoro, J. B., Pastor, C., Pou, L., and Sabin, P. Stability of ranitidine hydrochloride in total nutrient admixtures. *Am. J. Hosp. Pharm.* 45:1100, 1988.

31. Capron, J. P., Ginestron, J. L., Herve, M. A., and Braillon, A. Metronidazole in prevention of cholestasis associated with total parenteral nutrition. *Lancet* 1:1446, 1983.

32. Cerra, F. B., Cheung, N. K., Fischer, J. E., et al. Disease-specific amino acid infusion (F080) in hepatic encephalopathy: A prospective, randomized, double-blind, controlled trial. *J. Parenter. Enter. Nutr.* 9:288, 1985.

33. Chan, J., Malekzadeh, M., and Hurley, J. pH and titratable acidity of amino acid mixtures used in hyperalimentation. *J.A.M.A.* 220:1119, 1972.

34. Chen, M. F., Boyce, N. W., and Triplett, L. Stability of the B vitamins in mixed parenteral nutrition solution. *J. Parenter. Enter. Nutr.* 7:462, 1983.

35. Colding, H., and Anderson, G. E. Stability of antibiotics and amino acids in two synthetic L-amino acid solutions commonly used for total parenteral nutrition in children. *Antimicrob. Agents Chemother.* 13:555, 1978.

36. Colding, H., Moller, S., and Anderson, G. E. Continuous intravenous infusion of ampicillin and gentamicin during parenteral nutrition in 88 newborn infants. *Arch. Dis. Child.* 57:602, 1982.

37. Colding, H., Moller, S., and Anderson, G. E. Continuous intravenous infusion of ampicillin and gentamicin during parenteral nutrition to 36 newborn infants using a dosage schedule. *Acta Paediatr. Scand.* 73:203, 1984.

38. Cutie, M. R., and Waranis, R. Compatibility of hydromorphone hydrochloride in large-volume parenterals. *Am. J. Hosp. Pharm.* 39:307, 1982.

39. Cytosar product information. Kalamazoo, MI: Upjohn Laboratories, 1980.

40. D'Angio, R., Quercia, R. A., Treiber, N. K.,

McLaughlin, J. C., and Klimek, J. J. The growth of microorganisms in total parenteral nutrition admixtures. *J. Parenter. Enter. Nutr.* 11:394, 1987.

41. DeLuca, P. P. Binding of drugs into inline filters. (Letter) *Am. J. Hosp. Pharm.* 36:153, 1979.

42. Doherty, N. J. Sufian, S., Pavlides, C. A., and Matsumoto, T. Cimetidine in the treatment of severe metabolic alkalosis secondary to short bowel syndrome. *Int. Surg.* 63:140, 1978.

43. Dolcourt, J. L., Beightol, R. W., and Mutchie, K. D. Insulin delivery in neonatal parenteral nutrition solutions. Presented at the 8th clinical congress of the American Society for Parenteral and Enteral Nutrition, Las Vegas, NV, January 30, 1984.

44. Dolin, B. J., Davis, P. D., Holland, T. A., and Turner, J. A. Contamination rates of 3-in-1 total parenteral nutrition in a clinical setting. *J. Parenter. Enter. Nutr.* 11:403, 1987.

45. Driscoll, D. F., Baptista, R. J., Bistrian, B. R., and Blackburn, G. L. Practical considerations regarding the use of total nutrient admixtures. *Am. J. Hosp. Pharm.* 43:416, 1985.

46. Dudrick, S. J., Wilmore, D. W., Vars, H. M., and Rhoads, J. E. Long-term total parenteral nutrition with growth, development, and positive nitrogen balance. *Surgery* 64:134, 1968.

47. Dudrick, S. J., Wilmore, D. W., Vars, H. M., and Rhoads, J. E. Can intravenous feeding as the sole means of nutrition support growth in the child and restore weight loss in an adult? An affirmative answer. *Ann. Surg.* 169:974, 1969.

48. Echenique, M. M., Bistrian, B. R., Moldawer, L. L., Palombo, J. D., Miller, M. M., and Blackburn, G. L. Improvement in amino acid use in the critically ill patient with parenteral formulas enriched with branched chain amino acids. *Surg. Gynecol. Obstet.* 159:233, 1984.

49. Eggert, L. D., Rusho, W. J., MacKay, M. W., and Chan, G. M. Calcium and phosphorous compatibility in parenteral nutrition solutions for neonates. *Am. J. Hosp. Pharm.* 39:49, 1982.

50. Elleby, H., and Solhaug, J. H. Metronidazole, cholestasis, and total parenteral nutrition. *Lancet* 1:1161, 1983.

51. Elsborg, L. Inhibition of intestinal absorption of folic acid by phenytoin. *Acta Haematol.* 52:24, 1974.

52. Ennis, C. E., Merritt, R. J., and Neff, D. N. In vitro study of inline filtration of medications commonly administered to pediatric cancer patients. *J. Parenter. Enter. Nutr.* 7:156, 1983.

53. Fabri, P. J., Mirtallo, J. M., Ruberg, R. L., et al. Incidence and prevention of thrombosis of the subclavian vein during total parenteral nutrition. *Surg. Gynecol. Obstet.* 155:238, 1982.

54. Fagerman, K. E., and Dean, R. E. Daily digoxin administration in parenteral nutrition solution. *Am. J. Hosp. Pharm.* 38:1955, 1981.

55. Feigin, R. D., Moss, K. S., and Shackelford, P. G. Antibiotic stability in solutions used for intravenous nutrition and fluid therapy. *Pediatrics* 51:1016, 1973.

56. Fischer, J. E., and Baldessarini, R. J. False neurotransmitters and hepatic failure. *Lancet* 2:75, 1971.

57. Fitzgerald, K. A., and MacKay, M. W. Calcium and phosphate solubility in neonatal parenteral nutrient solutions containing TrophAmine. *Am. J. Hosp. Pharm.* 43:88, 1986.

58. Forster, F. J. Heparin insensitivity after prolonged total parenteral nutrition. *J.A.M.A.* 244:271, 1980.

59. Foyin-Fortunet, H., LeQuernec, L., Erlinger, S., Lerebours, E., and Colin, R. Hepatic alterations during total parenteral nutrition in patients with inflammatory bowel disease: A possible consequence of lithocholate toxicity. *Gastroenterology* 82:932, 1982.

60. Fraile, R. J., Baker, L. H., Buroker, T. R., Horwitz, J., and Voitkevicius, V. K. Pharmacokinetics of 5-fluorouracil administered orally, by rapid intravenous and by slow infusion. *Cancer Res.* 40:2223, 1980.

61. Freund, H. R., Atamian, S., and Fischer, J. E. Comparative study of parenteral nutrition in renal failure using essential and nonessential amino acid containing solutions. *Surg. Gynecol. Obstet.* 151:652, 1980.

62. Gilbert, L., Dean, R., and Karaganis, A. Iron-dextran administration via TPN solution in malnourished patients with low transferrin levels. *J. Parenter. Enter. Nutr.* 3:494, 1979.

63. Gilbert, M., Gallagher, S. C., Eads, M., and Elmore, M. F. Microbial growth patterns in a total parenteral nutrition formulation containing lipid emulsion. *J. Parenter. Enter. Nutr.* 10:494, 1986.

64. Gillis, J., Jones, G., and Pencharz, P. Delivery of vitamins A, D and E in total parenteral nutrition solutions. *J. Parenter. Enter. Nutr.* 7:11, 1983.

65. Glynn, M. F. X., Langer, B., and Jeejeebhoy, K. N. Therapy for thrombotic occlusion of long-term intravenous alimentation catheters. *J. Parenter. Enter. Nutr.* 4:387, 1980.

66. Goldberg, N. J., and Levin, S. R. Insulin adsorption to an in-line membrane filter. (Letter) *N. Engl. J. Med.* 298:1480, 1978.

67. Greene, H. L., Phillips, B. L., Franck, L., et al. Persistently low blood retinol levels dur-

ing and after parenteral feeding of very low birth-weight infants: Examination of losses into intravenous administration sets and a method of prevention by addition to a lipid emulsion. *Pediatrics* 79:894, 1987.

68. Halpin, T. C., Bertino, J. S., Rothstein, F. C., Kurczynski, E. M., and Reed, M. D. Iron-deficiency anemia in childhood inflammatory bowel disease: Treatment with intravenous iron-dextran. *J. Parenter. Enter. Nutr.* 6:9, 1982.

69. Hardin, T. C. Complex parenteral nutrition solutions. I. Drug additives. *Nutr. Supp. Serv.* 3:58, 1983.

70. Hardin, T. C., and Clibon, U. The stability of 5-fluorouracil in a crystalline amino acid solution. *Am. J. IV Ther. Clin. Nutr.* 9:39, 1982.

71. Hardin, T. C., Clibon, U., Page, C. P., and Cruz, A. B. Compatibility of 5-fluorouracil and total parenteral nutrition solutions. *J. Parenter. Enter. Nutr.* 6:163, 1982.

72. Hartline, J., and Zachman, R. Vitamin A delivery in total parenteral nutrition solution. *Pediatrics* 58:448, 1976.

73. Henann, N. E., and Jacks, T. T., Jr. Compatibility and availability of sodium bicarbonate in total parenteral nutrient solutions. *Am. J. Hosp. Pharm.* 42:2718, 1985.

74. Henry, R. S., Jurgens, R. W., Sturgeon, R. J., Athanikar, N., Welco, A., and Van Leunen, M. Compatibility of calcium chloride and calcium gluconate with sodium phosphate in a mixed TPN solution. *Am. J. Hosp. Pharm.* 37:673, 1980.

75. Hirsch, J. I., Fratkin, M. J., Wood, J. H., and Thomas, R. B. Clinical significance of insulin adsorption by polyvinylchloride infusion systems. *Am. J. Hosp. Pharm.* 34:583, 1977.

76. Hirsch, J. I., Wood, J. H., and Thomas, R. B. Insulin adsorption to polyolefin infusion bottles and polyvinylchloride administration sets. *Am. J. Hosp. Pharm.* 38:995, 1981.

77. Howard, L., Chu, R., Feman, S., Mintz, H., Ovesen, L., and Wolf, B. Vitamin A deficiency from long-term parenteral nutrition. *Ann. Intern. Med.* 93:576, 1980.

78. Hurtubise, M. R., Bottino, J. C., Lawson, M., and McGredie, K. B. Restoring patency of occluded central venous catheters. *Arch. Surg.* 115:212, 1980.

79. *Intralipid Admixture Manual.* Berkeley, CA: Cutter Laboratories, September 1982.

80. Isaacs, J. W., Millikan, W. J., Stackhouse, J., Hersh, T., and Rudman, D. Parenteral nutrition of adults with a 900 milliosmolar solution via peripheral veins. *Am. J. Clin. Nutr.* 30:552, 1977.

81. Jacobsen, S., Christenson, I., Kager, L., Kall-

ner, A., and Ljungdahl, I. Utilization and metabolic effects of a conventional and a single-solution regimen in post-operative total parenteral nutrition. *Am. J. Clin. Nutr.* 34:1402, 1981.

82. Jacobson, E. D., Prior, J. T., and Faloon, W. W. Malabsorptive syndrome induced by neomycin: Morphologic alterations in jejunal mucosa. *J. Lab. Clin. Med.* 56:245, 1960.

83. Jurgens, R. W., DeLuca, P. P., and Papadimitriou, D. Compatibility of amphotericin B with certain large-volume parenterals. *Am. J. Hosp. Pharm.* 38:377, 1981.

84. Kamen, B. A., Gunther, N., Sowinsky, N., Rizzo, J., Ball, W. D., and Marsik, F. Analysis of antibiotic stability in a parenteral nutrition solution. *Pediatr. Infect. Dis.* 4:387, 1985.

85. Kaminski, M. V., Harris, D. F., Collins, C. F., and Sommers, G. A. Electrolyte compatibility in a synthetic amino acid hyperalimentation solution. *Am. J. Hosp. Pharm.* 31:244, 1974.

86. King, J. C. *Guide to Parenteral Admixtures.* St. Louis, MO: Cutter Laboratories, 1982.

87. Kishi, H., Yamagi, A., Kataoka, K., et al. Vitamin A and E requirements during total parenteral nutrition. *J. Parenter. Enter. Nutr.* 5:420, 1981.

88. Knight, P., Heer, D., and Abdenour, G. Ca × P and Ca/P in the parenteral feeding of preterm infants. *J. Parenter. Enter. Nutr.* 7:110, 1983.

89. Knodell, R. G., Spector, M. H., Brooks, D. A., Keller, F. X., and Kyner, W. T. Alterations in pentobarbital pharmacokinetics in response to parenteral and enteral alimentation in the rat. *Gastroenterology* 79:1211, 1980.

90. Knodell, R. G., Steele, N. M., Cerra, F. B., Gross, J. B., and Soloman, T. E. Effects of parenteral and enteral hyperalimentation on hepatic drug metabolism in the rat. *J. Pharmacol. Exp. Ther.* 229:589, 1984.

91. Kobayashi, N. H., and King, J. C. Compatibility of common additives in protein hydrolysate/dextrose solutions. *Am. J. Hosp. Pharm.* 34:589, 1977.

92. Lambert, J. R., and Thomas, S. M. Metronidazole prevention of serum liver enzyme abnormalities during total parenteral nutrition. *J. Parenter. Enter. Nutr.* 9:501, 1985.

93. Leevy, C. M., Cardi, L., Frank, O., Gellene, R., and Baker, H. Incidence and significance of hypovitaminemia in a randomly selected municipal hospital population. *Am. J. Clin. Nutr.* 17:259, 1965.

94. Lemon, H. M., Modzen, P. J., and Mirchandani, R. Decreased intoxication by fluorouracil when slowly administered in glucose. *J.A.M.A.* 185:1012, 1963.

95. Lindsay, J., Thomas, R., and LaFrance, R.

Microbial growth patterns in parenteral nutrient solutions: An evaluative study. Presented at the 42nd annual meeting of ASHP, Reno, NV, June 3, 1985.

96. Longe, R. L. Stability of phytonadione in hyperalimentation fluids. (Letter) *Am. J. Hosp. Pharm.* 31:103, 1974.

97. Louie, N., and Stennett, D. J. Stability of folic acid in 25% dextrose, 3.5% amino acids, and multivitamin solution. *J. Parenter. Enter. Nutr.* 8:421, 1984.

98. Macias, J. M., Martin, W. J., and Lloyd, C. W. Stability of morphine sulfate and meperidine hydrochloride in a parenteral nutrient formulation. *Am. J. Hosp. Pharm.* 42:1087, 1985.

99. Macoviak, J. A., Melnik, G., McLean, G., et al. The effect of low dose heparin on the prevention of venous thrombosis in patients receiving short-term parenteral nutrition. *Curr. Surg.* 41:98, 1984.

100. Madiwale, M. S., Rao, S. S., and Dutta, N. K. Stability of folic acid in pharmaceutical preparations. *Ind. J. Pharm.* 27:113, 1965.

101. Malis, C. D., Racusen, L. C., Solez, K., and Whalton, A. Nephrotoxicity of lysine and of a single dose of aminoglycoside in rats given lysine. *J. Lab. Clin. Med.* 103:660, 1984.

102. Mansell, M. A., and Wing, A. J. Acetate or bicarbonate for haemodialysis? *Br. Med. J.* 287:308, 1983.

103. McFarlane, H., Reddy, S., Adcock, K. J., Adeshina, H., Cooke, A. R., and Akene, J. Immunity, transferrin, and survival in kwashiorkor. *Br. Med. J.* 4:268, 1970.

104. McKenna, M. C., and Bieri, J. G. Loss of vitamin A from total parenteral nutrition (TPN) solutions. (Abstract) *Fed. Proc.* 39:561A, 1980.

105. Mershon, J., Nogami, W., Williams, J. M., Yoder, E., Eitzen, H. E., and Lemons, J. A. Bacterial/fungal growth in a combined parenteral nutrition solution. *J. Parenter. Enter. Nutr.* 10:498, 1986.

106. Mirtallo, J. M., Caryer, K., Schneider, P. J., Ayers, L., and Fabri, P. J. Growth of bacteria and fungi in parenteral nutrient solutions containing albumin. *Am. J. Hosp. Pharm.* 38:1907, 1981.

107. Mirtallo, J. M., Rogers, K. R., Johnson, J. A., Fabri, P. J., and Schneider, P. J. Stability of amino acids and the availability of acid in total parenteral nutrition solutions containing hydrochloric acid. *Am. J. Hosp. Pharm.* 38:1729, 1981.

108. Mirtallo, J. M., Schneider, P. J., Mavko, K., Ruberg, R. L., and Fabri, P. J. A comparison of essential and general amino acid infusions in the nutritional support of patients with compromised renal function. *J. Parenter. Enter. Nutr.* 6:109, 1982.

109. Mirtallo, J. M., Schneider, P. J., and Ruberg, R. L. Albumin in TPN solutions: Potential savings from a prospective review. *J. Parenter. Enter. Nutr.* 4:300, 1980.

110. Mizock, B. A. Branched-chain amino acids in sepsis and hepatic failure. *Arch. Intern. Med.* 145:1284, 1985.

111. Moertel, C. G., and Reitemeier, R. J. *Advanced Gastrointestinal Cancer: Clinical Management and Chemotherapy.* New York: Harper & Row, 1969.

112. Moore, R. A., Feldman, S., Treuting, J., Bloss, R., and Dudrick, S. J. Cimetidine and parenteral nutrition. *J. Parenter. Enter. Nutr.* 5:61, 1981.

113. Moorhatch, P., and Chiou, W. L. Interactions between drugs and plastic intravenous fluid bags. *Am. J. Hosp. Pharm.* 31:72, 1974.

114. Mu-Chow, K. J., and Baptista, R. J. Cost-effectiveness of parenteral nutrient solutions containing cimetidine hydrochloride. (Letter) *Am. J. Hosp. Pharm.* 41:1321, 1984.

115. National Coordinating Committee on Large-Volume Parenterals. Recommendations to pharmacists for solving problems with large-volume parenterals. *Am. J. Hosp. Pharm.* 33:231, 1976.

116. Niemiec, P. W., Jr., and Vanderveen, T. W. Compatibility considerations in parenteral nutrient solutions. *Am. J. Hosp. Pharm.* 41:893, 1984.

117. Niemiec, P. W., Jr., Vanderveen, T. W., Hohenwarter, M. W., and Gadsden, R. H. Stability of aminophylline injection in three parenteral nutrient solutions. *Am. J. Hosp. Pharm.* 40:428, 1983.

118. Nolan, J. P. The role of endotoxin in liver injury. *Gastroenterology* 69:1346, 1975.

119. Norton, J., Peters, M., Wesley, R., Maher, M. M., and Brennan, M. F. Iron supplementation of total parenteral nutrition: A prospective study. *J. Parenter. Enter. Nutr.* 7:457, 1983.

120. Ostro, M. J., Russell, J. A., Soldin, S. J., Mahon, W. A., and Jeejeebhoy, K. N. Control of gastric pH with cimetidine: Boluses versus primed infusions. *Gastroenterology* 89:532, 1985.

121. Package Insert Information for ProcalAmine 3% Amino Acid/3% Glycerin Injection with Electrolytes. Irvine, CA: Kendall-McGaw, 1989.

122. Palmer, R. H. Bile acids, liver injury, and liver disease. *Arch. Intern. Med.* 130:606, 1972.

123. Pamperl, H., and Kleinberger, G. Morphologic changes of Intralipid 20% Liposomes in All-In-One solutions during prolonged storage. *Infusiontherapie* 9:86, 1982.

124. Parr, M. D., Bertch, K. E., and Rapp, R. P.

Amino acid stability in total parenteral nutrient solutions. *Am. J. Hosp. Pharm.* 42: 2688, 1985.

125. Paterson, W. L., and Richardson, C. T. Sustained fasting achlorhydria: A comparison of medical regimens. *Gastroenterology* 88:666, 1985.

126. Pestana, C. *Fluid and Electrolytes in the Surgical Patient* (3rd ed.). Baltimore: Williams & Wilkins, 1985.

127. Peterson, L., Caldwell, J., and Hoffman, J. Insulin adsorbance to polyvinylchloride surfaces with implications for constant-infusion therapy. *Diabetes* 25:72, 1976.

128. Petty, C., and Cunningham, N. L. Insulin adsorption by glass infusion bottles, polyvinylchloride infusion containers, and intravenous tubing. *Anesthesiology* 40:400, 1974.

129. Pomerance, N. H., and Rader, R. E. Crystal formation: A new complication of total parenteral nutrition. *Pediatrics* 52:864, 1973.

130. Poole, R. L., Rupp, C. A., and Kerner, J. A. Calcium and phosphorus in neonatal parenteral nutrition solutions. *J. Parenter. Enter. Nutr.* 7:358, 1983.

131. Quock, J. R., and Sakai, R. I. Stability of cytarabine in a parenteral nutrition solution. *Am. J. Hosp. Pharm.* 42:592, 1985.

132. Reed, M. D., Perry, E. B., Fennel, S. J., Brissie, E. O., and Ball, W. D. Antibiotic compatibility and stability in a parenteral nutrition solution. *Chemotherapy* 25:336, 1979.

133. Richards, R. H., Vreman, H. J., Zager, P., Feldman, C., Blaschke, T., and Weiner, M. W. Acetate metabolism in normal human subjects. *Am. J. Kidney Dis.* 2:47, 1982.

134. Riggli, M. A., and Brandt, R. B. Decrease of available vitamin A in parenteral nutrition solutions. *J. Parenter. Enter. Nutr.* 10:388, 1986.

135. Robinson, L. A., and Wright, B. T. Central venous catheter occlusion caused by body-heat-mediated calcium phosphate precipitation. *Am. J. Hosp. Pharm.* 39:120, 1982.

136. Roe, D. A., and Campbell, T. C. *Drug and Nutrients: The Interactive Effects.* New York: Marcel Dekker, 1984.

137. Rosen, H. M., Yoshimura, N., Hodgman, J. M., and Fischer, J. E. Plasma amino acid patterns in hepatic encephalopathy of differing etiology. *Gastroenterology* 72:483, 1977.

138. Rosenberg, H. A., Dougherty, J. T., Mayron, D., and Baldinus, J. G. Cimetidine hydrochloride compatibility. I. Chemical aspects and room temperature stability in intravenous infusion fluids. *Am. J. Hosp. Pharm.* 37:390, 1980.

139. Rowlands, B. J., Tindall, S. F., and Elliot, D. J. The use of dilute hydrochloric acid and cimetidine to reverse severe metabolic alkalosis. *Postgrad. Med. J.* 54:118, 1978.

140. Rusmin, S., and DeLuca, P. P. Effect of inline filtration on the potency of potassium penicillin G. *Bull. Parenter. Drug Assoc.* 30:64, 1976.

141. Rusmin, S., Welton, S., DeLuca, P., and DeLuca, P. P. Effect of inline filtration on the potency of drugs administered intravenously. *Am. J. Hosp. Pharm.* 34:1071, 1977.

142. Sayeed, F. A., Johnson, H. W., Sukumarad, K. B., et al. Stability of Liposyn II fat emulsion in total nutrient admixtures. *Am. J. Hosp. Pharm.* 43:1230, 1986.

143. Sayers, M. H., Johnson, D. K., Schumann, L. A., Ivey, M. F., Young, J. A., and Finch, C. A. Supplementation of total parenteral nutrition solutions with ferrous citrate. *J. Parenter. Enter. Nutr.* 7:117, 1983.

144. Scheckelhoff, D. J., Mirtallo, J. M., Ayers, L. W., and Visconti, J. A. Growth of bacteria and fungi in total nutrient admixtures. *Am. J. Hosp. Pharm.* 43:73, 1986.

145. Scheiner, J. M., Araujo, M. M., and DeRitter, E. Thiamine destruction by sodium bisulfite in infusion solutions. *Am. J. Hosp. Pharm.* 38: 1911, 1981.

146. Scheutz, D. H., and King, J. C. Compatibility and stability of electrolytes, vitamins, and antibiotics in combination with 8% amino acid solution. *Am. J. Hosp. Pharm.* 35:33, 1978.

147. Schilling, C. G. Compatibility of drugs with a heparin-containing neonatal total parenteral nutrient solution. (Letter) *Am. J. Hosp. Pharm.* 45:313, 1988.

148. Schneider, P. H. What drugs can be added to TPN solutions? *Infusion* 6:121, 1982.

149. Schneidlin, S., Lee, A., and Griffith, I. The action of riboflavin on folic acid. *J. Am. Pharmacol. Assoc.* (sci. ed.) 41:420, 1952.

150. Seifert, P., Baker, L. H., Reed, M. L., and Vaitkevicius, V. K. Comparison of continuously infused 5-fluorouracil with bolus injection in treatment of patients with colorectal adenocarcinoma. *Cancer* 36:123, 1975.

151. Shank, W. A., and Coupal, J. J. Stability of digoxin in common large-volume injections. *Am. J. Hosp. Pharm.* 39:844, 1982.

152. Shavelle, H. S., and Park, R. Postoperative metabolic alkalosis and acute renal failure: Rationale for the use of hydrochloric acid. *Surgery* 78:439, 1975.

153. Shenai, J., Stahlman, M., and Chytil, F. Vitamin A delivery from parenteral alimentation solution. *J. Pediatr.* 99:661, 1981.

154. Shenkin, A., Fraser, W. D., McLelland, A. J. D., Fell, G. S., and Garden, O. J. Maintenance of vitamin and trace element status in intravenous nutrition using a complete nutritive mixture. *J. Parenter. Enter. Nutr.* 11:238, 1987.

155. Smith, J. L., Canham, J. E., and Wells, P. A. Effect of phototherapy light, sodium bisulfite, and pH on vitamin stability in total par-

enteral nutrition admixtures. *J. Parenter. Enter. Nutr.* 12:394, 1988.

156. Stead, N., Curtis, M., and Grant, J. Changes in ferro-kinetics during parenteral nutrition. *J. Parenter. Enter. Nutr.* 4:585, 1980.

157. Suzuki, N. T. Heparin in peripheral parenteral nutrition. (Letter) *Drug Intell. Clin. Pharm.* 20:155, 1986.

158. Swenson, J. P., Edwards, D., Chamberlain, M., Rault, R., and Ivey, M. F. A total parenteral nutrition protocol. *Drug Intell. Clin. Pharm.* 11:714,1977.

159. Tansey, R. P., and Schneller, G. H. Studies on the stabilization of folic acid in liquid pharmaceutical preparations. *J. Am. Pharmacol. Assoc.* (sci. ed.) 44:34, 1955.

160. Tate, J. T., and Cowan, G. S. Insulin kinetics in hyperalimentation solution and routine intravenous therapy. *Am. Surg.* 43:811, 1977.

161. Trissel, L. A. *Handbook of Injectable Drugs* (5th ed.). Washington, DC: American Society of Hospital Pharmacists, 1988.

162. Trissel, L. A., and Flora, K. P. Stability studies: Five years later. (Commentary) *Am. J. Hosp. Pharm.* 45:1569, 1988.

163. Tsallas, G., and Allen, L. C. Stability of cimetidine hydrochloride in parenteral nutrition solutions. *Am. J. Hosp. Pharm.* 39:484, 1982.

164. Twardowski, Z. J., Nolph, K. D., McGary, T. J., and Moore, H. L. Influence of temperature and time on insulin adsorption to plastic bags. *Am. J. Hosp. Pharm.* 40:583, 1983.

165. Twardowski, Z. J., Nolph, K. D., McGary, T. J., et al. Insulin binding to plastic bags: A methodologic study. *Am. J. Hosp. Pharm.* 40:575, 1983.

166. Van Den Berg, L., and Soliman, F. S. Composition and pH changes during freezing of solutions containing calcium and magnesium phosphate. *Cryobiology* 6:10, 1969.

167. Vasilakis, P., and Apelgren, K. W. Answering the fat emulsion contamination question: Three-in-one admixture vs conventional total parenteral nutrition in a clinical setting. *J. Parenter. Enter. Nutr.* 12:356, 1988.

168. Walker, S. E., and Bayliff, C. D. Stability of ranitidine hydrochloride in total parenteral nutrient solution. *Am. J. Hosp. Pharm.* 42:590, 1985.

169. Wan, K. K., and Tsallas, G. Dilute iron dextran formulation for addition to parenteral nutrient solutions. *Am. J. Hosp. Pharm.* 37:206, 1980.

170. Weber, S. S., Wood, W. A., and Jackson, E. A. Availability of insulin from parenteral nutrient solutions. *Am. J. Hosp. Pharm.* 34:353, 1977.

171. Weinberg, E. D. Infection and iron metabolism. *Am. J. Clin. Nutr.* 3:1485, 1977.

172. Wells, P. An update on lipid compatibility issues. Presented at "Quality Nutrition Therapy on a Shrinking Budget," Clintec Nutrition, Cincinnati, OH, 1989.

173. Whalen, F. J., LeCain, W. K., and Lotiolais, C. J. Availability of insulin from continuous low-dose insulin infusions. *Am. J. Hosp. Pharm.* 36:330, 1979.

174. Will, G., and Groden, B. M. The treatment of iron deficiency anaemia by iron-dextran infusion: A radio-isotope study. *Br. J. Haematol.* 14:61, 1968.

175. Williams, R. R., Waterman, R. E., Kereszlesy, J. C., and Buchman, E. R. Studies of crystalline vitamin B_1. III. Cleavage of vitamin with sulfite. *J. Am. Chem. Soc.* 57:536, 1935.

176. Williams, S. K., Baptista, R. J., and Echenique, M. M. Dosing cimetidine HCl in a continuous infusion via parenteral nutrient solutions. *Infusion* 9:45, 1985.

177. Wolfe, B. M., and Ney, D. M. Lipid metabolism in parenteral nutrition. In J. L. Rombeau and M. D. Caldwell (eds.), *Parenteral Nutrition.* Philadelphia: W. B. Saunders, 1986. P. 79.

178. Wretlind, A. Parenteral nutrition. *Surg. Clin. North Am.* 58:1005, 1978.

179. Yuhas, E. M., Lofton, F. T., Mayron, D., Baldinus, J. G., and Rosenberg, H. A. Cimetidine hydrochloride compatibility. II. Room temperature stability in intravenous infusion fluids. *Am. J. Hosp. Pharm.* 38:879, 1981.

180. Yuhas, E. M., Lofton, F. T., Rosenberg, H. A., Mayron, D., and Baldinus, J. G. Cimetidine hydrochloride compatibility. III. Room temperature stability in drug admixtures. *Am. J. Hosp. Pharm.* 38:1919, 1981.

Education and a Hospital-Wide Program

Marsha E. Orr

The ideal condition would be, I admit, that men
should be right by instinct; but since we are all
likely to go astray, the reasonable thing is to
learn from those who can teach.

Sophocles

Modern health care has become increasingly specialized. Rapid advances in science and technology result in the need for specialists and experts whose area of practice is narrower in scope but has greater depth. The development of technology of the late 1960s that enabled patients to be fed totally by the parenteral route was the genesis of specialized nutrition support. Parenteral nutrition (PN), a therapy that can save lives, can also cause death or complications from metabolic, septic, and technical complications, especially in the hands of inexperienced personnel. Safe administration of PN requires knowledgeable health care professionals.

Early on, nutrition support was conceptualized as a team effort; involvement of a nurse, pharmacist, dietitian, and a physician was identified as the ideal approach for providing specialized nutrition support safely and effectively to patients.

Clinical studies have demonstrated that involvement of the nutrition support team (NST) in patient care, in either a consultative

or more direct role, does reduce the incidence of PN-related complications. Nehme [21] found significantly lower catheter-related sepsis rates and metabolic complications when patients were managed by an NST as compared to nonteam management. Dalton et al. [8] compared PN-related morbidity for a group of patients who were managed by their primary physicians and the NST acting in a consultative role, with a group of patients who were managed by both the NST and primary physicians. Significantly fewer mechanical and metabolic complications occurred with greater NST involvement. Keohane et al. [17] demonstrated a reduced rate of catheter-related sepsis from 33 to 4% when an NST nurse, compared to intensive care nurses, changed central venous PN catheter dressings. Traeger et al. [25] found that the NST improved the quality of patient care by preventing or repleting nutritional deficits and preventing PN-related complications. In Cincinnati the placement of nutritional support under the control of an NST has led to diminution of the sepsis rate from 28% before the team to the current 6.0%.

The concept of a team approach endures today, although the NST may have various configurations and organization structures. Education of the hospital staff has been, and continues to be, a major role of the NST. In order to operationalize the NST's role in a hospital-wide program, issues such as power and authority, the role of a consultant, and the role of a change agent must be considered.

CHARACTERISTICS OF THE NUTRITION SUPPORT TEAM

Power and Authority

Within any organization there are well-delineated formal lines of authority. The NST, as a part of an organization, is accountable to other departments, committees, or individuals for certain activities. Some of the activities for which the NST is accountable may be accomplished directly by NST members or by other personnel. For example, the NST may develop policies and procedures for the insertion and care of central venous lines, when the actual insertion and care are performed by other personnel. The NST may be responsible for developing policies and procedures and not have the responsibility for the enforcement aspects of policy. Likewise, the NST may have responsibility for **both** the development and enforcement of policies and procedures.

Hicks [14] defined authority as the right to act. To function effectively within an organization, the authority of the NST must be clearly established and recognized by others. Power has been defined as "the ability and willingness to affect the behavior of others" [5]. The NST must be given formal or authorized power within the institution. While an NST may function by endorsed power based on the recognition by others that the team possesses certain expertise, this type of power is often transient; as others develop additional skills, the team's power is lost. Formal, authorized power maintains the

team's right to act even as the team assists others to develop additional knowledge and skills.

Consultant Role

During the past decade, the use of PN and enteral nutrition (EN) therapies has become more commonplace. Patients are seldom congregated on specialized units and PN is used throughout most hospitals. Although some NSTs perform certain direct patient care (i.e., changing central venous catheter dressings, inserting central venous catheters or enteral feeding tubes), many of the NST's functions are in a consultative role. The NST provides expert resource personnel to other health care professionals who provide direct clinical care. For example, the NST nurse may teach staff nurses how to change the central venous dressing and determine that the staff nurses have developed competency in this skill.

Holtz [15] defined the consultant as a specialist who is retained to solve a problem. The NST, however, often intervenes in patient care when others do not recognize that there is a problem. Dealing with colleagues who do not recognize a problem requires the NST to exercise diplomacy and sensitivity. Most health care professionals function under the basic belief that they are helping patients and have the patient's welfare as a prime concern. Operating from a standpoint of respect for the other caregiver's concern for the patient, the NST can assist others to recognize that there is a problem in care delivery. Once the problem is identified, possible solutions can be proposed. The importance of the NST's ability to maintain a positive consultative relationship becomes apparent in situations where the NST is attempting to institute change.

As a Change Agent

Mauksch and Miller [20] defined change as "the process by which alterations occur in the function and structure of society . . . [and] impacts all behavior patterns." For the NST, the society of reference or target population is made up of those individuals who provide care to patients receiving PN and EN. The educational programs provided by the NST to other health care professionals often involve new skills or new behaviors; thus, the NST is introducing change. A working knowledge of change theory is helpful to the NST to maximize successful results.

Rogers [23] described seven functions of a change agent in the process of instituting change: (1) developing a need for change in the target population, (2) establishing a change relationship with the target population, (3) diagnosing the problem the change will correct, (4) identifying alternative courses of action for the target population and then creating the desire to change it, (5) translating the desire to change into action so that the target population actually makes changes, (6) stabilizing the change and attempting to prevent discontinuance, and (7) achieving a terminal relationship with the target population. Failure to consider all of the issues involved in the implementation of change can threaten success. The NST is most successful when the target population desires a change or perceives a need to change, the relationship between the NST and the target population is positive and trusting, problem behaviors have been clearly diagnosed from the **target population's perspective,** a variety of courses of action have been identified, new behaviors are implemented with support from the NST, feedback is given to the target population to confirm the change, and the target population is assisted to maintain the new behaviors independently.

Strategies used to achieve a change include coercion, persuasion, and reeducation. Although many of these strategies may be effective for different populations, in various circumstances, and for various goals, the NST may use persuasion and reeducation as predominant strategies given the nature of their consultant relationship with other health care professionals. If the NST encounters resistance to change, each step in the process of implementing change should be reexamined to determine whether issues have been over-

looked. Common reasons for resistance to change include problem behaviors of or prior poor rapport with the change agent, confusion about the nature of the change, external forces that favor or oppose the change, the desire of the target population to maintain the status quo, inadequate knowledge, negative past experiences with change, passive resistance, and lack of consensus about the goals or need for change [20].

In summary, the NST, in its role of educating and reeducating other health care professionals, is often instituting change. Inability to successfully implement change can be frustrating to the NST and can compromise the quality of care received by patients. Consideration of change theory and processes to implement change will enhance the NST's success in these endeavors.

DESIGNING EDUCATION PROGRAMS FOR ADULT LEARNERS

The NST's role in educating hospital staff has been well documented. Most of the literature describing the role of the NST include references to the team's role in staff education [3, 10, 16]. Even less formally structured nutrition support committees or resource persons incorporate staff education into their roles. The target audience for the NST includes health care professionals representative of the disciplines that make up the team and other health care personnel.

Designing educational programs for adult learners requires the NST to be cognizant of adult learning theories and to realize that most adult learners enjoy a self-directed or collaborative approach. In addition, health care professionals may have learning styles that are more similar than those of the general adult population because of the prevalence of the medical model (history, physical exam, diagnosis, treatment, and evaluation) in their formal education [11]. Green et al. [11] described characteristics of health care professionals as adult learners. The NST can integrate these characteristics into the design

Table 6-1. Health Care Professionals: Learning Characteristics and Implications for Designing Programs

Learning Characteristics	Implications for Program Design
Motivated to continue learning	Provide opportunities for self-assessment or peer review
Seek knowledge that has immediate and pragmatic application to current situations	Design continuing education that is relevant
Participation in educational programs is influenced by past experiences	Eliminate obstacles to learning and provide information applicable to current practice
Efforts to improve learning conditions can influence outcome of educational programs	Build on past experience and knowledge; incorporate adult learning principles
Must know how to continue learning to stay abreast of new developments, and adapt to new environments	Assist health care professionals to identify how they learn best
Enjoy a variety of learning formats	Provide a variety of learning formats for individuals and groups
Can be assisted toward more self-directed learning activities	Increase the learner's awareness of self-directed learning; provide appropriate resources

Adapted from Green, J. S., Grosswald, S. J., Suter, E., and Walthall, D. B. *Continuing Education for the Health Professions.* San Francisco: Jossey-Bass, 1984.

of educational programs to maximize learning for health care professionals (Table 6-1). A systematic process is used to identify the content for educational programs provided by the NST.

The steps in developing and implementing educational programs typically involve the following: (1) identifying the target audience, (2) determining the learning needs of the target audience, (3) setting educational goals and objectives, (4) designing learning situations, (5) implementing the program, and (6) evaluating the results of the program.

For the NST, the target audience can be a hospital-wide audience of various health care professionals, a smaller interdisciplinary audience, or individuals from one profession. The NST may be requested by another individual or group to provide the educational program, or the NST may initiate the program request. Determining the learning needs of the target audience is the next step.

Health care professionals receive their education in a variety of formal education programs: hospital-based training programs, technical schools, colleges, and universities. In addition, most health care professionals receive on-the-job training through in-service

and staff development programs. In determining a hospital-wide audience's learning needs in the area of specialized nutrition, the NST may wish to consider the nutrition component of the curricula of various health care professionals.

Nurses

During the early to mid 1990s (1900–1950), nutrition and dietetics were a discrete component of the curricula of most schools of nursing. However, when nutrition became "integrated" into the curricula, the number of hours offered became variable and the emphasis on nutritional aspects of illness decreased [9]. By the 1960s, bedside nurses rated nutrition as a low priority in patient care [22]. In a survey conducted in the early 1980s, Stotts et al. [24] found nutritional assessment to be the subject most frequently taught in 96% of baccalaureate schools of nursing. Other specific subjects taught less frequently were PN and EN therapy, diet counseling, and nutrition biochemistry, which were taught in 85, 84, and 71% of schools, respectively. Nutrition support nurses were seldom used as preceptors for students [24].

Baccalaureate education is the highest entry level of education for professional nurses. Associate degree and diploma programs may have less emphasis on nutrition in their curricula than that seen at the baccalaureate level. The NST can consider that approximately 15% of baccalaureate nurses will have had no course work on PN and EN, and 29% will have had no course work on nutritional biochemistry in their undergraduate programs. Any programs the NST offers to recent graduate nurses that require a strong **prior** background in PN and EN therapies or nutritional biochemistry may not be ideally suited to this target audience. The NST would need to provide programs that require a less extensive knowledge of nutrition biochemistry and perhaps introduce more basic principles of PN and EN to beginning nurses. At the University of Cincinnati Hospitals, an NST nurse participates in each orientation session for newly employed nurses by presenting a 1-hour program on specialized nutrition support therapies (see "Orientation" below).

Physicians

During the past few decades, attention has been focused on the nutrition curricula in medical schools. In 1963, a report by the Council on Foods and Nutrition of the American Medical Association stated that "In general, medical education and medical practice have not kept abreast of the tremendous advantages in nutritional knowledge" [6]. Recommendations to improve physicians' knowledge were presented by the Council and included expansion of programs on medical nutrition information, consideration of nutrition in intern and resident programs as one criteria for approval of hospital training programs, development of workshops on teaching nutrition at the postgraduate level, and expansion of short-term fellowships in clinical nutrition.

Cyborski [7] reported that 12 of 16 medical schools in the United States had nutrition courses in their curricula during 1958, but by 1977 only 19 of 100 medical schools had required courses in nutrition. Long [19] gave several reasons for the existence of impediments to nutrition education for physicians: (1) Nutrition is a vast field of study. (2) Nutrition curriculum is not an easy fit into other curricula. (3) Many institutions lack an advocate for nutrition curricula. (4) Nutrition does not fit into biochemistry where it may most logically belong. (5) Nutrition endures a large share of faddism and quackery. (6) Nutrition can be perceived as terribly boring. As a result of the omission or deficiency of nutrition curricula in their training, recent graduate physicians may be ill prepared to deal with complex nutritional problems in patient care. In developing a basic science component of clinical nutrition fellowships for physicians, Harper and Rosenberg [13] reported consensus on the assumption that few applicants will have had in-depth exposure to basic nutrition, and few will have had courses emphasizing whole-body and organ metabolic relationships. Bistrian [1] recently proposed two main types of clinical nutrition training programs: (1) a minimum of 1-year fellowships in nutrition support at a teaching institution, or (2) didactic training at an institution offering a graduate degree in nutrition.

Despite the attention that has been focused on nutrition education in medical schools, in 1985 only one school in five offered nutrition as a discrete, required course [4]. More than half of the schools offered less than 20 hours of basic nutrition and one in five offered less than 10 hours. Chamberlain et al. [4] conducted a survey of medical school faculty members who were asked to rate the importance of various nutrition competencies for medical students. The five most important competencies identified by the faculty were: (1) principles governing the use of EN and PN, (2) the appropriate use of PN and EN, (3) the effects of fluid and electrolyte imbalances, (4) management of conditions that involve fluid and electrolyte imbalances, and (5) the role of nutrition in the identification and management of selected disease states. Competencies in the use and understanding of PN and EN therapies were the areas rated highest by medical school faculty.

Because of their expertise in PN and EN, basic nutrition, clinical management of nutritional alterations, disease-specific nutritional consideration, and metabolism of nutrients, the NST is an excellent resource to medical students, residents, and staff physicians. Long [19] emphasized the importance of the role of the NST in providing continuing education about nutritional support.

Dietitians and Pharmacists

Unlike physicians and nurses, whose basic curricula do not focus on specific activities related to nutrition support, dietitians and pharmacists receive more focused course work in their basic educational programs.

Dietitians receive perhaps more nutrition curricula than any other member of the health care team. In fact, dietitians are appointed as faculty to some medical and nursing schools for the provision of nutrition-related curricula. Undergraduate and graduate education for dietitians, however, may not adequately prepare them for the complexities of specialized nutrition support. In particular, dietitians who have not been exposed to PN and EN in clinical practice may need additional knowledge about specialty formulas, enteral tubes and infusion pumps, parenteral solutions, access devices, absorption and use of parenterally administered nutrients, management of complications related to PN and EN, and drug-nutrient interactions. The NST and team dietitian are valuable resources to staff dietitians with whom they may often work collaboratively.

The undergraduate preparation of pharmacists typically includes courses focused on the preparation of large-volume parenteral solutions such as PN; compatibilities of intravenous admixtures; pharmacokinetics and pharmacotherapeutics; absorption, excretion, and metabolism of parenterally administered drugs; and drug interactions. Few pharmacists, however, receive nutrition courses in their undergraduate programs. Nutritional

assessment, nutrient metabolism, nutrient requirements, disease-specific nutritional alterations, enteral feeding techniques and equipment, and drug-nutrient interactions are focus areas for continuing education for pharmacists. Pharmacists who have not had clinical experience with specialized nutrition support may also not be knowledgeable about disease-specific parenteral and enteral formulations.

In summary, it is difficult at best to describe the educational needs of a wide group of health care professionals. Ideally, educational needs of a target audience are known prior to planning educational programs. An examination of undergraduate curricula for the various disciplines represented by NST members may be helpful as a starting point; however, the clinical experiences and expertise of a supposedly homogeneous group can be markedly variable. In implementing a hospital-wide program, the NST offers a variety of educational programs to meet the needs of beginning through advanced practitioners.

IMPLEMENTATION OF A HOSPITAL-WIDE PROGRAM

The NST focuses on six major areas related to staff education when planning and providing hospital-wide education: (1) orientation, (2) in-service programs, (3) staff development, (4) continuing education, (5) clinical rotations or preceptorships, and (6) other activities that are not primarily targeted toward education but have an educational component (Table 6-2). Each of these areas of focus is discussed with examples of how the NST can provide programs within the area.

Orientation

Orientation of hospital staff has the broad general purpose of acquainting the staff with personnel, policies, procedures, resources and resource persons, hospital layout, and the philosophical construct under which the system operates. Orientation programs are

Table 6-2. Components of a Hospital-Wide Education Program

Orientation
In-service programs
Staff development
Continuing education
Clinical rotations or preceptorships
Other activities

most frequently provided to a group of personnel within the same discipline, and are therefore directed toward that specific discipline's needs. Within the group, however, are health care personnel with diverse levels of experience and expertise. Generally, the experience level and expertise of the orientation group may not be known to the NST in advance, except for certain times in the year when a majority of new graduates attend orientation sessions.

Typically, orientation programs are coordinated by a specific department within the hospital: nursing staff development, department of surgery/medicine, department of pharmacy, department of dietetics/nutrition, or others. The sponsoring department can be of assistance to the NST in identifying the average experience and expertise level of the personnel who attend orientation and, in particular, those times of the year when the group is likely to be more homogeneous. The NST can also target those areas that are likely to meet the unique educational needs for the discipline related to nutritional support (see previous section). Evaluations of the program and direct feedback from the target population can help the NST or NST members to address more appropriately the group's needs in subsequent offerings. Finally, over time, the NST or NST member can identify educational needs by clinical observation of new orientees, discussion during the orientation session, and feedback from personnel who supervise orientees. Commonly, however, educational needs surpass the time allotment for orientation sessions.

Orientation sessions often represent the one period of time when the new employee is a "captive audience." Rarely in subsequent educational programs will the learner's attendance be guaranteed. For this reason, the NST or NST member is tempted to present "all one wants and needs to know about nutrition support" in an inadequate period of time.

A new employee is often inundated with facts, faces, and "don't forgets." Expecting that the orientee will have a high level of recall of information presented in marathon orientation sessions is unrealistic. Therefore, the NST should attempt to focus on information that will be most helpful to the orientee in the first few weeks of practice. Lengthier, more in-depth sessions (as an in-service or staff development session) can be postponed until the health care professional has had some experience in the system and is better equipped to retain information presented and formulate meaningful questions.

At the University of Cincinnati Hospitals, the nutrition support nurse clinician presents a 1-hour orientation session for newly employed nurses. The goals of the session are to: (1) identify the NST and NST nurses as resource persons; (2) state a rationale for each of the standing orders for PN and tube feeding; and (3) observe changing of the central venous dressing, PN bag, and tubing via a videotaped program. An outline of the content presented during this session is presented in Table 6-3.

In-service Programs

In-service programs generally focus on attainment of a skill or knowledge specific to an area of practice. Examples of in-service programs for nutrition support would include use of a specific enteral or parenteral infusion pump, insertion of a central venous catheter, performance of indirect calorimetry, obtaining a nutritional assessment, or preparing a total nutrient admixture. In-service programs are often presented by a member of the NST for other members of their discipline; thus, the nurse might provide inservice programs to nurses, the dietitian to dietitians, etc. Through these activities, NST

Table 6-3. Orientation Session for Nurses Presented by the Nutrition Support Nurse Clinician

I. Introduction
    A. The nutrition support team
        1. Roles and responsibilities
II. Enteral nutrition
    A. Equipment
    B. Formulas
    C. Complications
    D. Standing orders
    E. Nursing care
III. Parenteral nutrition
    A. Equipment
    B. Solutions
    C. Complications
    D. Standing orders
    E. Nursing care
IV. Changing central venous catheter dressing (videotape)
V. Changing bottle and tubing (videotape)

members enhance their visibility as resource persons to staff and demonstrate their expertise in the clinical arena. In-service programs are often used to introduce new supplies, equipment, procedures, and policies.

Staff Development

Staff development programs help to enhance health care professionals' skills and knowledge in areas that are broader and more comprehensive than in-service programs. Thus, rather than instructing staff in the use of a specific piece of equipment or performance of a procedure, a staff development program may have a goal of enhancing the health care professional's knowledge of principles or concepts relating to the care of a patient receiving specialized nutrition support. Staff development programs can be provided to a single discipline or interdisciplinary audience by the NST or team members; however, the target audience is usually limited to staff from the NST's hospital.

Continuing Education

Most education programs offered by the NST could be called continuing education pro-

grams; however, in the context of this chapter, continuing education is defined as educational programs that focus on acquisition of skills and knowledge and are given on a local, regional, or national basis. Therefore, continuing education is often directed at audiences both within and outside the hospital. The NST may offer a program as the sole sponsor, or network within the community or region to cosponsor a program with other NSTs, colleagues, or groups. Continuing education programs can be offered and marketed as workshops, seminars, conferences, and postgraduate courses.

Local and regional programs increase the NST's visibility within the institution, the community, and the region. In addition, regional conferences enable the NST to develop networks with other colleagues. Continuing education for team members is also an important feature of enriching the NST's expertise.

Preceptorships and Clinical Rotations

Many NSTs develop liaisons with schools of medicine, dietetics, nursing, and pharmacy for preceptorships or clinical rotations for graduate or undergraduate schools. NST members may have adjunct faculty appointments. At the University of Cincinnati Medical Center, NST members have preceptor arrangements with the College of Medicine, College of Pharmacy, and College of Nursing, and dietetic interns at the Medical Center. Medical students can choose nutrition support as an elective (clinical rotation). The NST acts as educator and facilitator for students who wish to learn more about the clinical management of patients receiving PN and EN. Typically, students from the various colleges attend NST rounds and work side-by-side with the NST member of their profession.

In July 1989, the Department of Surgery of the University of Cincinnati Medical Center began offering a 1-month clinical rotation with the NST to first- and second-year surgical residents. The residents act as team physician under the supervision of the director of

Table 6-4. Nutrition Support Rotation for Surgical Residents

	NST Member
Sessions*	
Orientation to the NST	MD, RN
Placement of central venous catheters	MD
General nutrition overview	MD
Nutritional assessment/indirect calorimetry	RD
Parenteral solutions/specialty solutions	PharmD
Central venous catheter management	RN
Selected aspects of enteral nutrition	RD, RN
Hepatic complications of parenteral nutrition	MD
Enteral nutrition	MD
Disease-specific nutrition support	MD
Other activities	
Team rounds, staff meeting, research meetings, clinic, surgical grand rounds	

NST = nutrition support team; RD = registered dietitian.
*Sessions average 1 hour in duration and are presented during the first 2 weeks of the rotation.

the NST and work collaboratively with other members of the team. In addition to clinical responsibilities, the surgical residents participate in several didactic and discussion sessions with team members (Table 6-4). Hamaoui and Rombeau [12] described the importance and future benefits of "imprinting" interns by teaching them about good nutritional care. Eventually, these same interns will influence their colleagues and new generations of interns.

Other Activities

The NST engages in various activities that, while not primarily targeted toward education, have an educational component. These activities include quality assurance, development of policies and procedures, clinical rounds, publication of manuals, and research.

Kudsk et al. [18] described the medical audit as a tool to develop educational programs. As a result of problems identified by an audit of nutritional care, lectures, workshops, and conferences were implemented to improve the quality of care. Involving hospital staff in the quality assurance process enhances their knowledge of quality indicators, especially when patient outcome becomes the measure of quality. The NST can conduct quality assurance programs or act as a resource to other groups or committees whose primary responsibility is quality assurance.

Policies and procedures often become the focus of in-service programs. Ideally, the NST has the authority to develop both policies or procedures **and** in-service education programs for staff. Active involvement by the NST helps to ensure that the rationale for decisions is presented as well as the desired behaviors. The NST can assist staff to remain knowledgeable about current research findings that subsequently become the basis for changes in clinical practice.

Clinical rounds provide a forum for the NST and staff to collaboratively plan patient care. As previously mentioned, students attend rounds during clinical rotations and participate in discussions of patient management. The NST can also encourage the staff to join in "walk rounds" on individual hospital units, thus involving the staff in the collaborative process of planning care and obtaining important information from bedside caregivers. Walk rounds also increase the NST's visibility and accessibility to the hospital staff.

In 1986 the NST at the University of Cincinnati Medical Center published a manual entitled *Protocol for Nutritional Support* [2]. The manual was distributed to each nursing unit as a resource to personnel (nurses, pharmacists, dietitians, and physicians). A pocket-size version of the manual is distributed to interns. Information within the manual provides a core of knowledge about specialized nutrition support for the practitioner. Periodic review and revision of the manual ensure that it remains current. The *Protocol for Nutritional Support* provides a basis from which many educational programs originate.

The NST engages in research to test hypotheses and discover new truths. In general, the purpose of research activities is to add to the body of knowledge about the area of inquiry. By directing or participating in research activities, the NST demonstrates a dedication to enriching and enlarging the scientific background on which PN and EN are based.

SUMMARY

A traditional and enduring role of the NST is the implementation of a hospital-wide education program. As the NST organizes a hospital-wide program, issues such as the team's power and authority, role as a consultant, and role as an agent of change must be considered. Successful educational programs require a systematic planning process, skillful implementation, and careful evaluation. When successful, a hospital-wide education program enables health care professionals to readily identify the NST as expert resource personnel, as "those who can teach." The NST has a unique opportunity, through education of the staff, to enhance the quality of nutritional care within the hospital.

REFERENCES

1. Bistrian, B. R. Thoughts on training and employment opportunities in clinical nutrition. *Am. J. Clin. Nutr.* 49:180, 1989.
2. Bower, R. H., and Griggs, B. A. (eds.). *Protocol for Nutritional Support.* Cincinnati: University of Cincinnati Medical Center, 1986.
3. Burke, W. A., Burkhart, V. D., and Pierpaoli, P. G. *A Guide for a Nutritional Support Service.* Deerfield, IL: Travenol Laboratories, 1980.
4. Chamberlain, V. M., Mays, M. H., and Cummings, M. N. Competencies in nutrition that U.S. medical students should acquire. *Academic Med.* 64:95, 1989.
5. Claus, K. E., and Bailey, J. T. *Power and Influence in Health Care: A New Approach to Leadership.* St. Louis: C. V. Mosby, 1977.
6. Council on Foods and Nutrition, American Medical Association. Teaching of nutrition in schools of medicine. *J.A.M.A.* 183:955, 1963.
7. Cyborski, C. K. Nutrition content in medical curricula. *J. Nutr. Educ.* 9:17, 1977.
8. Dalton, M. J., Schepers, G., Gee, J. P., Alberts, C. C., Eckhauser, F. E., and Kirking, D. M. Consultative total parenteral nutrition teams: The effect on the incidence of total parenteral nutrition-related complications. *J. Parenter. Enter. Nutr.* 8:146, 1984.
9. Englert, D. M., Crocker, K. S., and Stotts, N. A. Nutrition education in schools of nursing in the United States. Part 1: The evolution of nutrition education in schools of nursing. *J. Parenter. Enter. Nutr.* 10:522, 1986.
10. Grant, J. P. A Team Approach. In J. P. Grant (ed.), *Handbook of Total Parenteral Nutrition.* Philadelphia: W. B. Saunders, 1980.
11. Green, J. S., Grosswald, S. J., Suter, E., and Walthall, D. B. *Continuing Education for the Health Professions.* San Francisco: Jossey-Bass, 1984.
12. Hamaoui, E., and Rombeau, J. L. The Nutrition Support Team. In J. L. Rombeau and M. D. Caldwell (eds.), *Parenteral Nutrition.* Philadelphia: W. B. Saunders, 1984.
13. Harper, A., and Rosenberg, I. Reports from the consensus workshops on the specific components of clinical nutrition fellowship training. *Am. J. Clin. Nutr.* 44:135, 1986.
14. Hicks, H. G. *The Management of Organizations: A Systems and Human Resources Approach* (2nd ed.). New York: McGraw-Hill, 1972.
15. Holtz, H. *How To Succeed as an Independent Consultant.* New York: John Wiley & Sons, 1983.
16. Jeejeebhoy, K. N. Organization of the Nutritional Support Team. In K. N. Jeejeebhoy (ed.), *Total Parenteral Nutrition in the Hospital and at Home.* Boca Raton: CRC Press, 1983.
17. Keohane, P. P., Jones, B. J. M., Attrill, H., et al. Effect of catheter tunnelling and a nutrition nurse on catheter sepsis during parenteral nutrition: A controlled trial. *Lancet* 2:1388, 1983.
18. Kudsk, K. A., Thompson, M., Tranbaugh, R. F., and Sheldon, G. F. Medical audit as an educational tool to improve intravenous nutritional support. *J. Med. Educ.* 57:336, 1982.
19. Long, J. M. Opening the closet door: The key to education. *J. Parenter. Enter. Nutr.* 6:280, 1982.
20. Mauksch, I. G., and Miller, M. H. *Implementing Change in Nursing.* St. Louis: C. V. Mosby, 1981.
21. Nehme, A. E. Nutritional support of the hospitalized patient: The team concept. *J.A.M.A.* 243:1906, 1980.
22. Newton, M. E., Beal, M. E., and Strauss, A. L. Nutritional aspects of nursing care. *Nurs. Res.* 16:46, 1967.

23. Rogers, E. M. Change agents, clients, and change. In G. Zaltman, P. Kotter, and I. Kaufman (eds.), *Creating Social Change*. New York: Holt, Rinehart and Winston, 1972.

24. Stotts, N. A., Englert, D., Crocker, K. S., Bennum, N. W., and Hoppe, M. Nutrition education in schools of nursing in the United States. Part 2: The status of nutrition education in schools of nursing. *J. Parenter. Enter. Nutr.* 11:406, 1987.

25. Traeger, S. M., Williams, G. B., Milliren, G., Young, D. S., Fisher, M., and Haug, M. T. Total parenteral nutrition by a nutrition support team: Improved quality of care. *J. Parenter. Enter. Nutr.* 10:408, 1986.

Nursing Care of Total Parenteral and Enteral Nutrition

Crystal L. Davis

Nursing care plays a pivotal role in nutritional therapy. Nurses are on the front lines of assessing, monitoring, and intervening on behalf of their patients receiving nutritional support. Butterworth and Blackburn [6] suggested that one-fourth to one-half of medical-surgical patients hospitalized for 2 weeks or more suffer protein-calorie malnutrition. *[Editor's Note:* It should be remembered that much of this study took place in a city hospital, with many indigent patients. Studies in a private hospital setting may also reveal malnutrition, although not likely in near as high a percentage.] The malnourished patient does not heal well or resist infection normally, thus predisposing to the development of sepsis. If a catabolic state occurs and results in greater than 30% of the lean body mass being lost, death may result. The goal is to prevent malnutrition, preserving body cell mass. Hopefully, this goal can be accomplished through increased oral intake. When this cannot be achieved, parenteral and enteral therapy may be warranted.

Because specialized nutritional support is a complex and potentially hazardous form of therapy, a multidisciplinary team approach is of benefit in reducing related complications.

ASSESSMENT

Baseline assessment parameters assist in determining the correct mode of therapy, avoiding complications related to therapy, detecting possible complications as a result of therapy, and determining the adequacy of the therapy provided. In this age of technology, we must keep focused on the patient as this is the key to any successful intervention.

An assessment is performed prior to initiation of therapy. The therapy is thus personalized to the patient's needs. There is a dynamic relationship between the disease state and the malnourished state, with each impacting on the other. For example, a malnourished patient with coagulopathy requiring total parenteral nutrition (TPN) would need correction of clotting abnormalities prior to insertion of the catheter.

This nursing assessment should include: (1) biographic data; (2) chief complaint; (3) present health status with a summary of current problems; (4) current health data (i.e., medications, allergies); (5) past health status; (6) family history; (7) review of all physiologic systems with general description, nutritional assessment, and a complete "head-to-toe" assessment of each physiologic system; (8) health maintenance efforts (i.e., exercise, stress management); and (9) environmental health (i.e., inhalants, stairs to climb).

TOTAL PARENTERAL NUTRITION

TPN is the administration of nutrients via the intravascular route. These nutrients include dextrose, amino acids, electrolytes, vitamins, minerals, and fat emulsions. TPN solutions are highly concentrated, containing 15 to 47% dextrose. To avoid metabolic complications of hyperglycemia or hypoglycemia, TPN formulations are gradually advanced until target calories are achieved, and then tapered prior to completion of therapy. At the University of Cincinnati Medical Center, the following infusion regimen is generally tolerated [5].

Those TPN solutions with final dextrose dilutions of 15 to 25% are normally begun at a rate of 40 ml/hr. The TPN rate is then adjusted 20 ml/hr/day until target calories are achieved unless hyperglycemia prohibits advancement efforts. If a patient's blood sugar level is greater than 200 mg/dl, the advancement of TPN is normally held and appropriate insulin supplementation is initiated. The changing of one variable at a time (the rate) makes glucose management less difficult.

Cardiac and renal solutions are given to patients with decreased fluid tolerance and contain greater than 25% dextrose. These solutions are initiated at a rate of 30 ml/hr and advanced by increments of 10 ml/hr/day until target calories are achieved in the absence of hyperglycemia. Due to the hyperosmolar nature of these solutions, a large-diameter blood vessel is required to reduce the likelihood of thrombophlebitis. Ideally, the catheter tip terminates in the superior vena cava. Borow and Crowley [4] concluded that "all catheters form thrombi and fibrin sheaths, but there is a wide range of thrombogenicity between catheter materials. The most thrombogenic catheter material is polyurethane, and the least thrombogenic is polyurethane coated with hydromer. The next least thrombogenic catheter is silicone."

The two main catheter designs are those inserted by needle venipuncture and threaded percutaneously and those inserted by surgical implantation. The focus of this chapter is on temporary, percutaneously placed catheters. Chapter 23 discusses indwelling and implanted catheters for ambulatory and home TPN.

The two most commonly used vessels for percutaneously placed catheters are the subclavian vein and the internal jugular vein. The subclavian vein is preferred; however, each access site has advantages and disadvantages. Both subclavian and jugular veins are easily accessible, and their large diameter can accommodate high-flow states. The anatomic position of the veins brings about the following advantages and disadvantages. The subclavian vein provides a stable insertion site for the catheter to be anchored. It allows the patient freedom of movement and ease of dressing care. The jugular approach is less suitable for maintenance of a sterile occlusive dressing because of neck movement and surrounding hair. Neck movement is also a problem relating to flow difficulty as well as increasing the potential for line separation. Catheters in patients with endotracheal tubes or tracheostomies are more easily contaminated when they are placed via the jugular approach.

Preparation and Insertion

When a TPN catheter is placed, it should be understood that this is an elective, not an emergency procedure. It is essential that adequate time be allowed for hydration, for clotting abnormalities to be corrected, and for the patient to be stabilized prior to insertion of the catheter.

Careful consideration by the physician as to the optimal site of insertion is necessary. Consideration is given to: (1) skin condition, (2) surrounding drainage or secretions, (3) history of thrombosis or of difficulty during cannulation, and (4) ventilatory status. "Positive end expiratory pressure (PEEP) in mechanically ventilated patients should not be greater than 5 cm at the time of venipuncture because of the increased risk of pneumothorax. If the PEEP cannot be reduced during insertion, sites other than the subclavian should be considered" [20]. Preferably, the TPN catheter is placed during the day to ensure availability of radiology, nursing, and medical staff if a complication should ensue.

The procedure and potential complications should be explained by a physician. Concerns of patient and family members should be addressed prior to the procedure or initiation of therapy. The patient should be informed of the catheter location, maintenance of sterility, positioning, and what he or she can expect to feel during the procedure. Explanations as to why it is necessary for patients to turn their head away from the selected area and the importance of lying quietly with arms to sides during the procedure should be given.

Baseline vital signs, weight, TPN laboratory studies, and a complete patient assessment including breath sounds should be obtained. The Valsalva maneuver should be practiced prior to insertion. The Valsalva maneuver is accomplished by asking the patient to take a deep breath ("hold it, hold it") while the patient bears down as if straining for a bowel movement. If a patient is unable to cooperate in performing the Valsalva maneuver (i.e., a patient with altered mental status), then breathing patterns should be monitored and exchanges of catheter tubing accomplished during end expiration. Proper hydration, Trendelenberg positioning, and appropriate practice of the Valsalva maneuver all reduce the risk of air embolism.

Before the procedure is initiated, individual patient needs should be assessed (i.e., bladder or bowel elimination, suctioning). The environment should be conducive to performing a sterile procedure with necessary provisions made as follows: (1) clean work area, (2) closed curtains and doors, and (3) a sign indicating a sterile procedure is in progress. A mobile insertion cart with all the necessary supplies (including extra supplies in case of contamination) is placed in the room to facilitate the procedure. A rolled sheet, infusion device, sedation, and 500 ml of 5% dextrose in water (D_5W) with tubing and Y ports primed by a nurse should be available. It is important that tubing does not contain backflow valves as one may not be able to obtain a blood return when lowering the bag to check for reflux of blood. The assessment of a blood return is important in preventing the complication of infusing the solution into the pleura.

A general description of nursing responsibilities is discussed here. A detailed description of the insertion procedure can be found in Chapter 3. During catheterization of the subclavian or jugular vein, everyone except the patient should be masked. A rolled sheet should be placed at the base of the neck extending to the small of the back, allowing the shoulders to move back against the mattress, simulating a "soldier at attention." The bed is placed in Trendelenberg position to distend and increase the pressure within the vein, promoting venous return.

The physician administers appropriate sedation, then washes his or her hands, and prepares to "gown and glove." The nurse assists in this process. The nurse is available to assist in the pouring of preparation solutions and opening the catheter package so that the physician can maintain sterility. The physician then prepares the area utilizing a "clean-to-dirty" technique. The preparation is done with 70% alcohol, followed by povidone-iodine solution with a 2-minute contact time. The povidone-iodine solution is then removed with alcohol. The nurse should time this interval. Sterile towels are then placed around the area where the catheter is to be inserted. Local anesthesia is then injected at the site of the proposed insertion tract. The nurse may assist in raising the drape slightly to allow the patient more comfortable ventilation.

A small 22-gauge needle and 3-ml syringe are used to locate the vein. The needle and syringe are then removed after carefully noting the direction of the needle and the depths of the vein. This practice assists the physician in determining the precise location of the vein using a smaller, less traumatic needle.

Having established the location of the vein, the physician reenters the tract with a 14-gauge Intracath needle (Deseret, Sandy, UT) with a 3-ml syringe attached. On locating the vein, the syringe fills with dark blood. The patient is asked to perform the Valsalva maneuver (after practicing a few times) prior to detachment of the syringe. The Intracath with stylet is inserted through the needle and is threaded into the superior vena cava. The needle and catheter are withdrawn as a unit until the tip of the needle comes out of the skin, whereupon the catheter needle clip is applied and a single suture placed at the catheter insertion site. The subclavian catheter hub should be positioned in the direction of the mid-nipple line, **not** out toward the shoulder, because mobility of the shoulder can loosen dressing, increase the risk of line separation, and facilitate the entry of organisms into the catheter insertion site.

The patient is again requested to perform the Valsalva maneuver, and the infusion set is attached by the nurse. The roller clamp is opened to establish free flow and the solution bag is lowered to check for reflux of blood. Once blood return is observed, a bag of D5W is placed on the infusion device and the rate is regulated to 40 ml/hr. The dressing is then applied by the nurse and a portable chest x ray is obtained immediately to verify appropriate location of the catheter tip. The chest x ray is portable to allow for greater monitoring of the patient, should a complication ensue. After the physician has documented that the catheter tip is located in the superior vena cava or brachiocephalic vein, the infusion of TPN may be initiated.

The above summarized version of the "through-the-needle technique" reflects one protocol utilized by the University of Cincinnati Nutrition Support Department [5]. An alternative method of placement is the Seldinger or "over-the-guidewire" technique, as follows: (1) The vein is cannulated. (2) A soft J-tipped wire is passed through the needle into the superior vena cava (one should never lose control of the guidewire). (3) The needle is withdrawn. (4) The catheter is slid over the guidewire. (5) A single suture is placed at the catheter insertion site. (6) The guidewire is removed and the infusion begun. (7) Placement is verified radiographically. (8) The nurse applies the dressing. Since no needle is remaining, no needle guard or clip is needed. This reduces kinking of the catheter at the guard and is advantageous when cleaning the skin surface.

Dressing Care

It is common knowledge that washing one's hands is the single most effective measure for the prevention of nosocomial disease. It is interesting to note that the organisms that generally cause catheter-related sepsis (i.e., *Candida albicans*, *Staphylococcus epidermidis*, *Staphylococcus aureus*, and *Klebsiella*) are all organisms commonly found on the hands of hospital caregivers [19]. Maki [11], when tabulating data of investigators reporting the incidence of mortality due to endemic nosocomial bacteria from 1935 to 1976, found that on the average, 20 to 40% of the patients did not survive. On reviewing the investigations of Rose, Spengler, and McGowan, Maki [11] also suggested that nosocomial bacteremias account for $280 to $863 million in excess health care costs each year in the United States.

The skin is believed to be the body's first line of defense against infection. It does not seem surprising that Bjornson et al. [3] found an association between microorganism growth at the catheter insertion site and colonization of the catheter in patients receiving TPN.

There are many variations in skin care at the catheter insertion site that are effective and practical. Differences do exist within the literature concerning the type of dressing material to be used and the frequency of dressing changes required. It appears that the key to successful dressing management is an educated nursing staff who monitor and maintain a sterile, dry, occlusive dressing.

The summarized protocol used at the University of Cincinnati [23] is as follows:

1. The following supplies are brought to bedside: prepackaged sterile custom dressing kit, masks, one bottle of alcohol, paper towels, and extra sterile gloves. A sign indicating that a sterile procedure is in progress is placed on the door.
2. The procedure is explained to the patient.
3. The patient is positioned with the arm on same side of catheter is abducted. Proper positioning promotes better adherence of dressing.
4. The bedside table is cleansed with alcohol and the surface dried with paper towels.
5. The nurse puts on a mask and masks the patient. If the mask causes respiratory difficulty, a sterile towel may be utilized as a substitute.
6. The hands are washed.
7. The dressing kit is opened and gloves are placed to side.
8. After ascertaining that the catheter hub and intravenous tubing are secure, the tape securing junction is removed.
9. The intravenous tubing below the hub is taped to the patient; this stabilizes the catheter during the procedure.
10. The old dressing is removed with care so as not to dislodge the catheter. The nurse inspects the site, suture, and surrounding area.
11. Sterile gloves are placed. The area is then prepared with three alcohol swabsticks utilizing a "clean-to-dirty" technique. Defatting of the catheter insertion site with acetone is not done. Maki and McCormack [13] concluded that defatting did not reduce the incidence of catheter-related infection, but did increase skin in-

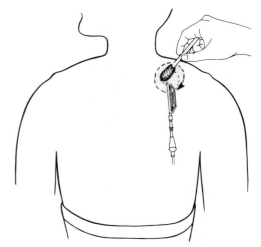

Figure 7-1. The area is aseptically prepared utilizing a "clean-to-dirty" technique. Preparation begins at the insertion site moving outward to the periphery with wider concentric circles.

flammation and patient discomfort. The "clean-to-dirty" technique begins at the insertion site with the swab held perpendicular to the skin and moving outward to the periphery with wider concentric circles (Fig. 7-1). One never returns to the center with the same swabstick that has touched the periphery. The entire dressing area, catheter, needle guard, and hub are cleansed with this process. Sitges-Serra et al. [21] found that catheter-related sepsis can have its origin at the catheter hub.

12. The alcohol is allowed to air-dry thoroughly before proceeding. The combination of alcohol and iodophor may liberate a strong tincture of iodine that may cause the skin to burn.
13. In the same manner, the area is prepared with the iodophor swabsticks for 2 full minutes. The iodophor is allowed to air-dry completely.
14. The iodophor ointment is applied to the center of the 2 × 2 in. gauze (Fig. 7-2). Maki and Band [12] suggested that "povidone-iodine ointment may be preferable for central venous catheters used

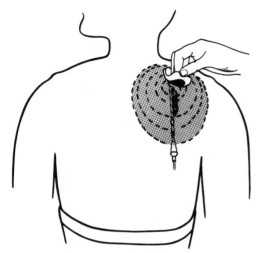

Figure 7-2. Application of a 2 × 2 in. gauze with iodophor ointment to the catheter insertion site.

for parenteral nutrition and arterial catheters where *Candida, Enterococci,* and resistant gram-negative bacilli are more frequently catheter pathogens, particularly when the patient is receiving systemic antimicrobial therapy." Further studies are needed in this area.

15. The insertion site is covered with the sterile 2 × 2 in. gauze sponges.
16. The skin surrounding the gauze is painted with tincture of benzoin. The benzoin is allowed to dry.
17. The elastic bandage dressing is applied to the area. Beginning half-way up the catheter hub, the dressing is placed by pulling with an upward motion until it covers the gauze and creates at least a 2.5-cm (1-in.) border around the gauze. Leaving half of the catheter hub uncovered by the basic dressing allows access for later intravenous tubing changes. The dressing should be contoured to the neck and shoulder area, consequently preventing the dressing from loosening with shoulder and neck movement.
18. The upper and lateral borders are then taped.
19. A slit piece of tape is placed under the

catheter hub, sealing the lower edge of the dressing.
20. One 2.5-cm (1-in.) piece of tape is applied above the ridge of the catheter hub.
21. The security of the catheter hub and intravenous tubing junction is rechecked via a push-and-twist motion to the right.
22. The catheter hub–tubing junction is sealed with a 10-cm (4-in.) long tape extending from the dressing, across the junction, and down the tubing. Tape is used in place of Luer lock connectors, which may not fit all catheter types. Tabbing this piece of tape distally to the patient facilitates easy removal when changing the tubing (Fig. 7-3).
23. The tubing is anchored to the shoulder with tape.
24. The dressing is labeled with the date, time, and initials of the nurse who changed the dressing. Transparent dressing is utilized if a patient has an endotracheal tube in place, tracheostomy, or any condition that may result in dressing contamination. Tape around the top and lateral borders is not necessary with transparent dressing and causes needless skin irritation (Fig. 7-4).

When the occlusiveness of the transparent dressing is assessed, if moisture is noted in the region of the 2 × 2 in. gauze, the dressing must be immediately changed as skin maceration can occur.

Dressing care is performed every Monday, Wednesday, and Friday, and when the dressing gets wet, loose, or soiled.

Documentation of dressing change should include: (1) type and location of the catheter; (2) dressing material used; (3) signs of infection, rash, or skin breakdown; and (4) description of the suture (i.e., number, loose, or intact). It is useful at the time of insertion to note the length of the catheter from the insertion site to the catheter hub and tubing junction so it can be used as a reference point in case the catheter is subsequently dislodged or pulls through the suture. If catheter dislodgement occurs, the physician needs to be

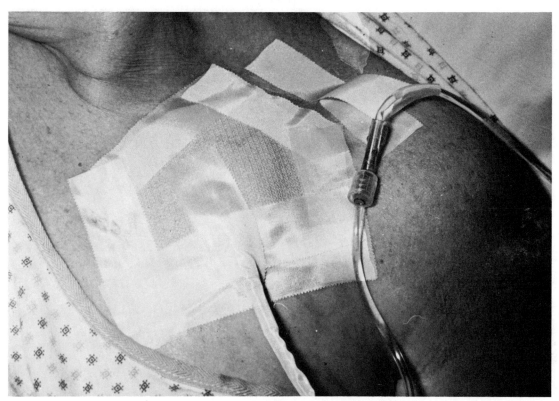

Figure 7-3. The elastic bandage dressing is applied, and all catheter hub and tubing junctions are secured with tape.

notified immediately and the catheter tip position verified radiographically.

Administration, Maintenance, and Monitoring

In addition to dressing changes, strict asepsis throughout the delivery system is necessary. To reduce manipulations of the delivery system, the catheter is used only for TPN except with approval of the nutrition support physician. In addition, single-lumen catheters are preferred unless limited venous access necessitates multilumen catheters.

Solutions are prepared under optimal conditions in the pharmacy after the catheter tip position in the superior vena cava or brachiocephalic vein is confirmed. Differing filtration systems exist. The microbial coverage ranges from 24 to 96 hours, thus dictating when tubing changes are required. This is a factor in cost and manipulations of the line. Ideally, the TPN system is spiked and primed with the filter by the pharmacy. Protocols for tubing changes should include maintenance of sterility of the catheter hub and tubing junction as well as observance of air embolism precautions.

The solution must be delivered at a constant rate via an infusion device to prevent metabolic complications. The infusion system must be checked frequently by the nurse to ensure proper functioning.

Urine sugar levels should be determined every 6 hours, or the fingerstick blood test for sugar levels performed as indicated, to establish patient tolerance to increased carbohydrate load. A blood sample is obtained immediately for 0.25% or greater glycosuria, and the physician notified. Glucose intolerance is sometimes the first indicator of

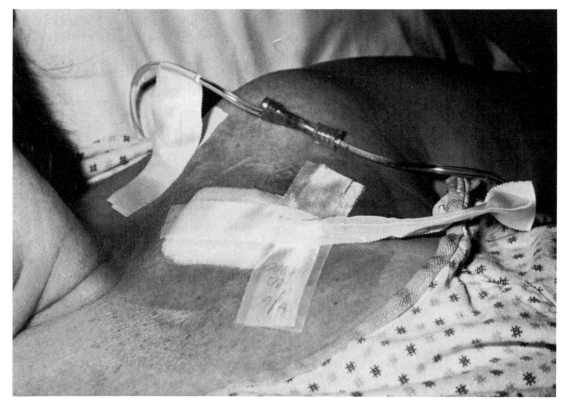

Figure 7-4. A transparent dressing is utilized when waterproofing of the site is required.

catheter-associated sepsis even before the temperature rises.

Weight measurements, although at times a cumbersome task, do provide important indicators of the adequacy of nutritional status and nutrients provided. Weights should be obtained daily at the same time of day, using the same scale.

Vital signs are monitored every 4 to 6 hours. Vital signs are assessed by examining trends and changes in clinical status, and by correlating data for indications of possible TPN-related complications.

Intake and output data are recorded and 24-hour trends are observed. Remember, 1 liter of fluid equals approximately 0.9 kg (2 lbs.), thus influencing significant changes in weight [10].

As the maintenance of a stable internal environment is essential to minimize the effects of overestimating or underestimating the body's requirements, TPN laboratory tests are performed twice weekly and as needed.

The malnourished patient has a loss of muscle mass and tone, decreased wound healing, decreased resistance to infection, and edema. Consequently, special attention must be given to hygienic needs including the skin, mouth, and hair. The nurse may be the first person to note hair loss caused by an essential fatty acid deficiency, the beginning of skin breakdown, or oral candidiasis (thrush). Occupational and physical therapy needs should also not be overlooked. Prevention and early detection are key to the patient's well-being.

COMPLICATIONS OF TOTAL PARENTERAL NUTRITION

The physician should be alerted to any technical, septic, or metabolic complications or problems related to TPN infusion. The following brief outline of complications can be used as an aid. Chapter 3 covers this subject matter in depth.

Technical Complications

Venous Thrombosis

Predisposing Factors
Stiff catheters, hypercoagulable states (i.e., sepsis), prolonged bed rest, dehydration, venous stasis, or certain malignancies.

Observations
Patient complains of shoulder, neck, back or arm pain; slight edema at the base of the neck; swelling of the arm or increased venous tributaries; internal jugular thrombosis; persistent headache; papilledema; sixth cranial nerve palsy; and double vision.

Intervention
Physician removes catheter; treat symptomatically with anticoagulants and local application of heat.

Septic Thrombosis (Life-Threatening)

Observations
As above; septic profile.

Intervention
Removal of catheter, anticoagulants; antibiotics for 6 weeks.

Lymphatic Injury

Predisposing Factors
A left subclavian approach in cirrhotic patients, as they have an enlarged thoracic duct.

Observations
Lymphatic drainage aspirated at time of insertion, lymph drainage at the insertion site, lymph drainage into the thoracic cavity or chest tube [20].

Intervention
Catheter removed, pressure applied; if continued leakage, operative procedure may be required.

Catheter Embolization (Life-Threatening)

Predisposing Factors
(1) Caused by pulling back the catheter or guidewire through the needle and subsequently shearing off. Always withdraw as a unit if difficulty threading. (2) Rupture of silicone catheter while attempting to flush occluded catheter. Do not apply pressure when meeting resistance; instead, attempt to aspirate. When performing routine heparinization of silicone catheter, use a syringe 10 ml or greater, as the smaller the syringe, the greater the pressure generated.

Observations
Catheter fragment on x-ray, cardiac arrhythmias, deteriorating patient status.

Intervention
Attempted retrieval under fluoroscopy, operative removal as indicated.

Arterial Laceration

Predisposing Factors
Occurs when needle is directed lateral to the subclavian vein.

Observations
Bright red blood, increased pressure of blood flow.

Intervention
Physician removes catheter immediately; constant direct pressure 10 minutes or longer; head of bed placed in high Fowler's position; frequent vital signs; repeated chest x ray for widened mediastinum; check arm and hand for impairment—numbness, decreased pulses, or temperature changes; notify physician.

Brachial Plexus Injury

Observations
Patient complains of excruciating pain down the arm, a tingling sensation in fingers, lack of movement, or paralysis of arms.

Intervention
Symptomatic treatment, physical therapy as indicated.

Carotid Artery Laceration (Jugular Approach)

Observations
Bright red blood, increased pressure of blood flow.

Intervention
Physician removes catheter immediately; pressure applied directly to puncture site for more than 5 minutes; head of bed in high Fowler's position; if unrecognized, can lead to expanding hematoma of neck causing tracheal compression or respiratory distress; apply direct pressure; notify physician immediately.

Arteriovenous Fistulas (Carotid, Internal Jugular)

Observations
Local protrusion, patient describes a feeling of vibration, may note a thrill or bruit, venous flow may be impeded.

Intervention
Physician removes catheter, pressure applied for longer than 5 minutes, may need operative intervention.

Air Embolism (Life-Threatening)

Predisposing Factors
(1) Improper hydration; (2) improper positioning; (3) insecure or loose catheter hub tubing junctions; (4) inadequate patient instruction of Valsalva maneuver; (5) lack of appropriate clamping of catheter.

Observations
Sharp pain, dyspnea, cyanosis, tachycardia, distended neck veins, hypotension, neurologic deficit, churning murmur.

Intervention
Stop inflow of air, place patient in Trendelenberg position, turn patient to a left lateral decubitus position, administer oxygen as ordered, have emergency equipment available.

Septic Complications

Line Sepsis

Predisposing Factors
Inadequate aseptic care of catheter.

Observations
Glucose intolerance, fever, chills, leukocytosis, deteriorating patient status, positive results on blood culture, septic shock.

Intervention
With catheter removal alone, sepsis usually resolves; administer antibacterial and systemic antifungal agents when warranted.

Septic Shock

Early Stage
Oliguria, sudden fever higher than 38.4C or 101°F, chills, nausea, vomiting, diarrhea, prostration.

Late Stage
Restlessness, apprehension, irritability, thirst, tachypnea, tachycardia, hypotension, altered sensorium, hyperventilation.

Late Signs
Hypothermia, anuria.

Intervention
Eliminate source of infection, reverse shock through volume expansion, monitor cardiac output, support ventilatory status as indicated, administer antibiotics to control infection, monitor intake and output strictly.

Candidiasis

Predisposing Factors
TPN patients receiving broad-spectrum antibiotics, steroids, radiation therapy, or immunosuppressants; diabetes mellitus; debilitating diseases; obesity; blood dyscrasias.

Observations of Superficial Candidiasis
(1) Skin: erythematous, exudate patches of varying size and shape, sometimes itchy; usually occurs in skin folds (i.e., below

breast, between fingers and toes, axilla, groin, or umbilicus). (2) Oral mucosa (thrush): creamy white patches on tongue, mouth, or pharynx. (3) Vaginal mucosa: white or yellow drainage with pruritus and local excoriation.

Observations of Systemic Candidiasis (Life-Threatening)
(1) Include same observations as with sepsis and septic shock, possibly including a rash. (2) Specific symptoms depend on the site of infection [7]. (a) Pulmonary: Hemoptysis, cough, fever. (b) Renal: fever, flank pain, dysuria, hematuria, pyuria. (c) Brain: headache, nuchal rigidity, seizures, focal neurologic deficits. (d) Endocardium: systolic or diastolic murmur, fever, chest pain, embolic phenomena. (e) Eye: endophthalmitis, blurred vision, orbital or periorbital pain, scotoma, exudate.

Intervention
Administration of antifungal medications; removal of TPN catheter with systemic candidiasis; control or elimination of precipitating factors if possible. When three sites are positive for *Candida* (e.g., urine, skin, esophagus), it is our practice to begin systemic amphotericin.

Metabolic Complications

Hypoglycemia

Precipitating Factors
Sudden withdrawal of nutritional support. Too much insulin.

Observations
Diaphoresis, nervousness, hunger, weakness, irritability, tremors, palpitations, headache, blurring or double vision, numbness of the lips or tongue.

Intervention
If TPN is discontinued, infuse a glucose solution; D5W administered at the same rate is usually adequate in preventing hypoglycemia. Adjust insulin in TPN.

Hyperglycemia

Precipitating Factors
Excess carbohydrate administration, glucocorticoids, insulin lack.

Observations
Thirst; fatigue; polyuria; dry, hot flushed skin.

Intervention
Change formulation as needed, change advancement regimen, provide insulin coverage, use hypoglycemic agent or antidiabetic agent.

Hyperosmolar Hyperglycemic Coma (Life-Threatening)

Precipitating Factors
Obtunded TPN and tube-fed patients unable to respond to thirst; diabetes; pancreatic disease; extensive burns; infections (especially respiratory); catastrophic illness; drugs—corticosteroids, diazoxide, phenytoin, epinephrine, diuretics (especially thiazides).

Observations
Dry skin, dry mucous membranes, fever, polydipsia, osmotic diuresis, hypovolemia, somnolence, seizures, coma.

Intervention
Gradual correction of hyperglycemia and hyperosmolality, fluid replacement and insulin therapy, administration of any deficient electrolytes.

TERMINATING TPN THERAPY

The transition from not eating to eating can be difficult for the patient. The patient may be fearful and the appetite poor. The nutritionist and nurse working together can help in making this transition easier. The nutritionist can assist in food selection and type of diet best suited for the patient. The nurse can assist the patient by providing a pleasant, clean atmosphere in which to eat. The nurse may need to assist in feeding the patient or merely opening packages, etc. Obtaining family support is oftentimes helpful, as partaking of food has many social and cultural implications. Families should be encouraged to bring special foods in. [Editor's Note: Getting a patient to eat may be one of the most difficult things in parenteral nutrition. It may be necessary to stop all glucose-containing infusions through the line and infuse normal saline solution until one can be certain the patient will eat.]

Accurately recording caloric intake is a necessary component to therapy. If caloric intake is not appropriately documented, it may result in prolonging a costly therapy and hospital stay.

Once it has been determined that the patient no longer requires TPN therapy, the catheter is removed and an occlusive dressing applied to the exit site.

ENTERAL FEEDING

The main advantages of enteral nutrition are cost, safety, patient tolerance, and maintenance of gastrointestinal integrity [22]. The stomach and jejunum are the two most common sites utilized for enteral feedings. The stomach has a large reservoir capacity and is less sensitive to volume and osmolality than the small intestine. Delivery of nutrients below the pylorus into the small intestine offers increased protection against aspiration by utilizing the barriers of the upper esophageal sphincter, lower esophageal sphincter, and the pylorus, but one sacrifices the ability to administer very concentrated solutions. Modes of therapy via these routes are: nasogastric, nasojejunal, gastrostomy, percutaneous endoscopic gastrostomy (PEG), jejunostomy, needle catheter jejunostomy, and double-lumen gastrostomy (jejunal tube); the latter tube allows for decompression of the stomach with simultaneous feeding into the intestine. The three methods of delivery of nutrients are: (1) bolus, (2) intermittent, and (3) continuous. Bolus feeding, the rapid

administration by syringe, is often poorly tolerated. Intermittent feeding with a prescribed amount administered over 20 to 30 minutes does not completely eliminate the problem of intolerance.

The most preferred method of delivery is continuous feeding over a 16- to 24-hour period via a feeding pump. It should be noted that delivery of nutrients into the small intestine usually requires continuous feeding, as the small intestine does not tolerate bolus feeding and sudden rate changes. The input of both physician and nutritionist is invaluable in providing a feeding regimen that will be best tolerated by the patient, including formula selection and advancement. General guidelines in feeding management include the following: (1) Introduce isotonic concentrations. (2) For intragastric feedings, increase strength first and then the rate, as the stomach tolerates higher osmolarities better than the small intestine by secreting enough gastric juices to render the solution iso-osmotic before transfer across the pylorus. (3) For feedings into the small bowel, increase the rate first and then the strength. (4) The variables of rate and concentration should not be changed simultaneously [14].

Although the enteral feeding route is generally a safe method of providing nutrients, potentially lethal complications can result from improper management and monitoring. Woodall and Winfield [24] reported complications of inadvertent tracheobronchial placement of small-bore feeding tubes with guidewires, and found that the presence of high-volume, low-pressure endotracheal cuffs did not preclude this complication. [Editor's Note: In our experience the Enteroflex tube seems much more prone to perforate the esophagus or bronchus than are other tubes.] Moustoukas and Litwin [16] described the unusual but lethal complication of intracranial placement of a nasogastric tube on a patient with a basilar skull fracture extending across the cribriform plate. These complications emphasize the need for proper selection of site, adequate training of staff, and radiographic verification.

Aspiration is a dreaded complication of enteral feeding, yet it is unfortunately one of the more common. Olivares et al. [18], in reviewing 720 neurologic autopsy cases, found that the use of gastric tubes (tube feeding) increases the risk of aspiration sixfold. Unfortunately, inflation of a tracheostomy tube cuff does not eliminate aspiration. To reduce the risk of aspiration, it is preferable to feed into the duodenum or jejunum in patients with gastroparesis or delayed gastric emptying, immediately postoperative patients, or those at increased risk for aspiration. Examples include the weak, debilitated, or comatose patient or those patients without an intact gag reflex. Meer's [15] retrospective study revealed that 40% of patients receiving nasoenteral tube feedings experienced inadvertent dislodgement of their feeding tubes, necessitating frequent monitoring and adequate methods of securing tubes.

The three major complications associated with enteral feeding are: (1) mechanical, (2) gastrointestinal, and (3) metabolic. Nursing care plays a pivotal role in prevention and early recognition of these complications.

COMPLICATIONS OF ENTERAL NUTRITION

Mechanical Complications

Tube Displacement/Aspiration Risk

Prevention/Observation/Management
Trained staff are used to place the tubes. Placement of the tube is verified radiographically prior to the initiation of feeding. The tube is secured, marked, and measured to obtain a future reference point. Using a 50-ml or larger syringe, the tube is aspirated and the amount of gastric contents recorded. Gastric fluid usually has a pH of 2 to 3 and will turn blue litmus paper red. Aspirating with a small syringe generates increased pressure within the tube, resulting in possible tube collapse or rupture of small-bore feeding tubes. Gastric contents are aspirated every 4 hours for continuous feeding and before each

intermittent feeding. If aspirates are less than 100 to 150 ml, return the aspirate to the stomach, then continue feeding. If the aspirate is greater than 100 to 150 ml, the aspirate is held and the physician notified. One would anticipate minimal aspirates in the jejunum due to its small reservoir capacity, unlike the stomach. Air injected into the stomach can be confused with the sound of air entering the bronchus, pharynx, or esophagus; therefore, it is not a reliable indicator of tube position.

The head of the bed should be elevated greater than 30 degrees during and for approximately 1 hour after intermittent feedings, and continuously for continuous feedings.

The tube feeding should be stopped ½ to 1 hour prior to suctioning, chest physical therapy, or placing a patient supine [9]. The patient is positioned on the right side to enhance gravity flow from the greater stomach curvature to the pylorus. Therefore, how a patient is positioned may affect the aspirate results. For example, placement on the right side decreases aspirates, while placement on the left side increases aspirates. Attempts are made to obtain gastric aspirates with the patient lying flat, with the head of the bed elevated greater than 30 degrees. Gastrointestinal intolerance such as increased abdominal girth, decreased bowel sounds, abdominal percussion of air, or abdominal pain is monitored. Tube feeding is stopped immediately if gastrointestinal intolerance, nausea, or vomiting occurs. If aspiration should occur, the tube feeding is immediately stopped and the following steps are performed: (1) endotracheal suctioning, (2) airway maintenance, (3) physician notification, (4) oxygen administration, and (5) patient status assessment. If one is not sure that the patient has aspirated, pulmonary secretions can be tested and will test positive for glucose if the patient has received a tube feeding with a glucose-containing base formula. The nurse should be aware that if blood is present in the secretions, a false-positive glucose measurement may occur. Regardless of the result, the physician should be notified of any suspected aspiration so that appropriate follow-up and intervention can be initiated.

Nasopharyngeal Irritation, Pressure Necrosis of Esophageal and Tracheal Wall

Prevention/Observation/Management
A small-bore polyurethane or silicone tube is used. If prolonged ventilatory support is necessary, consideration of a gastrostomy or jejunostomy tube may be warranted. Mouth care is provided every 4 hours. Ice chips, chewing gum, etc., are supplied to the patient if permitted. Vaseline is applied to the lips and a water-soluble lubricant is applied to the nose of the patient as needed. The tube is positioned in such a way as to avoid pressure on the nares, and the use of hypoallergenic tape is recommended. The nurse assesses for skin irritation and patient discomfort.

Otitis Media

Prevention/Observation/Management
A small-bore polyurethane or silicone tube is used. The patient is instructed to report symptoms of headache, earache, sinus pain, or sinus congestion [8]. The tube is removed and antibiotic therapy initiated as ordered by the physician. A new tube is inserted into the opposite nares if indicated.

Skin Irritation

Prevention/Observation/Management
The tube is secured to prevent undue stress on the tube. The length of the tube is noted to allow the nurse to check for displacement. The site is observed for drainage, redness, tenderness, or odor. The physician is notified of tube displacement or if skin irritation is observed.

Dressing Care (Gastrostomy or PEG Tube)
The skin surrounding the tube is washed with soap and water. The area is patted dry. Unless the tube is catching on clothing or drainage is present, the gauze dressing is not necessary.

Dressing Care (Jejunostomy/Needle Catheter Jejunostomy)
Cleanse the skin with a one-half water and one-half peroxide solution, using a cotton tip applicator. Rinse and allow to dry. Apply povidone-iodine ointment around the jejunostomy skin site. A split gauze pad is applied around the tube, with a second gauze pad going in the opposite direction; if the tubing is long, coil an extra length before placing on the second gauze pad. The dressing is taped to the skin with paper tape, or a transparent dressing is used.

Obstruction or Occlusion

The smaller the lumen of the tube, the greater the chance for obstruction. Consideration should be given to the formula selection, compatibility of medication, and method of administration (e.g., feeding pump for needle catheter jejunostomy). The feeding tube is irrigated every 4 hours with 30 ml of water. Crushed medications should not be administered via a small-bore feeding tube. The tube is irrigated before and after each medication. The following medications should **not** be crushed: enteric-coated tablets, sustained-release tablets and capsules, and sublingual and buccal tablets. Drugs are obtained in the liquid form if possible. If tablets must be used, they are crushed into a fine powder dissolved in approximately 30 ml of water. It should be realized that pharmaceutical syrups strongly acidic or buffered to pH values of 4 or below cause immediate clumping and other characteristics, and result in clogged tubes [1]. Tube feeding pump alarms should be responded to immediately. Feeding containers containing viscous formulas are shaken as needed because the formulas tend to separate. Curdling of a formula can result from bacterial contamination; therefore, perform the following: (1) Wash hands. (2) Maintain a clean system, preferably a closed system. (3) Never add new formula to the old. (4) Limit the hang time to 8 hours. (5) Change the administration set at least every 24 hours.

Intervention

A 50-ml syringe is used, alternating positive and negative pressure. Nicholson's work [17] using nine substances (pancrelipase [Pancrease, Viokase], pork pancreatin, bromelain, papain, cranberry juice, cola, chymotrypsin, and distilled water) to declog small-bore feeding tubes, revealed that none of the substances were effective within 4 hours. Therefore, prevention appears to be the key to managing this problem.

When medications are administered into feeding tubes, drug-nutrient interactions must also be considered.

Gastrointestinal Complications

Diarrhea

Prevention/Observation/Management

Intake and output and weight are recorded. The frequency, color, and consistency of stool are documented and assessed. The appropriate formula is administered and the rate is advanced slowly. The osmolarity of formula is reduced, and fat and lactose intolerances are avoided. Antibiotic therapy that results in superinfection with *Clostridium difficile* or *Staphylococcus aureus* is avoided or changed. Drugs commonly associated with diarrhea are avoided if possible: antiarrhythmic drugs (quinidine, propanolol), digitalis, potassium supplement, phosphorus supplements, magnesium-containing antacids, hypertonic oral electrolyte solutions, and cimetidine [2]. Continuous feedings are utilized via a pump as indicated. Medications are administered to restore bacterial flora. After an impaction is ruled out, antidiarrheal agents are administered.

Constipation

Prevention/Observation/Management

Intake and output and weight are recorded. The frequency, color, consistency, and amount of stool are documented and assessed. Prior history of laxative abuse is assessed. The nurse checks for impaction as in-

dicated. Fluid intake is increased and enema or laxative is administered as ordered.

Nausea/Vomiting

Prevention/Observation/Management

The tube feeding is stopped until the cause for intolerance is established. Bowel sounds, abdominal distention, and tenderness are evaluated. The aspirates are checked and their amounts recorded. The feeding is held as indicated. The abdominal girth is evaluated. The formula and rate of infusion are changed as ordered. Antiemetics may be prescribed.

Metabolic Complications

These are the same as for TPN. Refer also to Chapter 11.

CONCLUSION

TPN and enteral nutrition can be life-sustaining or life-threatening based on the care given.

Acknowledgments

The author wishes to thank the past and present members of the Nutritional Support Department, University of Cincinnati, for their support and encouragement. The valuable assistance of Jean Loos and Roger West for the preparation of figures, and that of Trenton Thomas and Steve Wiesner for preparation of the manuscript, is also appreciated.

REFERENCES

1. Altman, E., Cutie, A. J., and Schwartz, M. Compatibility of enteral products with commonly employed drug additives. *Nutr. Supp. Serv.* 4:8, 1984.
2. Anderson, B. J. Tube feeding: Is diarrhea inevitable? *Am. J. Nurs.* 86:704, 1986.
3. Bjornson, H. S., Colley, R. N., Bower, R. H., Duty, V. P., Schwartz-Fulton, J. T., and Fischer, J. E. Association between microorganism growth at the catheter insertion site and colonization of the catheter in patients receiving total parenteral nutrition. *Surgery* 92:720, 1982.

4. Borow, M., and Crowley, J. G. Evaluation of central venous catheter thrombogenicity. *Acta Anesthesiol. Scand.* Suppl. 81:59, 1985.

5. Bower, R. H., and Griggs, B. A. *Protocol for Nutritional Support.* Cincinnati: University of Cincinnati Hospital, 1986.

6. Butterworth, C. E., and Blackburn, G. L. Hospital malnutrition. *Nutr. Today* 10:8, 1975.

7. Hamilton, H. K. *Professional Guide to Diseases* (2nd ed.). Springhouse, PA: Springhouse, 1987.

8. Horbal-Shuster, M., and Irwin, M. Keeping enteral nutrition on track. *Am. J. Nurs.* 87:523, 1987.

9. Irwin, M. M., and Openbrier, D. R. Feeding ventilated patients. *Am. J. Nurs.* 85:544, 1985.

10. Lang, C. Providing Nutritional Support. In P. L. Swearigen, M. Sayer-Sommers, and K. Miller (eds.), *Manual of Critical Care.* St. Louis: C. V. Mosby, 1988.

11. Maki, D. G. Nosocomial bacteremia. *Am. J. Med.* 70:719, 1981.

12. Maki, D. G., and Band, J. D. A comparative study of polyantibiotic and iodophor ointments in prevention of vascular catheter-related infection. *Am. J. Med.* 70:739, 1981.

13. Maki, D. G., and McCormack, K. N. Defatting catheter insertion sites in total parenteral nutrition is of no value as an infection control measure. *Am. J. Med.* 83:833, 1987.

14. Matarese, L. E. Enteral Alimentation. In J. E. Fischer (ed.), *Surgical Nutrition.* Boston: Little, Brown, 1983.

15. Meer, J. A. Inadvertent dislodgement of nasoenteral feeding tubes: Incidence and prevention. *J. Parenter. Enter. Nutr.* 11:187, 1987.

16. Moustoukas, N., and Litwin, M. S. Intracranial placement of nasogastric tube: An unusual complication. *South. Med. J.* 76:816, 1983.

17. Nicholson, L. J. Declogging small-bore feeding tubes. *J. Parenter. Enter. Nutr.* 11:594, 1987.

18. Olivares, L., Segovia, A., and Revuelta, R. Tube feeding and lethal aspiration in neurological patients: A review of 720 autopsy cases. *Stroke* 5:654, 1974.

19. Ryan, J. A. Complications of Total Parenteral Nutrition. In J. E. Fischer (ed.), *Total Parenteral Nutrition* (1st ed.). Boston: Little, Brown, 1972.

20. Ryder, M. A. Parenteral Nutrition Delivery Systems. In J. A. Grant and C. Kennedy-Caldwell (eds.), *Nutritional Support in Nursing.* Philadelphia: Grune & Stratton, 1988.

21. Sitges-Serra, A., Linares, J., and Garau, J. Catheter sepsis: The clue is the hub. *Surgery* 97:355, 1985.

22. Torosian, M. H., and Rombeau, J. L. Feeding by tube enterostomy. *Surg. Gynecol. Obstet.* 150:918, 1980.

23. University of Cincinnati Hospital. *Nursing Care Policies and Procedures.* Cincinnati: University of Cincinnati, 1988.

24. Woodall, B. H., and Winfield, D. F. Inadvertent tracheobronchial placement of feeding tubes. *Radiology* 165:727, 1987.

Suggested Readings

Breach, C. L., and Saldanha, L. G. Tube feeding complications, Part I: Gastrointestinal. *Nutr. Supp. Serv.* 8:15, 1988.

Forlaw, L., and Torosian, M. Central Venous Catheter Care. In J. L. Rombeau and M. C. Caldwell (eds.), *Parenteral Nutrition.* Philadelphia: W. B. Saunders, 1986.

Haynes-Johnson, V. Tube feeding complications: Causes, prevention, and therapy. *Nutr. Supp. Serv.* 6:17, 1986.

Kennedy-Caldwell, C. *Nutrition Support Nursing.* Silver Spring: Aspen, 1985.

Nuwer-Konstantinides, N., and Shronts, E. Tube feeding: Managing the basics. *Am. J. Nurs.* 87:1312, 1983.

Rombeau, J. L., and Caldwell, M. D. *Clinical Nutrition,* Vol 1: Enteral and Tube Feeding. Philadelphia: W. B. Saunders, 1984.

Nutrition and Immunity

J. M. Tellado
Nicolas V. Christou

The immune system is fundamental to the survival of mammals. It is composed of a large and complex set of elements designed to protect against foreign pathogens, while not responding adversely to components of itself. The task confronting the immune system can be described by seven key words: **encounter, recognition, activation, deployment, discrimination, eradication,** and finally, **regulation.** The final outcome (i.e., elimination of an "invader"), be it a virus, a microbe, or a foreign protein, occurs via the inflammatory response. Specific immunity refers to that part of the immune defense system that is associated with responses that are antigen specific; that is, they are targeted to one and only one particular antigen. Strictly speaking, the immune system is degenerate and redundant, and thus one antibody may "cross-react" with a similar antigen and one antigen may unite with many antibodies, but in general a very high degree of specificity is maintained. In contrast, nonspecific immunity does not discriminate on the basis of antigen-antibody specificity. It is directed against a wide variety of "invaders." For example, a macrophage will phagocytose and kill an *Escherichia coli* bacterium as easily as it will kill a *Staphylococcus*, or a virus or a fungus, without regard to surface antigen expression on the invader, other than appropriate opsonization.

Immunity can further be characterized by its various components. An immune response involving primarily functional immune cells like lymphocytes and macrophages is referred to as cell-mediated. Noncellular elements such as antibodies, complement, immunoglobulins, and cytokines that exist in solution in body fluids are referred to as the humoral immune system. Optimal function of the immune system requires cooperation in that cellular elements as well as humoral elements must interact with each other.

LYMPHOCYTES

There are several distinct populations of morphologically indistinguishable lymphoid cells that can be identified by specific cell-surface markers. One class of lymphocytes, thymus-derived or T cells, mediates the cellular response, while another class of lymphocytes, B cells (bursa-derived), mediate the humoral immune response.

In mammals, primordial lymphocytes arise in the blood islands of the yolk sac and migrate to the embryonic liver and bone marrow. After birth and throughout the remainder of the organism's life, the bone marrow produces hematopoietic stem cells which have lymphocyte precursors among them.

These antigen-independent maturation processes give rise to populations of short-lived, antigen-specific T cells that migrate to peripheral lymphoid tissues. Here, contact with their target antigen results in the development of mature, long-lived circulating peripheral T cells that respond to further antigen stimulation by differentiating finally to effector cells. Effector T-cell populations include the cytotoxic or killer T cell, which eliminates foreign cells directly, and the cells responsible for delayed-type hypersensitivity, for helping B-cell proliferation and differentiation, for amplifying killer T-cell differentiation and proliferation, and for suppressing immune responses. Natural killer cells are a discrete population of cytotoxic lymphocytes capable of killing a variety of tumor cells.

A central feature of the immune system is its ability to recognize surface features of macromolecules and cells that are not constituents of the host organism—that is, that are "not self." This recognition is accomplished through cell-surface receptors present on lymphoid cells that are specific for a single foreign entity, or antigen. In the case of the B cell, the antigen receptor site is a portion of an immunoglobulin that can bind to the target antigen. The T-cell receptor has not been identified, but it may also involve immunoglobulin-like molecules. Regardless of the nature of the receptor, binding of antigen initiates the complicated processes leading to an immune response directed against the stimulating antigen. The immune system is capable of distinguishing very small differences in structures and can distinguish between single amino acid substitutions in a given protein molecule.

ANTIBODIES

While antigen activation of a T cell results in a cell-mediated elimination of the invading material, B-cell activation ultimately results in the production of an antibody response. Antibodies are protein molecules synthesized by B cells. They are highly specific for the stimulating antigen, and a given B-cell clone produces antibodies of a single specificity. Antibodies belong to a protein class called immunoglobulins. Immunoglobulins in mammalian serum can be divided into five classes on the bases of antigenic differences of their heavy-chain constant regions. The classes are designated IgG, IgM, IgA, IgD, and IgE.

CYTOKINES

Numerous hormone-like mediators are secreted in the course of an immunologic response. These mediators are globally referred to as **cytokines:** Those produced by lymphocytes are called **lymphokines** and those produced by monocytes and macrophages are called **monokines.** These mediators function as signals that can modulate immunity by directing the growth, differentiation, and mobility of various immune function cells. Among the important cytokines are the interleukins and interferon.

Interleukin-1 (IL-1) is synthesized and secreted by macrophages. All types of macrophages, including those from the peritoneal cavity, spleen, Kupffer cells, and lung, are capable of producing IL-1. IL-1 acts to promote the short-term proliferation of T cells. IL-2, also known as T-cell growth factor (TCGF), effects long-term proliferation of T cells. Current information suggests that antigen-induced IL-2 is made primarily by helper T cells (T4), although certain stimuli will induce IL-2 production by T8 (suppressor/cytotoxic lymphocytes).

Another mediator released by stimulated macrophage is cachectin or tumor necrosis factor (TNF) [11]. TNF is a hormone produced by stimulated macrophages with a molecular mass of approximately 17,000 d. It accounts for 1 to 2% of the total secretory product of macrophages. It appears in the circulation within minutes of macrophage stimulation and peaks after approximately 2 hours of the inciting activation insult. This can be bacterial lipopolysaccharide (LPS), activated components of complement such as C5a, whole bacteria, or antigen-antibody complexes. Its half-life is short, of the order of 6 minutes. TNF exhibits procoagulant activity, inhibition of thrombomodulin, and release of IL-1; it may act as an endogenous pyrogen, and it also activates polymorphonuclear neutrophils (PMNs). [*Editor's Note:* Much of what TNF is alleged to do solely and specifically is very dependent on the system in which the effect is elicited. After an initial burst of enthusiasm crediting TNF or cachectin with a central role in seemingly every response, a more balanced view has lately emerged, downgrading and making less likely a central role for TNF or cachectin.]

MALNUTRITION AND IMMUNOLOGIC RESPONSIVENESS

General Observations

The relation of immune function and nutritional status is a complex subject. It has been well established that malnutrition increases the incidence of infection and mortality rates [24, 26]. The study of kwashiorkor and marasmus in malnourished children of many Third World nations [21, 22, 25, 65, 72, 76, 77, 83] has served to focus the attention of nutritionists, as well as immunologists, on the interactions of diet and host defense mechanisms.

Malnutrition, defined by anthropometric and serum albumin measurements, has been estimated to be present in up to 50% of surgical patients. [*Editor's Note:* This estimate, in my opinion, is high. It may achieve that level in certain populations, such as the indigent or intensive care unit populations.] While some patients are malnourished on admission as a result of illness-induced inanition, others become malnourished subsequent to hypercatabolism associated with activation events such as trauma [30, 31, 55], infection [14, 19, 30, 35, 38], or surgery [13]. While the effects of infection on nutritional status and host immunocompetence have been more readily defined, it has proved difficult to ascertain the role of nutritional status **independent** of other environmental factors on host susceptibility to infection, by virtue of suppression of local and systemic immune responsiveness.

There is a significant "closeness" between malnutrition and diminished host resistance to sepsis, but a clear demonstration of cause and effect in either direction is lacking. A multitude of clinical and laboratory techniques are available for the assessment of nutritional status [44], but they are inconsistently used and many are semiquantitive at best. Malnutrition is due to many complex and interacting factors, both biologic and social. Alterations in host defense may be different when protein loss predominates compared to combined protein-calorie malnutrition [39] or when only a single nutrient deficiency is present [1, 3]. Our inability to rule out coexisting infection in patients who were studied to determine the influence of malnutrition on host defense compromises, to a degree, the establishment of a causal relationship, particularly since most studies in humans have been done on undernourished children from Third World nations. The interpretation of many of these clinical reports is rendered difficult and the applicability to the adult surgical population vague. Most likely, malnutrition and sepsis predispose to each other in some cases [10, 17] and coexist in a vicious cycle in others. The therapeutic objective, however, remains the same—improved patient survival with combined nutritional repletion and immunologic restoration.

B-Cell Function in Malnutrition

The exact location of the bursa-equivalent, or the primary lymphoid organ responsible for the development of the B-cell system in humans, is not known. However, secondary lymphoid tissue containing germinal centers responsible for some aspects of B-cell function are known to atrophy in malnutrition. Tonsillar size is decreased as is splenic weight [80]. Whether such a diminution in size is an immunologically specific effect of malnutrition or simply an overall effect of weight loss is unclear.

Bearing in mind the wide variability and a trend toward overestimation in early reports [52], the number of circulating B cells in the peripheral blood is probably normal [23, 49, 73] in malnourished patients. The relationship of the percentage of circulating B cells to the total body pool of cells actively or potentially capable of producing immunoglobulin is unknown.

Changes in serum immunoglobulin levels in malnutrition have been reported, but are inconsistent. In clinical and indeed in experimental studies, it is difficult to rule out recent and/or coexisting infection, which may increase immunoglobulin levels. Children with evident infection have elevated levels of IgG, but those without infection have reduced levels [23]. Most authors have found IgG, IgM, and IgA levels to be normal or elevated in malnourished children [18, 73, 81], adults [53], and guinea pigs [90], while in malnourished dogs the IgG level was reduced [34]. The finding that serum IgE level is elevated [65] in malnutrition is of interest, since in some primary immunodeficiency diseases the IgE level is correlated inversely with T-cell function [49].

Functional assays of the B-cell system in vivo—that is, measurements of the capacity to form specific antibody responses to antigens—require normal macrophage and helper T-cell function. A variety of antigens have been used in humans and animals, the responses to which are probably T-cell dependent. Subdivision of the antibody response into immunoglobulin types has rarely been done, even though this may be important in conditions of altered immunity. Using a hemagglutinin assay, which measures predominantly IgM titers, an early report described a reduced humoral immune response to killed *Salmonella typhosa* organisms in malnourished individuals [88]. In prisoners of war and other patients with malnutrition, response to tobacco mosaic virus and fawn red cells was also reduced [41]. Yellow fever vaccine produced a low response in malnourished children, while the response to polio and smallpox was normal [16]. In another study, anti–tetanus toxoid titers after immunization were normal, while titers to *Salmonella typhosa* were reduced [20]. In adults, response to diphtheria toxoid was normal [4, 5], but response to keyhold-limpet hemocyanin was impaired [52].

Animal studies have been more extensive. In rats immunized with sheep red blood cells (SRBCs) while protein deficient, lower spleen weights, lower splenic cell yields, and only one-third the normal number of direct plaque-forming cells were found [51]. Serum titers of antibody were also decreased, with similar findings reported by Mathur et al. [57]. In their study, simultaneous injection of syngeneic thymocytes was able to correct the number of plaque-forming cells almost to normal. Also using SRBCs in rats, Good et al. [43] established a dose-response curve with diets deficient in varying degrees of protein. Splenic cells from rats on a 6% diet yielded one-tenth the normal number of plaque-forming cells, while an intermediate diet in protein content produced an intermediate response for plaque formation. A similar dose-response effect was seen with another antigen, *Brucella abortus* [32]. Refeeding and the timing of immunization were studied by Law et al. [54]. Protein-depleted rats were refed 2 days before or 2 days after immunization with keyhold-limpet hemocyanin. Animals refed 2 days before immunization developed antibody titers significantly higher than those in persistently depleted rats and marginally higher than those in normal rats. Animals refed 2 days after immunization also showed an improved antibody response, but it was not as high as those refed before immunization. These experiments indicate that nutritional deprivation decreases humoral immune response and that refeeding can correct the abnormality.

The essence of these studies and speculations is the recognition that whereas B-cell abnormalities may occur in malnourished individuals, they are probably less severe than T-cell deficiencies. Our own work tends to support this hypothesis. The effects of short-term acute nutritional deprivation and refeeding on immune function were investigated in rats. Animals previously sensitized to keyhold-limpet hemocyanin were starved for 72 hours and refed for 7 days. Recall skin testing with keyhole-limpet hemocyanin and immunization with tetanus toxoid were used to assess delayed-type hypersensitivity (DTH) and humoral immune responses. DTH was maximally depressed late, after refeeding had begun. Anti–tetanus toxoid responses were depressed early during starvation. Neither DTH nor anti–tetanus toxoid responses had returned to normal after a period of refeeding sufficient to restore weight [66]. The effect of long-term protein deprivation, and refeeding, on DTH and humoral immune function was also investigated in rats. Animals previously sensitized to keyhole-limpet hemocyanin were placed on a 2% protein diet ad libitum for 8 weeks, after which some groups of animals were refed for up to 4 weeks. Control rats received normal rat chow. Recall skin testing with keyhole-limpet hemocyanin and immunization with tetanus toxoid were used to assess DTH and humoral immune responses. Weight, DTH, and antibody responses declined progressively with protein deprivation. Refeeding restored skin test responses and humoral immunity. There was a direct correlation between degree of malnutrition (as reflected by weight) and antibody responses, as well as between DTH and antibody responses. The data demonstrate that chronic protein deprivation modulates both DTH skin testing and

humoral immune responses, and there is a correlation between DTH responses and humoral immune function [67].

T-Cell Function in Malnutrition

In both humans and animals, primary and secondary lymphoid tissue is altered in malnutrition. In malnourished rats, the thymus is only one-sixth the normal weight [57]. In humans, it is also atrophic [80]. The spleen weight can be reduced to one-third of normal in rats and in humans; tonsillar size is grossly decreased [20, 80]. Histologic examination of lymph nodes shows diminished cellularity of both germinal centers and the T cell–dependent paracortical areas, but the latter are more severely affected [49, 80]. The etiology of this lymphoid tissue depletion is speculative; however, some have suggested it is due to an amino acid deficiency or an increase in adrenal corticosteroids [86], even though adrenalectomy failed to reverse lymphopenia in marasmic mice [6].

The percentage of T cells in peripheral blood lymphocyte preparations from malnourished individuals is below normal in children [23, 64, 73] but may be normal in adults. Studying North American children, Carney et al. [18] found a correlation between a decrease in the percentage of T lymphocytes and the number of infections that occurred during the subsequent hospital course; however, in adults with a marasmus-like condition, defined by weight loss and a serum albumin level below 3 g/dl, the percentage of T lymphocytes was normal [14].

Decreased response to phytohemagglutinin by peripheral blood lymphocytes from children [18, 20, 80], adults [53], guinea pigs [90], and dogs [34] has been reported. These data have to be interpreted knowing that assays done under suboptimal conditions may detect some "abnormalities" or, conversely, that assays done under suboptimal conditions will yield normal results. Pokeweed mitogen, which is a T cell–dependent B-cell mitogen, yielded better lymphocyte transformation than phytohemagglutinin did in malnourished animals [59], while in normals the converse occurred. This suggests a relatively more severe T-cell than B-cell deficit in malnutrition.

It is evident, then, that while some T-cell functions may be diminished by malnutrition, others are apparently enhanced—the same effect being noted with skin allograft rejection, where reports vary from a normal to an enhanced effect.

Nonspecific Immunity in Malnutrition

Early steps in circulating PMN activation seem to be altered in malnutrition. In protein-malnourished children as well as rats, phagocytic cell delivery to inflammatory lesions is reduced in both the number of delivered cells and the kinetics of the cellular influx [39, 84]. This failure of a prompt recruitment of phagocytic cells into a focus of infection could allow the establishment of local sepsis, which is followed by disseminated sepsis. In vitro phagocytic activity and bactericidal capacity of PMNs in malnutrition have been found to be normal.

Complement in Malnutrition

The prime function of the complement system is to mediate some aspects of inflammation and to facilitate ingestion of pathogens by phagocytes (opsonization) [37]. This action is nonspecific only in the **immunologic** sense; that is, antibodies to many types of antigens will trigger complement activation. The **biochemical** steps that constitute the sequence of complement interactions are highly specific. Most complement component proteins are present in serum in small amounts and are easily denatured. There is also the alternative complement pathway that is phylogenetically older than the antibody recognition mechanism and appears to play an important role in host defenses, particularly before antibody synthesis begins. The classic complement pathway is activated by antigen-antibody complexes, which leads to the generation of biologically important effector proteins.

Assay of most complement factors individually in children showed that in kwashiorkor, all factors except C4 were below normal, while in marasmus only C5, C6, and C3 proactivators were decreased [79]. This difference is likely due to different degrees of protein deficiency in the two groups, and corroborates other evidence of different alterations in host defense mechanisms in comparing protein versus protein-calorie malnutrition. C3 factor assay alone has frequently been performed; the factor was either decreased [89] or normal in children [73], but consistently decreased in dogs [34] and guinea pigs [90]. The relationship of altered serum levels of complement factors to altered function or patient outcome is not clear. Other serum proteins, collectively termed "acute-phase reactants," are often nonspecifically elevated in a variety of illnesses. In malnourished children, C-reactive protein levels were extremely elevated and fell to normal with treatment [58]. Several mechanisms may underlie those changes in the complement system; for example, decreased liver synthesis and macrophage production, and consumption of complement components by bacterial, parasites, and viral infections are seen frequently in these patients.

HOSPITALIZED PATIENTS: NUTRITIONAL ASSESSMENT AND OUTCOME

Hospitalization, Immunosuppression, and Sepsis

The contribution of malnutrition of hospitalized patients to immune compromise and mortality has been addressed in numerous studies in North America and Europe [12, 13, 46, 85]. Nearly 50% of severely ill and 24% of moderately ill patients in general wards can be characterized as having poor nutritional status. [*Editor's Note:* A word of caution. At least two of the studies were carried out in hospitals for indigent patients and their application to more economically advantaged patients must be at least questioned.] Diseases such as intestinal obstruction, and/or omission such as intravenous fluid support without calories for more than 3 days, play a common role in the development of hospitalized patients' malnutrition.

Numerous clinical studies have been conducted to identify the specific perturbations in immune function in malnutrition that increase patient susceptibility to infection and to mathematically interrelate such clinical markers in order to predict the outcome. Although malnutrition contributes to septic-related complications, and malnutrition is associated with immunosuppression in some patients, it is difficult to know, based on present data, what needs fixing—the malnutrition, the immunosuppression, both, or neither. In one animal experiment addressing this point, survival from peritonitis challenge was determined not by malnutrition per se, but by the adversely affected host immune state [47]. This study would indicate that what needs fixing is the immune suppression. Whether this can, or indeed, should be done independent of malnutrition remains to be proved.

DTH skin testing has been widely used in hospitalized patients as an assay to test global immune function. In a review of over 2000 patients, a statistically significant association was found between skin reactivity to five recall antigens and postsurgical septic complications [27]. Increased probability of patient mortality has also been shown to correlate with decreased skin reactivity, or anergy [28, 29, 56]. A multitude of factors may influence the DTH response, making it difficult to use this parameter to assess nutritional status [36]. Nutritional support of anergic patients has been demonstrated to restore reactivity in some but not all groups [45, 61].

A recent study [80b] examined several variables of immune function along with measures of the acute-phase response in 245 patients before surgery to determine which variables are associated with septic-related mortality following operation. Of the 14 deaths (5.7%), 12 were related to sepsis, and in 2, sepsis was contributory. The DTH response, age, serum albumin level, hemoglo-

bin, and total hemolytic complement were significantly different between those who died and those who lived. By logistic regression analysis, only the DTH skin test response and the serum albumin level were significantly and independently associated with mortality. The following equation can be used to estimate the probability of septic-related mortality in a preoperative patient given the serum albumin and the DTH skin test response:

$$P \mid death \mid = 1/\{1 + e^{(-3.45 + 1.75*(albumin) + 0.3*(\ln[DTH\ score])}\}$$

The resultant probability based on this mortality calculation equation was tested in a separate validation group of 519 patients and yielded a good predictive capability. [*Editor's Note:* It is striking how similar this equation is to the one derived by Mullen et al. [62]:

$$PNI = 158 - 16.6\ albumin - 0.78\ triceps\ skinfold - 0.20\ transferrin - 5.8\ DTH.]$$

It is difficult to establish the contribution of malnutrition to immunosuppression found in hospitalized patients since trauma, surgery, and other disease conditions can cause or contribute to impaired immunity. Thus, in postoperative patients, inadequate nutritional support contributing to a malnourished condition may or may not be the causal event in the development of immune system perturbation. Furthermore, reversal of the nutritional state of a patient may not be accompanied by a return of immune function. While some clinical studies demonstrated that nutritional support in the form of intravenous hyperalimentation can restore humoral, cellular, and phagocytic functions in previously malnourished subjects [34, 53, 63], other investigators failed to show a correlation between nutritional status and immune function [70]. The reasons for the observed differences among these studies may be related to factors such as differences in immune and nutritional parameters measured, therapeutic approach in treatment of the different patient populations studied, and differences in patient stratification both in terms of disease and severity [60, 69]. It is clear that nutritional support, both enteral and parenteral, can provide improved protein-sparing and decrease infection and mortality in malnourished patients. Whether this effect is primarily a result of improved host resistance is yet to be established.

AMINO ACIDS AND THE IMMUNE SYSTEM

The effects of inadequate dietary protein intake on the immune system have been described, but the role of individual amino acid deficiencies or excesses has not been well studied. The effect of alterations in amino acid pools within the cells involved in the immune system is unknown. Although there is a large body of information concerning the movement of amino acids into and out of tissues such as liver and muscle, little is known about the metabolic requirements and nutrient fluxes of immune system cells. It has been shown that during infections in protein-deficient humans, antibody synthesis and the synthesis of some complement components are maintained despite the reduction in synthesis of other serum proteins such as albumin [20]. Thus, there appears to be a mechanism to preserve host defense functions in order to enhance survival. The function of the immune system and other host defense mechanisms will ultimately depend on the availability of energy and the free amino acid sources within the body. Consequently, the quality and quantity of available nutrients play a vital role in determining the host's ability to maintain an effective defense mechanism.

Regulation of the host immune response by the quantity of dietary protein provided to an organism is important, but the quality or balance of the amino acid content of the protein is also important. The pattern of plasma amino acids and ultimately the tissue amino acid content will be determined by the proportion of individual amino acids in the protein source or in the infused fluids. Deficiencies of single amino acids in the diets of animals have been found to adversely affect lymphopoiesis and the anatomy of the lymphoid tissue [2]. A deficiency of isoleucine and especially of valine resulted in a reduced number of thymic and blood lymphocytes compared to animals consuming protein-deficient diets. Deficiencies of methionine and cysteine/cystine also adversely affect the thymus, lymph nodes, and spleen, and are similar to the effects observed in protein-deficient animals. A number of studies have demonstrated that deficiencies of some essential amino acids have variable effects on the humoral immune system. Tryptophan and phenylalanine deficiencies have been shown to reduce the primary and secondary responses of rats to SRCBs and to a synthetic antigen, and to impair phagocytic functions in mice [33, 42]. Further, the addition of tryptophan to diets deficient in this amino acid was found to stimulate the number of plaque-forming cells in the spleen and to increase serum hemolysin titers in adult rats [50]. Similar stimulation of IgG and IgM hemagglutinins during the primary response and IgG hemagglutinins during the secondary response was observed in young rats following tryptophan supplementation.

Supplemental arginine was found to increase thymic weights and lymphocyte counts in normal and traumatized rats [8, 9] and in obese mice [7]. Arginine supplementation was also shown to increase T-cell mitogenic responses in rats [9] and mice [7], and to promote wound healing in rats [78]. Furthermore, arginine supplementation was demonstrated to favor the host immune response to experimental tumor models [74, 75].

Mice fed diets deficient in tryptophan, phenylalanine-tyrosine, valine, threonine, methionine-cystine, and isoleucine had depressed titers of hemagglutinins and blocking antibodies when injected with allogeneic tumor cells [48]. Dietary restriction of leucine, isoleucine, or valine caused increased susceptibility to infection with *Salmonella typhimurium*, increased mortality, and increased spread of the microorganism in the livers and spleens of infected animals [71]. Lactating rats consuming methionine-deficient diets had reduced serum antibody levels and low blood plaque-forming cells to SRBCs, and their suckling offspring had increased rates of infection [40, 87].

Other studies have demonstrated the importance of the amino acid quality on maintenance of immune function. Addition of methionine to a soy protein diet, providing a mixture that was tryptophan-limiting, resulted in reduced IgG antibody titers. Mice fed diets of lactalbumin were found to have elevated humoral and cell-mediated responses when compared to animals fed casein hydrolysate diets [15]. There were no differences observed between the two groups of animals in body weights, total serum protein levels, white blood cell counts, or spleen weights. Mice receiving 28% lactalbumin diets had five times the number of plaque-forming cells to SRBCs in their spleens than did animals receiving casein diets. The major amino acid differences in these diets are the reduced content of phenylalanine and methionine in the lactalbumin diet (44% and 30%, respectively) compared to casein. Addition of phenylalanine to the lactalbumin diet sufficient to produce levels comparable to those found in casein resulted in a significant reduction in the numbers of plaque-forming cells to SRBCs and in a reduction of the phytohemagglutinin response following immunostimulation. This reduction in the immune response could not be attributed entirely to the added phenylalanine, since additional interactions with other amino acids were implicated.

The contribution of amino acid deficiencies to immune dysfunction observed in malnourished patients with various disease states had not been studied until recently. In a study of burn patients fed high (28%) or low (16.5%) protein diets, patients consuming the high protein diet gained weight, required fewer transfusions, and had improved survival rates [82]. This group of patients also had significantly elevated levels of total serum proteins, transferrin, C3, IgG, and serum opsonins. Further, specific amino acids correlated with the various improved parameters. For example, opsonic index positively correlated with lysine, arginine, alanine, and aspara-

gine, while IgG correlated with arginine, alanine, serine and glutamic acid. Nuwer et al. [68] found that stressed patients given hyperalimentation that was high in branched-chain amino acids had not only improved nitrogen retention, but also a marked improvement in skin test reactivity and absolute lymphocyte counts. Normal volunteers given arginine hydrochloride supplements for 1 week had a significant increase in lymphocyte blastogenic response to concanavalin A and phytohemagglutinin [7]. Thus, not only are the general catabolic requirements of malnourished individuals for energy and protein important, but also the requirements for individual nutrients that may have an important regulatory role for specific processes, such as immune function, must be considered.

CONCLUSION

Resistance to infection in patients after major surgery, with severe trauma, or with burn injury is of major clinical importance. Septic complications continue to be a leading cause of patient morbidity and mortality despite advances in surgical techniques, including antimicrobial therapy and extensive monitoring of the critically injured patient. Although much needs to be learned about the role of individual nutrients in the etiology of disease processes and subsequent susceptibility to infection, nutrition support that not only provides basic nutrient requirements but also provides nutrients with specific regulatory or pharmacologic-type effects could prove beneficial to patient recovery and outcome.

REFERENCES

1. Allen, J. I., Kay, N. E., and McClain, C. J. Severe zinc deficiency in humans: Association with a reversible T-lymphocyte dysfunction. *Ann. Intern. Med.* 95:154, 1981.
2. Aschkenasy, A. Dietary proteins and amino acids in leukopoiesis: Recent hematological and immunological data. *World Rev. Nutr. Diet* 21:151, 1975.
3. Axelrod, A. E. Immune processes in vitamin deficiency states. *Am. J. Clin. Nutr.* 24:265, 1971.
4. Balch, H. H. Relation of nutritional deficiency

in men to antibody production. *J. Immunol.* 64:397, 1950.

5. Balch, H. H. Antibody formation in malnourished patients. *Surg. Forum* 1:466, 1950.

6. Bang, B. G., Bang, F. B., and Foard, M. A. Lymphocyte depression induced in chickens in diets deficient in vitamin A and other components. *Ann. J. Pathol.* 68:147, 1972.

7. Barbul, A., Sisto, D. A., Wasserkrug, H. L., and Levenson, S. M. Arginine stimulates thymic immune function and ameliorates the obesity and the hyperglycemia of genetically obese mice. *J. Parenter. Enter. Nutr.* 5:492, 1981.

8. Barbul, A., Wasserkrug, H. L., Seifter, E., and Rettura, G. Immunostimulatory effects of arginine in normal and injured rats. *J. Surg. Res.* 729:228, 1980.

9. Barbul, A., Wasserkrug, H. L., Sisto, D. A., and Seifter, E. Thymic stimulatory actions of arginine. *J. Parenter. Enter. Nutr.* 4:446, 1980.

10. Beisel, W. R. Effect of infection on human protein metabolism. *Fed. Proc.* 25:682, 1966.

11. Beutler, B., and Cerami, A. Cachectin: More than a tumor necrosis factor. *N. Engl. J. Med.* 316:379, 1987.

12. Bistrian, B. R., Blackburn, G. L., Hallowell, E., and Heddle, R. Protein status of general surgical patients. *J.A.M.A.* 230:858, 1974.

13. Bistrian, B. R., Blackburn, G. L., Vitale, J., and Cochran, D. Prevalence of malnutrition in general medical patients. *J.A.M.A.* 235:1567, 1976.

14. Bistrian, B. R., Sherman, M., Blackburn, G. L., Marshall, R., and Shaw, C. Cellular immunity in adult marasmus. *Arch. Intern. Med.* 137:1408, 1977.

15. Bounous, G., and Kongshavn, P. A. L. Influence of dietary proteins on the immune response of mice. *J. Nutr.* 112:1747, 1982.

16. Brown, R. E., and Katz, M. Antigenic stimulation in undernourished children. *East Afr. Med. J.* 42:221, 1965.

17. Cannon, P. R., Wissler, R. W., Woolridge, R. L., and Benditt, E. P. The relationship of protein deficiency to surgical infection. *Ann. Surg.* 120:514, 1944.

18. Carney, J. M., Warner, M. S., Borut, T., et al. Cell-mediated immune defects and infection: A study of malnourished hospitalized children. *Am. J. Dis. Child.* 134:824, 1980.

19. Cerra, F. B., Siegel, J. H., Coleman, B., Border, J. R., and McMenamy, R. R. Septic autocannibalism: A failure of exogenous nutritional support. *Ann. Surg.* 192:570, 1980.

20. Chandra, R. K. Immunocompetence in undernutrition. *J. Pediatr.* 81:1194, 1972.

21. Chandra, R. K. Rosette-forming T-lymphocytes and cell-mediated immunity in malnutrition. *Br. Med. J.* 3:608, 1974.

22. Chandra, R. K. Lymphocyte subpopulations in human malnutrition: Cytotoxic and suppressor cells. *Pediatrics* 59:423, 1977.

23. Chandra, R. K. Cell-mediated immunity in nutritional imbalance. *Fed. Proc.* 39:3088, 1980.

24. Chandra, R. K. Nutritional regulation of immunity and infection in the gastrointestinal tract. *J. Pediatr. Gastroenterol. Nutr.* 2(Suppl. 1):S181, 1983.

25. Chandra, R. K. Numerical and functional deficiency in T helper cells in protein energy malnutrition. *Clin. Exp. Immunol.* 51:126, 1983.

26. Chandra, R. K., and Tejpar, S. Diet and immunocompetence. *Int. J. Immunopharmacol.* 5:175, 1983.

27. Christou, N. V. Host-defense mechanisms in surgical patients: A correlative study of the delayed hypersensitivity skin-test response, granulocyte function and sepsis. *Can. J. Surg.* 28:39, 1985.

28. Christou, N. V., Meakins, J. L., and MacLean, L. D. The predictive role of delayed hypersensitivity in preoperative patients. *Surg. Gynecol. Obstet.* 152:297, 1981.

29. Christou, N. V., and Yurt, R. W. Anergy testing in surgical patients. *Infect. Surg.* 2:692, 1983.

30. Clowes, G. H. A., George, B. C., Villee, C. A., Jr., and Saravis, C. A. Muscle proteolysis induced by a circulating peptide in patients with sepsis or trauma. *N. Engl. J. Med.* 308:545, 1983.

31. Clowes, G. H. A., Randall, H. T., and Cha, C. J. Amino acid and energy metabolism in septic and traumatized patients. *J. Parenter. Enter. Nutr.* 4:195, 1980.

32. Cooper, W. C., Good, R. A., and Mariani, T. Effects of protein insufficiency on immune responsiveness. *Am. J. Clin. Nutr.* 27:647, 1974.

33. Coovadia, H. M., and Soothill, J. F. The effect of amino acid restricted diets on the clearance of ^{125}I-labelled polyvinyl pyrrolidine in mice. *Clin. Exp. Immunol.* 723:562, 1976.

34. Dionigi, R., Zonta, A., and Dominioni, I. The effects of total parenteral nutrition on immunodepression due to malnutrition. *Ann. Surg.* 185:467, 1977.

35. Elia, M. Amino acid metabolism in trauma and sepsis. *Nutrition* 3:283, 1987.

36. Forse, R. A., Christou, N., Meakins, J. L., MacLean, L. D., and Shizgal, H. M. Reliability of skin testing as a measure of nutritional state. *Arch. Surg.* 116:1284, 1981.

37. Frank, M. D. *Complement in Current Concepts.* (Monograph) Kalamazoo, MI: Upjohn, 1985.

38. Freund, H. R., Ryan, J. A., and Fischer, J. E. Amino acid derangements in patients with sepsis: Treatment with branched-chain amino acid rich infusions. *Ann. Surg.* 188:423, 1978.

39. Freyre, E. A., Chabes, A. C., Poemape, O., and Chabes, A. Abnormal Rebuck skin window response in kwashiorkor. *J. Pediatr.* 82:523, 1973.
40. Gebhardt, B. M., and Newberne, P. M. Nutrition and immunological responsiveness: T cell function in the offspring of lipotrope- and protein-deficient rats. *Immunology* 26:489, 1974.
41. Gell, P. G., Parry, H., and Leitner, Z. A. Discussion on nutrition and resistance to infection. *Proc. R. Soc. Med.* 41:323, 1948.
42. Gershoff, S. N., Gill, T. J., Simonian, S. J., and Steinberg, A. I. Some effects of amino acid deficiencies on antibody formation in the rat. *J. Nutr.* 95:184, 1968.
43. Good, R. A., West, A., and Fernandes, G. Nutritional modulation of immune responses. *Fed. Proc.* 39:3098, 1980.
44. Grant, J. P., Custer, P. B., and Thurlow, J. Current techniques of nutritional assessment. *Surg. Clin. North Am.* 61:437, 1981.
45. Hak, L. J., Leffell, M. S., Lamanna, R. W., Teasley, K. M., Bazarre, C. H., and Mattern, W. D. Reversal of skin test anergy during maintenance hemodialysis by protein and calorie supplementation. *Am. J. Clin. Nutr.* 36:1089, 1982.
46. Hill, G. L., Blackett, R. L., Pickford, I., et al. Malnutrition in surgical patients: An unrecognised problem. *Lancet* 1:689, 1977.
47. Ing, A. F., Meakins, J. L., McLean, A. P., and Christou, N. V. Determinants of susceptibility to sepsis and mortality: Malnutrition vs. anergy. *J. Surg. Res.* 32:249, 1982.
48. Jose, D. G., and Good, R. A. Quantitative effects of nutritional essential amino acid deficiency upon immune response to tumors in mice. *J. Exp. Med.* 137:1, 1973.
49. Kahan, B. D. Nutrition and host defense mechanisms. *Surg. Clin. North Am.* 61:557, 1981.
50. Kenney, M. A., Magee, J. L., and Piedad-Pascual, F. Dietary amino acids and immune response in rats. *J. Nutr.* 100:1063, 1970.
51. Kenney, M. A., Roderuck, C. E., Arnrich, L., and Piedad, F. Effect of protein deficiency on the spleen and antibody formation in rats. *J. Nutr.* 95:173, 1968.
52. Kumagai, K., Abo, T., Sekizawa, T., and Sasaki, M. Studies of surface immunoglobulins on humans B lymphocytes. I. Dissociation of cell-bound immunoglobulins with acid pH or at 37°C. *J. Immunol.* 115:982, 1975.
53. Law, D. K., Dudrick, S. J., and Abdou, N. I. Immunocompetence of patients with protein-calorie malnutrition. *Ann. Intern. Med.* 79:545, 1973.
54. Law, D. K., Dudrick, S. J., and Abdou, N. I.

The effect of dietary protein depletion immunocompetence: The importance of nutritional repletion prior to immunologic induction. *Ann. Surg.* 179:168, 1974.
55. Long, C. L., Birkhahn, R. H., Geiger, J. W., and Blakemore, W. S. Contribution of skeletal muscle protein in elevated rates of whole body protein catabolism in trauma patients. *Am. J. Clin. Nutr.* 341:87, 1981.
56. MacLean, L. D. Delayed-type hypersensitivity testing in surgical patients. *Surg. Gynecol. Obstet.* 166:285, 1988.
57. Mathur, M., Ramalingaswami, V., and Deo, M. G. Influence of protein deficiency on 19S antibody-forming cells in rats and mice. *J. Nutr.* 102:841, 1971.
58. McFarlane, H. Cell-mediated immunity in clinical and experimental protein-calorie malnutrition. In R. M. Suskind (ed.), *Malnutrition and the Immune Response.* New York: Raven Press, 1977. P. 127.
59. McFarlane, I. I., and Hamid, J. Cell-mediated immune response in malnutrition. *Clin. Exp. Immunol.* 13:153, 1973.
60. McLoughlin, G. A., Wu, A. V., Saporoschetz, I., Nimberg, R., and Mannick, J. A. Correlation between anergy and a circulating immunosuppressive factor following major surgical trauma. *Ann. Surg.* 190:297, 1979.
61. Meakins, J. L., Pietsch, J. B., Bubenick, O., et al. Delayed hypersensitivity: Indicator of acquired failure of host defenses in sepsis and trauma. *Ann. Surg.* 186:241, 1977.
62. Mullen, J. P., Buzby, G. P., Matthews, D. C., Smale, B. F., and Rosato, E. F. Reduction of operative morbidity and mortality by combined preoperative and postoperative nutritional support. *Ann. Surg.* 192:604, 1980.
63. Mullin, T. J., and Kirkpatrick, J. R. The effect of nutritional support on immune competency in patients suffering from trauma, sepsis, or malignant disease. *Surgery* 117:266, 1981.
64. Neumann, C. G. Nonspecific host factors and infection in malnutrition. In R. M. Suskind, (ed.), *Malnutrition and the Immune Response.* New York: Raven Press, 1977. P. 355.
65. Neumann, C. G., Lawlor, G. J., Stiehm, E. R., et al. Immunologic response in malnourished children. *Am. J. Clin. Nutr.* 28:89, 1975.
66. Nohr, C. W., Tchervenkov, J. I., Meakins, J. L., and Christou, N. V. Malnutrition and humoral immunity: Short-term acute nutritional deprivation. *Surgery* 98:769, 1985.
67. Nohr, C. W., Tchervenkov, J. I., Meakins, J. L., and Christou, N. V. Malnutrition and humoral immunity: Long-term protein deprivation. *J. Surg. Res.* 40:432, 1986.
68. Nuwer, N., Cerra, F. B., Shronts, E. P., Lysne, J., Teasley, K. M., and Konstantinides,

F. N. Does modified amino acid total parenteral nutrition alter immune response in high level surgical stress? *J. Parenter. Enter. Nutr.* 7:521, 1983.

69. O'Mahony, J. B., Palder, S. B., Wood, J. J., et al. Depression of cellular immunity after multiple trauma in the absence of sepsis. *J. Trauma* 24:869, 1984.

70. Peterson, S. R., Kudsk, K. A., Carpenter, G., and Sheldon, G. E. Malnutrition and immunocompetence: Increased mortality following an infectious challenge during hyperalimentation. *J. Trauma* 21:528, 1981.

71. Petro, T. M., and Bhattacharjee, J. K. Effect of dietary essential amino acid limitations upon the susceptibility to *Salmonella typhimurium* and the effect upon humoral and cellular immune responses in mice. *Infect. Immun.* 32:251, 1981.

72. Purtilo, D. T., and Connor, D. H. Fatal infections in protein-calorie malnourished children with thymolymphatic atrophy. *Arch. Dis. Child.* 50:149, 1975.

73. Rafii, M., Hashemi, S., Nahani, J., and Mohagheghpour, N. Immune responses in malnourished children. *Clin. Immunol. Immunopathol.* 8:1, 1977.

74. Rettura, G., Padawer, J., Barbul, A., Levenson, S. M., and Seifter, E. Supplemental arginine increases thymic cellularity in normal and murine sarcoma virus-inoculated mice and increases the resistance to murine sarcoma virus tumor. *J. Parenter. Enter. Nutr.* 3:409, 1979.

75. Reynolds, J. V., Zhang, S., and Thom, A. Arginine as an immunomodulator. *Surg. Forum* 38:415, 1987.

76. Salimonu, L.S., Ojo-Amaize, E., Johnson, A. O. K., Laditan, A. A. O., Akinwolere, O. A. O., and Wigzell, H. Depressed natural killer cell activity in children with protein-calorie malnutrition. *Cell Immunol.* 82:210, 1983.

77. Schopfer, K., and Douglas, S. D. In vitro studies of lymphocytes from children with kwashiorkor. *Clin. Immunol. Immunopathol.* 5:21–30, 1976.

78. Seifter, E., Rettura, G., Barbul, A., and Levenson, S. M. Arginine: An essential amino acid for injured rats. *Surgery* 85:224, 1978.

79. Sirisinha, S., Suskind, R., Edelman, R., Charupatana, C., and Olson, R. E. Complement and C3-proactivator levels in children with protein-calorie malnutrition and effect of dietary treatment. *Lancet* 1:1016, 1973.

80. Smythe, P. M., Schonland, M., Brereton-Stiles, G. G., et al. Thymolymphatic efficiency and depression of cell-mediated immunity in protein-calorie malnutrition. *Lancet* 2:939, 1971.

80b. Solomkin, J. S., Dellinger, E. P., Christou, N. V., Busuttil, R. W. Results of a multicenter trial comparing imipenem/cilastatin to tobramycin/clindamycin for intra-abdominal infections. *Ann. Surg.*, 212:581, 1990.

81. Stiehm, E. R. Humoral immunity in malnutrition. *Fed. Proc.* 39:3093, 1980.

82. Stinnett, J. D., Alexander, J. W., Watanabe, C., et al. Plasma and skeletal muscle amino acids following severe burn injury in patients and animals. *Ann. Surg.* 195:75, 1982.

83. Suskind, R., Sirishinha, S., Vithayasai, V., et al. Immunoglobulins and antibody response in children with protein-calorie malnutrition. *Am. J. Clin. Nutr.* 29:836, 1976.

84. Tchervenkov, J. I., Latter, D. A., Psychogios, J., and Christou, N. V. The influence of long-term protein deprivation on in vivo phagocytic cell delivery to inflammatory lesions. *Surgery* 103:463, 1988.

85. Weinsier, R. L., Hunker, E. M., Krumdieck, C. L., and Butterworth, C. E. Hospital malnutrition: A prospective evaluation of general medical patients during the course of hospitalization. *Am. J. Clin. Nutr.* 32:418, 1979.

86. White, A., and Doughtery, T. F. The pituitary adrenotrophic hormone control of the rate of release of serum globulins from lymphoid tissue. *Endocrinology* 36:207, 1945.

87. Williams, E. A. J., Gebhardt, B. M., Morron, B., and Newberne, P. M. Effects of early marginal methionine-choline deprivation on the development of the immune system in the rat. *Am. J. Clin. Nutr.* 732:1214, 1979.

88. Wohl, M. D., Reinhold, J. G., and Rose, S. B. Antibody response in patients with hypoproteinemia. *Arch. Intern. Med.* 83:402, 1949.

89. Woodruff, J. F. Thymolymphatic deficiency and depression of cell-mediated immunity in protein-calorie malnutrition. (Letter) *Lancet* 1:92, 1972.

90. Wunder, J. A., Stinnett, J. D., and Alexander, J. W. The effect of malnutrition on variables of host defense in the guinea pig. *Surgery* 84:542, 1978.

9

Nutritional Assessment

Graham L. Hill

In the late 1960s, when effective means for the nutritional repletion of hospitalized patients became available, fresh interest developed in the objective evaluation of nutritional state. For years it was commonly taught that nutritional deficient states were rare and were mainly associated with specific micronutrient deficiencies secondary to gross dietary inadequacy. The new interest in hospital malnutrition revealed that macronutrient deficiency, in particular protein energy malnutrition, was much more common than previously thought and was often unrecognized and untreated. To properly treat patients with protein energy malnutrition, it was necessary to find objective, reliable, and clinically practical methods for the assessment of nutritional state. What was required were techniques that would not only diagnose, characterize, and quantify the form of malnutrition, but also provide a mechanism to monitor the therapeutic response to nutritional support. Even after much trial and error, and a considerable amount of research,

the science of clinical nutritional assessment is still in an early phase of development. Nevertheless, techniques that are now becoming available are proving to be of considerable help in hospital practice. Before these can be properly understood, it is first necessary to understand something of the pathophysiology of malnutrition in hospitalized patients.

PATHOPHYSIOLOGY OF MALNUTRITION IN HOSPITALIZED PATIENTS

Uncomplicated Starvation

The body mass comprises the fat mass and the fat-free body mass. The latter is composed of protein, water, minerals, and glycogen. In uncomplicated starvation where reduced food intake results in negative energy and protein balance, the consumption of host tissue results in loss of body weight. Very early in starvation, after liver glycogen stores

139

are depleted, body energy requirements are supplied by the catabolism of adipose tissue, triglyceride, and muscle protein. Later in starvation, as the brain adapts to the use of ketone bodies and no longer requires glucose, catabolism of muscle protein is reduced considerably [6]. The net change in body composition in uncomplicated starvation is therefore a reduction both in adipose tissue and in muscle tissue, although the latter is relatively preserved when starvation is prolonged. Total body water remains almost unchanged, although it is redistributed. As weight is lost, there is a relative expansion of extracellular water [38]. At the organ and tissue level, most organs have a percentage loss of mass roughly similar to that of the total body, with the exception of the brain [24]. Accompanying the loss of protein from vital structures are physiologic impairments. In one study, a loss of 25% of body weight over 6 months resulted in marked deterioration in maximum oxygen uptake, Harvard fitness test scores, and muscular strength [21]. More recently, fundamental impairments, including impairments in skeletal muscle function, respiratory muscle function, wound healing, and psychological function, were shown to occur when body weight was lost [14, 39]. When weight loss is accompanied by clinically obvious physiologic impairment, postoperative complications are increased and postoperative stay is prolonged [39].

Septic Starvation

The simple scheme depicting otherwise uncomplicated starvation becomes vastly more complex in patients with underlying disease. Severe stress and hypercatabolic states change the rate and pattern of tissue loss, even in uncomplicated semistarvation. When major trauma, sepsis, or metastatic neoplastic disease is present, protein catabolism occurs at a much higher rate, resulting in severe depletion of body protein stores [32]. The consequences of this on organ function are therefore greater. The altered metabolic and hormonal profile is such that renourishment

during the stress period is associated with little or no repletion of protein mass but excessive rates of glycogen and fat formation [35]. Thus, identifying the presence of metabolic stress is important in the proper assessment of nutritional state.

From this simplified presentation of the pathophysiologic basis of protein energy malnutrition, it will be seen that, for its proper assessment, information concerning energy and protein balance, body composition, organ function, and metabolic stress needs to be obtained.

PRINCIPLES OF NUTRITIONAL ASSESSMENT

In the clinical evaluation of nutritional state, the clinician aims to assess protein and energy balance, body composition, physiologic function, and the presence or absence of metabolic stress. A schema adapted from Heymsfield and Williams [16] is shown in Figure 9-1. The purpose of nutritional assessment is to find where the patient is in terms of body composition and function. Circle A is taken as the range of body composition and organ function compatible with health. Here energy, protein, and water balance are zero and body weight is stable. If energy and protein balance become negative, weight will decrease until circle B when all available stores of fat and protein are depleted and there is marked deterioration of organ function as a consequence. The patient then succumbs if negative energy and protein balance persist beyond circle B. A complication of malnutrition may intervene before circle B is reached, which will alter the natural history of the disease—point C. The aim of nutritional assessment is to find where the patient lies between points A, B, and C and to determine the direction and rate of change that is occurring. It is for this reason that protein energy balance, body composition, and organ function must be completely assessed whenever nutritional state needs proper evaluation. Because metabolic stress has such profound therapeutic implications, it must be carefully looked for as well. In broad terms,

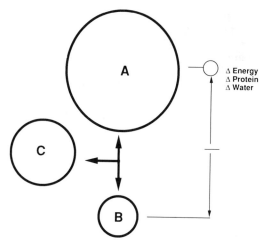

Figure 9-1. This model describes the components of the clinical assessment of nutritional state. Circle A represents the range of body composition and physiologic function found in health; weight is stable and the balance of energy, protein, and water is zero. If the patient sustains a period of negative metabolic balance, tissue stores of energy and protein become depleted and physiologic impairment occurs as a consequence. Circle B describes the minimal range of body composition and physiologic function that is compatible with survival. A malnutrition-related complication, C, may interrupt the course of the patient moving between points A and B. The clinical assessment is designed to find the patient's status in relation to points A, B, and C. (Adapted from Heymsfield, S. B., and Williams, P. J. Nutritional assessment by clinical and biochemical methods. In M. E. Shils and V. R. Young (eds.), *Modern Nutrition in Health and Disease* (7th ed). Philadelphia: Lea and Febiger, 1988.) Pp. 817–860.

each of these components can be adequately evaluated by clinical means [1, 18, 39]. The clinical methods are described first, and secondary assessment techniques that are sometimes used in specialized centers or for research are then briefly discussed.

CLINICAL ASSESSMENT OF ENERGY AND PROTEIN BALANCE

In many situations a full dietary assessment (as described below) can be most helpful, but

Table 9-1. Relationship between Meal Size and Loss of Body Weight over Time

Meal Size (% of Normal)	Weight Loss (%) over Time		
	3 Mo.	6 Mo.	12 Mo. or More
30	25	35	40
50	15	25	30
70	10	15	20

Adapted from the data of Keys, A., Brozek, J., Henschel, A., Mickelsen, O., and Taylor, H. L. *The Biology of Human Starvation*. Minneapolis: University of Minnesota Press, 1950.

the clinician can gain a fair idea of energy and protein balance by assessing the frequency and size of the patient's meals and comparing the results with an estimate of rate of loss of body weight. With data derived from the "Minnesota starvation experiment" [21], the relationship between reduced meal size and rate of weight loss can be seen (Table 9-1). Negative protein and energy balance may also occur in sepsis, trauma, or hypermetabolism and also when there are increased losses of fluids from the body. Bedside assessment of the magnitude of these losses is almost impossible.

SECONDARY ASSESSMENT TECHNIQUES

A more comprehensive assessment of energy and protein balance is performed by a dietitian, with three techniques available: the 24-hour recall with a food frequency crosscheck, analysis of a food record or diary, and a calorie count. Once collected, the diet information is processed by the use of food composition tables, and the amount and adequacy of total energy intake of carbohydrate, fat, and protein are assessed by comparison to recommended daily allowances. Abnormally large losses of energy and protein are identified from the history and by laboratory studies. Nausea, vomiting and diarrhea, and a history of intestinal disease, renal disease, diabetes, fever, or serious injury are all clues to the presence of increased losses of energy

Figure 9-2.   Clinical Methods for Assessing Total Energy Expenditure

Total energy expenditure (TEE) = Resting metabolic expenditure (RME)
                                 + Dietary-induced thermagenesis (DIT)
                                 + Activity energy expenditure (AEE)

RME: Calculate basal energy expenditure from tables and add disease-related thermal losses:

   Non-catabolic illness—Multiply BEE × 0.2
   Elective surgery   —Multiply BEE × 0.2
   Major trauma   —Multiply BEE × 0.3
   Serious sepsis   —Multiply BEE × 0.6

DIT: Multiply BEE × 0.2

AEE: Patient only sitting out of bed—*Add* duration × 0.1 BEE
       Up and about around the ward—*Add* duration × 1.4 BEE

or protein in chemical or thermal forms. The usual method for assessing total energy expenditure is to calculate approximate values for basal energy expenditure, thermic effect of food, physical activity, and fever or injury, as outlined in Figure 9-2. The calculation of energy and protein balance by more sophisticated techniques can only be done properly on a metabolic ward. Indirect calorimetry is often used clinically to assess resting metabolic expenditure and the thermal response to feeding, but energy expenditure due to physical activity is hard to assess accurately, thereby making assessment of total energy expenditure quite difficult at times.

ASSESSMENT OF BODY COMPOSITION

Clinical

Body Weight

It is important to stress that weight and height should be recorded in the chart of every hospitalized patient, and the weight of all patients undergoing nutritional support should be measured daily. Weight loss can be determined easily if the patient's weight is measured before and after the occurrence of the loss. Usually, however, patients have already lost weight when they are first seen, and then the size of the loss must be evaluated by comparing measured weight with some estimate of original weight. The accu-

racy of the result depends on the accuracy with which the original weight was measured. There is a substantial body of research on the measurement of original weight (well weight, ideal weight) and it is now clear that it is more reliable to estimate weight loss by using the patient's recalled well weight than using published tables of "ideal weight." Nevertheless, estimating weight loss can be quite misleading in individual cases and it is therefore important to relate this to the physical examination of the patient [26].

General Appearance

In simple starvation, 20% loss of body weight is associated with marked decreases in muscle tissue and subcutaneous fat, making the patient haggard and emaciated in appearance. The face is thin and cheekbones are prominent. The padding around the shoulder girdle is reduced and the skeleton is prominent. The wasting of soft tissue is particularly marked in the region of the buttocks, which are thin and flat. Hypermetabolic patients can be profoundly protein-depleted, yet without this classic appearance because they may have relative preservation of body fat mass and marked expansion of total body water.

Body Fat Stores

Gross loss of body fat can be observed not only from the patient's appearance, but also by palpating a number of skinfolds. When the dermis can be felt between the fingers on pinching the triceps and biceps skinfolds, considerable loss from body stores of fat will have occurred. In this situation, it has been shown that the body weight of the patient is composed of less than 10% fat. [*Editor's Note:* This is a useful bedside maneuver that seems largely to have escaped notice despite all the inappropriate publicity given the so-called measurement of triceps skinfold thickness (with dime-store plastic calipers).]

Body Protein Stores

In a similar manner, protein stores can be assessed by inspection and palpation of a number of muscle groups. The temporal muscles, deltoids, suprascapular and infrascapular muscles, the bellies of biceps and triceps, and the interosseous muscles should all be looked at and palpated. The long muscles in particular are considered to be profoundly protein-depleted when the tendons are prominent to palpation.

Secondary Assessment Techniques

Anthropometry

Body fat and fat-free mass can be assessed by anthropometry. Two types of measurement are usually made—skinfold thicknesses and limb circumferences. Measurement of a single skinfold thickness (usually triceps) can be used directly for comparison to reference tables and for longitudinal follow-up. A single skinfold thickness is a relatively poor predictor of the absolute amount and rate of change in total body fat [10]. Combining a limb skinfold thickness with a corresponding circumference allows the calculation of limb fat areas. It is also possible to measure a number of skinfolds (usually triceps, biceps, and subscapular) and to derive from them an estimate of total body fat [10]. The measurement of fat-free mass is also accomplished by the skinfold method. Total body fat is calculated and this is subtracted from body weight, giving a measurement for the fat-free body mass. There are considerable problems in using anthropometry because of large errors both in accuracy and in precision involved in individual patients [9]. Such measurements

may be very valuable, however, in patients undergoing long-term nutrition or follow-up over months or years, or in assessing the incidence of malnutrition in a hospital.

Chemical Methods

Other secondary techniques for assessing body composition include determining 24-hour urinary creatinine levels, creatinine height index, and serum proteins levels. Although albumin levels are more likely to be affected by things other than protein energy malnutrition, the short half-life plasma proteins such as prealbumin and retinol-binding protein are affected by recent changes in energy intake [20]. They can also be useful in following the patient longitudinally [3, 34].

Research Techniques

There are a host of research techniques for measuring body composition, including measurements of bioelectrical impedance [31] to measure body water and body fat, measurements of total body potassium to estimate the body cell mass [25], measurements of total body nitrogen by in vivo neutron activation analysis to measure body protein [2], and a number of isotopic dilution methods that are used to measure the compartments of body water [33]. These are all research techniques and as yet have no place in routine patient care.

ASSESSMENT OF PHYSIOLOGIC FUNCTION

Clinical

The question of functional impairment secondary to loss of body protein is the most important part of the assessment of nutritional state. The loss of function to be noted is that which occurred over the same time period as the loss of weight. The patient should be questioned about wound healing, easy tiredness, or changes in exercise tolerance. Weight loss without evidence of a functional abnormality probably is of no consequence [39]. Function is observed during the physical examination and by watching the patient's activity around the ward. Grip strength can be assessed by asking the patient to squeeze strongly the examiner's index and middle fingers for at least 10 seconds. Impairment is judged in light of the patient's age, sex, and body habitus. Respiratory muscle function is assessed by asking the patient to cough, holding a strip of paper 8 cm from the lips; this should normally be blown away with some force. Severe impairment is present when the paper does not move. Shortness of breath is noted at rest. Severe impairment is indicated when normal conversation is not possible. Excursion is noted by asking the patient to take as deep a breath as possible; when there is virtually no chest expansion, severe impairment exists.

Secondary Assessment Techniques

Objective measurements of wound healing [11, 41], grip strength [22], skeletal muscle function [29], and respiratory muscle function [40] have all received prominence recently, but they appear to have little more to add to a proper physical examination [39].

ASSESSMENT OF METABOLIC STRESS

Clinical

History and physical examination reveal evidence of metabolic stress. It is present if the patient has had major trauma or surgery in the previous week or any of the following criteria:

1. Highest temperature of greater than 38°C in the last 24 hours
2. Pulse rate greater than 100/min in the last 24 hours
3. Respiratory rate greater than 30/min in the last 24 hours

4. White blood cell count greater than 12,000 or less than 3000 in the last 24 hours
5. Positive blood culture in the last 24 hours
6. Active inflammatory bowel disease
7. Defined focus of infection

Secondary Assessment Techniques

In healthy subjects, the fat-free body mass is related closely to the basal energy expenditure [28]. Direct measurements of basal metabolic rate (by indirect calorimetry) and fat-free body mass (measured by anthropometry or by electric impedance) [31] will show a marked increase in this relationship if the patient has major metabolic stress.

NUTRITIONAL SYNDROMES

We have seen that hospitalized patients can be affected by both nutritional and metabolic processes. Semistarvation in patients with anorexia, vomiting, or partial obstruction results in gradual wasting of muscle and fat stores with lowered metabolic rate. Metabolic stress results in rapid breakdown of body tissues and an inability to preserve vital protein stores. Renourishment when the patient is stressed is not associated with a repletion of protein stores, but an excessive rate of glycogen and fat formation. From a combination of these two processes—semistarvation and metabolic stress—a number of nutritional syndromes can be identified.

Nutritional Depletion without Stress

Patients with this syndrome have an overall deficit in their intake and/or utilization of food. Weight loss is 10% or more and marked by clinical evidence of subcutaneous fat loss and wasting of muscle bellies. Metabolic rate is low and urinary nitrogen loss is small. Plasma proteins remain normal. Examples of this syndrome include cachexia as found in patients with strictures of the esophagus or cancer of the stomach. If the condition is severe, the patient looks like a walking skeleton.

Normal Nutritional State, but with Added Stress

These patients are usually quite easily picked out, as they are either septic or have recently been so. In surgical patients, apart from those who have undergone recent major surgery, the usual causes of this syndrome are acute attacks of inflammatory bowel disease and pancreatic abscess. Clinically, such patients may have near normal stores of muscle and fat, but there are clear signs of sepsis and plasma albumin levels are low. If this situation persists, muscle wasting follows although fat stores are relatively preserved.

Nutritional Depletion with Stress

This situation occurs in two ways: (1) depleted patients who have a metabolic insult such as sepsis or major operation, or (2) normally nourished patients who have severe metabolic stress and are rapidly depleted of nutritional reserves. Examples of the first situation are depleted patients with carcinoma of the esophagus or stomach who develop septic complications after esophagectomy or gastrectomy. Examples of the second situation occur in normally nourished patients with prolonged severe pancreatitis with sepsis or prolonged exacerbation of inflammatory bowel disease. These patients are obviously not well, with tachycardia, fever, and low intravascular volume. The degree of depletion, however, may not be apparent from the history and may be masked on physical examination by preservation of body fat stores or edema. However, muscle wasting, along with a low plasma albumin levels, is a constant feature of all these patients.

Major Trauma and Sepsis

Intensive care patients with major trauma and serious sepsis are often normally nourished at the outset. The metabolic changes outlined above result in a rapid erosion of body protein stores with hypoalbuminemia, wasting of muscle bellies, and erosion of visceral protein. Fat stores are relatively preserved and palpation of fat folds is not helpful in assessment, as these patients invariably have large excesses of body water [36].

Therapeutic Implications

Recognition of these nutritional syndromes is valuable in planning nutritional therapy. Figure 9-3 shows how patients who are nutritionally depleted without evidence of stress will gain body protein after a short course of intravenous nutrition, whereas intensive care patients with sepsis or trauma show no such response. These patients may lose considerable amounts of protein over a short time in spite of aggressive nutritional therapy [35].

FOLLOWING THE PATIENT ON TREATMENT

For nutritional therapy to be effective, it is necessary to ensure that the nutrients being provided are adequate and are being utilized effectively. A number of studies show that wound healing [15] and muscle function [7] may be measurably improved with intravenous nutrition, resulting in the clinical observation that the patient looks and feels better, and on examination appears to be physically stronger. On the laboratory side, nitrogen balance is sometimes used as a marker of dynamic nutritional assessment, but the technique must be meticulous so that results are meaningful; such standards are not generally available outside specialized units. As practical alternatives to nitrogen balance, four serum transport proteins have been suggested as markers of nutritional progress and are now being used in some nutritional assessment programs [3, 34]. These are: (1) albumin, (2) transferrin, (3) prealbumin, and (4) retinol-binding protein. Others have suggested that transferrin and prealbumin are good dynamic indices of nutritional state, and this was confirmed in a recent study [8]. It can be seen in Table 9-2 that in patients requiring intravenous nutrition for 2 weeks,

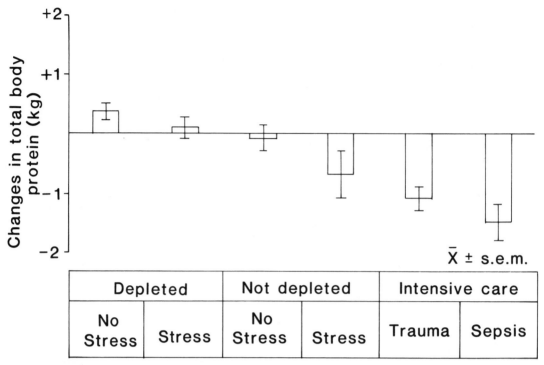

Figure 9-3. Changes in body stores of protein with 2 weeks of total intravenous nutrition for each of the nutritional syndromes. Only patients who are depleted, without evidence of metabolic stress, can be expected to gain body protein. (Adapted from Hill, G. L. Body composition research at the University of Auckland—some implications for modern surgical practice. *Aust. N. Z. J. Surg.* 58:131, 1988.)

a positive nitrogen balance was reflected by a rise in prealbumin in 88% of cases, whereas a negative nitrogen balance was associated with a falling prealbumin in 70%. Predictive values in the group indicate that 93% of patients with a rising prealbumin had a positive nitrogen balance.

ASSESSMENT OF NUTRITIONAL STATE PRIOR TO SURGERY

It is claimed that indices of nutritional state can identify patients at high risk of postoperative complications and that these indices are useful tools for the selection of candidates for

Table 9-2. Sensitivity, Specificity, and Predictive Values of a Weekly Rise in Plasma Protein Levels in Detecting Positive Nitrogen Balance in Patients Receiving Intravenous Nutrition for 2 Weeks

	Albumin	*Prealbumin*	*Transferrin*
Sensitivity (%)	61	88	67
Specificity (%)	45	70	55
Positive predictive value (%)	86	93	87
Negative predictive value (%)	17	56	27

Adapted from Church, J. M., and Hill, G. L. Assessing the efficacy of intravenous nutrition in general surgical patients: Dynamic nutritional assessment with plasma proteins. *J. Parenter. Enter. Nutr.* 11:135, 1987.

Table 9-3. Comparison of Nutritional Indices as Indicators of Surgical Risk[a]

	Indicator	Cutoff[b]	Sensitivity %	Specificity %	Positive Predictive Value %	Negative Predictive Value %	Overall Predictive Value %	Statistical Data[c] χ^2	p
Age	Age	> 73 yr	30	83	29	84	74	3.5	NS
Anthropometry	WL	> 16%	31	84	30	85	75	4.4	< 0.05
	BMI	< 3rd %ile	30	75	22	83	67	0.5	NS
	TSF	< 3rd %ile	21	80	19	84	70	0	NS
	MAMC	< 3rd %ile	26	83	25	87	73	1.1	NS
Indices of function	GS (males)	< 64 kPa	40	87	38	88	79	4.3	< 0.05
	GS (females)	< 47 kPa	30	83	21	89	76	0.3	NS
	Albumin	< 35 g/liter	33	82	29	85	73	4.2	< 0.05
	Transferrin	< 174 mg/dl	41	86	40	87	78	14.2	< 0.001
	Prealbumin	< 12 mg/dl	43	87	43	87	79	18.9	< 0.001
Prognostic indices	Philadelphia	> 45	35	83	32	85	75	6.5	< 0.05
	Boston	> −0.7	30	84	30	84	74	3.8	< 0.05
	Leeds	< −1.0	46	85	40	87	78	18.0	< 0.001
Clinical judgment	Surgeon's assessment	> 98 mm	32	83	27	86	75	2.0	NS
	Thorough clinical assessment	> 60%	41	85	32	89	78	6.3	< 0.025

WL = weight loss; BMI = body mass index; TSF = triceps skinfold; MAMC = midarm muscle circumference; GS = grip strength; kPa = kilopascals; NS = not significant.

[a] Note that in this retrospective study of 218 patients undergoing major abdominal surgery, grip strength, plasma proteins, and a thorough examination all pointed out a group of patients at increased risk.

[b] Each indicator was set such that 17–20% of patients were in high-risk group.

[c] Complication rates in high-risk versus low-risk groups.

From Pettigrew, R. A., and Hill, G. L. Indicators of surgical risk and clinical judgement: A prospective comparative study. *Br. J. Surg.* 73:47, 1986.

Table 9-4. Postoperative Course of the Three Clinical Categories of Patients*

Clinical Categories	Group I (n = 43) Weight Loss < 10% Normal Function	Group II (n = 17) Weight Loss > 10% Normal Function	Group III (n = 42) Weight Loss > 10% Abnormal Function	p
Major complications	6	3	15	< 0.05
Septic complications	8	4	18	< 0.02
Pneumonia	4	1	10	< 0.05
Wound infection	4	1	7	NS
Death	0	1	4	NS
Hospital stay (d; mean ± SEM)	15.9 ± 1.3 (NS)	12.7 ± 2.5 (p < 0.05)	19.2 ± 2.2 (p < 0.05)	

NS = not significant.
*Prospective trial conducted in order to determine whether clinical assessment of weight loss and physiologic function would identify patients with objective evidence of abnormal body composition and function, who were also at an increased risk of postoperative complications.
Adapted from Windsor, J. A., and Hill, G. L. Weight loss with physiologic impairment: A basic indicator of surgical risk. *Ann. Surg.* 207:290, 1988.

preoperative nutritional support. Profound weight loss [37], some anthropometric indices [17, 23], tests of muscle function [12, 23], and measurements of plasma proteins including albumin, [4, 22], transferrin [19], and prealbumin [27], as well as combinations of these (i.e., prognostic nutritional indices) [5, 13, 27], have all been used as indicators of risk of postoperative nutrition-associated complications. It is said by those who use them that these indicate the need for nutritional repletion prior to the operation itself. A comparison of these indicators of risk was recently made (Table 9-3) [27]. Measurements of weight loss and a variety of anthropometric indices are not clear indicators of risk, but

Table 9-5. Objective Validation of the Nutritional Status of the Three Clinical Patient Groups[a]

Clinical Categories	Group I Weight Loss < 10% Normal Function	Group II Weight Loss > 10% Normal Function	Group III Weight Loss > 10% Abnormal Function
Weight loss (%)	3.9 ± 0.7_____b_____13.4 ± 2.4_____NS_____14.8 ± 1.1		
Body fat stores Fat index (%)	117 ± 11_____NS_____102 ± 26_____NS_____84 ± 16		
Body protein stores Protein index (%)	88 ± 3_____NS_____78 ± 6_____NS_____68 ± 3		
Fat-free mass (kg)	51.4 ± 1.9_____NS_____47.8 ± 2.9_____NS_____41.3 ± 1.5		

NS = not significant; fat index = measured total body fat/predicted total body fat; protein index = measured total body protein/predicted total body protein.
[a]Values are given as mean ± SEM.
[b]p < 0.01.
[c]p < 0.05.
Adapted from Windsor, J. A., and Hill, G. L. Weight loss with physiologic impairment: A basic indicator of surgical risk. *Ann. Surg.* 207:290, 1988.

Table 9-6. Objective Validation of the Functional Status of the Three Clinical Patient Categories[a]

Clinical Categories	Group I Weight Loss < 10% Normal Function	Group II Weight Loss > 10% Normal Function	Group III Weight Loss > 10% Abnormal Function
Skeletal muscle function			
Grip strength (kg)	32.8 ± 1.8 —NS—	34.2 ± 1.9 —b—	22.9 ± 1.8
		⌊————b————⌋	
Relaxation time (msec)	104.5 ± 2.6 —NS—	100.4 ± 2.8 —b—	116.4 ± 2.8
		⌊————b————⌋	
Respiratory Function			
Respiratory muscle strength index (%)	106.9 ± 7.0 —NS—	98.1 ± 7.6 —b—	72.2 ± 8.6
		⌊————b————⌋	
FEV$_1$ (% predicted)	97.8 ± 33 —NS—	98.0 ± 5.7 —NS—	88.8 ± 5.3
		⌊————NS————⌋	
Vital capacity (% predicted)	108.8 ± 2.6 —NS—	108.7 ± 5.6 —b—	82.6 ± 3.6
		⌊————c————⌋	
FEV$_1$/VC (%)	75.9 ± 1.8 —NS—	78.3 ± 2.8 —NS—	73.8 ± 2.1
		⌊————NS————⌋	
PEFR (% predicted)	90.9 ± 2.5 —NS—	89.0 ± 4.9 —b—	75.2 ± 3.4
		⌊————b————⌋	
Maximum voluntary ventilation (% predicted)	81.1 ± 3.8 —NS—	84.4 ± 6.8 —NS—	63.5 ± 4.3
		⌊————c————⌋	
Psychological function			
POMS fatigue score	5.8 ± 1.5 —NS—	7.5 ± 1.8 —NS—	9.8 ± 1.4
		⌊————b————⌋	

NS = not significant; FEV$_1$ = forced expiratory volume in 1 sec; VC = vital capacity; PEFR = peak expiratory flow rate; POMS = profile of mood score.
[a]Values are given as mean ± SEM.
[b]$p < 0.05$.
[c]$p < 0.01$.
Adapted from Windsor, J. A., and Hill, G. L. Weight loss with physiologic impairment: A basic indicator of surgical risk. *Ann. Surg.* 207:290, 1988.

measurements of grip strength and low levels of plasma proteins are to some extent indicators of risk of postoperative complications. The various prognostic indices that are largely determined by plasma protein levels have little more to offer. It can be seen, however, that patients particularly at risk could be picked out by thorough physical examination and nutritional assessment. It was found in this study that a thorough clinical examination that assessed major-organ function proved to be as effective as any other indicator in identifying subjects at risk. *For clinical purposes, then, a fairly adequate assessment of malnutrition and its associated risks can be obtained from a good history of dietary intake and energy output, and a careful physical examination to assess the effects of protein depletion on each of the main-organ systems.*

Recently, a formal prospective trial was undertaken to determine if clinical assessment of weight loss and physiologic function could identify patients who had objective evidence of abnormal body composition and function, and who were also at increased risk of postoperative complications [39]. Of 101 patients awaiting gastrointestinal surgery, 42 had weight loss greater than 10% and also had clear evidence of physiologic dysfunction. These 42 patients had significantly more postoperative complications and a significantly longer hospital stay than the other pa-

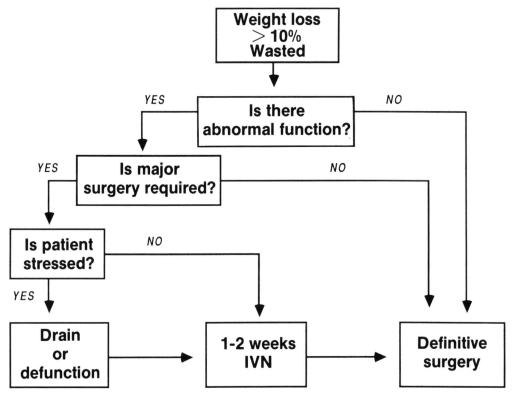

Figure 9-4. Indications for preoperative nutritional repletion: simple clinical protocol. Weight loss associated with clinically obvious physiologic impairment places the patient facing a very major surgical procedure at considerable risk. A period of nutritional repletion is indicated, providing the patient is not metabolically stressed. If metabolic stress is present, this must first be controlled before nutritional repletion will be effective. (Adapted from Hill, G. L., Malnutrition and surgical risk: Guidelines for nutritional therapy. *Ann. R. Coll. Surg. Engl.* 69:263, 1987.) IVN = intravenous nutrition.

tients, whether or not weight had been lost (Table 9-4). [*Editor's Note:* The lack of statistical significance in several categories in Table 9-4 appears to be due to a somewhat higher rate of complications in the normal (weight loss < 10%) group. This finding is similar to that in the study by Ryan and Taft [30] in which those patients with some weight loss appeared to fare best. Is it because with less fat, surgery is more straightforward?] Tables 9-5 and 9-6 show that objective measurements of body stores of fat and protein, psychological function, and respiratory and skeletal muscle function confirmed the validity of the classification into risk groups. Thus, it does appear that weight loss is a basic indicator of surgical risk, providing it is associated with clinically obvious organ dysfunction. Although a short course of nutritional repletion has been shown to decrease body protein stores and improve some aspects of organ function in depleted nonstressed patients (see Fig 9-3), it remains to be seen whether or not this results in fewer postoperative complications and a shorter hospital stay. Until that is known, a simple clinical protocol should be used (Fig. 9-4). Marked weight loss associated with clinically obvious physiologic impairment places the patient at a disadvantage, and, providing he or she is not stressed, it can be anticipated that nutritional repletion will be accompanied by protein gain and functional improvement. If such a patient faces a long and complicated operation, then a short period of nutritional repletion is recommended.

REFERENCES

1. Baker, J. P., Detsky, A. S., Whitwell, J., et al. A comparison of the predictive value of nutritional assessment techniques. *Hum. Nutr.: Clin. Nutr.* 36C:233, 1982.
2. Beddoe, A. H., and Hill, G. L. Clinical measurement of body composition using in vivo neutron activation analysis. *J. Parenter. Enter. Nutr.* 9:504, 1985.
3. Bourry, J., Milano, G., Caldani, C., and Schneider, M. Assessment of nutritional proteins during the parenteral nutrition of cancer patients. *Ann. Clin. Lab. Sci.* 12:158, 1982.
4. Brown, R., Bancewicz, J., Hamid, J., et al. Failure of delayed hypersensitivity skin testing to predict postoperative sepsis and mortality. *Br. Med. J.* 284:851, 1982.
5. Buzby, G. P., Mullen, J. L., Matthews, D. S., Hobbs, C. L., and Rosato, E. F. Prognostic nutritional index in gastrointestinal surgery. *Am. J. Surg.* 139:160, 1980.
6. Cahill, G. F. Starvation in man. *N. Engl. J. Med.* 282:668, 1970.
7. Church, J. M., Choong, S. Y., and Hill, G. L. Abnormalities of muscle metabolism and histology in malnourished patients awaiting surgery: Effects of a course of intravenous nutrition. *Br. J. Surg.* 71:563, 1984.
8. Church, J. M., and Hill, G. L. Assessing the efficacy of intravenous nutrition in general surgical patients: Dynamic nutritional assessment with plasma proteins. *J. Parenter. Enter. Nutr.* 11:135, 1987.
9. Collins, J. P., McCarthy, I. D., and Hill, G. L. Assessment of protein nutrition in surgical patients: The value of anthropometrics. *Am. J. Clin. Nutr.* 32:1527, 1979.
10. Durwin, J. V. G. A., and Womersley, J. Body fat assessed from total body density and its estimation from skinfold thickness: Measurements on 481 men and women aged from 16 to 72 years. *Br. J. Nutr.* 37:77, 1974.
11. Goodson, W. H., and Hunt, T. K. Development of a new miniature method for the study of wound healing in human subjects. *J. Surg. Res.* 33:394, 1982.
12. Grant, J. P. Clinical impact of protein malnutrition on organ mass and function. In G. L. Blackburn, J. P. Grant, and V. R. Young (eds.), *Amino Acids: Metabolism and Medical Applications.* Boston: John Wright, 1983. Pp. 347–358.
13. Harvey, K. B., Moldawar, L. L., Bistrian, B. S., and Blackburn, G. L. Biological measures for the formation of a hospital prognostic index. *Am. J. Clin. Nutr.* 34:2013, 1981.
14. Haydock, D. A., and Hill, G. L. Impaired wound healing in surgical patients with varying degrees of malnutrition. *J. Parenter. Enter. Nutr.* 10:550, 1986.
15. Haydock, D. A., and Hill, G. L. Improved wound healing response in surgical patients receiving intravenous nutrition. *Br. J. Surg.* 74:320, 1987.
16. Heymsfield, S. B., and Williams, P. J. Nutritional assessment by clinical and biochemical methods. In M. E. Shils and V. R. Young (eds.), *Modern Nutrition in Health and Disease* (7th ed.). Philadelphia: Lea and Febiger, 1988. Pp. 817–860.
17. Hickman, D. M., Miller, R. A., Rombeau, J. L., Twomey, P. L., and Frey, C. F. Serum albumin and body weight as predictors of postoperative course in colorectal cancer. *J. Parenter. Enter. Nutr.* 4:314, 1980.
18. Jeejeebhoy, K. N., Baker, J. P., Wolman, S. L., et al. Critical evaluation of the role of clinical assessment and body composition studies in patients with malnutrition and after total parenteral nutrition. *Am. J. Clin. Nutr.* 35:1117, 1982.
19. Kaminski, M. V., Fitzgerald, M. J., Murphy, R. J., et al. Correlation of mortality with serum transferrin and anergy. (Abstract) *J. Parenter. Enter. Nutr.* 1:27a, 1977.
20. Kelleher, P. C., Phinney, S. D., Sims, E. A. H., et al. Effects of carbohydrate-containing and carbohydrate-restricted hypocaloric and eucaloric diets on serum concentrations of retinol-binding protein, thyroxine-binding prealbumin and transferrin. *Metabolism* 32:95, 1983.
21. Keys, A., Brozek, J., Henschel, A., Mickelsen, O., and Taylor, H. L. *The Biology of Human Starvation.* Minneapolis: University of Minnesota Press, 1950.
22. Klidjian, A. M., Archer, T. J., Foster, K. J., and Karran, S. J. Detection of dangerous malnutrition. *J. Parenter. Enter. Nutr.* 6:119, 1982.
23. Klidjian, A. M., Foster, K. J., Kammerling, R. M., Cooper, A., and Karran, S. J. Relation of anthropometric and dynamometric variables to serious postoperative complications. *Br. Med. J.* 281:899, 1980.
24. Krieger, M. Ueber die Atrophie der menschlichen: Organe bei Inanition. 2. *Angew. Anat. Konstitutionsl.* 7:87, 1921.
25. Moore, F. D., Oleson, K. H., McMurrey, J. D., Parker, H. V., Ball, M. R., and Boyden, C. M. *The Body Cell Mass and Its Supporting Environment: Body Composition in Health and Disease.* Philadelphia: W. B. Saunders, 1963.
26. Morgan, D. B., Hill, G. L., and Burkinshaw, L. The assessment of weight loss from a single measurement of body weight: The problems and limitations. *Am. J. Clin. Nutr.* 33:2101, 1980.
27. Pettigrew, R. A., and Hill, G. L. Indicators of surgical risk and clinical judgement: A prospective comparative study. *Br. J. Surg.* 73:47, 1986.

28. Ravussin, E., Burnand, B., Schutz, Y., and Jequier, E. Twenty-four-hour energy expenditure and resting metabolic rate in obese, moderately obese, and control subjects. *Am. J. Clin. Nutr.* 35:566, 1982.

29. Russell, D. M., Leiter, L. A., Whitwell, J., Marliss, E. B., and Jeejeebhoy, K. N. Skeletal muscle function during hypocaloric diets and fasting: A comparison with standard nutritional assessment parameters. *Am. J. Clin. Nutr.* 37:133, 1983.

30. Ryan, J. A., Jr., and Taft, D. A. Preoperative nutritional assessment does not predict morbidity and mortality in abdominal operations. *Surg. Forum* 31:96, 1980.

31. Schroeder, D., Christie, P. M., and Hill, G. L. Bioelectrical impedance analysis for body composition: Clinical evaluation in general surgical patients. *J. Parenter. Enter. Nutr.* 14:129, 1990.

32. Shaw, J. H. F., and Wolfe, R. R. Energy and protein metabolism in sepsis and trauma. *Aust. N. Z. J. Surg.* 57:41, 1987.

33. Shizgal, H. M., Spanier, A. H., Humes, J., and Wood, C. D. The indirect measurement of total exchangeable potassium. *Am. J. Physiol.* 233:F253, 1977.

34. Smale, B. F., Muller, J. L., Hobbs, C. L., Buzby, G. P., and Rosato, E. F. Serum protein response to acute dietary manipulation. *J. Surg. Res.* 28:379, 1980.

35. Streat, S. J., Beddoe, A. H., and Hill, G. L. Aggressive nutritional support does not prevent protein loss despite fat gain in septic intensive care patients. *J. Trauma* 27:262, 1987.

36. Streat, S. J., and Hill, G. L. Nutritional support in management of critically ill patients in surgical intensive care. *World J. Surg.* 11:194, 1987.

37. Studley, H. O. Percentage of weight loss: A basic indicator of surgical risk in patients with chronic peptic ulcer. *J.A.M.A.* 10:458, 1936.

38. Windsor, J. A., and Hill, G. L. Protein depletion and surgical risk. *Aust. N. Z. J. Surg.* 58:711, 1988.

39. Windsor, J. A., and Hill, G. L. Weight loss with physiologic impairment: A basic indicator of surgical risk. *Ann. Surg.* 207:290, 1988.

40. Windsor, J. A., and Hill, G. L. Risk factors for postoperative pneumonia: The importance of protein depletion. *Ann. Surg.* 208:209, 1988.

41. Windsor, J. A., Knight, G. S., and Hill, G. L. Wound healing response in surgical patients: Recent food intake is more important than nutritional status. *Br. J. Surg.* 75:135, 1988.

Measurements of Relevant Nutrition Data for Determining Efficacy of Nutritional Support

Adrian Barbul

Once nutritional support has been instituted, sooner or later every clinician must question whether the prescribed therapy is efficacious. Efficacy means different things depending on clinical circumstances. Ideally, the best clinical index of efficacy is improved survival rate, lessened morbidity, and shorter hospital stay. These end points can be useful only in a retroactive manner. In addition, it is very difficult to correlate these outcome end points directly with the institution of nutritional support.

The metabolic aim of nutritional therapy is reversal of energy and protein catabolism. Clinically, there is a need for concurrent indices that are reflective of changes in nutritional state secondary to nutritional intervention. No single indicator reflects the metabolic efficacy of the nutritional support. However, a battery of tests together with careful clinical evaluations can help the clinician make decisions at the bedside regarding the adequacy of the nutritional therapy.

ADEQUACY OF CALORIC INTAKE

Excess caloric intake carries with it major risks of metabolic, hepatic, and respiratory complications, whereas provision of inadequate calories would lessen or abrogate the therapeutic effect of the nutritional support. Therefore, clinicians need to accurately measure and/or predict the energy requirements of hospitalized patients. These methods should be flexible enough to reflect changes in the clinical state of the patient. The obvious methodology for this is the energy balance technique. During positive energy balance, there will be glycogen and fat synthesis. For most hospitalized patients, the aim is to achieve zero energy balance.

ENERGY REQUIREMENTS

Daily energy requirements in healthy humans can be divided into three components. The resting energy expenditure (REE), accounting for 65 to 75% of energy expenditure, is the amount of energy required to support the body's metabolic processes. This equals about 20 to 25 kcal/kg/day. The second component of daily energy expenditure is related to the energy cost of physical activity. In sedentary individuals this accounts for 15 to 20% of daily energy needs, but it can increase drastically with intense physical exertion. The last component is the thermic effect of food or "specific dynamic action," which is the energy required to process ingested food. Although it accounts for about 10% of daily energy expenditure, it can vary greatly with the quantity and quality of the diet.

Energy expenditure can be measured directly or indirectly. Direct measurements require an enormously complex and expensive apparatus, which makes them unsuitable for routine clinical application. Indirect measurements or estimates of energy needs are in current clinical use.

Estimates of Energy Requirements

The values for REE are most commonly obtained from the regression equations of Harris and Benedict [28] who derived them from direct calorimetric measurements of basal metabolic rates (BMR). Since hospitalized patients expend energy moving around the bed, it is usual to add 10% to the BMR values obtained from nomograms in order to calculate the REE. Recently, the values predicted by these equations were found to overestimate energy needs in both lean and obese healthy humans by small but significant amounts [46]. In the hospitalized patient there is an additional component to the daily energy needs. This has been termed the "hypermetabolism of stress." There is great debate over the magnitude of this effect. Major fractures or peritonitis were noted to lead to 15 to 50% increases in REE [35, 37]. Although other workers have failed to note any significant increases in REE following major trauma and sepsis [47], these findings have not been reproduced. Apelgren and Wilmore [2] proposed the following formula for estimating energy requirements for maintenance in hospitalized patients: REE × 1.25 × stress

factor (thus allowing a 25% increase for physical activity and the stress of hospitalization and also correction for the disease process itself). If weight gain is desired, an additional 1000 cal/day are added to the regimen. From a practical point of view, the Harris-Benedict equations represent a good starting point for estimating energy requirements in patients.

Indirect Measurements of Energy Expenditure

The utilization of nutrients to produce heat proceeds by oxidation of carbon atoms, with ultimate production of carbon dioxide and water. Thus, by measuring the rate at which oxygen is consumed and carbon dioxide is produced, an estimate of total energy production can be obtained. In addition, estimates can be made of the proportion of energy production derived from the oxidation of various substrates.

Continuous Monitoring of Respiratory Gas Exchange

This technique requires that expired gas be collected and measurements of the individual gases be carried out. This entails numerous practical difficulties. Older techniques used the Douglas bag, which is uncomfortable and tends to leak. Kinney et al. [36] developed a system employing a transparent rigid canopy that encloses the patient's head and has a seal around the neck. Gas exchange is calculated via balance of inspired and expired gases. The system allows for long-term measurements, but it is not portable. Continuous monitoring of gas exchange is theoretically the best method because it measures energy expenditure directly. The disadvantages are the cost of the continuous monitoring system and the considerable inconvenience to the patient at having to be in an airtight canopy for many hours.

Spot Measurements

More recently, metabolic measuring carts (MMCs) have been developed and can be used at bedside. Some systems allow for measurements only in nonintubated patients by using a hood, while other systems can measure gas production on-line in endotracheally intubated patients. Measurements are made over periods of 10 to 20 minutes. The MMC measures the REE over the time of the actual measurement. To convert the REE to the total daily energy expenditure, it is necessary to integrate the spot measurement. This introduces errors as it assumes energy expenditure to be the same for 24 hours. The test costs about $100/patient.

Doubly Labeled Water Technique (DLW)
When $^2H_2^{18}O$ is given orally, it mixes with the body water in about 3 hours [50]. Deuterium (^2H) leaves the body as water, mainly in the urine, whereas ^{18}O leaves as both water and exhaled carbon dioxide. Therefore, the difference in loss rates of deuterium and ^{18}O is proportional to the rate of carbon dioxide production, from which the energy expenditure can be calculated. The loss rates for ^{18}O and deuterium are obtained by sampling body water at two time intervals from 3 to about 30 days apart. The total body water is obtained simultaneously by isotope dilution. The respiratory quotient (RQ) is needed to convert the carbon dioxide production rate in kilocalories. The principal advantages of the DLW method are its simplicity and applicability to studies of humans in their natural environment (a hospital is not a natural environment). It is best used for measuring the cumulative energy expenditure over periods of 0.5 to 3 half-lives of the body water pool, which is about 7 to 12 days. There is minimal inconvenience to the subject since either blood, urine, or saliva can be sampled. The principal sources of error with the DLW method are analytic errors and non–steady-state sampling of body fluids. The great disadvantage of the method is its expense (about $500/subject). While the DLW method cannot measure the BMR, it measures the cumulative energy expenditure over a period of days (> 2). The Harris-Benedict equation, which was derived from continuous monitoring data, correlates better with DLW mea-

surements than the "spot" MMC measurement [45].

Like continuous monitoring of respiratory gas exchange, the DLW method is likely to be of limited utility for clinical studies. Clinically, one cannot assume a constant background enrichment and a uniform rate of decline in the enrichment of the body water. Water that the patient drinks or is given intravenously in the hospital may have different background ^{18}O and deuterium enrichments than the patient's body water, which will represent the prevailing values in his home locality. The DLW method will continue to be important for highly specialized situations where fluid intake is highly controlled, the patient is hospitalized for extended periods, and in disease states where there is disagreement in the literature as to the energy expenditure. For example, there is great debate on whether elective surgery is associated with an increase in energy expenditure, since spot measurements by MMC suggest no significant increase and continuous gas exchange monitoring indicates an increase. Novick et al. [45] used the DLW method to determine the energy costs of elective surgery. The DLW method was feasible in this case because the study population involved patients with Crohn's disease who were receiving total parenteral nutrition (TPN) for a week or more before surgery, giving them time to equilibrate. Novick et al. found that elective surgery led to an approximately 15% increase in energy expenditure, in agreement with the continuous monitoring measurements.

Clinical and Practical Considerations

Neither continuous gas exchange monitoring nor the DLW method is suitable for routine use in the individual hospitalized patient. They are best regarded as research methodologies for validating the other two methods (the MMC and the Harris-Benedict equation).

In the clinical setting, it is essential to determine the individual patient's energy requirements rapidly and cheaply. If an actual measurement is required, MMC, which measures gas exchange values over a 10- to 15-

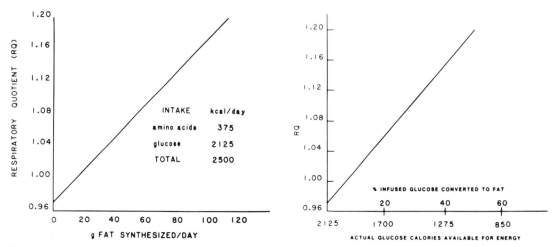

Figure 10-1. *A,* The effect of increasing lipogenesis from infused glucose on the respiratory quotient. *B,* As the proportion of glucose converted to fat increases, the amount of glucose available for energy decreases progressively (conditions same as in A). (From Stein, T. P. Why measure the respiratory quotient of patients on total parenteral nutrition? *J. Am. Coll. Nutr.* 4:501, 1985.)

minute period, is used. The problem with this method is that it gives the energy expenditure at that particular instance; thus, there is the question of whether it is worth the cost. Because of these problems, the MMC is not generally used alone to measure energy expenditure. [*Editor's Note:* In our own unit we tend to use MMC measurements, with appropriate corrections in conjunction with Harris-Benedict estimations, to get an accurate view of the energy needs of the critically ill.]

The alternative approach is to use the Harris-Benedict equation to estimate the REE (i.e., add 10%) and then multiply the REE by an activity coefficient corresponding to the degree of stress the patient is experiencing.

The principal utility of the MMC is to monitor the RQ for patients receiving TPN because it is the only way to ascertain whether the patient can actually use the calories given. A not infrequent problem with TPN is the development of fatty livers and subsequent liver dysfunction secondary to excess parenteral glucose [51].

For all fuel oxidation reactions, the RQ is less than 1.0, and only during fat synthesis is it greater than 1.0. Thus, if glucose is being

given as the sole caloric source, the RQ should be about 0.97. If it is over 1.0, the patient is making fat, and the amount of fat made can be considerable. An RQ greater than 1.0 is a signal to reduce the glucose dosage. Glucose that is converted into fat and deposited in the liver is not available for energy by the rest of the body; furthermore, as the amount of fat synthesized increases, the actual amount of the infused glucose available for energy decreases rapidly [55] (Fig. 10-1). Thus, for the patient with a RQ of 1.08, less than 70% of the glucose is available for immediate use as energy. The rest (1250 kcal/day) is being deposited as fat. Some of this shortfall is made up by oxidation of endogenous fat [34]. Depending on how much endogenous fat is mobilized, the patient will be in a semistarved state because only about two-thirds of the infused calories plus an unknown amount of endogenous fat are available for energy. In one study, a 60% substitution of glucose calories with fat resulted in a maintenance of the RQ below 1.0 for periods greater than 14 days [41].

An additional benefit of the MMC for patients receiving TPN is that it can detect potential respiratory distress secondary to excess glucose. TPN can aggravate respiratory dysfunction in some severely ill patients by increasing the ventilation rate [5]. This nutritionally induced increase comes at a time when the patient's pulmonary capacity is already compromised, with one consequence being an increased difficulty in weaning such patients from ventilators. [*Editor's Note:* As I have stated elsewhere in this volume, I believe the occurrence of this complication is greatly overestimated. It is wise to be aware of it, however.]

In summary, for most patients the combination of the Harris-Benedict equation and the appropriate activity coefficient is more than adequate for estimating a patient's energy requirement. However, for patients receiving TPN, the MMC allows the physician to determine whether the patient can actually use the TPN regimen given and, if not, to adjust it to meet the patient's metabolic capacity. The ability to do this is the most important and unique advantage of the MMC measurement of energy expenditure. The Harris-Benedict equation is sufficient, while understanding that calculating energy requirements does not necessarily mean that the patient is able to utilize that amount of calories in that particular form. Thus, judicious use of the RQ enables the physician to customize a nutrition regimen (TPN) to meet the patient's energy needs without exceeding the patient's capacity to utilize the energy in the form provided.

ADEQUACY OF PROTEIN SUPPORT

The recommended daily allowance for protein in adults is 0.8 g/k/day. This reflects the actual need of the body for amino acids in order to carry out normal synthetic processes and to compensate for obligatory nitrogenous losses. The amino acid requirements increase either in certain anabolic states (i.e., athletic training, growth, or pregnancy) or in catabolic states (stress and trauma) [56]. Simply stated, protein turnover represents the bal-

ance between synthesis and breakdown. Therefore, an increase in either protein synthesis or breakdown rates leads to higher amino acid requirements to maintain lean body mass and nitrogen equilibrium.

There are numerous techniques to evaluate protein stores or balance. All have theoretic or practical limitations. Many of these techniques are indirect and static, and do not reflect the evolution in protein metabolism that occurs in rapidly changing disease states or with constant nutritional support. Some of these techniques together with their clinical applicability are discussed below.

Nitrogen Balance Technique

Nitrogen balance technique has been widely used in patients on TPN as an index of protein requirements and of the efficacy of the nutritional therapy. Simply stated, nitrogen balance is the difference between the amount of nitrogen intake and output. Nitrogenous output or losses occur mainly in the urine, but the feces, skin, gastrointestinal tract, and other body secretions may contain significant amounts of nitrogen. Precise and accurate nitrogen balance studies are very difficult and demanding to perform, and therefore are reserved for research purposes. For most clinical situations, a determination of urinary nitrogen losses is sufficient to allow clinical judgments to be made about the adequacy of protein intake. Thus, 24-hour urinary urea nitrogen (the main component) can be measured by any clinical laboratory. Allowances are made for non-urea urinary nitrogen (approximately 2 g) and fecal and skin losses (approximately 2 g when diarrhea is absent) [7]. This provides a good estimate of nitrogen output for most patients.

An important point to consider is the relationship between nitrogen and energy inputs [59]. In the face of constant level of nitrogen input, increasing energy input leads to improved nitrogen balance. Conversely, at the same energy input, increases in nitrogen intake lead to increased nitrogen retention. Further, the efficiency of protein retention is greater in malnourished patients. Hypermetabolic, stressed patients have increased protein breakdown and retain less nitrogen at any given levels of protein and energy intake. Of most relevance to stressed patients, at higher energy levels (above calculated needs) increases in nitrogen intake lead to only modest improvements in nitrogen retention, and the extra caloric intake is utilized principally to synthesize fat, which may not be a desirable result. Most experts advocate increasing the nitrogen intake in stressed patients beyond theoretic calculations in order to achieve improvements in nitrogen retention, rather than increasing energy intakes beyond calculated needs.

Assessment of Somatic Protein Stores

Anthropometric Measurements

Muscle mass represents the largest concentration of body protein stores and also the major source of protein during starvation or increased metabolic needs. Therefore, anthropometric assessment of muscle mass has been used to estimate this component of body protein stores. The most widely used technique is the midarm muscle circumference. This is a derived calculation from the mid–upper arm circumference and the triceps skinfold thickness. The upper arm is not the perfect circle that this technique assumes it to be. However, the derived values correlate reasonably well with CT findings [29]. Of more concern are the great intraobserver and interobserver variations, which range from 10 to 33%, respectively [27]. Another limitation is that anthropometric values cannot reflect rapidly enough the changes in total body nitrogen stores brought about by nutritional intervention, stress, or immobility [15].

Another often used anthropometric measurement is body weight. In the nonhospitalized patient, changes in body weight are a reasonable measure of nutritional deficit. In patients receiving nutritional support, body weight changes cannot be used to assess efficacy. However, they are excellent for examining water balance.

Muscle Function Assessment

Since muscle protein stores are rapidly depleted with starvation, trauma, or sepsis, some researchers have tried to correlate muscle function with nutritional state. Active assessment is carried out by measuring grip strength. This correlates well with the level of preexisting malnutrition [60]. Diseases such as infection, severe illness, or use of sedatives influence hand grip directly and independent of nutritional status [17]. Another method utilizes stimulation of the ulnar nerve at the wrist with measurement of the force of contraction of the adductor pollicis muscle. Abnormalities of muscle function have been observed in severely depleted patients [38]. One study found little correlation between nutritional status as measured by isotopic body composition, nutritional support, and muscle function [53]. Glycolytic enzymes in muscle such as fructose bisphosphatase, phosphofructokinase, and hexokinase, are markedly reduced in undernourished patients in parallel with atrophy and loss of type II fibers [13]. After 14 days of TPN, only phosphofructokinase activity rose significantly in parallel with an increase in the size and number of type II fibers. All of these assessments are somewhat static and therefore cannot reflect rapid changes in energy or protein stores secondary to nutritional intervention.

Creatinine Excretion

Creatinine is an excretion product of creatine metabolism, the main compound of energy storage in muscle. Since creatinine is not reutilized, its urinary excretion is proportional to muscle creatine content and, therefore, to body muscle mass. This excellent correlation has been confirmed by isotope dilution or potassium-40 assessment of lean body mass [44, 57]. Many drawbacks exist to this assessment: (1) Creatinine excretion falls with age, particularly over the age of 55 years. (2) Urinary creatinine excretion is dependent on the creatine-creatinine content of the diet, not an important consideration in intravenously supported patients. (3) Severe trauma and infection increase creatinine excretion independently of changes in muscle mass. (4) Nonrenal clearance of creatinine increases in renal failure and in patients with serum creatinine values greater than 4 mg/dl %, and the correlation to body cell mass is poor. (5) Short-term (2–3 weeks) changes in body cell mass composition are not well reflected in the creatinine excretion measurements.

3-Methylhistidine Excretion

3-Methylhistidine (3-MH) excretion has been used extensively as an index of muscle protein breakdown. The theoretic advantages of using 3-MH are that it is present in myofibrillar protein, it is released during muscle protein breakdown, and it is not reutilized for protein synthesis but is excreted as such in the urine [63]. In cases of starvation or of nutritional support of nontrauma patients, urinary 3-MH excretion correlates well with extremity amino acid flux or whole-body protein breakdown [39, 40]. However, injury to the skin or gastrointestinal tract can contribute significant amounts of 3-MH to the total amount excreted in urine, thus giving disproportionately high estimates of muscle protein breakdown. In one study of patients undergoing major gastrointestinal surgery for tumors, urinary 3-MH excretion was increased by 40% while 3-MH arteriovenous differences from the lower extremity were reduced by 40% [48]. This indicates that tissues other than muscle can make substantial contributions to the total urinary excretion of 3-MH. Another drawback for most clinicians is that 3-MH measurements require an amino acid analyzer, which is not present in most hospitals. [*Editor's Note:* My opinion of urinary 3-MH excretion is that it probably is a reasonable reflection of protein **turnover,** rather than **breakdown.**]

Assessment of Visceral (Short-Turnover) Proteins

The liver synthesizes and secretes a variety of proteins. Nutrient supply is critical for the optimal synthesis of these proteins. Thus, although plasma levels of these proteins may or may not correlate with total body protein stores, their rapid turnover and short half-life make them attractive as biochemical indicators of changes in nutritional status. There are two main drawbacks to their use: (1) Plasma levels of these proteins decrease very quickly, independent of nutritional status in conditions such as trauma (including elective surgery) [3], sepsis [6], and severe illnesses [21] as a result of fluid shifts, alterations in capillary permeability or changes in rates of synthesis or degradation. (2) Plasma levels change slowly in response to nutritional intervention [10, 61].

Serum Albumin

This is the most abundant of liver-synthesized proteins. Albumin is not stored, but is secreted continuously into the plasma at a rate of 14 to 17 g/day. The half-life of albumin is rather long, about 20 days. Thus, changes in synthesis are reflected slowly by the plasma levels. Low albumin levels may reflect decreased liver function rather than nutrient deficiency. Fluid changes secondary to increased vascular permeability, increased catabolism, or losses from the gastrointestinal tract or burn wounds may all decrease plasma levels without a direct nutritional deficiency. [*Editor's Note:* It is thought that the degradation of albumin is directly correlated with the percentage that is extravascular.] Although albumin levels may have prognostic or diagnostic values [1], they have been found to be poor indicators of the adequacy of nutritional support [14, 54].

Serum Transferrin

Transferrin, which is synthesized in the liver, is a circulating glycoprotein with a short half-life (8–10 days) and a smaller extracellular pool than albumin. It is a carrier protein for iron and plays an important role in iron metabolism. Transferrin levels can be calculated from blood total iron-binding capacity or can be measured immunologically. Normal levels of transferrin range from 160 to 356 mg/dl (central 95 percentile) with a mean ± standard deviation of 258 ± 49 mg/dl [43]. The wide range of normal values is the main drawback to using transferrin levels. Low levels of transferrin have been found to correlate well with nutritional status as measured by isotopic total body composition studies [49], although there is a 60% false-positive rate and 31% false-negative rate. While in some studies transferrin level changes were found to be poor correlates of nutritional support efficacy as measured by nitrogen balance [14, 20] or body composition [49], others found a good correlation between transferrin and nitrogen balance in TPN-supported patients [22].

Prealbumin (Transthyretrin) and Retinol-Binding Protein

Retinol-binding protein is an alpha$_1$-globulin that carries retinol in plasma. It is synthesized mainly in the liver, and has a short half-life (10–12 hours) and a small circulating pool. Retinol-binding protein circulates in a 1:1 molar ratio with prealbumin, which is the thyroxine-binding protein. Prealbumin, which is also a carrier protein for retinol-binding protein, has a small body pool and a short half-life of 24 to 48 hours. The short half-life of prealbumin renders it a sensitive index of visceral protein status in critically ill patients [33], patients with cancer [9], or patients receiving TPN [16], although one study suggested that it is a better indicator of energy than of protein adequacy [26]. In one study of patients receiving TPN, in 90% of cases, rising prealbumin level were associated with a positive nitrogen balance, while in 70% of cases falling prealbumin levels were associated with negative nitrogen balance [14]. Retinol-binding protein also shows a good correlation with nitrogen balance in patients receiving TPN.

Plasma Amino Acid Levels

Alterations in plasma amino acid levels have been examined in several disease states. Uncomplicated starvation and weight loss correlate with low plasma valine levels [62]. Sepsis results in increases in aromatic and sulfur-containing amino acid levels [25], and these disturbances correlate with survival [24]. Furthermore, as the severity of sepsis increases,

exogenous nutritional support has no effect on muscle protein breakdown or alterations in plasma amino acids [11]. Acute hepatic failure leads to abnormal plasma amino acid levels that correlate with the presence of encephalopathy [18]. Normalization of the plasma amino acid levels reverses the encephalopathy [19]. Injury, such as surgery, is also associated with alterations in plasma and muscle amino acid levels [4].

Although the physiologic role of plasma amino acid alterations in various disease states remains an important research topic, monitoring of amino acid levels for current bedside care is not practical or useful at the present time.

Isotopic Determination of Body Composition

The body is composed of the body cell mass and the extracellular supporting component. Body cell mass is defined as the mitotically active, work-performing cells. The extracellular component can be determined from the measurement of extracellular water volume and total exchangeable sodium. The body cell mass bears a direct relationship to the intracellular volume and exchangeable potassium. Following injection of sodium 22 and tritiated water, one can determine total exchangeable sodium and total body water and derive total exchangeable potassium as indices of body composition [52]. The method has been used in very sick patients and in TPN-supported patients. Direct measurements of body exchangeable potassium have been carried out following injections of potassium 42 and using a total body counter [8].

An alternative method for determining body composition has been to use in vivo neutron activation and measuring total body nitrogen, potassium, sodium, chloride, and phosphorus [31]. From these values, body fat, protein, mineral, and water contents are calculated. This method has been applied to highly stressed and/or septic patients receiving TPN [30].

All body composition techniques involve the use of highly complex and expensive equipment that is not generally available. Their use is mainly as a research tool and not as a bedside standard application.

Immune Assessment

Since severe malnutrition leads to impairment in immune function, various tests have been used to diagnose the degree of malnutrition and to assess the rate of recovery. Discussed below are some of the more commonly used tests, although it should be pointed out that most of the tests are nonspecific in their ability to correlate with nutritional status alone.

1. Lymphocyte counts. A decrease in peripheral blood lymphocytes below 1200/mm^3 is often taken as a sign of malnutrition. Such values should be interpreted with caution, as many other nonnutritional factors can contribute to decreased lymphocyte counts. [*Editor's Note:* I would state it more strongly. I do not believe that total lymphocyte count is of any value with respect to nutritional status.]

2. Analysis of T lymphocyte and T lymphocyte subsets. T lymphocytes are divided into two major subgroups: T helper/effector cells (CD4) and T suppressor/cytotoxic (CD8). T lymphocytes and subsets can be quantified by use of monoclonal antibodies reacting with specific cell-surface antigens. Uncomplicated malnutrition is associated with a decrease in the number of T lymphocytes and is rapidly reversed by nutritional supplementation [12]. No consistent changes in T-lymphocyte subsets have been noted in uncomplicated protein-calorie malnutrition. In the hospitalized patient, many other factors, such as trauma, sepsis, and stress, may alter the number and ratios of T lymphocytes and subsets, thereby rendering these assays inaccurate for assessing the efficacy of nutritional intervention.

3. In vitro assays of lymphocyte immunoreactivity. Malnutrition is associated with a decrease of the in vitro immune responsiveness of T cells to a variety of lectins (such as concanavalin A, phytohemagglutinin,

pokeweed mitogen) or foreign antigens (as measured in a one-way mixed-lymphocyte reaction). There is no convincing evidence that nutritional support alone contributes to the restoration of lymphocyte immune responsiveness, which is often depressed in hospitalized patients. In addition, the tests are fraught with large intra-assay variability which makes day-to-day comparisons in individual patients difficult to interpret.

4. Delayed-type hypersensitivity responses. Delayed-type hypersensitivity (DTH) is a test that measures the erythematous indurated skin reaction in response to the intracutaneous administration of bacterial, fungal, or viral antigens to which the general population has been commonly exposed in the past. As performed today, DTH is measured to a panel of five to seven antigens; a response to at least two antigens is considered positive, a response to only one antigen is defined as partly anergic, and a lack of response is defined as anergy. The test measures both the afferent (recognition) and the efferent (responsive) arms of immune reactivity. All components of an intact immune system must function in order to obtain a positive DTH response. This test is commonly used to assess nutritional state, since malnutrition can be associated with decreased in vivo immune responses. This is not correct in so much as the test measures global immune reactivity, which may or may not be correlated solely to the nutritional state. For example, starvation for 10 days in normal humans failed to alter the DTH response [32]. Also, many nonnutritional factors, such as trauma, burns, hemorrhage, and general anesthesia, can contribute to a decrease in or lack of response [42]. Anergy has been associated with a marked increase in morbidity and mortality, although it is difficult to individualize the contribution of malnutrition to such an impaired response or to show a benefit of nutritional intervention in converting nonresponders to responders. The value of this assay as a test of the nutritional state or therapy is still unclear, and randomized studies need to be done to ascertain its value [23, 58].

CLINICAL RECOMMENDATIONS

From a clinical point of view, the nitrogen balance technique remains the simplest and most informative test of protein stores and the adequacy of the nutritional intervention. In interpreting the results, clinicians must be aware of the pitfalls in collecting accurate 24-hour urine samples. The test can be performed as often as desired, although from a practical point of view, once or twice a week is probably sufficient. All the other tests remain untested as tools of assessing the efficacy of nutritional therapy. However, in a clinically stable patient, a decrease in the values of short-turnover proteins from week to week is a strong indication that the nutritional regimen is inadequate. In patients with changing clinical pictures or intervening complications, the value of these tests remains to be determined. For now, body composition studies remain powerful research tools with little applicability at the bedside.

Acknowledgement

I wish to express my gratitude to Dr. T. P. Stein for useful and constructive advice during the writing of this chapter.

REFERENCES

1. Anderson, C. F., Moxness, K., Meister, J., and Burritt, M. F. The sensitivity and specificity of nutrition-related variables in relationship to the duration of hospital stay and the rate of complications. *Mayo Clin. Proc.* 59:477, 1984.
2. Apelgren, K. N., and Wilmore, D. W. Nutritional care of the critically ill patient. *Surg. Clin. North Am.* 63:497, 1983.
3. Aronsen, K. F., Ekelund, G., Kindmark, C. O., and Laurell, C. B. Sequential changes of plasma proteins after surgical trauma. *Scand. J. Clin. Lab. Invest. Suppl.* 29:127, 1972.
4. Askanazi, J., Elwyn, D. H., Kinney, J. M., Gump, F. E., Michelsen, C. B., and Stinchfield, F. E. Muscle and plasma amino acids after injury. *Ann. Surg.* 188:797, 1978.
5. Askanazi, J., Rosenbaum, S. H., Hyman, A. I., Silverberg, P. A., Milic-Emili, J., and Kinney, J. M. Respiratory changes induced by large glucose loads of total parenteral nutrition. *J.A.M.A.* 243:1444, 1980.
6. Beisel, W. R. Sepsis and metabolism. In R. A. Little and K. N. Frayn (eds.), *The Scientific Basis for the Care of the Critically Ill.* Manchester: Manchester University Press, 1986. P. 103.
7. Blackburn, G. L., Bistrian, B. R., Maini, B. S., Schlamm, H. T., and Smith, M. F. Nutritional and metabolic assessment of the hospitalized patient. *J. Parenter. Enter. Nutr.* 1:11, 1977.
8. Bocking, J. K., Holliday, R. L., Reid, B., Mustard, R., and Duff, J. H. Total exchangeable potassium in patients receiving total parenteral nutrition. *Surgery* 88:551, 1980.
9. Bourry, J., MIlano, G., Caldani, C., and Schneider, M. Assessment of nutritional proteins during the parenteral nutrition of cancer patients. *Ann. Clin. Lab. Sci.* 12:158, 1982.
10. Carpentier, Y. A., Barthel, J., and Bruyns, J. Plasma concentration in nutritional assessment. *Proc. Nutr. Soc.* 41:405, 1982.
11. Cerra, F. B., Siegel, J. H., Coleman, B., Border, J. R., and McMenamy, R. R. Septic autocannibalism: A failure of exogenous nutritional support. *Ann. Surg.* 192:570, 1980.
12. Chandra, R. K. Rosette-forming T lymphocytes and cell-mediated immunity in malnutrition. *Br. Med. J.* 3:608, 1974.
13. Church, J. M., Choong, S. Y., and Hill, G. L. Abnormalities of muscle metabolism and histology in malnourished patients awaiting surgery: Effects of a course of intravenous nutrition. *Br. J. Surg.* 71:563, 1984.
14. Church, J. M., and Hill, G. L. Assessing the efficacy of intravenous nutrition in general surgical patients: Dynamic nutritional assessment with plasma proteins. *J. Parenter. Enter. Nutr.* 11:135, 1987.
15. Collins, J. P., McCarthy, I. D., and Hill, G. L. Assessment of protein nutrition in surgical patients: The value of anthropometrics. *Am. J. Clin. Nutr.* 32:1527, 1979.
16. Douville, P., Talbot, J., and Lapointe, R. Potential usefulness of serum prealbumin in total parenteral nutrition. *Clin. Chem.* 28:1706, 1982.
17. Elia, M., Martin, S., and Neale, G. Effect of non-nutritional factors on muscle function tests. *Arch. Emerg. Med.* 1:175, 1984.
18. Fischer, J. E., Funovics, J. M., Aguirre, A., et al. The role of plasma amino acids in hepatic encephalopathy. *Surgery* 78:276, 1975.
19. Fischer, J. E., Rosen, H. M., Ebeid, A. M., James, J. H., Keane, J. M., and Soeters, P. B. The effect of normalization of plasma amino acids on hepatic encephalopathy in man. *Surgery* 80:77, 1976.
20. Fish, J., Konstantinides, F., Shronts, E., Mitchell, D., Li, J., and Cerra, F. Effect of nitrogen balance on visceral protein synthesis in polytrauma. (Abstract No. 1950) *F.A.S.E.B. J.* J:A632, 1988.
21. Fleck, A., Colley, C. M., and Myers, M. A. Liver export proteins and trauma. *Br. Med. Bull.* 41:265, 1985.
22. Fletcher, J. P., Little, J. M., and Guest, P. K. A comparison of serum transferrin and se-

rum prealbumin as nutritional parameters. *J. Parenter. Enter. Nutr.* 11:144, 1987.

23. Forse, R. A., Christou, N., Meakins, J. L., MacLean, L. D., and Shizgal, H. M. Reliability of skin testing as a measure of nutritional state. *Arch. Surg.* 116:1284, 1981.

24. Freund, H., Atamian, S., Holroyde, J., and Fischer, J. E. Plasma amino acids as predictors of the severity and outcome of sepsis. *Ann. Surg.* 190:571, 1979.

25. Freund, H., Ryan, J., and Fischer, J. E. Amino acid derangements in patients with sepsis. *Ann. Surg.* 188:423, 1978.

26. Golden, M. H. N. Transport proteins as indices of protein status. *Am. J. Clin. Nutr.* 35:1159, 1982.

27. Grant, J., Cyster, P. B., and Thurlow, J. Current techniques of nutritional assessment. *Surg. Clin. North Am.* 61:437, 1981.

28. Harris, J. A., and Benedict, F. G. Biometric study of basal metabolism in man. Publication no. 279. Washington, D.C.: Carnegie Institute of Washington, 1909.

29. Heymsfield, S. B., Olafson, R. P., Kutner, M. H., and Dixon, D. W. A radiographic method of quantifying protein-calorie malnutrition. *Am. J. Clin. Nutr.* 32:693, 1979.

30. Hill, G. L., and Beddoe, A. H. In vivo neutron activation in metabolic and nutritional studies. II: Clinical applications. *J. Clin. Surg.* 1:333, 1982.

31. Hill, G. L., McCarthy, I. D., Collins, J. P., and Smith, A. P. A new method for the rapid measurement of body composition in critically ill surgical patients. *Br. J. Surg.* 65:732, 1978.

32. Holm, G., and Palmblad, J. Acute energy deprivation in man: Effect on cell-mediated immunological reactions. *Clin. Exp. Immunol.* 25:207, 1976.

33. Ingenbleek, Y., Van der Schriek, H. G., DeNayer, P. H., and DeVisscher, M. Albumin, transferrin, and the thyroxine-binding prealbumin/retinol binding protein complex in assessment of malnutrition. *Clin. Chim. Acta* 63:61, 1975.

34. Jequier, E. Energy utilization in human obesity. *Ann. N.Y. Acad. Sci.* 499:73, 1987.

35. Kinney, J. M. Energy requirements in the surgical patient. In American College of Surgeons, *Manual of Surgical Nutrition.* Philadelphia: W. B. Saunders, 1975. P. 223.

36. Kinney, J. M., Morgan, A. P., Domingues, F. J., and Gildner, K. J. A method for continuous measurement of gas exchanges and radioactivity in acutely ill patients. *Metabolism* 12:205, 1964.

37. Long, C. L., Schaffel, N., Geiger, J. W., Schiller, W. R., and Blakemore, W. S. Metabolic response to illness: Estimation of energy and protein needs from indirect calorimetry and nitrogen balance. *J. Parenter. Enter. Nutr.* 3:452, 1979.

38. Lopes, J., Russell, D. M., Whitwell, J., and Jeejeebhoy, K. N. Skeletal muscle function in malnutrition. *Am. J. Clin. Nutr.* 36:602, 1982.

39. Lowry, S. F., Horowitz, G. D., Jeevanandam, M., Legaspi, A., and Brennan, M. F. Whole-body protein breakdown and 3-methylhistidine excretion during brief fasting, starvation and intravenous repletion in man. *Ann. Surg.* 202:21, 1985.

40. Lowry, S. F., Horowitz, G. D., Rose, D., and Brennan, M. F. Forearm amino acid metabolism following starvation and intravenous refeeding in normal man. *Surg. Forum* 34:93, 1983.

41. MacFie, J., Holmfield, J. H. M., King, R. F. G., and Hill, G. L. Effect of energy source on changes in energy expenditure and respiratory quotient during total parenteral nutrition. *J. Parenter. Enter. Nutr.* 7:1, 1983.

42. MacLean, L. D. Delayed type hypersensitivity testing in surgical patients. *Surg. Gynecol. Obstet.* 166:285, 1988.

43. Markowitz, H., and Fairbanks, V. F. Transferrin assay and total iron-binding capacity. *Mayo Clin. Proc.* 58:827, 1983.

44. Muldowney, F. P., Crooks, J., and Bluhm, M. M. The relationship of total exchangeable potassium and chloride to lean body mass, red cell mass and creatinine excretion in man. *J. Clin. Invest.* 36:1375, 1957.

45. Novick, W. M., Nusbaum, M., and Stein, T. P. Energy costs of surgery as measured by the doubly labelled water ($^2H_2^{18}O$) method. *Surgery* 103:99, 1988.

46. Owen, O. E. Resting metabolic requirements of men and women. *Mayo Clin. Proc.* 63:503, 1988.

47. Quebbeman, E. F., Ausman, R. K., and Scheneider, T. C. A re-evaluation of energy expenditure during parenteral nutrition. *Ann. Surg.* 195:282, 1982.

48. Rennie, M. J., Bennegard, K., Eden, E., Emery, P. W., and Lundholm, K. Urinary excretion and efflux from the leg of 3-methylhistidine before and after major surgical operation. *Metabolism* 33:250, 1985.

49. Roza, A. M., Tuitt, D., and Shizgal, H. M. Transferrin: A poor measure of nutritional status. *J. Parenter. Enter. Nutr.* 8:523, 1984.

50. Schoeller, D. A., and van Santen, E. Measurement of energy expenditure in humans by doubly labelled water method. *J. Appl. Physiol.* 63:955, 1982.

51. Sheldon, G. F., Scott, R. P., and Sanders, R. Hepatic dysfunction during TPN. *Arch. Surg.* 113:504, 1978.

52. Shizgal, H. M. Nutritional assessment with

body composition measurements. *J. Parenter. Enter. Nutr.* 11:42S, 1987.

53. Shizgal, H. M., Vasilevsky, C. A., Gardiner, P. F., et al. Nutritional assessment and skeletal muscle function. *Am. J. Clin. Nutr.* 44:761, 1986.

54. Starker, P. M., Gump, E. F., Askanazi, J., Elwyn, D. H., and Kinney, J. M. Serum albumin levels as an index of nutritional support. *Surgery* 91:194, 1982.

55. Stein, T. P. Why measure the respiratory quotient of patients on total parenteral nutrition? *J. Am. Coll. Nutr.* 4:501, 1985.

56. Stein, T. P. Protein metabolism and parenteral nutrition. In J. L. Rombeau and M. D. Caldwell (eds.), *Parenteral Nutrition.* Philadelphia: W. B. Saunders, 1986. P. 100.

57. Turner, W. J., and Cohn, S. Total body potassium and 24-hour creatinine excretion in healthy males. *Clin. Pharmacol. Ther.* 18:405, 1975.

58. Twomey, P., Ziegler, D., and Rombeau, J. Utility of skin testing in nutritional assessment: A critical review. *J. Parenter. Enter. Nutr.* 6:50, 1982.

59. Wilmore, D. W. Energy requirement for maximum nitrogen retention. In *Clinical Nutrition Update.* Chicago: American Medical Association, 1977. P. 47.

60. Windsor, J. A., and Hill, G. L. Grip strength: A measure of the proportion of protein loss in surgical patients. *Br. J. Surg.* 75:880, 1988.

61. Young, G. A., Collins, J. P., and Hill, G. L. Plasma proteins in patients receiving intravenous amino acids or intravenous hyperalimentation after major surgery. *Am. J. Clin. Nutr.* 32:1192, 1979.

62. Young, G. A., and Hill, G. L. Evaluation of protein-energy malnutrition in surgical patients from plasma valine and other amino acids, proteins, and anthropometric measurements. *Am. J. Clin. Nutr.* 34:166, 1981.

63. Young, V. R., and Munro, H. N. N^{τ}-methylhistidine (3-methylhistidine) and muscle protein turnover: An overview. *Fed. Proc.* 37:2291, 1978.

Metabolic Background

Daniel K. Lowe
Danny O. Jacobs
Douglas W. Wilmore

THE RESPONSE TO STARVATION

General Considerations

During long-term starvation, the body must adapt to substrate deprivation. While a normal adult can lose from 5 to 10% of body weight without a reduction in function, the loss of more than 40% of the normal body weight is not usually compatible with survival [51]. Ultimately, most of the energy requirements of the body are derived from stored fat, but the carbon skeletons of amino acids released from skeletal muscle are used to provide glucose for tissues that are obligate glucose consumers. An additional demand on the body during prolonged substrate deprivation is the elimination of potentially toxic substances such as organic acids that are produced in large amounts secondary to catabolic processes.

An understanding of the metabolic response to starvation is essential to understanding the effects of nutritional therapy. A hallmark of this response (i.e., the loss of ni-

trogen compounds in the urine) has been recognized since the early 1900s. These index studies demonstrated that the calories needed to support the body during a complete fast derived primarily (80–90%) from fat [13] (Table 11-1). Protein catabolism accounted for the remaining 20% of caloric needs.

Since the body stores only a small amount of calories as carbohydrate, it adapts to utilize fat deposits as energy. To conserve protein during an extended fast, most tissues in the body shift to fat oxidation to provide the energy required for metabolic processes. The brain cannot use free fatty acids as an energy source since these substances do not readily cross the blood-brain barrier. However, neuronal tissues do adapt and utilize "ketone bodies" (beta-hydroxybutyrate and acetoacetate). These end-products of fat metabolism rapidly enter the CNS for oxidation as a primary fuel.

Although body protein represents a large source of calories, there is no storage or de-

Table 11-1. Fuel Consumption during Short-Term Fasting

Day of Fast	Fuel Metabolized Carbohydrate (g)	Protein (g)	Fat (g)	Percentage of Total Metabolism Carbohydrate (%)	Protein (%)	Fat (%)
1	69	43	135	16.6	10.3	73.1
2	42	50	142	10.2	12.2	77.6
3	39	68	130	9.8	17.0	73.2
4	4	71	136	1.0	18.7	80.3
5	0	63	133	0	17.4	82.6
6	0	61	133	0	16.9	83.1
7	0	59	134	0	16.4	83.6

Adapted from Peters, J. P., and Van Syke, D. D. *Quantitative Clinical Chemistry.* Vol. I: Interpretations (2nd ed.). Baltimore: Williams & Wilkins, 1946, P. 649.

pot protein, per se. Each molecule of protein catabolized to provide energy has served some important structural, contractile, or enzymatic function. Therefore, protein must be conserved if normal organ and body function are to continue. Early in the course of starvation, skeletal muscle—the largest repository of body protein—is catabolized to provide some of the initial fuel for metabolic processes. The amino acids released as a result of skeletal muscle catabolism are the main sources of nitrogen released in the urine as urea. A mean urinary nitrogen output of 12 g/day during the first 3 to 5 days of starvation reflects the breakdown of these amino acids. If protein catabolism continued at this rate, which is equivalent to the loss of 75 g/day of protein or 300 g of hydrated muscle, approximately one-third of the total amount of body protein would be depleted in several weeks [13]. This loss would be incompatible with life. The caloric value of the tissue initially lost during starvation is much less than that lost later as starvation continues. Early on, the caloric equivalent of this catabolized tissue is approximately 2000 kcal/kg of wet weight. After ketoadaptation, the caloric equivalent of the lean body mass lost is approximately 8000 kcal/kg of wet weight—an amount that closely approximate the estimated caloric value of adipose tissue. Thus, the overriding effect of adaptation to long-term starvation is the sparing of body protein

and thereby the prolongation of survival. Urinary losses of nitrogen decline progressively to 3 or 4 g/day, an amount roughly equivalent to 20 to 25 g of protein and 98 g of wet muscle [13].

Metabolic Changes in Skeletal Muscle

The myocyte plays a critical role in maintaining glucose homeostasis. The low serum insulin levels that accompany prolonged starvation, combined with the characteristic high levels of growth hormone, minimize glucose uptake by skeletal muscle. Skeletal muscle extraction of free fatty acids depends primarily on concentration gradients. The high serum levels of free fatty acids that occur with fasting in combination with a diminished glucose uptake facilitate the use of fats as an energy source by the myocyte.

Skeletal muscle is the primary source of the amino acid moieties used in gluconeogenesis. However, muscle cannot directly provide new glucose molecules for use by other tissues since it lacks the enzyme systems necessary for gluconeogenesis. In addition, skeletal muscle glycogen stores, the largest in the body, cannot be metabolized to glucose by glucose-6-phosphatase. Without this key enzyme, the major product of glycogenolysis cannot be converted to glucose, which could traverse the cell membrane of the myocyte.

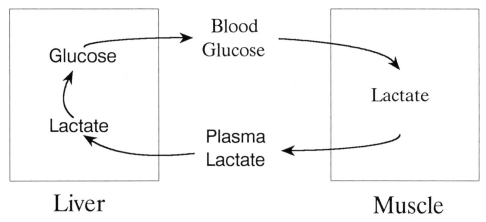

Figure 11-1. The Cori cycle. The liver uses lactate generated from skeletal muscle in the production of glucose via gluconeogenesis.

The lack of this enzyme effectively traps all of the glucose derived from glycogen inside the myocyte and forces the skeletal muscle cells to use glycogen stores for their own energetic needs. A minor but less efficient form of exported glucose carbons is found in the lactate produced by skeletal muscle.

In early fasting, the hormonal environment provides a strong stimulus for the oxidation of glucose derived from glycogen to lactate within the myocyte. Lactate is released into the circulation and delivered to the liver, where it is converted into glucose via the Cori cycle (Fig. 11-1). In addition, the low serum insulin concentrations combined with falling blood amino acid levels are powerful stimuli for amino acid release by skeletal muscle. Following deamination in the liver, the amino acids provide the three-carbon skeletons used to provide glucose via gluconeogenesis in the liver.

Metabolic Changes in Adipose Tissue and the Liver

During fasting, lipoprotein lipase activity is uninhibited since the insulin-glucagon ratio is low. As a result, lipolysis increases. The free fatty acids released from adipose tissue are then transported to the liver, skeletal muscle, and other tissues. The liver plays a central role as the modulator of most of the metabolic events during prolonged starvation and coordinates the production of glucose from gluconeogenesis and the synthesis of ketone bodies. Skeletal muscle supplies the precursors for gluconeogenesis. The energy required for gluconeogenesis is derived from the oxidation of free fatty acids released from the adipocyte. The glycerol remaining after triglyceride oxidation can also be used by the liver as a precursor for glucose production. Some of the free fatty acids are used to synthesize ketone bodies.

The synthesis of ketones and glucose in the liver is a multistep process. The hyperglucagonemia of fasting decreases the concentration of malonyl coenzyme A within the hepatocyte [13]. Lower levels of this substrate stimulate the oxidation of free fatty acids into acetoacetate and beta-hydroxybutyrate, or "ketones." With adaptation by the CNS, ketones are consumed as a major fuel source, thus decreasing the demand for glucose during starvation. Moreover, ketones, either directly or indirectly, signal skeletal muscle to reduce amino acid release and thereby conserve protein stores.

The production of glucose by the hepatocyte during prolonged starvation is a finely coordinated effort between the liver and skeletal muscle, involving the increased flux of carbon molecules for the synthesis of new glucose. Although many amino acids may be

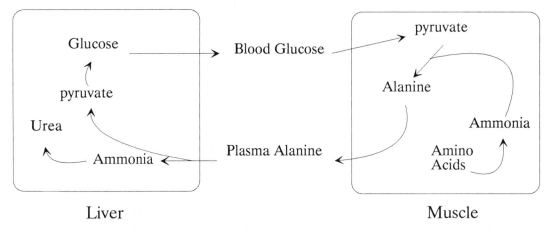

Figure 11-2. The alanine-glucose cycle. Carbon chains and ammonia are shuttled from skeletal muscle to the liver via the alanine-glucose cycle. The carbon skeleton is used for gluconeogenesis whereas the ammonia is used in the synthesis of urea.

used to provide carbon precursors for glucose, alanine serves as the major gluconeogenic amino acid. It is released from skeletal muscle in quantities that exceed the amounts found in skeletal muscle protein, which indicates that it may be produced within the cell. It is then exported via the bloodstream to the liver and, after deamination within the hepatocyte, the carbons are converted to glucose. The oxidative deamination of alanine by the hepatocyte provides energy for gluconeogenesis and allows muscle to rid itself of potentially toxic nitrogen end-products. A portion of the newly produced glucose is oxidized to pyruvate within the myocyte. Subsequently, the pyruvate is converted to alanine by transamination, with the nitrogen moiety being provided largely by the branched-chain amino acids (BCAAs)—leucine, valine, and isoleucine. The shuttling of alanine to the liver and glucose to muscle is known as the alanine-glucose cycle (Fig. 11-2).

This shuttle provides a precursor supply for new glucose; while glucose is metabolized within muscle, it is not oxidized but converted to lactate. This three-carbon compound is rapidly extracted by the liver and converted to glucose. The energy utilized for this process is derived from fatty acids. Carbons from fatty acids cannot be converted to glucose, but the **energy** provided by fat can

be used in the synthesis of new glucose. Finally, it is important to note that net glucose synthesis does not occur unless pyruvate is derived from other amino acids.

The Cori cycle (see Fig. 11-1) also produces glucose during starvation. Skeletal muscle and other tissues such as red blood cells, the renal medulla, and bone marrow do not completely oxidize glucose, but rather metabolize it to lactate and pyruvate during fasting. These intermediary metabolites are released into the bloodstream and are subsequently reconverted into glucose by the liver. The conversion of lactate into glucose by the liver requires energy, which is derived from fat oxidation. The newly synthesized glucose is delivered to peripheral tissue where it is then used as an energy source. The net effect is that the energy derived from fat oxidation in the liver is shuttled to those tissues requiring glucose as an energy source.

During starvation, the kidney excretes increased quantities of hydrogen ion to maintain body pH at normal levels and also eliminates nitrogen-containing waste products. Additionally, the kidney becomes a major source for glucose production. After 30 days of fasting, the kidney contributes almost one-half of the body's glucose requirements [40]. Most of the glucose synthesized by the kidney is derived from the glutamine cycle

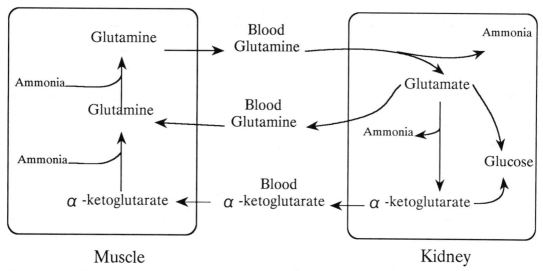

Figure 11-3. The glutamine cycle.

(Fig. 11-3). Glutamine, released by skeletal muscle, is metabolized to glutamate and ammonia within the renal parenchyma. The glutamate is deaminated to alpha-ketoglutarate, which becomes a part of the precursor pool for glucose production. The ammonia produced in these reactions neutralizes the acidic by-products of metabolism by accepting hydrogen ions. The latter is an important process during starvation, when significant amounts of base are needed to neutralize the 10 mEq of ketoacids produced each day.

In summary, the response to unstressed starvation is characterized by various biochemical and physiologic adaptations. In the postabsorptive state, some tissues can oxidize free fatty acids and use this substrate preferentially, although glucose production initially proceeds at normal levels. Alanine is a key amino acid used for gluconeogenesis by the liver and is synthesized from the transamination of glucose-derived pyruvate. Overall, the regulation of gluconeogenesis depends on the availability of substrate, numerous hormonal interactions, and changes in enzymatic activity. Gluconeogenesis is decreased or increased according to precursor availability or through changes in hepatic substrate extraction. Early in starvation, hepatic gluconeogenesis is accelerated secondary to an increased extraction of substrates and a hormonal environment favoring hepatic glucose production. Later, gluconeogenesis decreases progressively as a result of decreased precursor availability. In particular, alanine is released in reduced quantities from skeletal muscle. Furthermore, when the intake of nutrients is insufficient, a decline in insulin secretion appears to be an important signal for initiating the metabolic response to starvation. As starvation extends beyond 1 week, urinary excretion of nitrogen falls progressively. At this point, the major component of nitrogen excretion is urea. Other hormonal changes observed include an increase in circulating growth hormone levels and a decrease in the secretion of cortisol and serum triiodothyronine. These responses occur in association with a reduced level of catecholamines.

THE RESPONSE TO INJURY AND INFECTION

General Considerations

The response to injury and infection has been described since antiquity. The cardinal signs of inflammation—rubor, calor, dolor, and tumor (redness, heat, pain, and swelling)—

Table 11-2. Metabolic Changes in "Ebb" and "Flow" Phases

Ebb Phase	Flow Phase
Glucose elevated	Glucose normal or slightly increased
Glucose production normal	Glucose production greatly increased
Free fatty acids elevated	Free fatty acids normal or slightly elevated; flux increased
Insulin decreased	Insulin normal or elevated
Catecholamines elevated	Catecholamines high normal or elevated
Glucagon increased	Glucagon increased
Blood lactate elevated	Blood lactate elevated
Oxygen consumption depressed	Oxygen consumption elevated
Cardiac output decreased	Cardiac output increased
Core temperature decreased	Core temperature increased

were elucidated by Cornelius Celsus in his book, *De Re Medicinia: Book III,* sometime close to the birth of Christ. In the next century Galen added another sign to these: *functio laesa* (functional loss). As described by John Hunter in the late 1700s, these inflammatory responses were "an effect whose purpose is to restore the parts to their natural function." These early observations on inflammation have been broadened by observation and research in the last century to include the multitude of endocrine and metabolic responses of the patient with an injury or serious illness [19, 20]. Generalized symptoms of pain, fever and chills, myalgia, headache, and lethargy are the basic responses noted today. These responses are nonspecific, but when associated with a known insult, such as a burn, fracture, or infection, alterations of physiologic and metabolic parameters are expected within a certain time and a predictable magnitude.

The metabolic changes associated with illness or injury can be described in three consecutive phases occurring over time—acute, subacute, and chronic. The time course of these phases is from minutes to hours, days to weeks, and weeks to months, respectively. The duration of each phase is dependent on host determinants, magnitude of the insult, and occurrence of additional stresses such as operations or complications. The acute and subacute phases refer to the "ebb" and "flow" phases as originally described by

Cuthbertson. The body's maintenance of circulation and oxygenation to vital organs is the critical theme of the acute or "ebb" phase (Table 11-2). The metabolic changes that occur during this time period are primarily associated with the maintenance of sufficient glucose levels to support cardiorespiratory and CNS activity and other vital functions. Although the metabolic changes that occur during this phase are crucial for survival, they are generally of short duration because of the frequency of successful volume restoration.

With adequate circulating blood volume and support of tissue oxygenation, the patient progresses to the hypermetabolic or "flow" phase of injury. During this time period, the body provides circulating fuels and other metabolic substrate specifically to support organ function, prevent infection, and facilitate wound repair. A metabolic state that occurs mobilizes stored energy from adipose tissue and amino acids from skeletal muscle protein to ensure that metabolic substrate is provided for these essential functions. In contrast to starvation, the "flow" phase provides for accelerated mobilization of stored substrate. Conservation of body protein by adaptive metabolic processes does not occur.

Following the "flow" phase or hypermetabolic phase of illness, the patient eventually becomes anabolic and enters the recovery or rehabilitation phase. This period of convalescence frequently occurs at home or in a chronic care facility. The body's tissues rebuild using exogenous fuel, usually from enterally consumed nutrients. Repletion of adipose and skeletal muscle tissue occurs over time so that bodily function may return toward normal.

The Hypermetabolic or Flow Phase

The "ebb" phase of injury or infection resolves with stabilization of perfusion and tissue oxygenation. The "flow" phase then begins, and is characterized by increased requirements for metabolic substrate. Therefore, this phase is the time when nutritional support can be a factor in reducing body catabolism. At this time, the basal metabolic rate and overall body temperature rise. A catabolic state develops, with negative nitrogen balance, hyperglycemia, hyperinsulinemia, and accelerated lipolysis.

The graded elevation in the metabolic rate seen in patients following injury or illness is proportional to the magnitude of the stress. Typically in a simple elective operation, metabolism is increased by 10% [22], and following an uncomplicated long-bone fracture, energy expenditures may range between 15 to 25% above basal. Generalized sepsis is associated with elevations of oxygen consumption as high as 50 to 60% above normal levels, and patients with large thermal injuries may have levels of energy expenditure that are twice normal [51].

The time course of metabolic changes during injury and illness shows the basal metabolic rate to be decreased in the "ebb" phase, become maximal during the "flow" phase, and be increased in the "flow" phase. The peak change in basal metabolic rate occurs at 5 to 10 days after injury [18], with a gradual normalization during convalescence. Regional metabolic measurements have shown the hypermetabolism to be a generalized phenomenon with two-thirds of the heat produced in the viscera and one-third in the extremities [54, 55]. The hormonal mediation of this hypermetabolism has been duplicated in normal volunteers with a combined infusion of cortisol, glucagon, and epinephrine, and

also with sublethal infusions of cytokines [5, 36].

Following injury uncomplicated by invasive infection, the core temperature rises 1 to 2°C. Studies suggest that this occurs because of an upward adjustment of the central thermoregulatory setpoint [57]. The response is probably related to increased cytokine elaboration, which occurs in injured tissue or in the fixed macrophage population. The cytokines activate prostaglandin synthesis in the hypothalamus, resulting in fever, increased sympathetic outflow, and other centrally mediated metabolic changes [21].

A part of the hypermetabolic response can be associated with this elevated temperature, simply because chemical reactions are more robust at higher temperatures. However, it is difficult to explain increases in body oxygen consumption of greater than 25% using these conventional explanations alone (i.e., for every 1°C elevation in core temperature, there is a 10% increase in metabolic rate). The relationship between temperature and metabolic rate may represent a more complex interaction in the critically ill patient. The usual wisdom linearly relating these two variables may be incorrect. Recent evidence suggests that substrate cycling provides the heat for the hypermetabolism associated with burn injury, and this relates to the increased elaboration of glucagon [32, 59].

Protein Metabolism

The most significant feature of the hypermetabolic "flow" phase is the negative nitrogen balance and depletion of body protein that occurs in the critically ill patient. This is of great significance because protein represents functional tissue necessary for host repair and survival. Studies of patients with long-bone fractures demonstrate significant increases in urinary nitrogen loss, progressive wasting of skeletal muscle mass, and generalized weakness, changes that could not be accounted for by bedrest alone. These observations led Cuthbertson to attribute the nitrogen loss to a generalized and accelerated breakdown of skeletal muscle protein [17]. A variety of subsequent experiments related the extent of negative nitrogen balance to the severity of the injury, prior nutritional status, and prior skeletal muscle mass (as reflected by age, gender, and debility of the individual) [15].

Nitrogen balance is the difference between whole-body protein synthesis and breakdown. The negative nitrogen balance seen with severe injury or critical illness can result from various combinations of changes in synthesis and breakdown. In all these conditions, however, catabolism exceeds synthesis. Several studies of protein synthesis and catabolism in patients with injury, immobilization, or starvation demonstrate decreased rates of synthesis. However, increased rates of protein catabolism above normal were similarly demonstrated following injury and infection [16, 39]. Nutritional support augments protein synthesis during the hypermetabolic phase, but does not adequately compensate for the accelerated catabolism. Therefore, the negative nitrogen balance can be greatly reduced, but not totally eliminated, with nutritional support.

A major site of the increased protein catabolism in injured patients is skeletal muscle, as demonstrated by amino acid efflux from the extremity [2]. Serum levels of amino acids usually decline [1], and this alteration in serum concentration relates to increased uptake by the viscera in excess of the peripheral release. While this balance between peripheral amino acid release and visceral uptake is usually maintained, it may be altered with progressive illness. For example, a poor prognosis has been observed in patients with multiple-organ failure, generalized sepsis, and end-stage hepatic disease when both peripheral release and visceral uptake of amino acids return to or fall below normal [55].

The principal carriers of nitrogen from the skeletal muscle to the viscera are alanine and glutamine [44]. The liver converts alanine and other amino acids to glucose, and the nitrogen residue is used in the synthesis of acute-phase proteins or is disposed as urea. In the kidney, nitrogen from glutamine combines with hydrogen ions to form ammo-

nium, which is excreted in an effort to rid the body of the increased acid load associated with accelerated catabolism. In the gut, glutamine is a primary fuel for the enterocyte. This reaction yields some free ammonia, which is transported to the liver via the portal system, converted to urea, and excreted. Glutamine is also converted to alanine and then metabolized in the liver for gluconeogenesis and ureagenesis. All of these reactions favor the formation of nitrogen end-products, which are lost from the body in the urine, contributing to the accelerated ureagenesis and negative nitrogen balance associated with critical illness (see Figs. 11-2 and 11-3). [*Editor's Note:* One of the real questions concerning this process is the seemingly high wastage of nitrogen in the form of urea. This seems unwise in view of the importance of this metabolic intermediate. It may be that the glucose produced by gluconeogenesis in the liver gets to a critical area, but this has not been proved.]

The liver requires amino acids not only for gluconeogenesis but also for the synthesis of various proteins for inflammatory and immune functions during acute illness. These "acute-phase proteins" serve multiple functions in host defense and tissue repair [43], and are integral to recovery from serious illness.

Carbohydrate Metabolism

Patients with injury or illness generally have elevated blood glucose levels. The dependence of vital organs on glucose availability for energy production is thought to be the cause of this phenomenon. Originally the hyperglycemia was thought to be due to insulin deficiency, which could also have accounted for the protein catabolism. Subsequent studies have shown elevated insulin levels in the hypermetabolic state [34] and insulin resistance in normally sensitive tissues [12].

The source of the glucose produced during the initial phase of injury or illness is a result of hepatic glycogenolysis as well as accelerated gluconeogenesis. Infusion of exogenous glucose only partially diminishes hepatic glucose production in the septic or injured patient [11, 58]. This contrasts to studies in normal, unstressed individuals in which exogenous glucose almost totally attenuates hepatic glucose production. Hepatic venous catheterization studies and tracer kinetic investigations in injured and infected patients have documented the ability of the liver to increase glucose production up to twice the normal rates [55]. These same kinetic studies have shown increased rates of glucose utilization, compared to healthy control subjects. Patients with multisystem organ failure show a reduced ability to achieve this accelerated glucose production.

Evaluation of the source of the glucose suggests that 30% comes from lactate and pyruvate generated in peripheral tissue and cleared by the liver [54, 55]. Based on rates of urea production, an additional 30% of the glucose produced could be accounted for by amino acids contributing to hepatic gluconeogenesis. The remaining hepatic glucose comes from hepatic glycogen stores, which can be partially mediated by vigorous nutritional support.

Utilization of the increased glucose occurs in the wound and by inflammatory tissues. Fibroblasts, leukocytes, and epithelial cells (all those cells involved in tissue repair) are glycolytic and show a major capacity for anaerobic metabolism [53]. Glucose converts to lactate in the wound, which then recycles to the liver for synthesis into glucose. The oxidized glucose is replaced by glucose synthesized from amino acids originally from skeletal muscle and then transformed by hepatic gluconeogenesis.

The brain utilizes glucose at a normal rate following injury, whereas the kidney increases utilization [28]. The other major sources of increased glucose consumption are the cells involved in the reticuloendothelial system, particularly if they are stimulated by endotoxin or cytokines. Tissues that do not primarily require glucose, such as skeletal muscle, utilize fat as an alternative fuel. These tissues are traditionally regarded as insulin sensitive, but develop insulin resistance in the posttraumatic period [12]. One site of

insulin resistance was shown to be in uninjured forearm tissue, which is primarily composed of skeletal muscle. The uninjured forearm fails to increase glucose uptake in response to insulin infusion, which is in marked contrast to findings in normal individuals. These observations are important in terms of clinical management—hyperglycemia following injury rarely occurs in nondiabetics unless moderate quantities of glucose are administered. With infusion of glucose of more than 4 to 5 mg/min/kg of body weight, progressive hyperglycemia may occur because tissues that traditionally utilize the glucose become insulin resistant and thus do not extract this substrate from the bloodstream.

Fat Metabolism

The major source of fuel for oxidation following injury or critical illness is stored triglyceride. This endogenous fuel source is mobilized and oxidized at increased rates, as demonstrated by respiratory quotients approaching 0.7 during this time period [22, 45, 51]. Free fatty acid and glycerol levels may be elevated, reflecting increased lipolysis, but these concentrations may be normal or low in spite of accelerated turnover. Studies of glycerol turnover in injured and septic patients, and palmitate turnover in burn patients, confirm that increased release and clearance of fatty acids occur in these hypermetabolic states [14]. During the "flow" phase, fatty acids may be utilized by many tissues in the body, particularly cardiac and skeletal muscle. The lipid is mobilized from adipose stores by heightened sympathetic nervous stimulation as well as the development of resistance to the antilipolytic effects of insulin.

Mediators of the Flow-Phase Response

The stress response is associated with elevated blood levels of cortisol, glucagon, catecholamines, and growth hormone. The levels of these counterregulatory hormones are generally proportional to the magnitude of the insult and return to normal over time with wound closure or resolution of the infection. The effect of these hormones on a specific tissue is dependent on multiple factors. Perfusion defects, acidosis, fever, and hypoxia and other acute homeostatic defects alter tissue responses to these hormones and thereby modulate the metabolic expression of these agents.

One major component of the stress response is the activation of the sympathoadrenal axis. In response to injury, surgical operation, or sepsis, or in response to pain, fear, cold exposure, hypoxia, and other stresses, signals are transmitted through the splanchnic nerves to initiate circulatory release of epinephrine and other catecholamines [42]. The initial description of the "fight-or-flight" response characterizes the effects of sudden sympathoadrenal discharge. The organism experiences tachycardia, tachypnea, piloerector activity, and pupillary dilation. An organ's response to sympathetic nervous system activation is determined by the distribution of alpha- and beta-adrenergic receptors, the responsiveness of the end organ, and the absolute and relative concentrations of epinephrine and norepinephrine reaching the receptors. Epinephrine increases cardiac output, blood pressure, and splanchnic and muscle blood flow, and reduces renal and dermal blood flow. The beta-adrenergic effects of this agent are important in the stimulation of heat generation. Norepinephrine causes venoconstriction and increased peripheral resistance, resulting in increased blood pressure and coronary blood flow.

The metabolic effects of the catecholamines are additive to the other counterregulatory hormones in altering carbohydrate metabolism [5]. Epinephrine tends to elevate blood glucose concentration by accelerating hepatic glycogenolysis and gluconeogenesis, converting skeletal muscle glycogen to lactate, and enhancing glucagon elaboration. Additional metabolic effects include mobilization of free fatty acids by direct catecholamine effect on adipose tissue and indirectly by suppression of insulin [42].

CNS release of corticotropin from the anterior pituitary during major stress results in release of adrenocortical hormones, primarily cortisol. Although the level of cortisol is related to the severity of the stress, a decreased or low level may occur in premorbid states or acute adrenal insufficiency from adrenal hemorrhage [24, 25]. Glucocorticoids are necessary for the normal response to injury and infection, particularly to restore blood volume following hypovolemia. Although investigators are undecided on what specific level of cortisol is necessary to exert a sufficient effect on blood volume maintenance, absent or low levels usually result in death.

Cortisol has widespread effects on carbohydrate metabolism, acting primarily on the liver to maintain glucose availability in the acute phase of stress, and mediating skeletal muscle insulin resistance [5]. Other endocrine effects include potentiation of glucagon, epinephrine, and growth hormone; inhibition of insulin elaboration; stimulation of lipolysis; mediation of skeletal muscle proteolysis; and, in excess, inhibition of immunologic and inflammatory responses.

Blood glucagon concentrations are consistently elevated during stress states even in the presence of hyperglycemia or following the administration of glucose [49, 56]. Glucagon acts primarily to promote glycogenolysis and stimulate gluconeogenesis. These effects are short-lived, but become prolonged by the addition of cortisol. Glucagon may also stimulate lipolysis in hepatic and peripheral tissues. The resultant free fatty acids are used for hepatic gluconeogenesis. Following injury or serious illness, the host significantly increases the energy demand, primarily for glucose substrate. The acute-phase response to mobilize glucose stores is a critical part of immediate survival as well as subsequent wound healing, immune system recovery, and overall recovery.

Insulin levels show a diphasic response to acute illness or injury. Levels are frequently below normal during the acute phase despite elevated levels of blood glucose [52]. Following resuscitation, during the subacute phase of injury, insulin levels rise and are usually appropriate or even elevated for the degree of hyperglycemia. Progressive insulin resistance develops [11], primarily in skeletal muscle [12], although the hepatic response is also diminished. When administered with large quantities of glucose, insulin has major anabolic effects and has been shown to diminish urinary nitrogen losses in severely injured patients [30]. This reflects in part a reduction in the efflux of amino acids from skeletal muscle, which occurs during insulinization despite the insensitivity of skeletal muscle glucose uptake to insulin.

Cytokines

Many of the metabolic alterations that are known to occur during severe illness, inflammation, or injury (e.g., hypermetabolism, hyperglycemia, increased fat utilization, negative nitrogen balance, and weight loss) can be related to the elaboration of counterregulatory hormones such as cortisone, glucagon, and catecholamines [5]. However, other manifestations of the "acute-phase response," namely fever, malaise, increased C-reactive protein levels, leukocytosis, and redistribution of trace elements such as iron, are related to the elaboration of products known as cytokines produced by macrophages and T cells. These substances are elaborated and exert their effects locally, but can also be detected in the bloodstream. A number of cytokines have been identified and characterized. Of these, interleukin-1 (IL-1), tumor necrosis factor (TNF) or cachectin, and interferon gamma play important roles in the metabolic response to infection. In addition, many cytokines stimulate cyclo-oxygenase pathways, prostaglandins, and prostacyclins that may also influence systemic or local responses to injury. In particular, TNF is thought to mediate many of the systemic effects of infection and inflammation, and may act in concert with IL-1, leukotrienes, and platelet-activating factor [7].

Other experimental evidence suggests that TNF is an important central mediator of the response to infection and/or endotoxin challenge. Mice, which have a genetically determined inability to produce TNF, are resistant to the effects of endotoxin [8]. Furthermore, pretreatment of endotoxin-sensitive mice with a highly specific rabbit polyclonal antibody directed against mouse TNF protects against the lethal effects of endotoxin [10]. In a similar fashion, pretreatment of baboons with monoclonal antibody to TNF prevents death after lethal doses of live *Escherichia coli* bacteria [46]. In humans, endotoxin administration increases plasma TNF concentrations, the rise of which is temporally associated with physiologic and metabolic changes similar to those observed during sepsis [35], and TNF administration alone induces metabolic changes similar to those following endotoxin infusion [36].

Like TNF, IL-1 is a peptide or closely related group of peptides synthesized by tissue macrophages and circulating monocytes in response to invasion by microorganisms and their products [21]. It can induce fever, mobilize leukocytes from the bone marrow, stimulate acute-phase protein synthesis by the liver, redistribute trace metals, activate B cells, and enhance natural T-cell killer activity.

Effects on Glucose and Intermediary Metabolism

Cytokines such as TNF may play a very important role in the elevation of carbohydrate metabolism seen in sepsis. Rats infused with human recombinant TNF have increased glucose metabolism similar to that observed in gram-negative sepsis [3]. The infusion of TNF was associated with a transient increase in insulin levels in some studies [47], but had no effect in another [23]. It is unclear if TNF has direct effects on cellular metabolism or acts indirectly.

Other studies suggested that TNF helps regulate the utilization of energy stores within skeletal muscle. Cachectin increases glucose uptake and increases glycogenolysis and lactate production in myocyte cultures [33]. Effects of IL-1 on glucose metabolism are also described. A recent study of the effects of purified IL-1 in vitro showed that this cytokine reduces intracellular steroid receptors and decreases phosphoenol-pyruvate carboxykinase activity, which results in diminished gluconeogenesis and reduced blood glucose concentrations [29].

Effects on Skeletal Muscle

Cachectin may contribute to the anorexia and weight loss seen in severe illness [6]. Traditionally, loss of skeletal muscle protein in sepsis, in trauma, or after surgery was thought to be primarily mediated by changes in the catabolic and counterregulatory hormones. Studies that altered the hormonal environment by artificially raising cortisol and catecholamine levels showed that amino acid loss from skeletal muscle can be elicited in normal individuals, although not to the levels observed during critical illness. Although the effects of critical illness on the mobilization of skeletal muscle protein stores is mediated in part by prostaglandin E_2 (PGE$_2$), recent data indicate that cyclo-oxygenase pathways, prostaglandins, and prostanoids do not play a significant role in the regulation of protein homeostasis or regulate changes in protein balance in skeletal muscle [31, 37, 38].

As yet, it is not entirely clear what role TNF, IL-1, or other cytokines play in skeletal muscle protein balance. There are conflicting data on the effects of cytokines on skeletal muscle metabolism. In a recent study of the effects of pure recombinant IL-1 (alpha or beta) and a variety of other cytokines (including TNF and interferon alpha, beta, and gamma) on muscle proteolysis and prostaglandin production, none of these products administered singly had a demonstrable effect on skeletal muscle breakdown or PGE$_2$ production [27]. However, a large increase in net protein breakdown was induced in rat soleus muscle by polypeptides released from porcine monocytes or by serum from febrile cattle that had been injected with *Pasteurella haemolytica* or bovine rhinotracheitis virus. From these data, the authors concluded that there are still as yet unidentified cytokines which contribute to the negative nitrogen balance that accompanies severe illness.

In another animal study, net skeletal mus-

cle protein breakdown was increased by infusion of TNF-alpha but not by infusion of IL-1 [41]. However, together the two cytokines acted synergistically to increase skeletal muscle protein breakdown and to reduce skeletal muscle protein content.

Thus, it may be the interaction of various cytokines that mediates protein homeostasis during sepsis and injury. TNF, when administered chronically, could alter protein balance by secondary hormone production or other cytokine-mediated events [48]. For example, cachectin stimulates the release of corticotropin [4]. Patients [50] and canines [23] given TNF have increased circulating levels of cortisol. IL-1 also stimulates glucocorticoid release through effects on the hypothalamus and on the adrenal gland [4].

Effects on Fat Metabolism

As discussed previously, fat stores are mobilized during times of stress and starvation, which ultimately facilitates protein conservation and carbohydrate sparing. Infection is associated with a decreased clearance of circulating lipids through effects on membrane lipoprotein lipase. TNF- or cachectin-induced changes in fat metabolism may contribute to the mobilization of lipid stores as an alternative fuel source during critical illness. TNF in vitro decreases the clearance of lipids, increases fatty acid synthesis, and increases cellular lipolysis by suppressing membrane lipoprotein activity [9]. The administration in vivo of lethal doses of TNF reproduces the hyperlipidemic conditions of severe illness. Dogs given sublethal quantities of TNF have elevated serum triglyceride and free fatty acid levels [47]. The rise in serum triglyceride levels observed in primates given infusions of live gram-negative bacteria is blocked when the apes are pretreated with monoclonal antibodies against TNF [26].

SUMMARY

Although the hormonal changes observed after an injury are well described and the nature of the alteration of target tissues to these changes is known, the precise signals that alter the hormonal and tissue responses constituting the stress response have not been determined. More recent studies suggest that cytokines, the products of cyclo-oxygenase pathways, prostacyclines, and prostanoids, all play important roles in regulating the body's response to trauma.

REFERENCES

1. Askanazi, J., Carpentier, Y. A., Michelsen, C. B., et al. Muscle and plasma amino acids following injury: Influence of intercurrent infection. *Ann. Surg.* 192:78, 1980.
2. Aulick, L. H., and Wilmore, D. W. Increased peripheral amino acid release following burn injury. *Surgery* 85:560, 1979.
3. Bagby, G. J., Lang, C. H., Hargrove, D. M., Thompson, J. J., Wilson, L. A., and Spitzer, J. J. Glucose kinetics in rats infused with endotoxin-induced monokines or tumor necrosis factor. *Circ. Shock* 24:111, 1988.
4. Besedovsky, H., Delrey, A., Sorkin, E., and Dinarello, C. A. Immunoregulatory feedback between interleukin-1 and glucocorticoid hormones. *Science* 233:652, 1986.
5. Bessey, P. Q., Watters, J. M., Aokim, T. T., and Wilmore, D. W. Combined hormonal infusion stimulates the metabolic response to injury. *Ann. Surg.* 200:264, 1984.
6. Beutler, B., and Cerami, A. Cachectin and tumor necrosis factor as two sides of the same biological coin. *Nature* 320:584, 1986.
7. Beutler, B., and Cerami, A. Cachectin: More than a tumor necrosis factor. *N. Engl. J. Med.* 316:379, 1987.
8. Beutler, B., Krochin, N., Milsark, I. W., Leudke, C., and Cerami, A. Control of cachectin (tumor necrosis factor) synthesis: Mechanisms of endotoxin resistance. *Science* 232:977, 1986.
9. Beutler, B., Mahoney, J., Le Trang, N., Pekala, P., and Cerami, I. Purification of cachectin, a lipoprotein lipase-suppressing hormone secreted by endotoxin induced RAW 264.7 cells. *J. Exp. Med.* 161:984, 1985.
10. Beutler, B., Milsark, I., and Cerami, A. Passive immunization against cachectin/tumor necrosis factor protects mice from the lethal effects of endotoxin. *Science* 229:869, 1985.
11. Black, P. R., Brooks, D. C., Bessey, P. Q., Wolfe, R. R., and Wilmore, D. W. Mechanisms of insulin resistance following injury. *Ann. Surg.* 196:420, 1982.
12. Brooks, D. C., Bessey, P. Q., Black, P. R., Aoki, T. T., and Wilmore, D. W. Posttraumatic insulin resistance in uninjured forearm tissue. *J. Surg. Res.* 37:100, 1984.
13. Cahill, G. F., Jr. Starvation in man. *N. Engl. J. Med.* 282:668, 1970.
14. Carpentier, Y. A., Askanazi, J., Elwyn, D. H., et al. Effects of hypercaloric glucose infusion on lipid metabolism in injury and sepsis. *J. Trauma* 19:649, 1979.
15. Cohn, S. H., Vartsky, D., Yasumura, S., et al. Compartmental body composition based on total-body nitrogen, potassium, and calcium. *Am. J. Physiol.* 239:E524, 1980.
16. Crane, C. W., Picou, D., Smith, R., and Waterlow, J. C. Protein turnover in patients before and after elective orthopaedic operations. *Br. J. Surg.* 64:129, 1977.
17. Cuthbertson, D. P. The disturbance of metabolism produced by bone and non-bony injury, with notes on certain abnormal conditions of bone. *Biochem. J.* 24:1244, 1930.
18. Cuthbertson, D. P. Post-shock metabolic response. *Lancet* 1:433, 1942.
19. Cuthbertson, D. P. Alterations in metabolism following injury: Part I. *Injury* 11:175, 1980.
20. Cuthbertson, D. P. Alterations in metabolism following injury: Part II. *Injury* 11:286, 1980.
21. Dinarello, C. A. Interleukin-1. *Rev. Infect. Dis.* 6:51, 1984.
22. Duke J. H., Jr., Jorgensen, S. B., Broell, J. R., Long, C. L., and Kinney, J. M. Contribution of protein to calorie expenditure following injury. *Surgery* 68:168, 1970.
23. Evans, D. A., Jacobs, D. O., Revhaug, A., and Wilmore, D. W. The effects of tumor necrosis factor and their selective inhibition by ibuprofen. *Ann. Surg.* 209:312, 1988.
24. Finley, W. E. I., and McKee, J. I. Serum cortisol levels in severely stressed patients. (Letter) *Lancet* 1:1414, 1982.
25. Foley, F. D., Pruitt, B. A., Jr., and Moncrief, J. A. Adrenal hemorrhage and necrosis in seriously burned patients. *J. Trauma* 7:863, 1967.
26. Fong, Y., Lowry, S. F., and Cerami, A. Cachectin/TNF: A macrophage product that induces cachexia and shock. *J. Parenter. Enter. Nutr.* 12(6):72s, 1988.
27. Goldberg, A. L., Kettelhut, I. C., Furono, K., Fagan, J. M., and Baracos, V. Activation of protein breakdown and prostaglandin E_2 production in rat skeletal muscle in fever is signaled by a macrophage produced distinct from interleukin-1 or other known monokines. *J. Clin. Invest.* 81:1378, 1988.
28. Goodwin, C. W., Jr., Aulick, L. H., Powanda, M. C., Wilmore, D. W., and Pruitt, B. A., Jr. Glucose dynamics following severe injury. *Eur. Surg. Res.* 12(Suppl. 1):126, 1980.
29. Hill, M. R., Stith, R. D., and McCallum, R. E. Interleukin-1: A regulatory role in glucocorticoid regulated hepatic metabolism. *J. Immunol.* 137:858, 1986.
30. Hinton, P., Allison, S. P., Littlejohn, S., and

Lloyd, J. Insulin and glucose to reduce catabolic response to injury in burn patients. *Lancet* 1:767, 1971.

31. Hulton, N. R., Johnson, D. J., and Wilmore, D. W. Limited effects of prostaglandin inhibitors in *Escherichia coli* sepsis. *Surgery* 98:291, 1985.

32. Jahoor, F., Herndon, D. N., and Wolfe, R. R. Role of insulin and glucagon in the response of glucose and alanine kinetics in burn-injured patients. *J. Clin. Invest.* 78:807, 1986.

33. Lee, M. D., Zentella, A., Vine, W., Pekala, P. H., and Cerami, A. Effect of endotoxin-induced monokines on glucose metabolism in the muscle cell line L6. *Proc. Natl. Acad. Sci. USA* 84:2590, 1987.

34. Long, C. L., Spencer, J. L., Kinney, J. M., and Geiger, J. W. Carbohydrate metabolism in man: Effect of elective operations and major injury. *J. Appl. Physiol.* 31:110, 1971.

35. Michie, H. R., Manogue, K. R., Spriggs, D. R., et al. Detection of circulating tumor necrosis factor after endotoxin administration. *N. Engl. J. Med.* 318:1481, 1988.

36. Michie, H. R., Spriggs, D. R., Manogue, K. R., et al. Tumor necrosis factor and endotoxin induce similar metabolic responses in humans. *Surgery* 104:280, 1988.

37. Moldawer, L. L., Svaninger, G., Gelin, J., and Lundholm, K. Interleukin 1 (alpha or beta) and tumor necrosis factor do not regulate protein balance in skeletal muscle. *Am. J. Physiol.* 253:C766, 1987.

38. Odessey, R. Effect of inhibitors of proteolysis and arachidonic acid metabolism on burn-induced protein breakdown. *Metabolism* 34:616, 1985.

39. O'Keefe, S. J. D., Sender, P. M., and James, W. P. T. "Catabolic" loss of body nitrogen in response to surgery. *Lancet* 2:1035, 1974.

40. Owen, O. E., Felig, P., Wahren, J., and Cahill, G. F. Liver and kidney metabolism during prolonged starvation. *J. Clin. Invest.* 48:574, 1969.

41. Pomposelli, J. J., Flores, E. A., and Bistrian, B. R. Role of biochemical mediators in clinical nutrition and surgical metabolism. *J. Parenter. Enter. Nutr.* 12:212, 1988.

42. Porte, D., Jr., and Robertson, R. P. Control of insulin secretion by catecholamines, stress, and the sympathetic nervous system. *Fed. Proc.* 32:1792, 1973.

43. Powanda, M. C., and Moyer, E. D. Plasma protein alterations during infection: Potential significance of these changes to host defense and repair systems. In M. C. Powanda and P. G. Canonico (eds.), *Infection: The Physiologic and Metabolic Responses of the Host.* Amsterdam: Elsevier/North Holland Biomedical Press, 1981.

44. Ruderman, N. B. Muscle amino acid metabolism and gluconeogenesis. *Annu. Rev. Med.* 26:245, 1975.

45. Stoner, H. B., Little, R. A., Frayn, K. N., Elebute, A. E., Tresadern, J., and Gross, E. The effect of sepsis on the oxidation of carbohydrate and fat. *Br. J. Surg.* 70:32, 1983.

46. Tracey, K. J., Fong, Y., Hesse, D. G., et al. Anti-cachectin/TNF monoclonal antibodies prevent septic shock during lethal bacteremia. *Nature* 330:662, 1987.

47. Tracey, K. J., Lowry, S. F., Fahey, T. J., et al. Cachectin/tumor necrosis factor induces lethal shock and stress hormone responses in the dog. *Surg. Gynecol. Obstet.* 164:415, 1987.

48. Tracey, K. J., Wei, H., Manogue, K. R., et al. Cachectin/tumor necrosis factor induces cachexia, anorexia, and inflammation. *J. Exp. Med.* 167:1211, 1988.

49. Unger, R. H. Glucagon and the insulin:glucagon ratio in diabetes and other catabolic illnesses. *Diabetes* 20:834, 1971.

50. Warren, R. S., Starnes, H. F., Gabrielove, J. L., Oettgen, H. F., and Brennan, M. F. The acute metabolic effects of tumor necrosis factor administration. *Arch. Surg.* 122:1396, 1987.

51. Wilmore, D. W. *The Metabolic Management of the Critically Ill.* New York: Plenum Medical, 1977.

52. Wilmore, D. W. Carbohydrate metabolism following injury. In K. G. M. B. Alberti (ed.), *Clinics in Endocrinology and Metabolism.* London: W. B. Saunders, 1976. P. 731.

53. Wilmore, D. W., and Aulick, L. H. Metabolic changes in burn patients. *Surg. Clin. North Am.* 58:1173, 1978.

54. Wilmore, D. W., Aulick, L. H., Mason, A. D., Jr., and Pruitt, B. A., Jr. Influence of the burn wound on local and systemic responses to injury. *Ann. Surg.* 186:444, 1977.

55. Wilmore, D. W., Goodwin, C. W., Aulick, L. H., et al. Effect of injury and infection on visceral metabolism and circulation. *Ann. Surg.* 192:491, 1980.

56. Wilmore, D. W., Lindsey, C. A., Moylan, J. A., Faloona, G. R., Pruitt, B. A., and Unger, R. H. Hyperglucagonaemia after burns. *Lancet* 1:73, 1974.

57. Wilmore, D. W., Orcutt, T. W., Mason, A. D., Jr., and Pruitt, B. A., Jr. Alterations in hypothalamic function during thermal injury. *J. Trauma* 15:697, 1975.

58. Wolfe, R. R., Durkot, M. J., Allsop, J. R., and Burke, J. F. Glucose metabolism in severely burned patients. *Metabolism* 28:1031, 1979.

59. Wolfe, R. R., Herndon, D. N., Jahoor, F., Miyoshi, H., and Wolfe, M. Effect of severe burn injury on substrate cycling by glucose and fatty acid. *N. Engl. J. Med.* 317:403, 1987.

II

Specific Aspects

12

Energy Requirements for Parenteral Nutrition

John M. Kinney

The energy requirements for parenteral nutrition depend on three factors: the energy expenditure of the patient; the clinical diagnosis that prevents adequate enteral nutrition; and the underlying metabolic state of the patient, which will influence the effectiveness with which any nutrition is utilized. Therefore, each physician and/or nutrition specialist must have definite nutritional objectives when starting parenteral nutrition and utilize whatever methods of nutritional assessment are available to monitor the response of the patient.

CALORIMETRY: DEVELOPMENT AND APPLICATION

The term calorimetry derives from heat metabolism, which is measured by the methodology of direct calorimetry. Unfortunately, direct calorimetry is cumbersome, expensive, and difficult to apply to acutely ill or injured patients. Therefore, the measurement of oxygen consumption and carbon dioxide production, when corrected for nitrogen excretion, allows the calculation of the energy expenditure and the proportion of fat, carbohydrate, and protein in the metabolic fuel mixture. This method provides unique information, is noninvasive, and can be applied to acutely ill and bedridden patients.

The principles of gas exchange were introduced in the late 1700s, but were not refined for nutritional use until a century later by Voit and Rubner [13]. Basal metabolism was studied in various medical conditions by Lusk [19] and DuBois [6], but such measurements were seldom used for clinical management except for thyroid disease between 1925 and 1950. At that time, thyroid disease began to be evaluated by chemical measurements on blood or urine, and calorimetry disappeared as part of the clinical care of patients. After neglect for 20 years, a resurgence of interest in gas exchange for indirect calorimetry began during the 1970s as a result of three factors: (1) a renewed interest in the energy imbalance represented by obesity, (2) a growing interest in sports medicine and stress testing, and (3) the desire to utilize energy expenditure for calculating the appropriate caloric intake of patients receiving total parenteral nutrition (TPN).

The decade of the 1980s has produced both new products for parenteral nutrition and the commercial availability of various instruments that can be taken to the bedside for measurements of gas exchange. The increasing availability of such measurements has emphasized the clinical circumstances in which knowing the resting energy expenditure (REE) can improve the nutritional care of hospital patients.

The total energy expenditure (TEE) is usually expressed as kilocalories per unit of time, which is the sum of three factors:

$$TEE = BMR + DIT + ACT$$

The basal metabolic rate, or BMR, is the gas exchange measured under postabsorptive conditions (no food for the previous 8–10 hours), under resting conditions (formerly measured on awakening before any activity) in a thermoneutral environment. Hospital measurements of indirect calorimetry for nutritional purposes have commonly been made as the resting metabolic rate, performed at various times during the waking day rather than under basal conditions. Diet-induced thermogenesis, or DIT, usually represents only approximately 10% of the energy expenditure during caloric equilibrium. The energy expenditure of activity (ACT) is usually the most variable of the three components of the TEE, and the daily cost of activity is difficult to measure by most methods of calorimetry. Measurements in a respiration chamber or with doubly labeled water provide improved estimates of ACT, but as yet are not widely available. The ACT in ambulatory hospitalized patients can be expected to add 15 to 25% of the REE, and can be reduced to 5% or less in bedridden or early postoperative patients.

MEASUREMENT OF INDIRECT CALORIMETRY

Indirect calorimetry is based on the accurate measurement of gas exchange for a specific interval. The traditional approach to such a bedside measurement in the hospital involves the use of a mask or mouthpiece for a period of perhaps 15 minutes. Transparent head enclosures can avoid the spurious hyperventilation that may occur with a tight-fitting mask or mouthpiece when used with an acutely ill patient [5]. Such head enclosures may function by a negative pressure at the air outlet, drawing room air into the enclosure. It is possible to isolate the patient from room air by ventilating the head enclosure with a continuous stream of outside air. This may become important if the patient is surrounded by medical staff or family in a poorly ventilated area in which the ambient air no longer has the composition of ordinary room air.

The desire to measure energy expenditure over prolonged periods that simulate daily life has led to increasing attention to 24-hour measurements in a room-sized chamber calorimeter where the subject can be measured continuously while sleeping, awake, and resting; during and after meals; or during periods of activity on a treadmill or cycle ergometer [12]. The 24-hour energy expenditure of any given adult individual is surprisingly constant. However, interpersonal variations are considerable.

A variety of indirect methods have been utilized to assess TEE without the usual measurements for calorimetry. These have been based on (1) physiologic measurements such as ventilation or heart rate, (2) a measurement of REE by calorimetry plus the energy cost of activity estimated from a diary, (3) REE plus the output of an activity meter, or (4) the isotopic dilution of doubly labeled water. The assumptions and problems with each of these methods have been compared with those of conventional indirect calorimetry by Jequier et al. [11]. The first three methods are often not applicable to an ill or injured patient who might require parenteral nutrition.

However, the use of doubly labeled water may offer important clinical information regarding TEE when averaged over intervals that vary from 5 to 12 days in the free-living state.

The method of measuring energy expenditure in free-living animals was extended by Schoeller et al. [24, 25] to the study of humans in various conditions of normal life. A loading dose of water labeled with deuterium and ^{18}O is administered to the individual, and the difference in the rate of elimination of the two isotopes in urinary water is taken to represent the average daily excretion of carbon dioxide. The relative advantages and disadvantages have been reviewed [11]. This method has the advantages of utilizing a nonradioactive isotope, which allows the study of infants and pregnant women, a determination over many days, a simple and convenient technique with simultaneous information regarding total body water, and the simultaneous study of many individuals. The disadvantages are the expense of the isotope and mass spectrometry, the estimates are only of carbon dioxide production (with its greater potential error than measuring oxygen uptake), it requires correction factors that include fractionation of the isotope, and it cannot indicate variations in energy expenditure from day to day. The method has been used to study parenteral nutrition [21] and studies of sports medicine [30]. Studies in various forms of disease and injury are currently underway.

METABOLIC BODY SIZE

It has been recognized for over a century that energy expenditure does not vary as a linear function of body weight. Rubner [1] found that when the metabolic rate was expressed per square meter of body surface area, the effect of body size disappeared. This indicated to him that fasting homeotherms have a daily heat production of 1000 kcal/m². He believed that this was consistent with the idea that oxygen comes into the body and heat leaves the body through surfaces that are proportional to the body surface area. Kleiber [16] presented a spirited critique of the body surface area being a primary physiologic variable for energy expenditure, and strongly argued for the use of body weight to the ¾ power. He noted, however, that using such a power function to express energy expenditure was of greatest importance when comparing large weight differences between species and was of much less importance when comparing the energy expenditure over the weight range of adult men and women.

A series of investigators developed equations to express normal energy expenditure based on height and weight corrected for age and gender. The most popular of these has been the Harris-Benedict equations, which give heat production in kilocalories per day [18]. Daly et al. [4] reported data on 201 adult men and women and noted that the Harris-Benedict equations overestimated the energy expenditure by 10 to 15%. These authors also reported on 15 other studies in which measured basal energy expenditure in healthy, lean individuals could be compared with a value predicted from the Harris-Benedict equations, and found results to vary from +19% to −14%. The reasons for this variability could not be determined, but it did emphasize the importance of standardized measurement procedures with carefully calibrated equipment.

Cunningham [2] analyzed the subject data for the Harris-Benedict equations, using the predicted body water for their weight and sex from the equations of Moore et al. [20]. This allowed the estimation of the lean body mass, which was found to be the best single predictor of BMR, while the influence of sex and age added little to the estimation. These findings suggested that estimations of BMR based on body surface area owed their usefulness to a hidden correlation with lean body mass in each sex. This would be in agreement with Benedict's suggestion, made in 1915, that the "active body mass" determined the BMR.

Roza and Shizgal [22] reanalyzed the data from Harris and Benedict, converting body weight, age, and sex to total body water, then to extracellular and intracellular water, then to total exchangeable potassium, and finally to body cell mass, utilizing the regression equations of Moore et al. [20]. These authors found that the Harris-Benedict equations predicted the REE with a precision of 14% in normally nourished individuals, but were unreliable in the malnourished patient. The REE appeared to be directly related to the body cell mass and was independent of age and sex. Shizgal [27] divided the lean tissues of the body into the extracellular and intracellular portions by examining the ratio of total exchangeable sodium to total exchangeable potassium. This method has a particular advantage: Under various pathologic conditions, the extracellular phase tends to undergo relative or absolute expansion as represented by increases in exchangeable sodium, while the body cell mass tends to shrink; therefore, the ratio of exchangeable sodium to exchangeable potassium increases as a result of both changes. Shizgal et al. considered this ratio to approximate 1.0 in normal adults and values above 1.2 as representing malnutrition. Recent work from this group showed that mortality is associated in sigmoid fashion with values between 1.5 and 2.2 [28].

There is widespread interest in finding more convenient and inexpensive methods for measuring body composition in hospitalized patients, particularly measuring total body water by physical methods such as total body conductivity or body impedance. Validation studies of such methods are being conducted in many centers.

Body weight or total body mass encompasses two major compartments: body fat and lean body mass. Grande [9] noted that for both males and females from 20 to 60 years old, a single value of 4.4 ml of oxygen per minute (or about 1.3 kcal/hr) per kilogram of fat-free body weight can be used instead of the customary tables and graphs based on the artificial concept of surface area as a determinant of basal metabolism. The fat-free mass is usually determined by measuring body water by isotope dilution, un-

derwater weighing, or multiple skinfold measurements.

RELATIONSHIP OF ENERGY INTAKE TO NITROGEN BALANCE

The daily nitrogen balance is dependent on both the nitrogen and the energy intake. If either is insufficient, there will be a net loss of nitrogen or a negative nitrogen balance. Excess energy intake can be expected to cause a positive nitrogen balance within the hereditary limits of an individual's body build, and assuming there is no increase in catabolic stimuli that tend to increase muscle proteolysis and thus increase urea synthesis and excretion. One of the difficulties of knowing the amount of calories to provide a patient receiving TPN is to recognize the clinical situations where increasing the extent of a positive calorie balance will improve the nitrogen balance without producing undesirable side effects such as hepatic steatosis, reduced immune function, or major increases in carbon dioxide production in the presence of serious pulmonary compromise.

In the absence of nitrogen balance measurements, it has been common to provide parenteral nutrition with a ratio of 100 to 120 cal/g of nitrogen. This ratio is somewhat lower than that consumed in an average American diet, on the assumption that an increased nitrogen intake will perhaps be of benefit in the acutely ill or injured patient.

DIET-INDUCED THERMOGENESIS

The thermic responses to food, or DIT, were formerly thought to be independent of the thermogenic response to cold. However, both forms of thermogenesis are mediated by the sympathetic nervous system, and blunted thermogenesis has been suggested as the basis for certain cases of obesity. Landsberg and Young [17] presented evidence that diet-induced changes in the sympathetic nervous system may underlie some of the changes in tissue function which accompany alterations in nutritional status. DIT can be divided into obligatory thermogenesis (formerly known as specific dynamic action), which is the energy cost of handling specific substrates. This is in contrast to adaptive thermogenesis (formerly known as luxuskonsumption), which is the apparent discrepancy between estimates of energy intake and utilization. Adaptive thermogenesis is stimulated by the ingestion of a meal, a part of which is oxidized to produce this heat, and may account for as much as 10 to 15% of the energy expenditure. Unfortunately, most of the human studies on DIT have not involved actual measurements of energy balance.

PHYSICAL ACTIVITY

The mid–19th century saw a change in the attitude toward bedrest for the treatment of many kinds of illness. Earlier there had been a general reluctance to remain in bed unless there was literally no choice. Later it was concluded that if immobilization could heal a broken bone, then it should be helpful in treating other medical problems. Thus, patients began to have enforced bedrest for weeks and even months when progressive movement out of bed would have been beneficial. During the 1940s certain physicians began to question the common practice of having 4 to 6 weeks of bedrest following an operation or a myocardial infarction, pointing out the clinical risks of prolonged bedrest, such as pulmonary embolism.

Skeletal muscle has been recognized as a target tissue in the weight loss that accompanies illness and injury. The negative nitrogen balance of these conditions is directly correlated with muscle proteolysis. However, the alterations in metabolic and nutritional behavior of muscle tissue due to the catabolic influences are difficult to separate from the changes that occur from the associated bedrest and inactivity. Previous healthy volunteers had metabolic balance studies performed while they ate a normal diet and were encased in a whole-body plaster cast [5]. This enforced bedrest was associated with a nega-

tive nitrogen balance of approximately 2 g/day. However, studies with the astronauts showed impressive muscle protein loss in the weightless state. Fong et al. [8] studied normal volunteers after 10 days of total starvation and reported that daily exercise did not improve the utilization of hyperalimentation given for repletion.

Waterlow [29] reviewed the question of metabolic adaptation to low intakes of energy and protein, separating the efficiency of physical work into mechanical efficiency and physiologic efficiency. The mechanical efficiency of work on an ergometer is usually between 26 and 30%, with some variation related to differences in the pattern of fiber types being utilized at different speeds of work. The physiologic efficiency of activity may be considered as the energy expended during work, minus the energy expended at rest, divided by the total energy expended while working. The energy cost is expressed as a multiple of BMR with no indication of the absolute mechanical work that is done. Efficiency of real-life activities may be influenced by unnecessary movements, and abolishing such movements may be an important form of adaptation to decreased food intake. Finding the optimum speed for a given activity may also be part of adaptation.

It is common medical experience to have patients return to the physician's office 2 to 4 weeks after leaving the hospital following a major illness or injury, and volunteer that they feel fine when they arise in the morning but are limp by noontime. The last thing to return in convalescence is the ability to work a full day without fatigue. This may relate to the extent of muscle proteolysis that occurred in the hospital as a result of some combination of catabolic stimuli and undernutrition.

The metabolic changes of bedrest and associated cardiovascular changes require new knowledge in order to treat them better when they occur and to minimize them in future management. Can particular forms of nutritional support lessen the impact of catabolic stimuli on muscle work capacity, particularly when coupled with properly designed low-level exercise programs? There is new interest in the role of proper diet and exercise to achieve physical fitness [10]. Sports medicine has become a formal specialty with increasing attention to muscle work capacity and muscle efficiency. At the same time the space program has stimulated new research on the physiologic effects of inactivity and bedrest [23]. Current nutritional support is often directed toward avoiding a negative balance of calories and nitrogen. Presumably avoiding a negative balance by dietary means should be associated with a decrease in net muscle proteolysis. However, data on a correlation between the preservation of muscle protein and the preservation of the muscle work capacity are not available. It seems reasonable to believe that the coming decade will see application of new concepts and better methods to monitor the combined effects of diet and activity on muscle energetics and particularly on muscle work capacity.

ENERGY EXPENDITURE OF HOSPITALIZED PATIENTS

Malnutrition is a condition having a familiar connotation to the physician of weight loss, hypoalbuminemia, anemia, and weakness. However, the relation between malnutrition and energy metabolism is understood in only the most general terms, which offer little guidance as to the optimum energy intake that should be provided when a patient requires TPN. Uncomplicated undernutrition generally is associated with a fall in energy expenditure, yet clinical conditions with weight loss do not always have an REE lower than the predicted normal value. Therefore, one must differentiate between weight loss with the hypometabolism of partial starvation and other examples of weight loss where the energy expenditure is within a normal range (relative hypermetabolism) or increased above the normal range (absolute hypermetabolism) despite the weight loss.

The BMR in health and various medical diseases was extensively studied by DuBois [6] before World War I. The two most dramatic increases in BMR were found with hy-

perthyroidism (increases in BMR of up to 80%) and with fever (increases in BMR of up to 50%). The large nitrogen losses shown by Cuthbertson [3] following long-bone fracture were interpreted by some surgeons as evidence of very large expenditures after injury in which body protein was required as additional fuel beyond that supplied by body fat. The idea of extremely high energy expenditures with injury led to a sense of resignation on the part of many surgeons because no means of high-calorie nutritional support was available. This was later compounded by the idea that the catabolic breakdown of body tissue after injury was triggered by hormones from the adrenal cortex and that this response was an obligatory part of the metabolic response to injury.

During the 1960s, Kinney et al. [14] undertook the study of the REE in various types of surgical disease and injury. There was considerable surprise to learn that after major surgical operations, the REE varied from no change to a change of no more than +10%. Convalescence from multiple injury, particularly if fractures of the extremities or pelvis were involved, was associated with increases in REE of 10 to 25% that lasted for 2 to 3 weeks in parallel with the increase in nitrogen excretion. The presence of fever with bacteremia was found to increase the REE approximately 7% for each Fahrenheit degree (13% for each Celsius degree) above the normal temperature, just as had been demonstrated by DuBois [6]. However, if the infection involved an extensive inflammatory response, such as acute peritonitis or empyema, the REE might be increased from 30 to 50% with correspondingly large increases in nitrogen excretion. Extensive third-degree burns were found to have the largest increases, being from 40 to 100% above the predicted normal. Burned patients were commonly treated during the 1960s with open exposure to normal ambient temperatures and surface antibacterial ointments for prolonged periods. The radiative as well as the evaporative cooling of these patients was increased. The severe hypermetabolism in the extensively burned patient appeared to be some combination of obligatory increases in heat loss and increased heat production of internal organs as a result of strong catabolic stimuli. The management of such patients has made considerable progress in the last 25 years, with a corresponding increase in the survival of patients with large burns. Resuscitation is usually prompt, pulmonary injury is recognized and treated, the environment is warmed, excision of the burn surface is started soon after resuscitation, and closed dressings are often used to prevent evaporative cooling. With such modern techniques, the burned patient seldom has elevations of REE greater than 70% above normal, and is often in the range of +50% or less. [*Editor's Note:* The discrepancies between the data obtained two decades ago and the considerably smaller increases in REE measured today is still a matter of speculation. The reason for discrepancies between these two careful sets of studies is not clear.]

The REE of every patient represents a balance between increases due to catabolic influences and decreases due to whatever tissue depletion may have occurred. The range of REE encouraged in surgical patients during the 1960s extended from +100% for patients with large burns to −40% for patients with advanced cachexia. Just as improvements in burn care have reduced the upper end of this range, corresponding improvements in hospital nutrition have made advanced cachexia a rare condition such that the hypometabolism of undernutrition seldom has associated decreases of more than 20% below the predicted REE.

Since the range of abnormalities in the REE of hospital patients is much smaller than that of 25 years ago, some physicians have questioned whether measuring energy expenditure remains of use in patient care. Any increase in REE, even if only modest, has importance as a "metabolic marker." Hypermetabolism in the cells of involved tissues is probably much more marked than is evident from a whole-body measurement. Furthermore, the measurement of a population of patients with any particular diagnosis nearly always shows a much wider range of values

about the mean than in the distribution of normal subjects, and patients above the mean often cannot be distinguished by conventional clinical evaluation.

ENERGY INTAKE: TWO DECADES OF CHANGE

TPN was introduced by Wretlind and associates [31] in Sweden during the early 1960s. A safe and effective lipid emulsion allowed caloric equilibrium with a normal proportion of the macronutrients supplied via the intravenous route. Dudrick et al. [7] introduced "hyperalimentation" in the late 1960s as high glucose, lipid-free intravenous nutrition with the intent of providing a positive balance of calories and nitrogen at a time when the nutrient balance was usually negative in association with some form of gastrointestinal failure. The idea of giving enough calories to ensure a positive calorie balance was considered to be important for two different reasons. Some physicians believed that a very high energy expenditure was present and needed to be offset. Others believed that the extra nitrogen loss was because protein was being oxidized for fuel and that an excess of administered calories might somehow reduce this protein degradation.

During the first decade of hyperalimentation, the recommended calorie intakes were relatively high by current standards. Factors contributing to these initial high calorie (and high glucose) intakes were:

1. The persistent belief that the rapid weight loss of acute catabolic conditions was associated with large increases in REE.
2. When the increases in REE were measured and found to be less than previously thought, an additional amount was added as a "stress factor" that might raise the caloric intake to twice the energy expenditure of that individual under normal conditions.
3. The high glucose loads were usually reduced as intravenous lipid became available, but lipid was sometimes added to

the usual glucose intake as a sort of calorie "bonus."

4. There was a delayed recognition that a strongly positive calorie balance might be associated with undesirable side effects such as abnormal liver enzyme levels, hepatic steatosis, diet-induced stimulus to the sympathetic nervous system, and decreases in pulmonary diffusing capacity and in cellular immune function. It appeared that these undesirable effects were more evident when high calorie loads were given during the acute catabolic phase of illness or injury, and much less evident during the later anabolic phase of convalescence.

Thus, the recommended calorie intake during the acute catabolic phase has changed toward giving only what is required for energy equilibrium, and gradually increasing the intake to a positive balance during the subsequent anabolic phase. In other words, a positive balance of calories and nitrogen is to achieve tissue synthesis, and this is not a major priority for the body during the acute catabolic phase.

FUTURE OBJECTIVES IN ENERGY METABOLISM AND TOTAL PARENTERAL NUTRITION

The careful selection of candidates for TPN in the future will require improvements in our methods for nutritional assessment. Such methods must include more and better methods of assessing tissue or cellular function, which will almost certainly involve energy supply and utilization. Once candidates for TPN have been identified, specific goals must be established and progress toward these goals must be documented on a regular basis. The use of TPN (and the length of time it is employed) will increasingly depend on collecting persuasive data to show the clinical risk of a given level of malnutrition and how much TPN is required to lower this level of risk.

Measurements of energy expenditure are

performed on the whole body, and we know little of the correlation of abnormal rates of energy expenditure with changes in the energetics of cells and tissues. We need to know whether the DIT seen in normal individuals may be accentuated in the acutely catabolic patient, and thus modify the efficiency with which calories and nitrogen are utilized.

The past two decades since the introduction of TPN have been devoted primarily to learning how much of the conventional nutrients to give, particularly as to how many calories. The coming decade can be expected to have a change of emphasis with the introduction of new types of fuels that are directed to the needs of specific cellular function rather than juggling the composition and amount of solutions composed of conventional nutrients.

The appropriate nutrition for any patient depends not only on his or her clinical diagnosis but also on the underlying metabolic state [26]. The future care of patients on TPN will involve improved ways to evaluate the underlying metabolic state, particularly with regard to energy utilization. It seems possible that the metabolic state will come to be evaluated in the future by measuring a particular metabolic response to a small controlled nutritional challenge.

REFERENCES

1. Blaxter, K. *Energy Metabolism in Animals and Man.* Cambridge: Cambridge University Press, 1989. P. 123.
2. Cunningham, J. J. A reanalysis of the factors influencing basal metabolic rate in normal adults. *Am. J. Clin. Nutr.* 33:2372, 1980.
3. Cuthbertson, D. P. Observations on disturbance of metabolism produced by injury to limbs. *Q. J. Med.* 25:233, 1932.
4. Daly, J. M., Heymsfield, S. B., Head, C. A., et al. Human energy requirements: Overestimation by widely used prediction equation. *Am. J. Clin. Nutr.* 42:1170, 1985.
5. Dietrick, J. E., Whedon, G. D., and Shorr, E. Effects of immobilization upon various metabolic and physiologic functions of normal men. *Am. J. Med.* 4:3, 1948.
6. DuBois, E. F. *Basal Metabolism in Health and Disease.* Philadelphia: Lea & Febiger, 1924.

7. Dudrick, S. J., Wilmore, D. W., Vars, H. M., and Rhoads, J. E. Long-term parenteral nutrition with growth, development, and positive nitrogen balance. *Surgery* 64:134, 1968.

8. Fong, Y., Hesse, D. G., Tracey, K. J., et al. Submaximal exercise during intravenous hyperalimentation of depleted subjects. *Ann. Surg.* 207:297, 1988.

9. Grande, F. Body weight, composition and energy balance. In R. E. Olson (ed.), *Present Knowledge in Nutrition*. Washington, DC: The Nutrition Foundation, 1984. P. 7.

10. Horton, E. S., and Terjung, R. L. *Exercise, Nutrition, and Energy Metabolism*. New York: Macmillan, 1988.

11. Jequier, E., Acheson, K., and Schutz, Y. Assessment of energy expenditure and fuel utilization in man. *Am. Rev. Nutr.* 7:187, 1987.

12. Jequier, E., and Schutz, Y. Long-term measurements of energy expenditure in humans using a respiration chamber. *Am. J. Clin. Nutr.* 38:989, 1983.

13. Kinney, J. M. Food as fuel: The development of concepts. In M. E. Shills and V. R. Young (eds.), *Modern Nutrition in Health and Disease* (7th ed.). Philadelphia: Lea & Febiger, 1988. P. 516.

14. Kinney, J. M., Duke, J. H., Long, C. L., and Gump, F. E. Tissue fuel and weight loss after injury. *J. Clin. Pathol.* 23(Suppl. 4):65, 1970.

15. Kinney, J. M., Morgan, A. P., and Dominguez, F. J., and Gildner, K. J. A method for continuous measurement of gas exchange and expired radioactivity in acutely ill patients. *Metabolism* 13:205, 1964.

16. Kleiber, M. *The Fire of Life: An Introduction to Animal Energetics*. Huntington, NY: Krieger, 1975.

17. Landsberg, L., and Young, J. B. Autonomic regulation of thermogenesis. In L. Girardier and M. J. Stock (eds.), *Mammalian Thermogenesis*. London: Chapman & Hall, 1983. P. 99.

18. Lusk, G. *The Elements of the Science of Nutrition* (4th ed.). Philadelphia: W. B. Saunders, 1928.

19. Lusk, G. *The Science of Nutrition* (4th ed.). New York: Johnson Reprint Corporation, 1976.

20. Moore, F. D., Oleson, K. H., McMurrey, J. D., Parker, H. V., Ball, M. R., and Boyden, C. M. *The Body Cell Mass and Its Supporting Environment: Body Composition in Health and Disease*. Philadelphia: W. B. Saunders, 1963.

21. Riumallo, J. A., Schoeller, D., Barrera, G., Gattas, V., and Uauy, R. Energy expenditure in underweight free-living adults: Impact of energy supplementation as determined by doubly labeled water and indirect calorimetry. *Am. J. Clin. Nutr.* 49:239, 1989.

22. Roza, A. M., and Shizgal, H. M. The Harris-Benedict equation reevaluated: Resting energy requirements and the body cell mass. *Am. J. Clin. Nutr.* 40:168, 1984.

23. Sandler, H., and Vernikos, J. *Inactivity: Physiological Effects*. New York: Academic Press, 1986.

24. Schoeller, D. A., Kushner, R. F., and Jones, P. J. H. Validation of doubly labeled water for measuring energy expenditure during parenteral nutrition. *Am. J. Clin. Nutr.* 44:291, 1986.

25. Schoeller, D. A., Ravussin, E., Schutz, Y., Acheson, K. J., Baertschi, P., and Jequier, E. Energy expenditure by doubly labeled water: Validation in humans and proposed calculation. *Am. J. Physiol.* 250:R823, 1986.

26. Shaw, J. H. F., and Holdaway, C. M. Protein-sparing effect of substrate infusion in surgical patients is governed by the clinical state, and not by the individual substrate infused. *J. Parenter. Enter. Nutr.* 12:433, 1988.

27. Shizgal, H. M. Nutritional failure. In J. Tinker and M. Rapin (eds.), *Care of the Critically Ill Patient*. Berlin: Springer-Verlag, 1983.

28. Tellado, J. M., Garcia-Sabrido, J. L., Hanley, J. A., Shizgal, H. M., and Christou, N. V. Predicting mortality based on body composition analysis. *Ann. Surg.* 209:81, 1989.

29. Waterlow, J. C. Metabolic adaptation to low intakes of energy and protein. *Annu. Rev. Nutr.* 6:495, 1986.

30. Westerterp, K. R., De Boer, J. O., Saris, W. H. M., Schoffelen, P. F. M., and Ten Hoor, F. Measurement of energy expenditure using doubly labeled water. *Int. J. Sports Med.* 5(Suppl.):74, 1984.

31. Wretlind, A. Development of fat emulsion. *J. Parenter. Enter. Nutr.* 5:230, 1981.

Acute Renal Failure

Shujun Li

Total parenteral nutrition (TPN) has been advocated as a part of normal therapy for acute renal failure during the past 10 years. Sophisticated nutritional therapy must be based on thorough knowledge of the biologic disturbances of renal failure, including the hypercatabolism, proteolysis, retention of nitrogenous waste products, water, and electrolytes. Clearly, better understanding of this critical pathologic process should result in appropriate therapy.

The purpose of nutritional therapy in acute renal failure is to provide nutrients via a parenteral or (when possible) an enteral route to improve the nutritional status and to enhance wound healing and resistance to infection. In addition, the provision of nutritional support may help correct impaired biochemical homeostasis, as will be detailed. Finally, specialized nutritional support may promote healing of the renal lesion.

Although the use of TPN for the treatment of acute renal failure has been controversial since its inception nearly 20 years ago, the major issues remain: What kind of solution is appropriate? How do we evaluate the clinical result? Here I argue that a basic principle of parenteral nutrition in the treatment of acute renal failure is that the nutritional regimen should reduce the workload of renal excretion, and nutritional support should ameliorate the biochemical consequences of renal failure.

HISTORICAL PERSPECTIVES

Nutritional support in uremic patients has been a subject of clinical and research interest for many years. Early investigators were concerned with the quality and form of exogenous nitrogen that could safely be administered to patients with renal failure and the amount of energy required to obtain nitrogen balance, using a diet high in calories and low in protein. In 1947, Gamble [20] indicated that at least 100 g/day of dietary carbohydrate was needed in healthy male volunteers to reduce protein breakdown. This was called a protein-sparing effect, and gave impetus to the administration of high doses of carbohydrate to patients in acute renal failure. The dietary regimens, which were thus changed to high carbohydrate and fat, and free of protein, were designed to provide sufficient calories to reverse gluconeogenesis and thus reduce the concomitant production of potentially toxic substances. However, this regimen soon lost favor because many patients with acute renal failure had severe gastrointestinal symptoms and could not tolerate the oral intake.

In 1954, Rose et al. [46] published their milestone work, classifying the amino acids into two categories—essential amino acids. (EAAs) and nonessential amino acids (NEAAs). They found that nitrogen equilibrium could not be maintained unless the eight EAAs were present in a diet. The quantitative amino acid experiments of Rose et al. formed the foundation on which all subsequent synthetic amino acid diets were based. In later work, Rose and Dekker also showed that urea could be a source of nonprotein nitrogen for maintenance of nitrogen equilibrium [48]. (Urea cannot be used by mammals, but the gut bacteria can split urea to ammonia which, when energy is supplied, can be incorporated into amino acids.) This experimental investigation was confirmed by the clinical observations of Giordano [22] that in a group of normal and uremic patients, endogenous urea could be utilized as a source of nitrogen for protein synthesis. He administered a diet of "high biologic value" (high percentage of EAAs) and observed decreased azotemia and positive nitrogen balance. The Giordano-Giovannetti diet was proved to be effective in improving uremic symptoms and decreasing the elevation of urea nitrogen concentration [8]. The provision of adequate calories with EAAs and "recycling of endogenous urea" for protein synthesis have become the major goals of treatment in acute renal failure. [*Editor's Note*: Although much of the original work was carried out on the premise of "urea recycling," subsequent work has suggested that de-

creased urea emergence because of the EAAs is the major mechanism of decreases in BUN. "Urea recycling" does occur, but only to about 25% of the effect, and probably less than that.]

The success of diet in the treatment of acute renal failure brought TPN to the forefront of modern medicine. Growing out of their experience with general TPN, Wilmore and Dudrick [58] first reported using a solution of EAAs and hypertonic dextrose in a patient with acute renal failure. During the period of TPN, the patient's body weight and serum albumin levels increased, while serum phosphorus levels and uremic symptoms decreased. More interestingly, by day 5 of administration of this special formulation, positive nitrogen balance was obtained. A new era in the treatment of acute renal failure with TPN was thus begun. In the early 1970s, many investigators confirmed these findings of stabilized BUN and significant decreases in serum levels of potassium, magnesium, and phosphate [1, 2]. These lower serum electrolyte levels could be obtained without evidence of increased loss in urine and feces. Abel et al. [3] suggested that the decrease in electrolyte concentrations and stabilization of BUN could have reflected incorporation of these ions and nitrogen waste products into tissue structural or secretory protein. The patients with acute renal failure treated by EAAs and hypertonic dextrose solution showed hypokalemia rather than hyperkalemia, and required rather large amounts of additional potassium during the course of treatment. Also, marked hypophosphatemia and hypomagnesemia occurred, requiring supplementation. Abel et al. [4] subsequently published the first prospective, double-blind, controlled clinical trial in which a solution composed of EAAs and dextrose was given to 53 patients with acute renal failure, demonstrating higher survival of patients and perhaps more rapid recovery from renal failure in patients receiving this regimen (75%) as compared with patients receiving isocaloric dextrose solutions alone (44%). However, another report did not show significant differences in patients' survival between study groups and control groups [33], although patient populations were very different. By the mid-1970s, the renal formulation for acute renal failure had been established and accepted as part of medical practice.

In 1975, Baek et al. [6] introduced solutions containing hypertonic glucose and commercially prepared fibrin hydrolysate which contained both EAAs and NEAAs. Patients receiving hemodialysis while on the study solutions had a significantly greater survival rate compared with those receiving isocaloric glucose alone. The incidence of hyperkalemia in patients receiving the amino acid and dextrose solution was lower than that in the control group, and a majority of the study group patients required potassium supplementation. This finding challenged the concept that EAAs plus hypertonic glucose was the only formula for acute renal failure, as the authors demonstrated that these patients could be treated effectively with a complete amino acid solution (i.e., a balanced amino acid solution with EAAs and NEAAs).

In recent years, investigators have focused on the comparison between EAA-dextrose solutions and EAA-NEAA–dextrose solutions. Mirtallo et al. [38] reported on a study in which they administered either EAA-dextrose solution or EAA-NEAA–dextrose solution to two groups of patients with impaired renal function. None of the patients underwent dialysis, and the BUN levels decreased at the same rate in both groups. In addition, there was no significant difference in net protein use, urea appearance rate, or nitrogen balance in either group. BUN levels were reduced and positive nitrogen balance was achieved using both solutions. Interestingly, they also found that the decreases in serum creatinine values were not associated with concomitant decreases in BUN levels during the study period. It was suggested that the effect on BUN was probably secondary to a decrease in the rate of catabolism and not due to urea reutilization. Feinstein et al. [17] found no difference between an EAA solution and one containing both EAAs and NEAAs, but the number of patients was small.

Similar results were reported by Pelosi et al. [41] and Proietti et al. [44]. It is worth mentioning that in the latter study [44], all patients received hemodialysis at 24- to 48-hour intervals during the 12-day study period. All patients were in negative nitrogen balance, but those receiving balanced amino acid solutions were in less negative nitrogen balance. Proietti et al. [44] concluded that: (1) "Rational" nutritional support should include a balanced protein intake with an EAA–total nitrogen ratio of greater than 4.0 and a branched-chain amino acid–EAA ratio of greater than 0.5. (2) The combined use of parenteral and enteral nutrition appeared to be the treatment of choice. Their observation that patients with acute renal failure can be treated with balanced amino acid solutions in appropriate concentrations was a significant departure from the classic thinking, and this may be related to the increasing application of dialysis therapy in acute renal failure. It is reasonable that once the patient in acute renal failure regains some kidney function (albeit through dialysis), he or she should be benefited by conventional parenteral nutritional support, which provides balanced amino acids and sufficient calories.

Perhaps a reasonable approach is as follows: In patients in whom the necessity for dialysis has not become apparent, we would utilize an EAA solution since we continue to believe that EAA solutions are superior to mixed EAA-NEAA solutions in preventing the rise of BUN [19], and dialysis (which has its own intrinsic complications and mortality) may be avoided. Once dialysis has been initiated, both EAAs and NEAAs are being lost and should be replaced.

METABOLIC DISTURBANCES—SEVERE CATABOLISM

A rising BUN is a clinical hallmark of acute renal failure, reflecting the loss of renal excretory function. However, in recent years, clinical observations and experimental studies have demonstrated that nitrogen retention was greatly exaggerated by coexisting catabolic processes in acute renal failure. This hypercatabolic status is related to acute renal failure and the underlying primary diseases, such as sepsis and severe trauma. Although much work has been done in this area, the underlying pathologic process is not clear. In general, the implicating factors can be classified in three categories: (1) circulating proteolytic enzymes, (2) hormonal disturbances, and (3) nitrogen and calorie deficiency.

Proteases that promote protein degradation have been found in the blood of patients with catabolic disorders. Clowes et al. [14] described a circulating peptide in patients with sepsis and surgical patients during the postoperative period. Horl and Heidland [26] and Heidland et al. [25] reported increased circulating protease activity in the catabolic response to acute renal failure. They showed that serum fractions obtained from patients with acute renal failure who were markedly catabolic had increased proteolytic activity as determined by enhanced proteolytic effect. Interleukin-1 (IL-1) was postulated as the factor that led to the release of protease [7], but the responsible factor has not been definitely identified as yet.

Hormonal disturbances may be present in postoperative, septic, or trauma patients and may contribute to the changes in muscle protein metabolism in these patients. Bessey et al. [9] recently pointed out the importance of multiple hormonal perturbations in the generation of metabolic derangements seen after injury. Normal human subjects received infusions of hydrocortisol, glucagon, and epinephrine, which reproduced blood concentrations likely to be found in a stressed patient; these infusions resulted in increased urea nitrogen appearance rates, negative nitrogen balance, enhanced basal energy expenditures, increased protein catabolism, insulin resistance, and hyperinsulinemia.

In acute renal failure, several hormones may contribute to the catabolic response. Insulin resistance and glucose intolerance occur in acute renal failure. The plasma glucose level may be elevated in patients with acute renal failure due to reduced uptake of glu-cose by skeletal muscle [39], while blood levels of glucagon [29] and growth hormone [30] are also elevated. Parathyroid hormone is another hormone that is elevated in acute renal failure [34].

In 1957, Sellers et al. [50] reported that urea synthesis in liver slices was reduced after feeding glucose to uremic rats. Spreiter et al. [54] showed that administration of calories was important in reducing urea generation in patients with acute renal failure, and that as much as 50 kcal/kg/day may be required to control negative nitrogen balance. The importance of deficient nitrogen substrate is suggested by the observations of Toback et al. [56]. They found that the level of free leucine in renal cells was decreased in rats with acute renal failure and was restored to normal with amino acid infusions, and the rate of protein synthesis rose after such infusions. In a recent study of energy balance, Mault et al. [35] found that the resting energy expenditure in patients with acute renal failure in an intensive care unit was 37% above normal level. They even indicated that the major contribution to mortality in acute renal failure might be starvation. Based on these observations, one can postulate that if energy and nitrogen intake can be sufficiently supplied, the catabolic status may be improved.

The hypercatabolic status in acute renal failure, as in any stress situation, may have positive effects on survival. Shear [51] reported that in rats with acute renal failure, the liver and cardiac muscle had increased rates of protein synthesis, while skeletal muscle protein synthesis was reduced. Toback et al. [55, 56] studied the rate of protein and phospholipid synthesis in renal tissue from rats with mercuric chloride–induced acute renal failure and found that the regeneration of renal tissue, as indicated by increased [^{14}C] choline incorporation into membrane phospholipids, is markedly increased as compared to normal renal tissue. This suggests that during hypercatabolic periods, muscle protein breakdown provides endogenous nitrogen and energy to the body to ensure continued survival.

BASIC TOTAL PARENTERAL NUTRITION FORMULATION FOR ACUTE RENAL FAILURE

The provision of EAAs plus hypertonic dextrose is associated with salutary clinical and biochemical effects, and may result in improved survival rates and more rapid return of renal function in patients with acute renal failure. After nearly 20 years, application of this renal formulation has successfully withstood clinical trials, and is still the principal regimen of TPN for patients with acute renal failure. The content of this solution is shown in Table 13-1. The dextrose concentration is approximately 47% and the administration of

Table 13-1. Composition of Total Parenteral Nutrition Solution for Acute Renal Failure

Ingredient	Amount
Water	750 ml
Amino acids	
Isoleucine	1.4 g
Leucine	2.2 g
Lysine	2.0 g
Methionine	2.2 g
Phenylalanine	2.2 g
Threonine	1.0 g
Tryptophan	0.5 g
Valine	1.6 g
Total	12.75 g
Glucose	350 g
Vitamins	
A	5000 USP U
B_1 (thiamine hydrochloride)	25 mg
B_2 (riboflavin)	5 mg
B_6 (pyridoxine hydrochloride)	7.5 mg
Niacinamide	50 mg
Panthenol	12.5 mg
C (ascorbic acid)	1.5 g
D_2 (ergocalciferol)	500 USP U
E (dl-alpha-tocopheryl acetate)	2.5 IU
Electrolytes	
Sodium	1.2 mEq
Calories	
Nonnitrogen	1190 kcal
Total	1240 kcal
Osmolarity	2100 mOsm/liter
pH	6.4
Alpha-amino nitrogen	1.3 g
Total nitrogen	1.46 g
Fat emulsion (optional)	250 ml (20%)

a single unit of this formulation as prepared provides approximately 13 g of EAAs, which is the level recommended by Rose [47], and about 1200 kcal. If one adds a 20% fat emulsion (250 ml), the total calorie supply is increased up to 1700 kcal.

MONITORING AND MANAGEMENT

Because most patients with acute renal failure are in critical condition with impaired immune function, line sepsis has been a major problem especially when multiple-lumen, central venous catheters are used. Line sepsis rates as high as 19% have been reported [42]. [*Editor's Note:* Our own policy is not to use anything other than single-lumen catheters for hyperalimentation. If double- and triple-lumen catheters must be used, most are agreed that sepsis rates are higher.] Strict attention must be paid to line placement, nursing care, and preparation and administration of the solution. Because of the high osmolarity of this solution, it is mandatory to insert the central line directly into the internal jugular or subclavian vein, and the tip of the catheter should be in the superior vena cava.

Blood Sugar Monitoring

The infusion of renal formula should normally begin slowly, at approximately 30 ml/hr. This provides a total of approximately 700 ml/day of fluid, which can be tolerated even by anuric patients without excessive fluid losses. Although this rate of administration should be within the limits of glucose utilization, hyperglycemia is fairly common after the initiation of TPN in patients with acute renal failure. This may be related to underlying diseases, such as diabetes mellitus, pancreatic insufficiency, generalized sepsis, steroid administration, or concomitant peritoneal dialysis utilizing glucose as the osmotic agent. Above all, the insulin resistance may be caused by acute renal failure itself, as discussed above. As the catabolic state of acute renal failure varies from mild to marked, so the glucose intolerance may also be mild to severe. Urinary glucose is unreliable in renal failure, so that determination of blood glucose concentration every 6 hours during the initial phase of treatment is mandatory. The blood glucose level should be maintained at approximately 250 mg/100 ml or below.

In order to control blood sugar, one may use insulin subcutaneously on a schedule mandated by the blood sugar value, or add regular insulin to the TPN solution. The dosage range has been extremely wide, from 15 to 100 U/bottle of solution. If the addition of insulin to the TPN solution still cannot control hyperglycemia, control may be achieved by an intravenous insulin drip (1–6 U/hr) or (less satisfactory) sliding-scale subcutaneous insulin injections (3–12 U/injection). The actual dosage of insulin is completely dependent on the blood sugar monitoring. One of our patients consumed 242 U of insulin in 24 hours.

It is noteworthy that when a patient's condition improves, the insulin resistance may suddenly vanish and the insulin supplement must be withdrawn accordingly. In patients with acute renal failure, we sometimes advance the TPN rate and insulin dose at the same time. In certain unusual cases in which the addition of even large amounts of insulin directly in the TPN solution or intravenously does not control hyperglycemia, it may be unwise to increase insulin without limitation; rather, maintenance of a low infusion rate and dependence on lipid as an energy source may be the better choice.

Some have suggested that insulin suffers a significant loss of activity when placed directly into intravenous solutions; the addition of a small amount of protein (albumin) to the intravenous solution may reduce insulin adsorption to the glass and plastic tubing to insignificant levels [57].

Energy Expenditure Monitoring

The calorie requirement usually depends on the severity of acute renal failure and the un-

derlying disorder. Abitbol and Holliday [5] treated anuric children with calorie intakes that ranged from 20 to 70 kcal/kg/day, and noted improvement in negative nitrogen balance at the higher calorie intake. Blackburn et al. [10] studied adults using treatment regimens with either 37.5% or 52.2% glucose concentrations. The urea nitrogen appearance decreased to a greater extent with higher calorie intake. A direct correlation of calorie intake and estimated nitrogen balance in adults with acute renal failure was reported by Spreiter et al. [54]. While it is not possible to separate the effects of calorie intake alone from total nutrient intake, it does suggest that the sufficient provision of calories to patients with acute renal failure is very important in decreasing protein breakdown. Clinical studies have demonstrated that patients who received more calories had better survival and recovery of renal function than those who did not [17], but this is not universal [19]. The survival rate was higher in those patients whose accumulative caloric balance was positive when compared with those patients in whom it was negative [17].

Energy expenditure can be estimated by calculations based on clinical findings. More recently, indirect calorimetry measurement was used to obtain accurate estimations of actual energy needs of patients with acute renal failure [37]. According to the energy expenditure, the basic formulations can be adjusted and the infusion rate and total volume chosen for calorie and nitrogen intake. If patients show glucose intolerance, the ratio of lipid to glucose in the total energy supply of the TPN regimen can be increased. We normally provide as high as 30% and rarely as high as 60% of total calories as lipid.

Nitrogen Monitoring

Negative nitrogen balance can be recognized by many clinical manifestations, such as weight loss; muscle wasting; and lowered serum levels of total protein, albumin, transferrin, etc. [17]. Total nitrogen analysis of excreta is no longer a routine measurement for patient monitoring except for research purposes. However, one should remember that urea nitrogen appearance may be the simplest and most useful measurement for estimating nitrogen balance (mainly nitrogen output) in uremic patients, since nitrogen excretion in forms other than urea tends to be nearly constant [32], and low values of urea nitrogen appearance indicate effective nitrogen conservation. The urea nitrogen appearance can be easily calculated during a 24-hour time interval using the following equations [15]:

1. Urea nitrogen appearance (g/day) = change in body urea nitrogen content + urinary urea nitrogen + dialysate urea nitrogen.
2. Change in body urea nitrogen (g/day) = [change in BUN (g/liter) × initial body weight (kg) × 0.6 liter/kg] + [change in body weight (kg) × final BUN (g/liter) × 1 liter/kg].
3. Nitrogen output = 0.97 (urea nitrogen appearance) + 1.93.

Signs and symptoms of uremic toxicity have long been known to correlate with the level of blood urea. The accumulation of toxic products of protein catabolism is correlated with the accumulation of urea. In fact, urea itself is not thought to be toxic at levels below 100 mg/dl of urea nitrogen. This has been demonstrated by the absence of uremic symptoms in subjects with normal kidneys who continuously ingest enough protein to maintain BUN over 60 mg/dl [45] or who are given urea as a diuretic [36]. At higher concentrations (150 mg/dl), urea is toxic, and patients usually show uremic symptoms such as nausea, vomiting, itching, lethargy, and tremors. Clinically, we prefer to have the urea level below 80 to 100 mg/dl. At this point, urea level monitoring is for the severity of uremia rather than nitrogen metabolism. However, BUN levels do not reflect directly the level of endogenous protein breakdown or (in TPN) exogenous amino acid consumption. A continuing rise of BUN during treatment with the renal formula means either deteriorating renal function, in-

creasing protein catabolism, or overload of exogenous amino acids, especially if patients are undergoing dialysis.

With the renal TPN formula, 12 to 24 g/day of amino acids is usually administered. We consider that, along with sufficient energy supply, this amount of amino acids may induce the reutilization of endogenous nitrogen sources (25%) and decrease muscle protein breakdown (75%). Although the renal TPN formula has a fixed amino acid composition, we do consider energy and nitrogren supply separately and vary dextrose concentrations and energy sources (lipid and glucose) to meet the patient's specific requirement.

It is important to remember that patients with acute renal failure have more negative nitrogen balance when they are on dialysis therapy [12]. Some investigators have shown that dialysis patients had negative nitrogen balance on days of dialysis therapy regardless of whether the patient ingested low or high protein intakes, but had positive nitrogen balance on other days. One of the reasons for the dialysis-associated catabolism may be related to the loss of protein and amino acids across the dialysis membrane [59]. During peritoneal dialysis, protein losses are around 12.9 ± 4.4 (SD) g/10 hours (8.5 g of albumin) [11], and the amino acid losses are 3.4 ± 1.2 (SD) g/24 hours [31]. As an approximation, 1 g of amino acids is lost for each hour of hemodialysis [24]. This loss should be replaced by TPN. The other possible reason for dialysis-associated catabolism is the release of granulocyte proteinases after contact of the blood with the dialysis membrane [27]. It is logical that the lost amino acids may include EAAs and NEAAs, and thus the balanced amino acids may be provided at this time via TPN. Since the amount of loss is so small, some may argue the necessity of the change of amino acid composition.

Biochemical Monitoring

Urine output is still one of the best criteria of renal function and body fluid balance. The best way to treat fluid retention in acute renal failure is some form of dialysis therapy or hemofiltration. Once dialysis is initiated, fluid management becomes easy. The fluid volume removed by dialysis on the previous day and the change of total body weight are the main references for the volume of total fluid replacement including TPN and other therapeutic solutions. It should be noted that when some physicians attempt to remove more water via dialysis, they usually increase the glucose concentration in the dialysate (200–400 mg/dl). In this way, some glucose is absorbed by the body, which may serve as an extra glucose load and cause hyperglycemia.

Hyponatremia develops in acute renal failure due to inability of the kidneys to excrete free water, cellular metabolism products, and therapeutic solutions administered to these patients. Elevations in total body sodium are associated with water retention. Caution should be utilized in administering sodium, since this may lead to extracellular fluid load and pulmonary edema. There is no sodium in the renal formula. In dialyzed patients, a small amount of sodium supplement may be needed, depending on fluid balance.

Hyperkalemia is the most serious complication of acute renal failure that may lead to sudden death [40]. It is the result of impaired renal excretion and increased release of potassium from intracellular sources. Extensive catabolism or continued administration of potassium-containing intravenous fluid or antibiotics, such as penicillin K, aggravates the rise in serum potassium level. Emergent treatment of hyperkalemia is sometimes necessary. However, when the renal TPN formula is utilized, hypokalemia is often seen; the fall in serum potassium level is ascribed to the movement of potassium intracellularly as anabolism ensues or glucose moves [2]. In the management of hypokalemia associated with this therapy, it should be remembered that since renal excretion of potassium is minimal, small amounts of exogenous potassium will result in wide variations in serum concentrations. Besides, endogenous potassium is still abundant because of the continuous

release of potassium from tissues in ongoing hypercatabolism. Unless cardiac arrhythmias exist at low to normal serum potassium concentrations (3.5–4.0 mEq/liter), no potassium should be given intravenously. Once the patient becomes anabolic in association with TPN, the addition of small amounts of potassium is recommended. Needless to say, dialysis is one of the best ways to control serum potassium levels, but urgent therapy for hyperkalemia is rarely needed.

Hypocalcemia and hyperphosphatemia are common findings in acute renal failure. The rise of serum phosphate levels results from decreased renal excretion and may be exacerbated by increased cellular release of phosphate. The serum calcium concentration falls concurrently with the development of hyperphosphatemia and leads to elevated parathyroid hormone levels [34]. Also, low levels of vitamin D metabolites are found and may contribute to hypocalcemia [43]. Hyperphosphatemia, as well as hypermagnesemia, does not have strong clinical significance. Along with TPN or dialysis, these problems are usually corrected; replacement of phosphate and magnesium to prevent hypophosphatemia and hypomagnesemia may be required. Exceedingly low concentrations of serum phosphate have been associated with a significant alteration in red blood cell glycolytic intermediates and thus in oxygen transport capacity [28]. Levels below 0.5 mg/dl are associated with changes in mentation and coma.

In acute renal failure, the metabolic acidosis associated with a hypercatabolic state is often present. TPN with the renal formulation usually does not result in any improvement of persistent metabolic acidosis, nor would one expect such improvement since even if protein breakdown is decreased, the patient is unable to excrete acid by-products. Acid-base monitoring is necessary. Routine buffering agents can be used to correct significant acidosis, but dialysis may rarely be necessary to correct metabolic acidosis. Sodium bicarbonate should be administered with caution to patients with oliguric acute renal failure, as sodium overload may cause congestive heart failure. The use of potassium acetate has been helpful in certain instances of concomitant hypokalemia.

In summary, careful blood chemistry monitoring is essential, and careful planning for replacement therapy is necessary.

BALANCED AMINO ACID SOLUTIONS

Dialysis has become a key element in modern management of acute renal failure, with some even advocating early or prophylactic dialysis. There are two components to dialysis: (1) removal of fluid, and (2) diffusion of solute. Thus, BUN and serum potassium levels can be well controlled by frequent dialysis. In some patients who require large volumes of nutritional solutions in addition to antibiotics, blood, and other fluid intake, daily dialysis or continuous hemofiltration may be necessary. Dialysis does not ameliorate and can aggravate the catabolic response; it may actually exaggerate the negative nitrogen balance because of the associated nitrogen loss.

Balanced amino acid solutions combined with hypertonic glucose are sometimes used as the TPN regimen for acute renal failure, as discussed earlier. Feinstein [16] designed a renal formulation in which both EAAs and NEAAs are provided and the calorie intake is approximately 35 to 50 kcal/kg of body weight/day. The criteria by which we determine when to place a patient on a complete TPN solution utilizing both EAAs and NEAAs are: (1) The patient is on daily dialysis, and volume and BUN are no longer problems. (2) The patient has poor nitrogen reserve (i.e., is already severely malnourished). (3) The patient's blood amino acid profile shows low levels of many amino acids, including EAAs and NEAAs. With standard TPN formulations, we can supply 2500 to 3000 kcal and 60 to 90 g of amino acids. It is worth mentioning that when larger amounts of mixed amino acid solutions are administered, BUN sometimes stays elevated, in part due to the increased nitrogen load.

ENTERAL NUTRITION IN ACUTE RENAL FAILURE

In the past 10 years, enteral feeding has made significant progress due to the development of enteral feeding formulas and advances in tube-feeding techniques [53]. It became generally agreed that whenever possible, nutrition should be provided at least in part via the gastrointestinal tract. Bower et al. [13] found no difference in nitrogen balance, body weight change, or serum protein levels between postoperative patients receiving TPN and those receiving tube feedings. The TPN group had higher transaminase levels than did the enteral feeding group. In addition to the potential increase of hepatic complications of TPN [23], intestinal atrophy is another major problem of TPN, perhaps increasing the absorption of gut bacterial products [49]. In these two aspects, enteral feeding has potential advantages. For patients with acute renal failure, the main obstacles for enteral nutrition have been the severe gastrointestinal symptoms of nausea, vomiting, and even gastrointestinal bleeding. If these symptoms can be successfully controlled, enteral nutrition would be possible. Frequent dialysis may decrease gastrointestinal side effects.

Patients with persistent severe insulin resistance and hyperglycemia associated with sepsis during TPN may be more easily controlled with enteral feedings, or at least this has been our impression.

We are not aware of any large series reporting enteral nutritional support of patients with acute renal failure. We do recommend switching to enteral feeding when TPN is not well tolerated by patients with acute renal failure or whenever enteral feeding can be tolerated.

The most common enteral formula used for acute renal failure is AminAid (Kendall-McGaw), a concentrated dextrose solution with EAAs. If the patient is on frequent dialysis, other enteral formulas may be appropriate, such as Isocal, Isocal-HCN, and Osmolyte. The general management of acute renal failure with enteral nutrition is similar to treating the patient with TPN.

DIALYSIS THERAPY AS NUTRITIONAL SUPPORT

Feinstein et al. [18] added additional glucose (5%) and amino acids (0.4%) to hemodialysate solutions, using a low flow rate (27 ml/min). Seventy percent of the nutrients in the dialysate were absorbed, up to 49 g/hr of glucose and 4 g/hr of amino acids. Recently, Geronemus and Schneider [21] and Sigler and Teehan [53] also performed continuous arteriovenous hemodialysis with a dialysate containing 1.5% glucose; the mean glucose uptake was 107 mg/min or 154 g/day, or approximately 500 cal. However, this could serve as a supplement to borderline enteral feeding, for example. This area needs to be further investigated. It should be noted that when the dialysate flow rate is lowered, the efficiency of dialysis is reduced and the patient may need longer dialysis time.

SUMMARY

Although remarkable progress has been made in the nutritional support of patients with acute renal failure over the past 15 years, it is still not entirely satisfactory. TPN remains an important part of management of patients with acute renal failure. Successful treatment depends on close monitoring of metabolic changes and individually adjusting the TPN formulation and rate of delivery. Better survival is expected when nutritional support is correctly delivered.

REFERENCES

1. Abbott, W. M., Abel, R. M., and Fischer, J. E. Treatment of acute renal failure insufficiency after aortoiliac surgery. *Arch. Surg.* 103:590, 1971.
2. Abel, R. M., Abbott, W. M., and Fischer, J. E. Acute renal failure: Treatment without dialysis by total parenteral nutrition. *Arch. Surg.* 103:513, 1971.
3. Abel, R. M., Abbott, W. M., and Fischer, J. E. Intravenous essential L-amino acids and hypertonic dextrose in patients with acute renal failure: Effects on serum potassium, phosphate and magnesium. *Am. J. Surg.* 123:632, 1972.
4. Abel, R. M., Beck, C. H., Jr., Abbott, W. M., Ryan, J. A., Jr., Barnett, G. O., and Fischer, J. E. Improved survival from acute renal failure after treatment with intravenous essential L-amino acids and glucose: Results of a prospective, double-blind study. *N. Engl. J. Med.* 288:695, 1973.
5. Abitbol, C. L., and Holliday, M. A. Total parenteral nutrition in anuric children. *Clin. Nephrol.* 5:153, 1976.
6. Baek, S. M., Makabali, G. G., Byran-Brown, C. W., Kusek, J., and Shoemaker, W. C. The influence of parenteral nutrition on the course of acute renal failure. *Surg. Gynecol. Obstet.* 141:405, 1975.
7. Baracos, V., Rodermann, H. P., Dinarello, C. A., and Goldberg, A. L. Stimulation of muscle protein degradation and prostaglandin E release by leukocyte pyrogen: A mechanism for the increased degradation of muscle proteins during fever. *N. Engl. J. Med.* 308:553, 1983.
8. Berlyne, G. M., Bazzasd, F. J., Booth, E. M., Janabi, K., and Shaw, A. B. The dietary treatment of acute renal failure. *Q. J. Med.* 35:59, 1967.
9. Bessey, P. O., Watters, J. M., Aoki, T. T., and Wilmore, D. W. Combined hormone infusion stimulates the metabolic response to injury. *Ann. Surg.* 200:264, 1984.
10. Blackburn, G. L., Etter, G., and Mackenzie, T. Criteria for choosing amino acid therapy in acute renal failure. *Am. J. Clin. Nutr.* 31:1841, 1978.
11. Blumenkrantz, M. J., Gahl, G. M., Kopple, J. D., et al. Protein losses during peritoneal dialysis. *Kidney Int.* 19:593, 1981.
12. Borah, M. F., Schoenfeld, P. Y., Gotch, F. A., Sargent, G. J., Wolfson, M., and Humphreys, M. H. Nitrogen balance during intermittent dialysis therapy of uremia. *Kidney Int.* 14:491, 1978.
13. Bower, R. H., Talamini, M. A., Sax, H. C., Hamilton, F., and Fischer, J. E. Postoperative enteral vs. parenteral nutrition: A randomized controlled trial. *Arch. Surg.* 121:1040, 1986.
14. Clowes, G. H. A., Jr., George, B. C., Villee, C. A., Jr., and Saravis, C. A. Muscle proteolysis induced by a circulating peptide in patients with sepsis or trauma. *N. Engl. J. Med.* 308:545, 1983.
15. Feinsten, E. Nutrition in acute renal failure.

In J. L. Rombeau and M. D. Caldwell (eds.), *Parenteral Nutrition.* Philadelphia: W. B. Saunders, 1986. Pp. 586–601.

16. Feinstein, E. I. Total parenteral nutritional support of patients with acute renal failure. *Nutr. Clin. Pract.* 3:9, 1988.

17. Feinstein, E. I., Blumenkrantz, M. J., Healy, M., et al. Clinical and metabolic responses to parenteral nutrition in acute renal failure: A controlled double-blind study. *Medicine* 60:124, 1981.

18. Feinstein, E. I., Collins, J. F., Blumenkrantz, M. J., Roberts, M., Kopple, J. D., and Massry, S. G. Nutritional hemodialysis. In K. Atsumi, M. Maekawa, and K. Ota (eds.), *Progress in Artificial Organs.* Cleveland: ISAO Press, 1984. Pp. 421–426.

19. Freund, H., and Fischer, J. E. Comparative study of parenteral nutrition in renal failure using essential and nonessential amino acid containing solutions. *Surg. Gynecol. Obstet.* 151:652, 1980.

20. Gamble, J. L. Physiological information gained from studies on the life raft ration. *Harvey Lect.* 42:247, 1947.

21. Geronemus, R., and Schneider, N. Continuous arteriovenous hemodialysis: A new modality for treatment of acute renal failure. *Trans. Am. Soc. Artif. Intern. Organs* 30:610, 1984.

22. Giordano, C. Use of exogenous and endogenous urea for protein synthesis in normal and uremic subjects. *J. Lab. Clin. Med.* 62:231, 1963.

23. Grant, J. P., Cox, C. E., Kleinman, L. M., et al. Serum hepatic enzyme and bilirubin elevation during parenteral nutrition. *Surg. Gynecol. Obstet.* 145:573, 1977.

24. Hak, L. J., and Raasch, R. H. Use of amino acids in patients with acute renal failure. *Nutr. Clin. Pract.* 3:19, 1988.

25. Heidland, A., Weipert, J., Schaefer, R. M., Heidbreder, E., Peter, G., and Hörl, W. W. Proteases and other catabolic factors in renal failure. *Kidney Int.* 32:S94, 1987.

26. Horl, W. H., and Heidland. A. Enhanced proteolytic activity cause of protein catabolism in acute renal failure. *Am. J. Clin. Nutr.* 33:1423, 1980.

27. Horl, W. H., and Heidland, A. Evidence for the participation of granulocyte proteinases in intradialytic catabolism. *Clin. Nephrol.* 21:314, 1984.

28. Johnson, W. J., Hagge, W. W., Wagoner, R. D., Dinapoli, R. P., and Rosevear, J. W. Effects of urea loading in patients with far advanced renal failure. *Mayo Clinic Proc.* 47:21, 1972.

29. Kokot, F. The endocrine system in patients with acute renal failure. *Proc. Eur. Dial. Transplant. Assoc.* 18:617, 1981.

30. Kokot, F., and Kuska, J. The endocrine system in patients with acute renal insufficiency. *Kidney Int.* 10(suppl.):26, 1981.

31. Kopple, J. D., Blumenkrantz, M. J., Jones, M. R., Moran, J. K., and Coburn, J. W. Plasma amino acid levels and amino acid losses during continuous ambulatory peritoneal dialysis. *Am. J. Clin. Nutr.* 36:395, 1982.

32. Kopple, J. D., and Coburn, J. W. Metabolic studies of low protein diets in uremia. I. Nitrogen and potassium. *Medicine* 52:583, 1973.

33. Leonard, C. E., Luke, R. G., and Siegel, R. R. Parenteral essential amino acids in acute renal failure. *Urology* 6:154, 1975.

34. Massry, S. G., Arieff, A. L., and Coburn, J. W. Divalent ion metabolism in patients with acute renal failure: Studies on the mechanism of hypocalcemia. *Kidney Int.* 5:437, 1974.

35. Mault, J. R., Bartlett, R. H., Dechert, R. E., Clark, S. F., and Swartz, R. D. Starvation: A major contribution to mortality in acute renal failure? *Trans. Am. Soc. Artif. Intern. Organs* 29:390, 1983.

36. Miller, H. R., and Feldman, A. Prolonged use of massive doses of urea in cardiac dropsy. *Arch. Intern. Med.* 49:964, 1932.

37. Miller, R. L., Taylor, W. R., Gentry, W., and Day, A. T. Indirect calorimetry in postoperative patients with acute renal failure. *Am. Surg.* 49:494, 1983.

38. Mirtallo, J. M., Schneider, P. J., and Mavko, K. A comparison of essential and general amino acid infusions in the nutritional support of patients with compromised renal function. *J. Parenter. Enter. Nutr.* 6:109, 1982.

39. Mondon, C. E., Dolkas, C. B., and Reaven, G. M. The site of insulin resistance in acute uremia. *Diabetes* 27:571, 1978.

40. Moore, F. D. *Metabolic Care of the Surgical Patient.* Philadelphia: W. B. Saunders, 1960.

41. Pelosi, G., Proietti, R., Arcageli, A., Magalini, S. I., and Bondoli, A. Total parenteral nutrition infusate: An approach to its optimal composition in post-trauma acute renal failure. *Resuscitation* 9:45, 1981.

42. Pemberton, L. B., Lyman, B., Lander, V., and Convinsky, J. Sepsis from triple vs single-lumen catheters during total parenteral nutrition in surgical or critically ill patients. *Arch. Surg.* 121:591, 1986.

43. Pietrek, J., Kokot, F., and Kuska, J. Serum 25-hydroxyvitamin D and parathyroid hormone in patients with acute renal failure. *Kidney Int.* 13:178, 1978.

44. Proietti, R., Pelosi, G., Santori, R., et al. Nutrition in acute renal failure. *Resuscitation* 10:159, 1983.

45. Richards, P., and Brown, C. L. Urea metabolism in an azotaemic woman with normal renal function. *Lancet* 2:207, 1975.

46. Rose, W. C., Coon, M. J., and Lambert, G. F. The amino acid requirements of man: The role of lysine, arginine and tryptophan. *J. Biol. Chem.* 206:421, 1954.

47. Rose, W. C., Wixom, R. L., Lockhart, H. B., et al. The amino acid requirements of man: XV. The valine requirement; Summary and final observations. *J. Biol. Chem.* 217:987, 1955.

48. Rose, W. C., and Dekker, E. E. Urea as a source of nitrogen for the biosynthesis of amino acids. *J. Biol. Chem.* 223:107, 1956.

49. Sax, H. C., Talamini, M. A., Brackett, K., and Fischer, J. E. Hepatic steatosis in total parenteral nutrition: Failure of fatty infiltration to correlate with abnormal serum hepatic enzyme levels. *Surgery* 100:697, 1986.

50. Sellers, A. L., Katz, J., and Marmorstein, J. Effect of bilateral nephrectomy on urea formation in rat liver slices. *Am. J. Physiol.* 191:345, 1957.

51. Shear, L. Internal redistribution of tissue protein synthesis in uremia. *J. Clin. Invest.* 48:1252, 1967.

52. Sigler, M., and Teehan, B. P. Solute transport in continuous hemodialysis: A new treatment for acute renal failure. *Kidney Int.* 32:562, 1987.

53. Silk, D. B. A. Future of enteral nutrition. *Gut* 27:116, 1986.

54. Spreiter, S. C., Myers, B. D., and Swenson, R. S. Protein energy requirement in subjects with acute renal failure and receiving intermittent hemodialysis. *Am. J. Clin. Nutr.* 33:1433, 1980.

55. Toback, F. G. Amino acid enhancement of renal regeneration after acute tubular necrosis. *Kidney Int.* 12:193, 1977.

56. Toback, F. G., Dodd, R. C., Mayer, E. R., and Havener, L. J. Amino acid administration enhances renal protein metabolism after acute tubular necrosis. *Nephron* 33:238, 1983.

57. Weisenfeld, S., Podolsky, X., Goldsmith, L., and Ziff, L. Absorption of insulin to intravenous bottles and tubing. *Diabetes* 17:766, 1968.

58. Wilmore, D. W., and Dudrick, S. J. Treatment of acute renal failure with intravenous essential L-amino acids. *Arch. Surg.* 99:669, 1969.

59. Wilfson, M., Jones, M. R., and Kopple, J. D. Amino acid losses during hemodialysis with infusions of amino acids and glucose. *Kidney Int.* 21:500, 1982.

Nutritional Support in Cardiac and Pulmonary Diseases

Herbert R. Freund

The patient with cardiac and/or pulmonary diseases in need of nutritional support presents similar problems to the clinician, problems for which physicians have, as yet, only limited solutions. Both kinds of patients may need moderate to severe fluid restriction, and both may be severely depleted because of their basic cardiac-pulmonary disorder or due to a second affliction such as pulmonary infection, cardiac decompensation, related or unrelated surgical intervention, respiratory failure, and critical care therapy, causing increased catabolism and hypermetabolism.

A second aspect of extreme interest when discussing cardiopulmonary patients is the interaction between the different nutrients and the cardiac muscle and lung. Namely, what do the heart and lung, under various pathophysiologic conditions, prefer as nutrients to improve their function and which nutrients might, in turn, prove detrimental to these organs in certain other pathophysiologic situations? For the sake of brevity, however, this chapter does not deal with the dietary implications of atherosclerotic cardiovascular disorders, in particular coronary artery disease. These topics are well covered in excellent, recently published reports [7, 31].

CARDIAC

The myocardium metabolizes glucose, fatty acids, triglycerides, lactate, pyruvate, ketones, and amino acids. In general, glucose and fatty acids are the primary sources of fuel for the myocardium. Under different pathophysiologic conditions, some of these fuel substrates are clearly preferred to the others. For example, under resting conditions, free fatty acids are utilized, whereas during ischemia the utilization of carbohydrate will increase manyfold.

Various Aspects of Malnutrition and Cardiac Cachexia

Malnutrition among general hospital patient populations and in patients undergoing sur-

203

gery has been reported to be common [15, 16] and a major contributory factor in the development of postoperative morbidity and mortality [73]. [*Editor's Note:* These studies [15, 16] were carried out in a city or county type of hospital with a greater percentage of indigent patients. In other types of hospitals the percentage of malnourished patients, while still present, is probably considerably smaller.] Starvation, malnutrition, and the inability of patients to receive adequate nourishment during the course of severe illness may have far-reaching detrimental effects on host defense mechanism, wound healing, respiratory and cardiac function, and many other vital organ systems, obviously carrying a grave prognosis.

Not long ago, the heart was believed to be spared during starvation [96, 97]. However, more recent studies demonstrated that starvation can result in atrophy of the human heart; in decrease in heart rate, arterial and venous pressures, stroke volume, and cardiac output and index [59, 60]; in a 20 to 30% decrease in myofibrillar diameter [5]; in a chamber volume reduction proportional to body weight loss [50]; and in distinct morphologic changes, mainly myocardial atrophy and interstitial edema [83, 84]. Functionwise, reduction in left ventricular compliance, force velocity, peak developed pressure, cardiac contractility, and stroke volume were reported in starving hearts [5, 62]. Myocardial atrophy was presumably associated with decreased contractility, whereas myocardial edema resulted in left ventricular stiffness [5].

In the cardiac patient, we as physicians might encounter two different types of malnutrition states. The first is the classic cardiac cachexia seen in patients with long-standing congestive heart failure. In the etiology of cardiac cachexia, several factors were named and included anorexia, an elevated metabolic rate, cellular hypoxia due to hypoperfusion and impaired delivery of nutrients to the tissues, deranged removal of cellular waste products, and possibly increased urinary and fecal nutrient losses [52]. The second form of malnutrition is iatrogenic as the result of

complicated cardiac or any other type of complicated major surgery in the cardiac patient.

Considerations of nutritional support are very different in these two types of cardiac cachexia. In the first form, we are dealing with patients in long-standing congestive heart failure, due mainly to rheumatic valvular disease or congenital heart malformations, in need of corrective cardiac surgery. In the second group of patients, which has grown to a considerable number in recent years, we are dealing with an excessive metabolic response to major surgery and ensuing postoperative complications in patients who initially presented in a satisfactory nutritional status, mainly patients undergoing coronary artery bypass grafts for ischemic heart disease or patients with ischemic heart disease undergoing any other major surgical intervention. To this we have to add a much smaller group of patients with a severe myocardial infarction, necessitating resuscitation and critical care therapy, with cardiac failure, renal failure, the need for mechanical ventilation, and an intra-aortic balloon. This complex combination is a strong catabolic stimulus and, coupled with the inability to eat, constitutes another strong indication for total parenteral nutrition (TPN).

In the past, perioperative nutritional support in the form of parenteral or enteral nutrition was attempted for primary cardiac cachexia. In a study of 44 malnourished patients undergoing cardiac surgery, Abel et al. [4] observed a higher rate of sepsis and respiratory failure, a longer stay in the intensive care unit, greater hospital cost, and increased mortality compared to normally nourished operated controls. This incidence of complications and higher mortality rate were not improved by a postoperative 5-day course of TPN. Blackburn et al. [17] described reduced morbidity and mortality in three patients undergoing triple valve replacement following 3 weeks of preoperative TPN. [*Editor's Note:* Of course, a three-patient anecdotal study is hardly conclusive, although the 3-week preoperative parenteral nutrition preparation is probably more of the order of magnitude needed to begin to reverse cardiac cachexia.]

Keys et al. [59, 60] reported a prolonged period of disability following nutritional repletion in starving normal volunteers. Animal data from Abel [1] suggested that despite nutritional repletion of malnourished dogs, significant depression of ventricular performance still existed. Our own data in the Langendorff preparation of a rat model of starvation and refeeding demonstrated that although a constant heart–body weight ratio was maintained during both starvation and refeeding, developed force and force velocity decreased during protein malnutrition as compared to control rats, and returned to control levels during refeeding [37]. These changes were less obvious at low heart rates, but reached statistical significance at paced heart rates of 300 and 400 beats/min (Fig. 14-1). We thus clearly demonstrated that experimental protein malnutrition induced derangements in myocardial function, in particular at times of increased demands as is the case during higher heart rates. These derangements reversed almost completely to normal on prolonged refeeding [37]. These observations gain special clinical significance in view of recent studies reporting a high incidence of protein-calorie malnutrition in general hospital populations, particularly among severely injured and/or elderly patients. Nutritional support, aimed at the maintenance of lean body mass and other vital functions, has the potential to reverse the starvation-induced derangements in cardiac function and its ensuing morbidity.

Very similar considerations exist when dealing with infants with congenital heart diseases (CHD), in whom failure to thrive and growth retardation are common. This in turn delays the surgical correction of their anomalies and again, in a vicious cycle, impedes catch-up growth due to the development of pulmonary hypertension. Moreover, poor nutrition increases surgical risk and delays recovery. Bougle et al. [18] treated 13 children for 40 days with enteral feeding via nasogastric tubes of 137 kcal/kg/day and were able to show weight gain and growth, and to safely accomplish cardiac surgery in 9 of these patients. A similar report was pub-

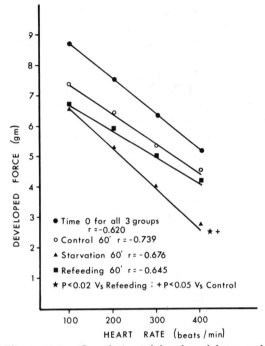

Figure 14-1. Correlation of developed force and heart rate in control, starving, and refed isolated rat hearts at time zero (same line for all three groups) and after 60 minutes of Langendorff perfusion. Note the stronger decline in developed force of starving animals compared to the control and the refed groups ($p < 0.02$–0.05). (From Freund, H. R., and Holroyde, J. Cardiac function during protein malnutrition and refeeding in the isolated rat heart. *J. Parenter. Enter. Nutr.* 10:470, 1986.)

lished by Vanderhoof et al. [95], allowing for earlier and safer surgical intervention in 11 tube-fed infants.

As short-term preoperative nutritional support appears to be inadequate and long-term support seems not to be feasible because of the severity of the heart condition necessitating surgery, we and others advocate 1 to 2 weeks of preoperative nutritional support continued into the postoperative period, with simultaneous early and guided postoperative resumption of oral feeding. [*Editor's Note:* On the basis of Abel's data, this period might well be required to be longer, probably up to 4 weeks.]

Previously well-nourished cardiac patients, usually those undergoing coronary artery bypass surgery and with any major operative or postoperative complications resulting in a prolonged and complicated postoperative course, should be put on TPN or, if tolerated, enteral nutrition, early, usually within the first 3 to 5 days postoperatively. Here the indications for TPN do not differ from those for any other patient undergoing major surgery and developing severe postoperative complications. Abel et al. [3] estimated that approximately 3% of patients undergoing cardiac surgery require TPN postoperatively, which corresponds to the expected census of 3 to 5% of general hospital populations requiring TPN.

Total Parenteral Nutrition for the Cardiac Patient

The following is a brief discussion of the special nutritional requirements of the heart during various pathophysiologic conditions, and whether the cardiac patient behaves differently in response to, and during, TPN.

Glucose, Insulin, and Glucagon

Some data exist as to the positive inotropic effects of hypertonic glucose [61], a carbohydrate–amino acid mixture [6], and insulin [32, 56]. Our own results in the Langendorff preparation of the normal and septic heart indicate that neither insulin nor glucagon affects the function of the normal heart, and that insulin and, to a lesser degree, glucagon have positive inotropic effects on the isolated septic heart, although these are not dose-response effects [69].

In a recent interesting study, Lolley et al. [66] performed preoperative nutritional manipulations in 312 patients who were to undergo elective coronary artery bypass surgery. It was possible to alter myocardial glycogen stores and thus offer better myocardial protection by the preoperative supplementation of a combination of oral fat and intravenous hypertonic glucose.

Fat

Fat emulsions were reported to be detrimental to the canine myocardium and to its systemic vascular resistance [47]. However, these observations were not confirmed in patients recovering from coronary bypass surgery in whom no adverse hemodynamic changes occurred with the infusion of relatively high doses of fat [34]. Only enormous amounts of fat (5.25 mg/kg/min), which are never used in clinical practice, resulted in the depression of myocardial contractility [2]. Thus, there seems to be no contraindication to the use of fat emulsions in the cardiac patient, either as part of the glucose system or as part of the "all-in-one" system.

Branched-Chain Amino Acids in Sepsis and Ischemia

Recent work with the use of branched-chain amino acids (BCAAs) in the septic [35] and ischemic [89] heart offers new insight into possible nutritional and metabolic manipulations of the heart. Protein turnover in cardiac and skeletal muscle is affected by the provision of amino acids, particularly the BCAAs. This effect on cardiac and skeletal muscle not only is related to their role as an energy substrate via oxidation and gluconeogenesis, but also involves their ability to regulate turnover by accelerating protein synthesis and inhibiting protein degradation [22, 25, 26, 43, 72, 75]. The effects on protein turnover are particularly apparent under conditions of elevated BCAA concentration, and even metabolites of the BCAAs modify protein turnover in cardiac and skeletal muscle [93]. In vivo studies in a rat injury model [38, 39, 41, 42] and recent clinical studies [23, 24, 38, 40] confirmed these nitrogen-sparing effects of BCAAs. [Editor's Note: By and large, studies on the use of BCAA solutions in patients with sepsis have been as yet disappointing [19]. The reason for this appears to be that the BCAAs do not decrease catabolism in muscle from septic animals [49].]

It is generally agreed that myocardial depression and ultimately failure occur in sepsis [53, 77], but their possible contributory role to the development of septic shock is still in question. Suggested causes for the heart failure observed in sepsis include structural damage to the myocardium [77, 90], increased circulatory requirements resulting in

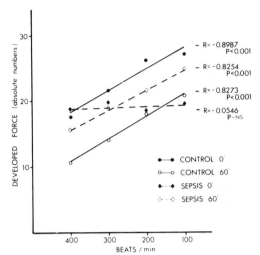

Figure 14-2. Regression lines for developed force and heart rate in control and septic animals at time zero and after 60 minutes of Langendorff perfusion. Note similar slopes for control animals at time zero and 60 minutes while septic animals exhibited significantly ($p < 0.05$) different slopes. At time zero in septic animals, developed force did not decrease with increasing heart rate as observed in control animals. After 60 minutes of perfusion, septic animals regained this negative linear correlation of developed force and heart rate ($p < 0.001$), with developed force being significantly improved at 60 minutes compared with time zero. (From Freund, H. R., Dann, E. J., Burns, F., Gotsman, M. S., and Hasin, Y. The effect of branched chain amino acids on systolic properties of the normal and septic isolated rat heart. *Arch. Surg.* 120:488, 1985. Copyright 1985, American Medical Association.)

hypotension and inadequate coronary perfusion [90], intracardiac fluid and ionic disturbances [53], or a toxic phenomenon in the form of a myocardial depressant factor [46, 64]. In our series of experiments with the isolated rat-heart Langendorff preparation [36, 48], we were able to demonstrate significant reductions of both developed force and force velocity during sepsis (Fig. 14-2). These deranged systolic properties improved during perfusion with all solutions tested, suggesting a mechanical washout effect of a "toxic" substance. In addition, there was a distinct improvement in systolic properties when utilizing an amino acid formulation containing 42% BCAAs, suggesting that a

significant and important improvement in cardiac function can be achieved by supplying balanced BCAA-enriched amino acid solutions [36, 68].

Just a brief note summarizing our recent experimental work looking into the myocardial protection effects of BCAA during ischemia and reperfusion of the Langendorff and working heart preparations [89]. Perfusion with BCAAs resulted in prolongation of the time to initiation of ischemic contracture and improvement of postischemic recovery. However, the most striking beneficial effects, in both hemodynamic and biochemical parameters, were observed in the ischemia-depleted heart when BCAAs and glucose were added to the oxygenated crystalloid cardioplegia solution (Fig. 14-3). The mechanism of BCAA-enhanced postischemia cardiac recovery is not yet sufficiently clear. It seems possible that glucose and amino acids in the oxygenated cardioplegia solution bring about increases in tissue levels of amino acid and Krebs cycle intermediates necessary for oxygenation, protein synthesis, and repletion of adenine nucleotides. Thus, BCAAs exhibit beneficial biochemical and hemodynamic effects on the ischemic heart [89].

Special Considerations

There are really only minor modifications in the management and TPN protocols of cardiac patients compared to ordinary patients. The major difference in the management of TPN in cardiac patients is the need to restrict total volume (approximately 1500 ml/day) and sodium (approximately 1.5 g/day) administration. For this purpose, we advocate the use of formulations prepared with more concentrated amino acid (10%) and glucose (70%) solutions, the final formulation containing 5% amino acids in 35% glucose. If fat is added, either separately or in the "all-in-one" system, the 20% emulsion should be used to offer a higher caloric density. The use of higher glucose concentrations is one reason for the higher rate of hyperglycemia seen in these patients, necessitating more frequent monitoring of blood glucose levels and the

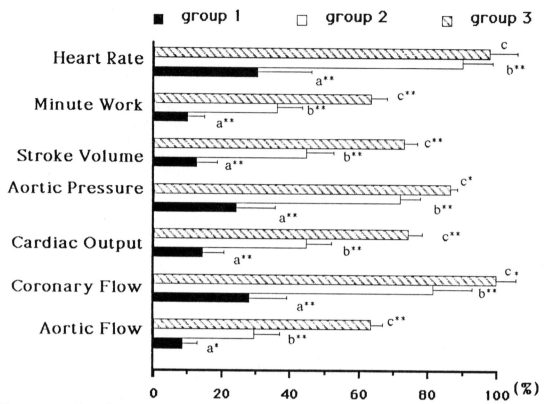

Figure 14-3. The effect of oxygenated crystalloid cardioplegic solution enriched by glucose and branched-chain amino acids (BCAAs) on the hemodynamic recovery in postischemic reperfused rat hearts (mean ± SEM): Group 1, cardioplegia solution without glucose; Group 2, cardioplegia solution with 11.1 mmol glucose; Group 3, cardioplegia solution with 11.1 mmol glucose and 3.5 mmol BCAA. (a, Group 1 vs. Group 2; b, Group 1 vs. Group 3; c, Group 2 vs. Group 3; *$p < 0.05$, **$p < 0.01$; by Mann-Whitney test.) (From Schwalb, H., Freund, H. R., and Uretzky, G. Role of amino acids in myocardial protection during ischemia and reperfusion. In J. M. Kinney and P. R. Borum (eds.), Perspectives in Clinical Nutrition. Baltimore/Munich: Urban and Schwarzenberg, 1989. Pp. 57–69.)

addition of higher amounts of insulin to the TPN formulation. Two other reasons to explain the glucose intolerance in these patients are that ischemic heart disease in our patient population is often related to diabetes mellitus and that congestive heart failure causes low flow to the muscle, liver, and pancreas, all of them involved in glucose metabolism.

Other minor considerations are that diuretic therapy might bring about the need for additional potassium, magnesium, and possibly zinc supplementation. Additional potassium might also be needed for the process of anabolism. Monitoring of potassium levels is particularly important in patients on digitalis therapy. No increased technical compli-

cations or TPN-related infections were reported for TPN in cardiac patients.

Most patients will well tolerate fluid and gas exchange loads imposed by continuous enteral and parenteral nutrition. However, some patients, particularly those who are severely malnourished with limited cardiac and/or pulmonary reserve, might develop the "refeeding syndrome" [51, 59, 60]. These patients may develop dyspnea, hypercapnia, tachycardia, elevated venous pressure, and congestive heart failure or cardiac arrest. It thus seems necessary not only to closely monitor volume and electrolyte intake and balance, but also to carefully adjust caloric input and source, depending on an appropriate mixture of carbohydrate and fat calories.

PULMONARY

Surgical patients with acute respiratory failure can be categorized into two major groups: (1) those with chronic lung disease on top of which an acute event is superimposed, and (2) those patients with essentially normal pulmonary function developing acute respiratory failure following injury or sepsis. Nutritional support is indicated for both patients previously malnourished as a result of their chronic lung disease, as well as for patients inflicted with a severe hypermetabolic-catabolic stimulus such as injury, trauma, complicated surgery, and severe infection. Early and appropriate nutritional support helps to sustain the function of various essential organ systems, including the respiratory system.

Starvation, Malnutrition, and the Respiratory System

Malnutrition is a relatively common development in critically ill patients who are being mechanically ventilated [28], more so in patients who previously had chronic obstructive pulmonary disease (COPD) in whom weight loss and a deranged nutritional status are common [54]. Patients with severe airflow obstruction tend to weigh less than patients with less severe COPD [72], while those patients with excessive weight loss have a lower survival rate than patients with COPD who maintain their weight [94]. Moreover, patients with COPD who develop acute respiratory failure tend to be more malnourished than patients who do not develop complications [29].

Both essentially normal patients and patients with preexisting pulmonary disease develop protein-calorie malnutrition when they are critically ill and mechanically ventilated. This in turn results in further abnormalities of pulmonary function and structure (loss of pulmonary connective tissue, reduced lung weight, development of emphysema), reduced expiratory and inspiratory muscle contractility, deranged ventilatory control, reduced production of surfactant, and abnormal pulmonary defense mechanisms resulting in increased incidence of respiratory infections [30, 33, 45, 80, 87, 92, 99].

Respiratory Muscle Function

Muscle wasting as a result of malnutrition also affects respiratory muscle mass and function, inducing muscle atrophy and decreased muscle force output. These in turn reduce the capacity of patients to sustain adequate levels of ventilation. The loss of muscle strength is evenly distributed between inspiratory and expiratory muscles [9]. The reduction in diaphragmatic muscle mass (dry weight, wet weight, and muscle thickness) during nutritional deprivation was claimed to be proportional to the decrease in body weight and limb muscle weight loss [30]. However, in an autopsy study, the diaphragm weight of emphysematous patients was decreased out of proportion to the reduction in body weight [92]. Not only are the diaphragmatic muscle mass and thickness reduced, but the contractile strength of the remaining muscle fibers at any given fiber length or stimulus frequency is also [58, 81]. However, this is accompanied by a paradoxic increase in diaphragmatic endurance [80]. There seems to occur a greater decrease in diaphragmatic cross-sectional area for fast-twitch (fast oxidative) fibers than for slow-twitch (slow oxidative) fibers [58, 65]. ATP levels measured in intercostal and quadriceps muscles have been similarly decreased in patients with COPD, and were restored following appropriate nutritional therapy [45].

Malnutrition-associated reduction in inspiratory muscular strength, which might reach levels as low as 30% of normal, results in hypercapnic respiratory failure [20]. A good correlation was reported between maximum inspiratory mouth pressure and body cell mass [57]. In poorly nourished patients with COPD, an even greater degree of respiratory muscle weakness is apparent [30], and might reach critical levels and eventual hypercapnic respiratory failure when injury or infection are superimposed.

Pulmonary Parenchyma

Mild starvation or protein deficiency does not change the morphology or composition of connective tissue of the lung. However, severe starvation causes decreased internal surface area and number of alveoli, increased alveolar size, and minimal or no change in pulmonary compliance [30]. These morphometric findings are consistent with the definition of emphysema. Starvation also increases surface forces in the lung by loss of pulmonary surfactant, the result of an imbalance between production and degradation of surfactant [33, 87]. Biochemical changes include a decrease in lung lipid content due to a decrease in lipogenesis [88], net protein loss because of decreased synthesis [44], and derangements of hydroxyproline and elastin metabolism. Other important nutritional elements that can affect lung connective tissue are copper, zinc, pyridoxine, ascorbic acid, and vitamin A. Many of these may also cause impaired immunocompetence, resulting in an increased tendency for pulmonary infection and further respiratory compromise.

Lung Defenses

Two major mechanisms are to be considered when one discusses lung defense mechanisms. The first is the antioxidant defense system, which, for example, is severely impaired by prenatal and postnatal nutritional deprivation [30]. In the newborn, this results in deranged oxygen tolerance [30]. Other nutritional deficiencies that can impair antioxidant protective mechanisms are reduced levels of sulfur-containing amino acids, copper, selenium, iron, vitamin E, carotenes, ascorbic acid, fatty acid saturation in lipid, and caloric intake.

The second defense mechanism to be considered is immunologic competence. Nutritional deficiency causes an increase in the number of lymphatic cells in alveolar and bronchial washings, a decrease in the T helper–T suppressor cell ratio, decreased ciliary movement, and increased bacterial ad-

herence to epithelial cells [74]. Furthermore, protein-calorie malnutrition interferes with the conversion of monocytes to active alveolar macrophages, compromising phagocytosis and cell-mediated immunity [55, 70].

Ventilatory Drive

Starvation- or semistarvation-induced malnutrition can reduce oxygen consumption, basal metabolic rate, minute ventilation, mean inspiratory flow rate, and ventilatory response to hypoxia in normal volunteers [8, 27, 98]; all of these are mediated by sympathetic suppression of the neural ventilatory drive [78]. The data are less clear with regard to the hypercapnic drive. Also lacking are data to define how malnutrition affects the respiratory control system in patients with chronic lung disease, with or without an acute injury.

Nutritional Support in Patients with Acute Respiratory Failure

Acute respiratory failure is very often the result of injury or sepsis, resulting in severe catabolism, hypermetabolism, and eventual protein-calorie malnutrition, if no early nutritional intervention is being undertaken. The problem can be even more complex and urgent in critically ill patients with baseline chronic lung disease accompanied by chronic nutritional depletion.

Amino Acids

In addition to serving as substrate for protein synthesis, amino acids were reported to increase minute ventilation, oxygen consumption, and ventilatory response to hypoxia and hypercarbia [99, 100]. Askanazi et al. [12], in eight patients with weight loss greater than 10%, infused 7.5 mg of nitrogen/kcal resting energy expenditure or 15 mg of nitrogen/kcal resting energy expenditure and found, with the high nitrogen infusion, a significant reduction in arterial carbon dioxide tension ($PaCO_2$) with increased sensitivity and enhanced ventilatory response to carbon dioxide. Recently it was demonstrated that the BCAAs have a specific stimulatory effect on the ventilatory drive, an observation that might carry a promising therapeutic modality in certain cases of respiratory failure [91].

Carbohydrate

Hypocaloric amounts of glucose administered to normal volunteers resulted in a low metabolic rate, decreased minute ventilation, and decreased response to hypoxia. The administration of glucose to cover resting energy expenditure increased minute ventilation in proportion to the increase in carbon dioxide production [82] and increased the ventilatory response to hypoxia [100]. This increased respiratory work in response to the increased carbon dioxide production caused by carbohydrate oxidation is one of the major reasons for the current common practice of using mixed glucose-fat fuel in the critically ill patient, particularly when mechanically ventilated. Excessive carbohydrate intake in mechnically ventilated patients was reported to result in the accumulation of excess carbon dioxide and difficulty in weaning off the respirator [11]. This is probably the case in only a minority of patients, particularly in those with previous pulmonary problems with marginal respiratory function and reserve. [Editor's Note: As stated elsewhere in this volume, this occurs only in very few patients. The setting is a depleted, septic patient to whom a sudden excessive carbohydrate load is administered.]

Lipids

Intravenous fat emulsions were reported to cause impairment of pulmonary function in healthy adults, premature infants, patients with preexisting pulmonary disease, and experimental animals. The lung function abnormalities usually involve increases in diffusion capacity inequalities. However, arterial oxygen and carbon dioxide tension changes never proved of any clinical significance [48]. Despite these human and experimental animal data suggesting deteriorating pulmonary function with the use of intravenous fat emulsions, lipid emulsions are well tolerated by patients with respiratory insufficiency or patients who are mechanically ventilated. A recent study even indicated that the use of lipid emulsions improves pulmonary mechanical properties and surfactant production in the injured rat [13]. Moreover, recent extensive work from Kinney's group indicated that intravenous fat emulsions are a preferred fuel source for the injured and septic patient [10, 79].

Effect of Nutritional Support on Weaning off Mechanical Ventilation

Very little data exists as to the efficacy of nutritional support on the treatment of respiratory failure and in particular on the weaning of ventilated patients. In starved rats, short-term nutritional repletion normalized surfactant concentrations with no change in tissue elasticity and airspace abnormalities [86]. Russell et al. [85] reported that nutritional support improves peripheral muscle function, well before repletion of muscle mass. One month of TPN in 11 youngsters with cystic fibrosis significantly improved maximum inspiratory and expiratory pressures [67]. Keys et al. [59] observed decreased vital capacity and respiratory efficiency after 12 and 24 weeks of semistarvation. Twelve weeks of refeeding resulted in a slow reversal to control levels.

Another retrospective study reported an 86% extubation rate in patients receiving TPN compared to only 22% in patients treated with routine glucose-electrolytes therapy [71]. [Editor's Note: Such data are tantalizing, but why can't such studies be done on a prospective, randomized basis? They not only do not provide the outcome data we need, but also may actually prevent the performance of properly designed clinical trials.] A similar study in a larger group of patients revealed a 93% weaning rate in a nourished group compared to 54% in a routine intravenous therapy group [14]. A recent study reported that patients' ability to breathe spontaneously was dependent on their nutritional intake; with increasing caloric intake, the percentage of spontaneously breathing patients increased from 11 to 79% [63]. Kelly et al. [57] demonstrated that in 21 of 29 critically ill patients receiving TPN for 2 weeks, inspiratory muscle strength as well as body cell mass improved significantly.

Special Considerations in the Nutritional Management of the Patient with Pulmonary Insufficiency and Mechanical Ventilation

Patients with pulmonary insufficiency share many of the problems encountered in cardiac patients, mainly the need for sodium and volume restriction. As interactions between nutrients and respiration have been repeatedly suggested, special care should be taken in selecting the amounts and composition of nutrients to be infused in the catabolic patient with compromised respiratory function. As mentioned earlier, the ventilatory response to hypoxia and particularly to hypercarbia is enhanced with an increasing intake of amino acids [12]. These effects are even more enhanced when using BCAAs [91]. This stimulation of respiratory function might well have beneficial effects by improving the ventilatory efficiency. However, it might also induce muscle fatigue and difficulty in weaning. These potential advantages and disadvantages of amino acid infusions need further study. Thus, the amount of protein supplied should be advanced slowly and its possible detrimental effect on respiration closely monitored.

A similar situation exists as to the supply of calories to this type of patient. In general, the catabolic patient in need of ventilatory support should receive up to 1.5 × resting energy expenditure while the respiratory rate, vital capacity, minute ventilation, and blood gases are carefully monitored. Nonprotein calories should be provided as equal proportions of carbohydrate and fat, in an attempt to avoid excessive carbon dioxide production as a result of excess glucose. It was recommended to limit glucose intake to a maximum of 4 to 5 mg/kg/min [21], although even this amount and rate might prove excessive in patients with limited respiratory reserve. In an attempt to make weaning easier, it was also recommended, although has not

been proved in a clinical study, to reduce the caloric intake to about 50% of needed calories in patients with marginal respiratory function. This reduction in protein and caloric intake fits well with the need for a gradual return of the sodium pump function deranged by malnutrition [76]. With excessive refeeding of malnourished patients, large amounts of sodium shift from the intracellular into the extracellular compartment, contributing to the development of edema with further difficulty in weaning. Thus, it is important at this stage to limit protein, calories, fluids, and sodium.

Once the patient has been weaned off mechanical ventilation, caloric and protein intake should be gradually increased to the full desired nutritional support regimen, attempting to achieve positive balance and repletion. Later, with the improvement in the patient's general and disease status, enteral feeding with one of the commercially available formulas should be initiated. A transition period of combined enteral and parenteral nutrition will ultimately lead, with the return of appetite, to complete enteral or oral nutrition.

If fluid restriction is a limiting factor for nutritional support, more concentrated formulations should be prepared, with 10% amino acids, 20% lipid emulsion, and 70% glucose. Adequate amounts of electrolytes, minerals, vitamins, and trace elements should be provided since some deficiencies, such as phosphate and magnesium impair myocardial and diaphragmatic contractility.

TPN-associated complications to which the pulmonary patient is more prone include pneumothorax from the introduction of a subclavian catheter in the COPD patient, injury-induced hyperglycemia, and line sepsis if and when a TPN line is in close proximity to a tracheostomy and nursing care is suboptimal.

REFERENCES

1. Abel, R. M. Nutrition and the heart. In J. E. Fischer (ed.), *Surgical Nutrition*. Boston: Little, Brown, 1983. Pp. 619–641.
2. Abel, R. M., Fisch, D., and Grossman, M. L.

Hemodynamic effects of intravenous 20% soy oil emulsion following coronary bypass surgery. *J. Parenter. Enter. Nutr.* 7:534, 1983.

3. Abel, R. M., Fischer, J. E., Buckley, M. J., and Austen, W. G. Hyperalimentation in cardiac surgery: A review of sixty-four patients. *J. Thorac. Cardiovasc. Surg.* 67:294, 1974.

4. Abel, R. M., Fischer, J. E., Buckley, M. J., Barnett, G. O., and Austen, W. G. Malnutrition in cardiac surgical patients: Results of a prospective randomized evaluation of early postoperative parenteral nutrition. *Arch. Surg.* 111:45, 1976.

5. Abel, R. M., Grimes, J., Alonso, D. R., Alonso, M. L., and Gay, W. A. Biochemical, adverse hemodynamic and ultrastructural changes in dog hearts subjected to protein-calorie malnutrition. *Am. Heart J.* 97:733, 1979.

6. Abel, R. M., Subramanian, V. A., and Gay, W. A., Jr. Effects of an intravenous amino acid nutrient solution on left ventricular contractility in dogs. *J. Surg. Res.* 23:201, 1977.

7. AHA Nutrition Committee: Rationale of the Diet-Heart Statement of the American Heart Association. *Arteriosclerosis* 4:177, 1982.

8. Angelillo, V. A., Bedi, S., Durfee, D., et al. Effects of low and high carbohydrate feedings in ambulatory patients with chronic obstructive pulmonary disease and chronic hypercapnia. *Ann. Intern. Med.* 103:883, 1985.

9. Arora, N. S., and Rochester, D. F. Respiratory muscle strength and maximal voluntary ventilation in undernourished patients. *Am. Rev. Respir. Dis.* 126:5, 1982.

10. Askanazi, J., Carpentier, Y. A., and Elwyn, D. H. Influence of total parenteral nutrition on fuel utilization in injury and sepsis. *Ann. Surg.* 191:40, 1980.

11. Askanazi, J., Rosenbaum, S. H., Hyman, A. L., Silverberg, P. A., Milic-Emili, J., and Kinney, J. M. Respiratory changes induced by the large glucose loads of total parenteral nutrition. *J.A.M.A.* 243:1444, 1980.

12. Askanazi, J., Weissman, C., LaSala, P. A., Milic-Emili, J., and Kinney, J. M. Effect of protein intake on ventilatory drive. *Anesthesiology* 60:106, 1984.

13. Bahrami, S., Strohmaier, W., Redl, H., and Schlag, G. Mechanical properties of the lungs of posttraumatic rats are improved by including fat in total parenteral nutrition. *J. Parenter. Enter. Nutr.* 11:560, 1987.

14. Bassili, H. R., and Dietel, M. Effect of nutritional support on weaning patients off mechanical ventilators. *J. Parenter. Enter. Nutr.* 5:161, 1981.

15. Bistrian, B. R., Blackburn, G. L., Hallowell, E., and Heddle, R. Protein status of general surgical patients. *J.A.M.A.* 230:858, 1974.

16. Bistrian, B. R., Blackburn, G. L., Vitale, J., and Cochran, D. Prevalence of malnutrition of general medical patients. *J.A.M.A.* 235:1567, 1976.

17. Blackburn, G. L., Gibbons, G. W., Bothe, A., Benotti, P. N., Harken, D. E., and McEnany, T. M. Nutritional support in cardiac cachexia. *J. Thorac. Cardiovasc. Surg.* 73:489, 1977.

18. Bougle, D., Iselin, M., Kahyat, A., and Duhamel, J. F. Nutritional treatment of congenital heart disease. *Arch. Dis. Child* 61:799, 1986.

19. Bower, R. H., Muggia-Sullam, M., Vallgren, S., et al. Branched chain amino acid-enriched solutions in the septic patient: A randomized, prospective trial. *Ann. Surg.* 203:13, 1986.

20. Braun, N. M. T., Arora, N. S., and Rochester, D. F. Respiratory muscle and pulmonary function in polymyositis and other proximal myopathies. *Thorax* 38:616, 1983.

21. Burke, J. F., Wolfe, R. R., Mullany, C. J., Mathews, D. E., and Bier, D. M. Glucose requirements following burn injury. *Ann. Surg.* 190:274, 1979.

22. Buse, M. G., and Reid, S. S. Leucine: A possible regulator of protein turnover in muscle. *J. Clin. Invest.* 56:1250, 1975.

23. Cerra, F. B., Blackburn, G. L., Hirsch, J., Mullen, K., and Luther, W. The effect of stress level, amino acid formula and nitrogen dose on nitrogen retention in traumatic and septic stress. *Ann. Surg.* 205:282, 1987.

24. Cerra, F. B., Upson, D., Angelico, R., et al. Branched chains support postoperative protein synthesis. *Surgery* 92:192, 1982.

25. Chua, B. H. L., Siehl, D. L., and Morgan, H. E. Effect of leucine and metabolites of branched chain amino acids on protein turnover in heart. *J. Biol. Chem.* 254:8358, 1979.

26. Chua, B. H. L., Siehl, D. L., and Morgan, H. E. A role for leucine in regulation of protein turnover in working rat hearts. *Am. J. Physiol.* 239:510, 1980.

27. Doekel, R. C., Zwillich, C. W., Scoggin, C. H., Kryger, M., and Weil, J. V. Clinical semistarvation: Depression of hypoxic ventilatory response. *N. Engl. J. Med.* 295:358, 1976.

28. Driver, A. G., and LeBrun, M. Iatrogenic malnutrition in patients receiving ventilatory support. *J.A.M.A.* 244:2195, 1980.

29. Driver, A. G., McAlevy, M. T., and Smith, V. L. Nutritional assessment of patients with chronic obstructive pulmonary disease and acute respiratory failure. *Chest* 82:26, 1982.

30. Edelman, N. H., Rucker, R. B., and Peavy, H. H. Nutrition and the respiratory system. *Am. Rev. Respir. Dis.* 134:347, 1986.

31. The Expert Panel: Report of the National

Cholesterol Education Program Expert Panel on Detection, Evaluation and Treatment of High Blood Cholesterol in Adults. *Arch. Intern. Med.* 143:36, 1988.

32. Farah, A. E., and Alousi, A. A. The actions of insulin on cardiac contractility. *Life Sci.* 29:975, 1981.

33. Faridy, E. E. Effect of food and water deprivation on surface activity of lungs of rats. *J. Appl. Physiol.* 29:493, 1970.

34. Fisch, D., and Abel, R. M. Hemodynamic effects of intravenous fat emulsions in patients with heart disease. *J. Parenter. Enter. Nutr.* 5:402, 1981.

35. Freund, H. R. Effects of malnutrition and sepsis on systolic properties of isolated rat heart. In J. M. Kinney and P. R. Borum (eds.), *Perspectives in Clinical Nutrition.* Baltimore/Munich: Urban and Schwarzenberg, 1989. Pp. 43–56.

36. Freund, H. R., Dann, E. J., Burns, F., Gotsman, M. S., and Hasin, Y. The effect of branched chain amino acids on systolic properties of the normal and septic isolated rat heart. *Arch. Surg.* 120:483, 1985.

37. Freund, H. R., and Holroyde, J. Cardiac function during protein malnutrition and refeeding in the isolated rat heart. *J. Parenter. Enter. Nutr.* 10:470, 1986.

38. Freund, H. R., Hoover, H. C., Atamian, S., and Fischer, J. E. Infusion of the branched chain amino acids in postoperative patients: Anti-catabolic properties. *Ann. Surg.* 190:18, 1979.

39. Freund, H. R., James, J. H., and Fischer, J. E. Nitrogen sparing mechanisms of singly-administered branched chain amino acids in the injured rat. *Surgery* 90:237, 1981.

40. Freund, H. R., Ryan, J. A., and Fischer, J. E. Amino acid derangements in patients with sepsis: Treatment with branched chain amino acid rich infusions. *Ann. Surg.* 188:423, 1978.

41. Freund, H. R., Yoshimura, N., and Fischer, J. E. The effect of branched chain amino acids and hypertonic glucose infusions on post-injury catabolism in the rat. *Surgery* 87:401, 1980.

42. Freund, H. R., Yoshimura, N., Lunetta, L., and Fischer, J. E. The role of the branched chain amino acids in decreasing muscle catabolism in vivo. *Surgery* 83:611, 1978.

43. Fulks, R. M., Li, J. B., and Goldberg, A. L. Effects of insulin, glucose and amino acids on protein turnover in rat diaphragm. *J. Biol. Chem.* 250:290, 1975.

44. Gacad, G., Dickie, K., and Massaro, D. Protein synthesis in lung: Influence of starvation on amino acid incorporation into protein. *J. Appl. Physiol.* 33:381, 1972.

45. Gertz, I., Hedenstierna, G., Hellers, G., and Wahren, J. Muscle metabolism in patients with chronic obstructive lung disease and acute respiratory failure. *Clin. Sci. Mol. Med.* 52:395, 1977.

46. Goldfarb, R. D., Weber, P., and Eisenman, J. Isolation of a shock-induced circulating cardiodepressant substance. *Am. J. Physiol.* 237:168, 1979.

47. Grimes, J. B., and Abel, R. M. Hemodynamic effects of fat emulsion in dogs. *J. Parenter. Enter. Nutr.* 3:40, 1979.

48. Hageman, J. R., and Hunt, C. E. Fat emulsions and lung function. *Clin. Chest Med.* 7:69, 1986.

49. Hasselgren, P. O., LaFrance, R., Pedersen, P., James, J. H., and Fischer, J. E. Infusion of a branched chain amino acid enriched solution and alpha-ketoisocaproic acid in septic rats: Effects on nitrogen balance and skeletal muscle protein turnover. *J. Parenter. Enter. Nutr.* 12:244, 1988.

50. Heymsfield, S. B., Bethel, R. A., Ansley, J. D., Gibbs, D. M., Felner, J. M., and Nutter, D. O. Cardiac abnormalities in cachectic patients before and during nutritional repletion. *Am. Heart J.* 95:584, 1978.

51. Heymsfield, S. B., Caspar, K., and Funfar, J. Physiologic response and clinical implications of nutrition support. *Am. J. Cardiol.* 60:75G, 1987.

52. Heymsfield, S. B., Smith, J., Redd, S., and Whitworth, H. B. Nutritional support in cardiac failure. *Surg. Clin. North Am.* 61:635, 1981.

53. Hinshaw, L. B. Myocardial function in endotoxin shock. *Circ. Shock* 1:43, 1979.

54. Hunter, A. M. B., Carey, M. A., and Larsh, H. N. The nutritional status of patients with chronic obstructive pulmonary disease. *Am. Rev. Respir. Dis.* 124:376, 1981.

55. Jackab, G. I., Warr, G. A., and Astry, C. L. Alteration of pulmonary defense mechanisms by protein depletion diet. *Infect. Immun.* 34:610, 1981.

56. Kao, R. L., Christman, E. W., Lun, S. L., Krauks, J. M., Tyers, G. F. O., and Williams, E. H. The effect of insulin and anoxia on the metabolism of isolated mature rat cardiac myocytes. *Arch. Biochem. Biophys.* 203:587, 1980.

57. Kelly, S. M., Rosa, A., Field, S., Coughlin, M., Shizgal, H. M., and Macklem, P. T. Inspiratory muscle strength and body composition in patients receiving total parenteral nutrition therapy. *Am. Rev. Respir. Dis.* 130:33, 1984.

58. Kelsen, S. G., Ference, M., and Kapoor, S. Effects of prolonged undernutrition on structure and function of the diaphragm. *J. Appl. Physiol.* 58:1354, 1985.

59. Keys, A., Brozek, J., Henschel, A., Mickel-

sen, O., and Taylor, H. L. *The Biology of Human Starvation.* Minneapolis: The University of Minnesota Press, 1950. P. 494.

60. Keys, A., Henschel, A., and Taylor, H. L. The size and function of the human heart in semi-starvation and in subsequent rehabilitation. *Am. J. Physiol.* 50:153, 1947.

61. Ko, K. K., and Paradise, R. R. The effects of substrate on contractility of rat atria depressed with halothane. *Anesthesiology* 31:532, 1969.

62. Kyger, E. R., Block, W. J., Roach, G., and Dudrick, S. J. Adverse effects of protein malnutrition on myocardial function. *Surgery* 84:147, 1978.

63. Laaban, J. P., Lemaire, F., Baron, J. F., et al. Influence of caloric intake on the respiratory mode during mandatory minute volume ventilation. *Chest* 87:67, 1985.

64. Lefer, A. M. Role of a myocardial depressant factor in the pathogenesis of circulatory shock. *Fed. Proc.* 29:1836, 1978.

65. Lewis, M. I., Sieck, G. C., Fournier, M., and Belman, M. J. Effect of nutritional deprivation on diaphragm contractility and muscle fiber size. *J. Appl. Physiol.* 60:596, 1986.

66. Lolley, D., Myers, W. O., Ray, J. E., Sautter, R. D., and Tewksbury, D. A. Clinical experience with preoperative myocardial nutrition management. *J. Cardiovasc. Surg.* 26:236, 1985.

67. Mansell, A. L., Andersen, J. E., Muttart, C. R. Short-term pulmonary effects of total parenteral nutrition in children with cystic fibrosis. *J. Pediatr.* 104:700, 1984.

68. Markovitz, L. J., Hasin, Y., Dann, E. J., Gotsman, M. S., and Freund, H. R. The different effects of leucine, isoleucine and valine on systolic properties of the normal and septic isolated heart. *J. Surg. Res.* 38:231, 1985.

69. Markovitz, L. J., Hasin, Y., and Freund, H. R. The effect of insulin and glucagon on systolic properties of the normal and septic isolated rat heart. *Basic Res. Cardiol.* 80:377, 1985.

70. Martin, T. R., Altman, L. C., and Alvares, O. F. The effect of severe protein calorie malnutrition on antibacterial defense mechanisms in the rat lung. *Am. Res. Respir. Dis.* 128:1013, 1982.

71. Mattar, J. A., Velasco, I. T., Esgail, A. S., and Takaoka, F. Parenteral nutrition as a useful method for weaning patients from mechanical ventilation. *J. Parenter. Enter. Nutr.* 2:50, 1978.

72. Morgan, H. E., Chua, B. H. L., and Boyd, T. A. Branched chain amino acids and the regulation of protein turnover in heart and skeletal muscle. In M. Walser and J. R. Williamson (eds.), *Metabolism and Clinical Implica-* tions of Branched Chain Amino and Keto-Acids. New York: Elsevier North-Holland, 1981. Pp. 217–226.

73. Mullen, J. L., Gernver, M. H., and Buzby, G. P. Implications of malnutrition in the surgical patient. *Arch. Surg.* 114:121, 1979.

74. Niederman, M. S., Merrill, W. M., Ferranti, R. D., Pagano, K. M., Palmer, L. B., and Reynolds, H. Y. Nutritional status and bacterial binding in the lower respiratory tract in patients with chronic tracheostomy. *Ann. Intern. Med.* 100:795, 1984.

75. Odessey, R. Amino acid and protein metabolism in the diaphragm. *Am. Rev. Respir. Dis.* 119:107, 1979.

76. Patrick, J., and Golden, M. H. N. Leukocytes, electrolytes and sodium transport in protein-energy malnutrition. *Am. J. Clin. Nutr.* 30:1478, 1977.

77. Postel, J., and Schloerb, P. R. Cardiac depression in bacteremia. *Ann. Surg.* 186:74, 1977.

78. Renzetti, A. D., McClement, J. H., and Litt, B. D. The Veterans Administration Cooperative study of pulmonary function: Mortality in relation to respiratory function in chronic obstructive pulmonary disease. *Am. J. Med.* 41:115, 1966.

79. Robin, A. P., Nordenström, J., Askanazi, J., Carpentier, Y. A., Elwyn, D. H., and Kinney, J. M. Influence of parenteral carbohydrate on fat oxidation in surgical patients. *Surgery* 95:608, 1984.

80. Rochester, D. F. Body weight and respiratory muscle function in chronic obstructive pulmonary disease. *Am. Rev. Respir. Dis.* 134:646, 1986.

81. Rochester, D. F., Arora, N. S., and Braun, N. M. T. Maximum contractile force of human diaphragm muscle, determined in vivo. *Trans. Am. Clin. Climatol. Assoc.* 93:200, 1981.

82. Rodriguez, J. L., Askanazi, J., Weissman, C., Hensle, T. W., Rosenbaum, S. H., and Kinney, J. M. Ventilatory and metabolic effects of glucose infusions. *Chest* 88:512, 1985.

83. Rossi, M. A., Pissaia, O., Cury, Y., and Oliveira, J. S. M. Noradrenaline levels and morphologic alterations of myocardium in experimental protein-calorie malnutrition. *J. Pathol.* 131:83, 1980.

84. Rossi, M. A., and Zucoloto, S. Ultrastructural changes in nutritional cardiomyopathy of protein-calorie malnourished rats. *Br. J. Exp. Pathol.* 63:242, 1982.

85. Russell, D. M., Walker, P. M., Leiter, L. A., et al. Metabolic and structural changes in skeletal muscle during hypocaloric dieting. *Am. J. Clin. Nutr.* 39:503, 1984.

86. Sahebjami, H., and Vassallon, C. L. Effects of starvation and refeeding on lung mechan-

ics and morphometry. *Am. Rev. Respir. Dis.* 119:443, 1979.

87. Sahebjami, H., Vassallo, C. L., and Wirman, J. A. Lung mechanics and ultrastructure in prolonged starvation. *Am. Rev. Respir. Dis.* 117:77, 1978.

88. Scholz, R. W. Lipid metabolism by rat lung in vitro: Utilization of citrate by normal and starved rats. *Biochem. J.* 126:1219, 1972.

89. Schwalb, H., Freund, H. R., and Uretzky G. Role of amino acids in myocardial protection during ischemia and reperfusion. In J. M. Kinney and P. R. Borum (eds.), *Perspectives in Clinical Nutrition.* Baltimore/Munich: Urban and Schwarzenberg, 1989. Pp. 57–69.

90. Siegel, J. H., Cerra, F. B., Coleman, B., et al. Physiological and metabolic correlations in human sepsis. *Surgery* 86:163, 1979.

91. Takala, J. Branched chain amino acids and respiratory function in man. In J. M. Kinney and P. R. Borum (eds.), *Perspectives in Clinical Nutrition.* Baltimore/Munich: Urban and Schwarzenberg, 1989. Pp. 221–229.

92. Thurlbeck, W. M. Diaphragm and body weight in emphysema. *Thorax* 33:483, 1978.

93. Tischler, M. E., Desautels, M., and Goldberg, A. L. Does leucine, leucyl tRNA, or some metabolite of leucine regulate protein synthesis and degradation in skeletal and cardiac muscle? *J. Biol. Chem.* 257:1613, 1982.

94. Vandenburg, E., Van de Woestigne, K., and Gyselen, A. Weight changes in the terminal stages of chronic obstructive lung disease. *Am. Rev. Respir. Dis.* 96:556, 1967.

95. Vanderhoof, J. A., Hofschire, P. J., Balluff, M. A., et al. Continuous enteral feedings: An important adjunct to the management of complex congenital heart disease. *Am. J. Dis. Child* 136:825, 1982.

96. Vasquez, H. *Diseases of the Heart.* Laidlaw, G. F. (ed.). Philadelphia: W. B. Saunders, 1924.

97. Voit, C. Uber die Verschiedenheiten der Eiweiszersetzung beim Hungern. *Z. F. Biol.* 2:308, 1866.

98. Weissman, C., Askanazi, J., Rosenbaum, S., Hyman, A. I., Milic-Emili, J., and Kinney, J. M. Amino acids and respiration. *Ann. Intern. Med.* 98:41, 1983.

99. Wilson, D. O., Rogers, R. M., and Hoffman, R. M. Nutrition and chronic lung disease. *Am. Rev. Respir. Dis.* 132:1347, 1985.

100. Zwillich, C. W., Sahn, S. A., and Weil, J. V. Effects of hypermetabolism upon respiratory gas exchange in normal man. *J. Clin. Invest.* 66:900, 1977.

Preoperative Total Parenteral Nutrition

James D. Luketich
James L. Mullen
Gordon P. Buzby

The use of total parenteral nutrition (TPN) in the preoperative period is controversial in malnourished surgical patients. Such use in well-nourished patients has never been rational or widespread. This application refers to the prophylactic use of TPN to reduce nutrition-related postoperative complications. A typical preoperative TPN plan includes parenteral nutrient delivery during both the preoperative and the postoperative period: 3 to 7 days of preoperative TPN, continued for 7 to 10 days postoperatively until the gastrointestinal tract is functionally adequate. The objective of preoperative TPN is to reduce nutritional dysfunction in the days immediately before and after operation. Although improved nutrition-associated organ function may be a legitimate objective in and of itself, in most cases it is not sufficient to justify the potential morbidity and expense of preoperative parenteral feeding unless there is a direct clinically apparent benefit to the patient. If such a direct benefit exists, it will most likely be a reduction in postoperative morbidity and/or mortality. One can justify the use of preoperative TPN only if one can provide convincing evidence that this therapy reduces postoperative complications or death. Preoperative nutritional support has been supposedly successful in reducing postoperative morbidity and mortality in subsets of surgical patients. Reportedly, those patients who had improved outcome were those with moderate to severe preoperative malnutrition, which encompasses less than 10% of operative candidates in most general surgery populations.

The interest in preoperative nutritional intervention developed as a logical consequence of several important observations. First, patients with certain "nutritional deficits" were found to have an increase in nutrition-related mortality and morbidity. Second, patients at risk for nutrition-related complications had definable characteristics that allowed prospective characterization or identification. Third, once such patients were identified, preoperative nutritional intervention seemed to be beneficial in early sketchy reports.

Much recent controversy revolves around the question of how to best identify the nutritionally high-risk operative candidates who are likely to benefit from TPN in the preoperative period [14]. Less important questions involve how much TPN to give, the nutrient composition, the timing, and the duration of treatment. In the future, more selective prospective identification of appropriate candidates for preoperative parenteral nutrition will be possible, facilitating administration of the most beneficial nutrient prescription.

The multiple objectives of this chapter are: (1) to define "clinically relevant malnutrition" in the context of a quantitative relationship between "malnutrition" severity and clinical outcome; (2) to provide an overview of the clinical utility of preoperative nutritional status testing; (3) to survey the effects of short-term TPN on nutritional status measures; (4) to review the results of early preoperative TPN trials, and to determine if any nutritional status measures improve along with a positive clinical outcome; (5) to objectively critique the study design of early trials; (6) to review the preliminary results of the recent Veterans Administration (VA) randomized controlled trial; and (7) to present our practical approach to the prospective identification of patients who should receive prophylactic preoperative TPN.

In this chapter, we do **not** discuss patients who will **eventually** require a major operative procedure but who are **not** candidates for immediate operation and who cannot consume an adequate oral diet. In this setting, the goal of TPN is to avoid development or progression of nutritional deficits while a patient awaits surgery.

Given the morbidity and mortality associated with preoperative malnutrition [5], it is unacceptable to permit malnutrition to develop or progress during a period of preoperative starvation in a patient who cannot undergo immediate operation. The efficacy of nutritional support in this setting has not been proved conclusively in a randomized clinical trial, but it is unlikely that such a trial

can or should be undertaken. Common sense and ethical concerns dictate against permitting development or progression of a documented operative risk factor when this can be prevented by a safe and proven technology. It is not clear precisely how long one can permit a patient to starve before significant nutritional deficits develop. Within 5 days in an unstressed patient, or 3 days in a stressed setting, changes in levels of circulating proteins with short half-lives are detectable. It seems reasonable to provide nutritional support in those circumstances when the duration of preoperative "starvation" is likely to exceed these limits. Such limits are consistent with guidelines of the American Society of Parenteral and Enteral Nutrition in which nutritional support is suggested if a period of starvation in excess of 5 to 7 days is anticipated in a previously well-nourished or mildly malnourished patient [1]. These guidelines suggest a more aggressive approach in severely malnourished patients with institution of nutritional support within 1 to 3 days. The guidelines are based on extensive collective clinical experience and provide a reasonable approach to the use of nutritional support when the alternative is prolonged "starvation" in the preoperative period.

DO "MALNOURISHED" PATIENTS HAVE INCREASED OPERATIVE MORBIDITY AND MORTALITY?

Numerous reports have documented the association between "malnutrition" and operative clinical outcome. In 1936, Studley [68] reported an increased mortality in patients with extreme weight loss who were undergoing major surgery for peptic ulcer disease. If preoperative weight loss exceeded 20%, operative mortality was 33%; in contrast, if weight loss was less than 20%, postoperative mortality was less than 5%. Rhoads et al. [52] and Thompson et al. [69] identified a relationship between hypoproteinemia and wound healing and infection in animals. Rhoads and Alexander [51] later confirmed the importance of this association in a retrospective study of surgical patients, showing a high incidence of postoperative complications in patients with hypoproteinemia.

These early findings were repeatedly confirmed and expanded. Bistrian et al. [5] found an increased surgical mortality associated with an albumin level of less than 3.0 g/dl. In 1975, MacLean et al. [36] reported increased septic complications and mortality in anergic trauma patients. Cannon et al. [15] reported increased rates of infection in patients with protein deficiency. Hickman et al. [28] retrospectively studied preoperative albumin levels and postoperative morbidity and mortality in 83 patients undergoing colorectal surgery. If the albumin level was less than 3.5 g/dl, the postoperative mortality rate was 28% and the overall complication rate was 61%. In patients with an albumin level greater than 3.5 g/dl, the mortality and morbidity rates were 4.1 and 31%, respectively.

Although most early studies were retrospective, they provided extensive evidence that there was an association between preoperative malnutrition and postoperative outcome. It became apparent that a single test lacked sensitivity and specificity in predicting clinical outcome and that not all patients with an abnormal result on a single nutritional test had a severe enough degree of malnutrition to impact on clinical outcome. We [46] examined a barrage of nutritional tests in 64 general surgical patients: 97% had at least one abnormal nutritional test result. Not all abnormal nutritional test results were associated with poor outcome. This study demonstrated that an isolated abnormal nutritional test result did not equal "clinically relevant malnutrition."

A number of multiparameter indices have been developed to improve the clinician's ability to identify "clinically relevant malnutrition." This involves comparing the outcome results with a large number of nutritional test results and statistically choosing those that combine for the best predictive model. For example, our Prognostic Nutritional Index (PNI) was developed to predict postoperative complications linked to preoperative nutritional assessment parameters and was based on an initial retrospective analysis [45]. Four parameters were identified by discriminant analysis and a computer-based stepwise regression, and then incorporated into a linear predictive model:

$$PNI(\%\,risk) = 158 - 16.6(ALB\ g/dl) \\ - 0.78(TSF) - 0.2(TFN,\ mg/dl) - 5.8(DH)$$

where ALB is serum albumin level, TSF is triceps skinfold, TFN is serum transferrin level, and DH is delayed hypersensitivity. [*Editor's Note:* The bulk of predictive value resides in albumin, making clear once again the importance of serum albumin level as a prognostic sign. Albumin has been a major feature of all prognostic indices.]

To test the predictive accuracy of PNI, the linear regression model assigned each of 121 patients to one of three predicted risk groups for comparison to actual outcome (Fig. 15-1). The predictive model accurately and quantitatively identified patients with subsequent postoperative morbidity and mortality.

In a follow-up validation study, the PNI was applied to 100 consecutive patients undergoing major nonemergency gastrointestinal surgery [13]. Patients were assessed preoperatively and assigned to low-, intermediate-, or high-risk nutritional groups. A highly significant increase in the actual incidence of death, complications, and sepsis was noted as the predicted risk increased (Fig. 15-2).

Other investigators developed alternative predictive indices using a combination of objective and subjective data, with similar good predictive results [10, 16, 20, 25, 39, 40, 62]. The most able predictors seem to be serum protein levels despite many factors that should preclude their utility.

The clinical concept of prospectively identifying those individuals who will suffer the consequences of malnutrition defines "clinically relevant malnutrition": a nutritional deficit that is associated with an increased risk of adverse clinical events, such as morbidity or death, and associated with a de-

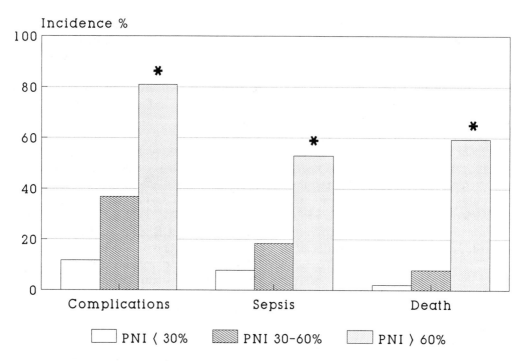

*Denotes p⟨0.05
Figure 15-1.   Prognostic Nutritional Index (PNI) development.

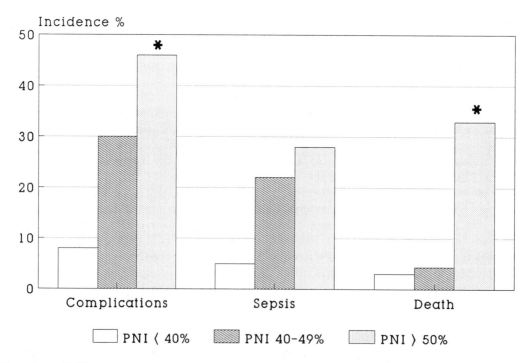

*Denotes p⟨0.05
Figure 15-2.   Prognostic Nutritional Index (PNI) for 100 patients undergoing major nonemergency gastrointestinal surgery.

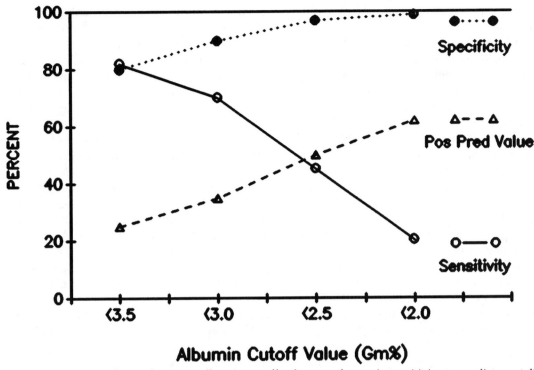

Figure 15-3.   The effects of varying albumin cutoff values on the test's sensitivity to predict mortality.

creased risk of such events when the nutritional deficit is corrected.

HOW DOES ONE SPECIFICALLY IDENTIFY INDIVIDUAL PATIENTS WHO HAVE SUCH AN INCREASED OPERATIVE RISK BECAUSE OF THEIR "MALNUTRITION"?

The subset of patients having "clinically relevant malnutrition" within different populations varies in size depending on several factors. For example, tertiary care institutions may demonstrate true differences in the prevalence of malnutrition and associated outcomes, compared to a community program or an outpatient setting. In a study of adult intensive care patients [2], a serum albumin level of less than 2.5 g/dl was associated with close to 100% mortality. [*Editor's Note:* One must be careful, in demographic studies such as this, to measure albumin levels at a specific time such as at admission

rather than after 3 weeks with multiple complications in the intensive care unit, in which case an albumin of 2.5 g/dl or less would indicate severe complications.] When the same albumin cutoff value was applied to a hospitalized pediatric population, a mortality rate of only 3.5% was present [26].

Equally important is the effect of varying the cutoff point of the test being used to diagnose "clinically relevant malnutrition" within a given population: Changing this cutoff point can markedly affect test specificity and sensitivity. To illustrate the importance of this concept, Reinhardt et al. [50] defined "malnutrition" by a serum albumin level in a single group of patients. As the cutoff point for albumin was increased from 2.0 to 3.5 g/dl, the sensitivity to predict mortality increased from 20 to 82%, but the specificity fell from 99 to 80% (Fig. 15-3).

The perfect nutritional test would prospectively identify all individuals who subsequently have a nutritionally related complication, and would not falsely identify anyone.

In clinical practice, no test is perfect at discriminating the normonourished from the malnourished. From a practical standpoint in clinical nutritional assessment, an ideal test must have a very high sensitivity. To achieve this goal, one may have to lower the cutoff point for an abnormal result even if it is at the expense of losing a degree of specificity. This is justified considering that nutritional intervention is associated with minimal morbidity; we would prefer to overtreat some patients as opposed to missing and undertreating a malnourished patient who would clinically benefit from intervention.

These points emphasize that any definition of "clinically relevant malnutrition" must be developed and evaluated carefully in populations similar to which it is to be applied; most cannot be universally adopted. Despite these problems, some nutritional parameters have emerged as having significant ability to predict a patient's clinical outcome: serum protein levels, body weight, anthropometrics, and the multiparameter indices.

Serum albumin measurement is generally regarded as the single best nutritional test to predict outcome. In most reports, the cutoff used to define "clinically relevant" malnutrition ranges from 3.0 to 3.5 g/dl%. We reviewed the performance of albumin to predict postoperative outcome in six studies [9, 24, 28, 46, 49, 57]. The sensitivity of a serum albumin level of less than 3.0 to 3.5 g/dl% to predict outcome was variable, ranging from 21 to 91%; specificity was in the 80 to 90% range.

Most circulating serum proteins made in the liver can identify patients at risk of complications following surgery. To assess the relative value of albumin, prealbumin, transferrin, and retinol-binding protein as predictors of outcome, 319 consecutive patients undergoing surgery at the Philadelphia Veterans Administration Medical Center (VAMC) had serum protein levels measured on admission and were monitored for complications until death or discharge [7]. Decreased mean values of all proteins were found in patients who had complications or who died versus those who had an uneventful course. Using an albumin cutoff at 4 g/dl%, the differences in complication rates (28 versus 11%) and deaths (9 versus 1%) was substantial. For a transferrin cutoff of 200 mg/dl, the reduction in complications and deaths (15 versus 3%) was substantial. Similar results were found for retinol-binding protein and prealbumin. This study strongly supports the use of serum protein levels to identify patients in the high-risk group.

Extremes of weight loss have a clear correlation with outcome. Seltzer et al. [56] reported that a 4.5-kg (10-lb.) preoperative weight loss was associated with a 19-fold increase in postoperative mortality. A number of other studies evaluated weight loss in the range of 5 to 10% and documented an association with outcome. In general, weight loss does not have enough sensitivity to function as the sole criteria in the nutritional assessment. However, its predictive abilities have been verified in many studies employing multivariate analysis.

Few studies reported predictions of postoperative outcome based solely on anthropometric measurements. Friedman [24] reported triceps skinfold measurements as a predictor of outcome and found a significant correlation only in females; arm muscle area was a better predictor. While this measure has been useful in population studies, the very wide 95% confidence interval suggests that application in this area is not useful.

The multiparameter indices maintain sensitivity even as specificity is improved, compared to single tests of nutritional status. When the prevalence of nutrition-related complications is above 25 to 30%, 80 to 90% sensitivity is achieved, with greater than 60% specificity in predicting clinical outcome in surgical populations [6, 20, 21]. As expected, at lower prevalence rates of nutrition-related complications in more well-nourished populations, the performance of these nutritional indices declines. No single test of nutritional status is 100% effective in prospectively diagnosing clinically relevant malnutrition. Nutritional indices have the best performance as predictors in sick complex patient populations, although clearly many rely heavily on

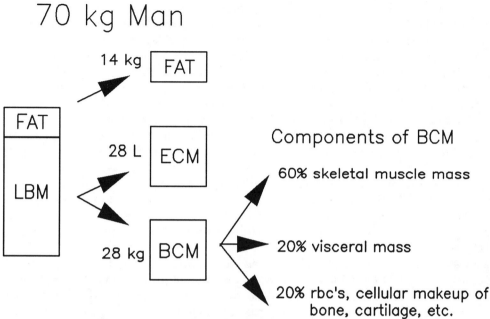

Figure 15-4. Body composition analysis quantitates the size of specific body compartments: lean body mass (LBM) and fat mass. ECM = extracellular mass; BCM = body cell mass; rbc's = red blood cells.

serum albumin and transferrin levels as the major component. These objective criteria must be combined with clinical judgment in the decision-making process.

DOES SHORT-TERM PREOPERATIVE TPN PROVIDE MEASURABLE CHANGES IN NUTRITIONAL STATUS?

Body weight increases with preoperative TPN [34, 47, 65], but this change is not a reliable indicator of improvement in nutritional status. Most of the increase in weight associated with less than several weeks of parenteral nutrition is primarily due to an increase in the extracellular mass and total body water and fat; little is due to increases in total body nitrogen [29, 58–60].

Since changes in body weight alone may simply represent changes in total body water, increasing emphasis has been placed on body composition analysis for evaluating the effects of TPN. Anthropometrics are a noninvasive method to assess fat stores, but we found only one study [65] that claimed im-

provement in skinfold thickness with less than 2 weeks of TPN. Most agree [8, 53] that this measure does not change reliably with short-term TPN.

Detailed body composition analysis quantitates the size of specific body compartments [35]: lean body mass and fat mass (Fig. 15-4). Lean body mass can be further subdivided into the extracellular mass and a cellular component, the body cell mass. Moore et al. [42, 43] defined the body cell mass as the sum of all cellular components of the body including the oxygen-exchanging, glucose-oxidizing, work-performing tissues of the body. The body cell mass constitutes 40% of the body weight of a normal adult and is composed of 60% skeletal muscle mass; 20% red blood cells and the cellular makeup of cartilage, bone, tendons, and adipose tissue; and 20% visceral cell mass such as liver and kidney. Maintenance and repletion of the body cell mass should be the goal of nutritional intervention.

A sustained decrease in nutrient intake results in a depletion of the body cell mass [43]. Shizgal and colleagues [58–60] showed that short-term TPN can increase the body cell mass in some patients. However, when Hill et al. [29] studied the effects of 11 to 40 days of intravenous nutrition on total body protein, only two of 20 surgical patients gained significant protein. Most of the weight gain observed in the other patients was due to an increase in total body water. Differences between studies may result from different TPN regimens and different measurement techniques.

Serial nitrogen balance measurements can be a useful guide to the clinician when monitoring the patient's response to TPN. The provision of adequate protein intake by preoperative TPN generally results in a positive nitrogen balance within 2 to 4 days [23, 41].

Commonly used proteins in nutritional assessment are serum albumin, transferrin, and prealbumin. Their serum levels are dependent on both nutritional and nonnutritional factors. Levels of these serum proteins have been found to decline in response to starvation and increase with nutritional repletion. Their response to short-term TPN has been variable.

Most studies have shown little or no improvement in the level of serum albumin during preoperative TPN because of albumin's long half-life. In 1977, Holter et al. [31] showed an increase in albumin with 3 days of preoperative TPN and 10 days of postoperative TPN. Heatley et al. [27] failed to show any improvement after 7 to 10 days of preoperative TPN, but did observe that the decline in serum albumin level was less in the TPN-treated group than in the matched control group. Other studies showed little or no change in the serum albumin level with 10 days of preoperative TPN [31, 48], or up to 14 days of TPN repletion in animal models [64]. Still others indicated that any change in albumin with short courses of TPN is probably secondary to diuresis [67].

Transferrin and prealbumin have shorter half-lives of 8 and 2 days, respectively. The serum levels of these proteins have been shown to change with relatively short durations of TPN. In one study, prealbumin was a more accurate indicator of positive nitrogen

balance and nutritional repletion than albumin or transferrin [17]. Several studies monitored transferrin levels in patients receiving TPN and demonstrated an increase following 4 to 10 days of TPN [11, 35, 47, 48]. In our monkey study [64], serial transferrin levels were monitored during 7 days of starvation and subsequent 14 days of TPN. Transferrin responded rapidly to both depletion and repletion, with a significant increase after 5 days of TPN. This increase in serum transferrin level has not been a uniform finding with short courses of TPN in the clinical setting. Roza et al. [54] reported no change in serum transferrin level with 2 weeks of TPN in spite of documented increases in the body cell mass. Similarly, Smith and Hartemink [65] found no improvement in transferrin levels, despite improvement in other nutritional parameters following 10 days of preoperative TPN.

Some early reports [35, 38] suggested that an abnormal delayed cutaneous hypersensitivity reaction found in malnourished surgical patients could be changed in some patients with short courses of TPN. Patients demonstrating this improvement in skin testing reactivity had improved outcome, compared to those who remained anergic. Subsequent evaluation criticized these earlier reports based on lack of control for age, antigen variability, prior antigen exposure, and other design problems [71]. Alterations in skin reactivity may be secondary to concurrent disease and/or sepsis, with no definite causal relationship to malnutrition and/or repletion. In spite of interesting results, one cannot enthusiastically recommend delayed cutaneous hypersensitivity as an end point of efficacy of short-term TPN.

WHAT DID EARLY PREOPERATIVE TPN TRIALS SHOW?

Early retrospective reports were optimistic and suggested that TPN use in the preoperative setting in a wide variety of patients might provide good results.

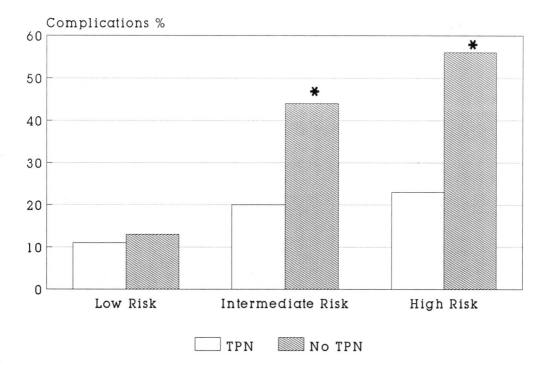

•Denotes p<0.05

Figure 15-5. The effect of a preoperative trial of total parenteral nutrition (TPN) on the incidence of complications.

Copeland et al. [18] reported that pre- and postoperative TPN was effective in reducing complications in cancer patients. Further support for the efficacy of TPN in cancer patients undergoing major surgery was noted by Daly et al. [19] in esophageal cancer patients treated with TPN compared to an untreated group and historical control subjects. These and other preliminary clinical reports suggested that preoperative TPN might improve postoperative outcome.

Other investigators began to look closer at standardizing the TPN regimen and stratifying patients according to preoperative nutritional status. In these follow-up studies, less uniform and less optimistic improvements in outcome were noted [34, 55, 63].

In 1978 we studied a heterogeneous group of surgical patients who received a standardized regimen of TPN [44]. Only patients who received at least 7 days of preoperative TPN (> 35 kcal/kg/day and > 1.5 g of protein/kg/day) were included in the treatment group

and were compared to a similar group that received no preoperative nutritional support. Groups were comparable in their degree of malnutrition. Preoperative TPN did not improve clinical outcomes in the treatment group, compared to the untreated group, if preoperative malnutrition was mild to moderate as defined by our PNI. Only those patients with severe malnutrition who received preoperative TPN had a significant reduction in complications (Fig. 15-5), major sepsis (Fig. 15-6), and mortality (Fig. 15-7), compared to the severely malnourished control group. Preoperative TPN seemed to have a dramatic clinical effect, but only in the severely malnourished.

During the development of the VA randomized controlled trial, we systematically reviewed prospective, randomized studies on the efficacy of preoperative TPN in reducing postoperative complications [14]. Of the eight trials reviewed [27, 31, 34, 41, 47, 48, 55, 61], only two demonstrated a significant

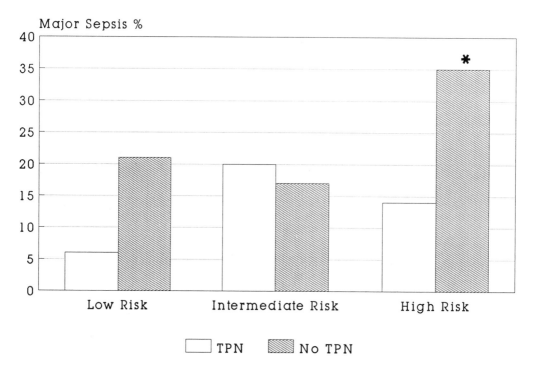

Figure 15-6. The effect of a preoperative trial of total parenteral nutrition (TPN) on the incidence of major sepsis.

reduction in operative complications and only one, a reduction in mortality. The remaining studies failed to demonstrate any beneficial effect of preoperative TPN on ultimate incidence of complications and/or death. Serious questions, which will be addressed later, have been raised about these early studies.

In another review from a different perspective, Detsky et al. [22] derived a quantitative meta-analysis based on 18 controlled trials that were designed to measure the effectiveness of preoperative parenteral nutrition. In this analysis a small benefit to TPN was suggested, but the 95% confidence interval for the difference in major surgical complication rates between treatment groups was wide, ranging from 12.8 percentage points better for TPN-treated patients to 2.3 percentage points worse. The authors concluded that any possible benefit of preoperative TPN in well-nourished patients must be small and is probably not clinically important, while the

efficacy in mildly or severely malnourished patients may be greater, but requires further confirmation.

While the VA randomized controlled trial was ongoing, several more recent studies approached this question. Smith and Hartemink [65] reported on a randomized prospective trial in 34 patients and found only a trend to reduction in morbidity and mortality in those who were moderately malnourished. Bellantone et al. [4] prospectively randomized 100 patients to preoperative TPN or a control group. The treatment group received at least 7 days of preoperative TPN, which included 30 kcal/kg/day and 200 mg of nitrogen/kg/day. Analysis of the entire group showed a septic complication rate of 30% in the TPN group and 35% in the control group, which was not statistically different. A subanalysis of only patients who were moderately malnourished showed a significant decline in the septic complication rate in the TPN group compared to the control group (21 versus

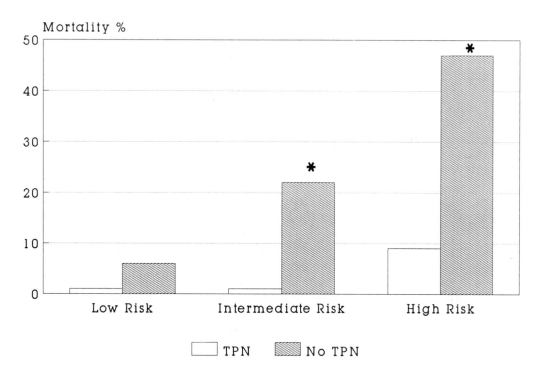

*Denotes p⟨0.05

Figure 15-7. The effect of a preoperative trial of total parenteral nutrition (TPN) on mortality.

53%, $p < 0.05$). In a different approach, Woolfson and Smith [72] prospectively randomized 122 patients to postoperative TPN or no treatment. Neither group received preoperative nutritional support, and patients were not stratified according to their nutritional status. There were no differences in the complication rates between the TPN and control groups. However, the authors acknowledged that due to the small sample size in each group, there was a 95% chance of missing a 20% improvement.

DID THE REPORTED IMPROVED POSTOPERATIVE OUTCOME REQUIRE THE PREOPERATIVE CHANGE OF MEASURABLE NUTRITIONAL STATUS PARAMETERS?

Few studies have looked carefully at this question using currently available tests of nutritional status.

Meakins et al. [38] studied delayed skin hypersensitivity in patients receiving preoperative TPN. In patients who remained anergic after preoperative TPN, there was a 75% death rate compared to a 5% mortality in those patients who responded to TPN with improved skin test results.

In another study of surgical patients [66], anergy was associated with the erosion of body cell mass. The administration of TPN improved the body cell mass in some patients, and an improvement in both delayed hypersensitivity reaction and clinical outcome was demonstrated. In those patients in whom the body cell mass did not improve with TPN, anergy was persistent and clinical outcome remained poor.

Moghissi et al. [41] studied nitrogen balance and clinical outcome in a small group of patients with esophageal cancer who received preoperative TPN. Patients who converted to a positive nitrogen balance prior to surgery had an improved postoperative course.

In a study of preoperative TPN in cancer patients, we reported a five-fold reduction in operative deaths when a significant increase in preoperative transferrin levels occurred [2].

Blackburn et al. [6] reported that transferrin levels increased in survivors, compared to nonsurvivors in whom transferrin levels failed to improve. Mckone et al. [37] studied the effects of TPN in a group of patients with postoperative complications. In patients in whom an improved serum fibronectin response could be demonstrated with TPN, survival was improved, compared to those in whom the fibronectin level remained low.

It has become obvious that changes in the currently measured nutritional parameters resulting from short courses of TPN should not be universally expected and are not an absolute prerequisite for improved clinical outcome. Likewise, with short courses of TPN, multiparameter indices do not change. The administration of preoperative TPN on a short-term basis improves clinical outcome long before there is a consistent significant change in most nutritional status parameters. Major changes in body composition should also not be expected, yet the metabolic changes are exceedingly important. Jeejeebhoy [32] stated that "giving TPN for the purpose of increasing lean body mass or body nitrogen is neither necessary nor desirable on a short-term basis." His recent studies [33] suggested that changes in certain muscle function parameters may precede body composition changes during periods of nutritional depletion and repletion, and are likely to play an increasingly important role in evaluating the efficacy of TPN in the future.

WERE EARLY STUDIES DESIGNED APPROPRIATELY TO ADEQUATELY ASSESS THE EFFICACY OF PREOPERATIVE TPN?

Failure to achieve consistent results from previous trials could be due to any of at least three factors: (1) Preoperative TPN does not reduce complications in any group. (2) Preoperative TPN does reduce complications in some patients which have not yet been well identified. (3) There are defects in the study design and/or execution. We [14] and Detsky et al. [22] reviewed these studies extensively. Substantial defects in design and analysis were present in many. One cannot prove with any reasonable certainty the null hypothesis that no difference exists in most clinical settings between malnourished surgical patients who receive preoperative TPN and those who do not.

The study defects can be grouped into four major categories: (1) defects in statistical design—inadequate sample size, inappropriate procedures for randomization; (2) inappropriate patient selection—presence or severity of malnutrition not being a study entry criterion; (3) inappropriate treatment regimens—inadequate TPN regimen in treated patients, use of forced enteral feedings in control subjects; and (4) inadequate definition of end points—lack of objective criteria defining presence and severity of complications (Tables 15-1 and 15-2).

Statistical design defects were almost universal. The most common violation was a lack of sufficient sample size and inappropriate randomization techniques. For example, even if TPN effected a 50% reduction in complication rates, there were insufficient numbers of patients studied to provide an 80% chance of correctly demonstrating this large difference (power < 0.80). Clearly, this defect in design introduces a high risk of both type I and type II errors. A second common statistical problem was in the randomization procedures. Several of the trials did not state their method of randomization and others used methods that had the potential to introduce bias.

The second area of criticism includes inappropriate selection criteria for patient entry into the study. If the inclusion criteria that define the "malnourished groups" are too liberal (high sensitivity, low specificity), a dilution of the true high-risk pool occurs and a low complication rate is reported. If the cutoff points for "malnutrition" are too strict

Table 15-1. Design Consideration of Previous Randomized Clinical Trials of Perioperative Total Parenteral Nutrition (TPN)

Study	Organ System	Nutritional Eligibility Criteria	Randomization Technique	No. of Days Preop.	No. of Days Postop.	Daily Caloric Goal	Complications Monitored	Complication Defined
Holter et al. [31]	GI tract	4.5-kg weight loss	Random number table	3	10	2000 kcal	Multiple major and minor	No
Heatley et al. [27]	Stomach, esophagus	None	Year of birth (odd, even)	7–10	0–5	40 kcal/kg	Wound and other infections and anastomotic leaks	Yes and no
Holter and Fischer [30]	GI tract	4.5-kg weight loss	Random number table	2	10	2000 kcal	Multiple major and minor	No
Moghissi et al. [41]	Esophagus	Severe dysphagia	Alternate patients	5–7	6–7	35 kcal/kg	Wound healing and infection	Yes
Simms et al. [61]	Stomach, esophagus	None	Not stated	7–10*	7–10	30 kcal/kg	Not stated	No
Lim et al. [34]	Esophagus	Severe dysphagia	Not stated	21–28	Not stated	60 kcal/kg	Wound infections, anastomotic leaks, and respiratory failure	No
Schildt et al. [55]	Stomach	None	Not stated	14	7	Not stated	Not stated	No
Müller et al. [47]	GI tract	None	Not stated	10	?	35 kcal/kg	Multiple major and minor	No

*Also reported a group receiving postoperative TPN not included here.

Table 15-2. Results of Previous Clinical Trials of Perioperative Total Parenteral Nutrition (TPN)

Study	Organ System	No. of Patients		Morbidity (%)		Mortality (%)		Required Sample Size*		Statistically Proved Benefits Observed in TPN Groups
		TPN	Control	TPN	Control	TPN	Control	Morbidity	Mortality	
Holter et al. [31]	GI tract	30	26	13	19	6.6	7.6	195	420	Less weight loss; increased serum albumin
Heatley et al. [27]	Stomach, esophagus	38	36	7.7	31	15	22	120	195	Significant reduction in wound
Holter and Fischer [30]	GI tract	13	13	16	18	0	0	195	N/A	Less weight loss
Moghissi et al. [41]	Esophagus	10	5	0	20	0	0	195	N/A	Improved nitrogen retention
Simms et al. [61]	Stomach, esophagus	20	20	—	—	0	10	N/A	420	Improved nitrogen retention
Lim et al. [34]	Esophagus	10	9	30	50	10	20	57	195	Weight gain
Schildt et al. [55]	Stomach	8	7	38	57	0	0	42	N/A	Weight gain
Müller et al. [47]	GI tract	66	59	11	19	3	11	195	420	Significant reduction in mortality and rate of major complications (intraabdominal abscess, peritonitis, anastomotic leak, ileus)

N/A = not available.
*Approximate sample size required per group for power 0.80.

(low sensitivity, high specificity), this gives a high complication rate but misses some patients at high risk. This critical issue of the presence, absence, or degree of malnutrition in study participants was overlooked in a number of studies. Only three of 11 randomized studies included any findings of "malnutrition" as screening criteria for entry. One cannot test the effectiveness of a treatment (preoperative TPN) if the study patients do not have the disease (malnutrition).

To expect efficacy of TPN, patient criteria should include: (1) requirement of an operation associated with a sufficiently high morbidity and mortality that a reduction in these numbers would be both clinically important and statistically demonstrable using a realistic sample size; (2) presence of malnutrition as defined by objective, reproducible measures and the severity of the malnutrition of the degree to provide an association with increased risks of complications or death above the level expected in well-nourished patients in whom the measurements are not abnormal; (3) study patients free of nonnutritional comorbidities that substantially increase operative risk due to unequivocally nonnutritional factors that might obscure any potential benefit achieved by reduction of nutrition-related risk.

The duration of preoperative TPN has been very variable between studies. In many instances, insufficient data were available to determine composition, quantity, duration, and route of administration. Clearly, some studies employed treatment regimens that were too short in duration and inadequate in caloric and nitrogen intake. In five of 11 randomized trials reviewed, there was less than 5 days of preoperative TPN.

To be effective, preoperative nutritional support must correct the nutrition-related defect or physiologic dysfunction that predisposes the patient to increased complications. The precise nutrient prescription in terms of composition or duration to optimize clinical outcome remains unclear. Currently, there is no standard nutritional test available to act as an indicator that adequate nutritional status

and function with an associated normal outcome have been attained preoperatively.

A final criticism of many previous trials was the lack of a precise definition of complications or other end point criteria. Studies with high complication rates often included morbidities such as superficial wound infections, minor atelectasis, and lower urinary tract infections. It would be more relevant to include only those complications that affect survival or significantly prolong hospitalization (e.g., major sepsis, death). In at least half of the studies reviewed, complications monitored were not adequately defined or included minor complications of questionable significance.

VA RANDOMIZED CONTROLLED TRIAL

Our early work and review and recommendations led to the development of the VA randomized controlled trial of preoperative TPN in malnourished surgical patients. This study was carefully designed to address and avoid the major criticisms of previous studies [14]. The goals of the VA study were: (1) to determine if preoperative TPN is effective in reducing operative morbidity and/or mortality in malnourished surgical patients or subsets thereof, (2) to define parameters that are able to prospectively identify which patients will be most likely to benefit from preoperative TPN versus those in whom benefit is highly unlikely, (3) to identify the clinical and laboratory studies that indicate adequate nutritional repletion before undergoing surgery to facilitate objective end points for preoperative TPN, (4) to determine the cost of an adequate period of preoperative TPN, and (5) to determine if preoperative TPN is cost-effective.

The study population included all patients undergoing major nonemergency intraperitoneal or intrathoracic operation who met certain criteria for study eligibility (Table 15-3). After meeting initial eligibility criteria, patients underwent nutritional assessment and

Table 15-3.   Criteria for Study Eligibility: VA Randomized Controlled Trial

Preliminary Eligibility Criteria	Specific Exclusions	Nutritional Eligibility Criteria
≥ 21 yr old	Contraindication to delaying surgery for 10 d	NRI ≤ 100, where NRI = (15.9 × ALB) + (0.147 × % UBW)
Life expectancy > 90 d if patient survives operation	Contraindication to TPN	**Or:** Any two of the following are present:
Major nonvascular abdominal or noncardiac thoracic operation anticipated on nonemergency basis	Perioperative TPN essential	Current weight ≤ 95% ideal ALB ≤ 39.2 g/liter
No previous major abdominal or thoracic operation in 30 d before screening	Severe organ system derangement(s)	Prealbumin ≤ 0.186 g/liter

TPN = total parenteral nutrition; NRI = Nutritional Risk Index; ALB = albumin; UBW = usual body weight.

were randomized only if they were "malnourished" based on a previously validated multiparameter nutritional index, focused on weight loss and serum albumin level. Patients were randomized to one of two treatment groups. The TPN-treated group received TPN for a minimum of 7 days and a maximum of 15 days before operation and 3 days after operation. The control group received no preoperative TPN. Patients were monitored for the occurrence of complications related to their operation, disease, and the administration of TPN from time of randomization until postoperative day 90.

Based on the initial preliminary analysis, the incidence of major noninfectious complications was significantly reduced in the moderately to severely malnourished patients who received preoperative TPN compared to control subjects. These noninfectious complications were primarily related to failure to heal wounds: fascial dehiscence, anastomotic leak, and bronchopleurocutaneous fistula. This improvement in outcome in the most severely "malnourished" patients was seen whether malnutrition was defined using subjective global assessment [3] or the Nutrition Risk Index, an objective measure based on serum albumin level and weight loss [14]. TPN-treated patients with milder degrees of malnutrition experienced no reduction in the incidence of these complications below the already low level observed in control patients.

The preliminary analysis also showed a higher infection rate in all malnutrition groups of patients who received preoperative TPN. This increased infection rate was not completely due to the presence of a central venous catheter but more to the increased incidence of other postoperative infections such as pneumonia and wound infections. In the severely malnourished patients (the worst 5–6% of the population studied), the substantial improvement in noninfectious complications still outweighed the minimal increase in infections and was still sufficient to yield a substantially better overall complication rate in patients who received preoperative TPN (26% for TPN patients versus 47% for controls). In mildly and moderately malnourished patients by either assessment criteria, this increase in infectious complications was more substantial and negated any benefit achieved by the decrease in noninfectious complications.

It is unclear whether the TPN was causally related to the increased incidence of infections seen in the TPN-treated patients. TPN-treated patients were hospitalized 5 days longer prior to operation than were control subjects, perhaps providing greater opportunity for colonization. The ingredients of TPN may have predisposed the host to these clinically apparent infections. This may be similar to results observed in the randomized trial of preoperative TPN by Müller et al. [47]. In that trial, patients receiving preoperative TPN in which lipid supplied 50% of the calories experienced more major complications and deaths than did control subjects and significantly more deaths than patients receiving lipid-free TPN. This observation may suggest some causative role for lipid in this process, although this is only speculative.

The mean daily caloric intake (oral plus parenteral) in TPN patients approached 3000 kcal and exceeded 4000 kcal for some. Although this level of caloric intake was considered optimal in the early 1980s when the study was designed, it is substantially greater than what is considered appropriate today, and this caloric oversupply may have had a deleterious effect. Other investigators postulated that the lower oral intake in TPN patients (400 kcal/day less than that in controls) permitted greater gut mucosal atrophy and bacterial translocation, explaining the higher rate of infections. [*Editor's Note:* There is small evidence at present in humans or even in experimental animals that the increased evidence of bacteria in mesenteric lymph nodes seen in animals on TPN is clinically significant. Translocation does not appear to be clinically significant unless there is a **major** insult such as a major burn.]

Preoperative TPN may be a "double-edged sword" requiring selective use for specific subgroups. If immediate operation is clinically feasible, patients with mild to moderate preexisting malnutrition may have more complications if an operation is delayed to provide preoperative TPN. These patients are best served by prompt operation. In contrast, an operative delay to provide preoperative nutritional support is justified in patients with severe nutritional deficits based on the substantial reduction in postoperative complications. The differential results observed in the VA trial between the impact of preoperative TPN on patients with mild to moderate degrees of malnutrition and those with more severe deficits underscore the importance of careful preoperative nutritional as-

sessment as the first step in clinical decision making. One can effectively use either a subjective approach or a more objective assessment. The beneficial effect of preoperative TPN was confined to patients who were nutritionally the worst 6% of patients requiring laparotomy or thoracotomy. It should be emphasized that this VA trial did not assess efficacy in patients who were not candidates for prompt operation. Regardless of nutritional status on admission, those patients should receive nutritional support if it is necessary to prevent development or progression of malnutrition while they await delayed operation.

PRACTICAL APPROACH TO THE IDENTIFICATION OF PATIENTS WHO REQUIRE PREOPERATIVE TPN

Based on all currently available information, we recommend the following practical approach in decision making regarding the preoperative use of TPN. The first decision involves whether the intrathoracic or intraabdominal operation is an emergency or a nonemergency situation.

Obviously, if the patient's problem requires an emergency operation, there is no indication for preoperative TPN, and the operation should proceed immediately.

If the surgical therapy is of a nonemergency nature, then one needs to decide whether the patient is ready to undergo the surgery immediately or whether there is a necessary period of delay to optimize critical organ function and to perform other preoperative diagnostic tests or therapeutic regimens. If there will be a delay of this nonemergency operation, one needs to nutritionally assess the patient. If the patient is well nourished to moderately malnourished, and if the operation will occur within 5 days, there is no need for preoperative TPN. If the delay will exceed 5 days in these patients, one should use preoperative TPN. On the other hand, if the patient is severely malnourished by nutritional assessment measures and the delay is going to exceed 3 days, then preoperative TPN should be utilized. If the delay in the severely malnourished patient is only several days, there is no reasonable indication to use preoperative TPN.

Finally, if the patient can undergo elective surgery without delay, nutritional assessment should be performed. In those patients who are well nourished or are only mildly to moderately malnourished, the operation should proceed without delay for preoperative TPN. Only in the patient with severe malnutrition as determined by nutritional assessment should the use of preoperative TPN occur. Nutritional assessment should utilize serum proteins primarily and weight loss secondarily. If any or all of serum proteins are depleted (albumin < 3.0 g/dl, transferrin < 200 mg/dl, prealbumin < 10 mg/dl) without an obvious source of distortion and/or the amount of weight loss has exceeded 5%, one should consider the patient severely malnourished and proceed with preoperative TPN. One should be sure that the disposal systems of the kidneys and liver can handle the nutrient load before initiating this approach. Preoperative TPN should be used for 1 week and one should not expect any measurable changes in nutritional assessment parameters in this short time period. This approach clearly does not replete muscle or fat stores; however, a positive nitrogen balance or serum protein response might well be attained. As a general rule, we would supply calories in a range of 130 to 150% of the patient's measured resting energy expenditure and 2 g of protein/kg of ideal body weight. [Editor's Note: In my opinion, the excessive caloric intake used in the VA cooperative trial may have contributed to the increased infections. Thus, I would use sufficient calories to meet the patient's requirements.]

SUMMARY

The ultimate decision to use preoperative TPN is influenced by the prognosis and anticipated course of the patient's primary disease, additional planned therapies, and the estimated impact of the nutritional status on the outcome of these events. The decision to force feed must be in concert with and adjunct to the clinical treatment plan of the patient's primary diseases and/or disorders.

In the specific circumstances of a patient ready for a nonemergent major procedure, one must remember that substantial nutritional defects are associated with poorer postoperative outcome, including complications and death. Preoperative short-term TPN, by providing adequate nutrient intake, improves the postoperative clinical course in the patients with severe degrees of malnutrition.

REFERENCES

1. American Society of Parenteral and Enteral Nutrition Board of Directors. Guidelines for use of total parenteral nutrition in the hospitalized adult patient. *J. Parenter. Enter. Nutr.* 10:441, 1986.
2. Apelgren, K. N., Rombeau, J. L., Twomey, P. L., and Miller, R. A. Comparison of nutritional indices and outcome in critically ill patients. *Crit. Care Med.* 10:305, 1982.
3. Baker, J. P., Detsky, A. S., Wesson, D. E., et al. Nutritional assessment: A comparison of clinical judgment and objective measurements. *N. Engl. J. Med.* 306:969, 1982.
4. Bellantone, R., Doglietto, G. B., Bossola, M., et al. Preoperative parenteral nutrition in the high-risk surgical patient. *J. Parenter. Enter. Nutr.* 12:195, 1988.
5. Bistrian, B. R., Blackburn, G. L., Hallowell, E., and Heddle, R. Protein status of general surgical patients. *J.A.M.A.* 230:858, 1974.
6. Blackburn, G. L., Bistrian, B. R., and Harvey, K. Indices of protein-calorie malnutrition as predictors of survival. In S. M. Levenson (ed.), *Nutritional Assessment: Present Status, Future Directions and Prospects.* Columbus, OH: Ross Laboratories, 1981. P. 131.
7. Boraas, M., Peterson, O., Knox, L., Mullen, J. L., and Buzby, G. P. Serum proteins and outcome in surgical patients. (Abstract) *J. Parenter. Enter. Nutr.* 6:585, 1982.
8. Bozzetti, F., Ammatuna, M., Migliavacca, S., et al. Total parenteral nutrition prevents further nutritional deterioration in patients with cancer cachexia. *Ann. Surg.* 205:138. 1987.
9. Braga, M., Baccari, P., Scaccabarozzi, S., et al. Prognostic role of preoperative nutritional and immunological assessment in the surgical patient. *J. Parenter. Enter. Nutr.* 12:138, 1988.
10. Brenner, U., Müller, J. M., Keller, H. W., et al. Nutritional assessment in surgical planning. *Clin. Nutr.* 7:225, 1988.

11. Buzby, G. P., Forster, J., Rosato, E. F., and Mullen, J. L. Transferrin dynamics in total parenteral nutrition. (Abstract) *J. Parenter. Enter. Nutr.* 3:34, 1979.
12. Buzby, G. P., and Mullen, J. L. Nutritional assessment. In M. Caldwell and J. Rombeau (eds.), *Clinical Nutrition*. Vol. I: Enteral and Tube Feeding. Philadelphia: W. B. Saunders, 1984.
13. Buzby, G. P., Mullen, J. L., Matthews, D. C., Hobbs, C. L., and Rosato, E. F. Prognostic nutritional index in gastrointestinal surgery. *Am. J. Surg.* 139:160, 1980.
14. Buzby, G. P., Williford, W. O., Peterson, O. L., et al. A randomized clinical trial of total parenteral nutrition in malnourished surgical patients: The rationale and impact of previous clinical trials and pilot study on protocol design. *Am. J. Clin. Nutr.* 47:357, 1988.
15. Cannon, P. R., Wissler, R. W., Woolridge, R. L., and Benditt, E. P. Relationship of protein deficiency to surgical infection. *Ann. Surg.* 120:514, 1977.
16. Ching, N., Grossi, C. E., Angers, J., et al. The outcome of surgical treatment as related to the response of the serum albumin level to nutritional support. *Surg. Gynecol. Obstet.* 151:199, 1980.
17. Church, J. M., and Hill, G. L. Assessing the efficacy of intravenous nutrition in general surgical patients: Dynamic nutritional assessment with plasma proteins. *J. Parenter. Enter. Nutr.* 11:135, 1987.
18. Copeland, E. M., Daly, J. M., and Dudrick, S. J. Nutrition as an adjunct to cancer treatment in the adult. *Cancer Res.* 37:2451, 1977.
19. Daly, J. M., Massar, E., Giacco, G., et al. Parenteral nutrition in esophageal cancer patients. *Ann. Surg.* 196:203, 1982.
20. Dempsey, D. T., and Mullen, J. L. Prognostic value of nutritional indices. *J. Parenter. Enter. Nutr.* 11(Suppl.):109s, 1987.
21. Dempsey, D. T., Mullen, J. L., and Buzby, G. P. The link between nutritional status and clinical outcome: Can nutritional intervention modify it? *Am. J. Clin. Nutr.* 47:352, 1988.
22. Detsky, A. S., Baker, J. P., O'Rourke, K. O., and Goel, V. Perioperative parenteral nutrition: A meta-analysis. *Ann. Intern. Med.* 107:195, 1987.
23. Elwyn, D. H., Gump, F. E., Munro, H. N., Iles, M., and Kinney, J. M. Changes in nitrogen balance of depleted patients with increasing infusions of glucose. *Am. J. Clin. Nutr.* 32:1597, 1979.
24. Freidman, P. J. A prospective comparison of methods to identify lethal wasting malnutrition. *Nutr. Res.* 6:139, 1986.
25. Grimes, C. J. C., Younathan, M. T., and Lee, W. C. The effect of preoperative total parenteral nutrition on surgery outcome. *J. Am. Diet. Assoc.* 87:1202, 1987.
26. Hay, R. W., and Whitehead, R. G. Serum-albumin as a prognostic indicator in edematous malnutrition. *Lancet* 2:427, 1975.
27. Heatley, R. V., Williams, R. H. P., and Lewis, M. H. Preoperative intravenous feeding: A controlled trial. *Postgrad. Med. J.* 55:541, 1979.
28. Hickman, D. M., Miller, R. A., Rombeau, J. L., Twomey, P. L., and Frey, C. F. Serum albumin and bodyweight as predictors of postoperative course in colorectal cancer. *J. Parenter. Enter. Nutr.* 4:314, 1980.
29. Hill, G. L., Bradley, J. A., Smith, R. C., et al. Changes in body weight and protein with intravenous nutrition. *J. Parenter. Enter. Nutr.* 3:215, 1979.
30. Holter, A. R., and Fischer, J. E. The effects of preoperative hyperalimentation on complications in patients with carcinoma and weight loss. *J. Surg. Res.* 23:31, 1977.
31. Holter, A. R., Rosen, H. M., and Fischer, J. E. The effects of hyperalimentation on major surgery in patients with malignant disease: A prospective study. *Acta Chir. Scand. Suppl.* 466:86, 1977.
32. Jeejeebhoy, K. N. The functional basis of assessment. In J. M. Kinney, K. N. Jeejeebhoy, G. Hill, and O. E. Owen (eds.), *Nutrition and Metabolism in Patient Care*. Philadelphia: W. B. Saunders, 1988.
33. Jeejeebhoy, K. N. Bulk or bounce: The object of nutritional support. *J. Parenter. Enter. Nutr.* 12:539, 1988.
34. Lim. S. T. K., Choa, R. G., Lam, K. H., Wong, J., and Ong, G. B. Total parenteral nutrition versus gastrostomy in the preoperative preparation of patients with carcinoma of the oesophagus. *Br. J. Surg.* 68:69, 1981.
35. Lukaski, H. C. Methods for the assessment of human body composition: Traditional and new. *Am. J. Clin. Nutr.* 46:537, 1987.
36. MacLean, L. D., Meakins, J. L., Taguchi, K., Duignan, J. P., Dhillon, K. S., and Gordon, J. Host resistance in sepsis and trauma. *Ann. Surg.* 182:207, 1975.
37. Mckone, T. K., Davis, A. T., and Dean, R. E. Fibronectin: A new nutritional parameter. *Am. J. Surg.* 51:336, 1985.
38. Meakins. J. L., Pietsch, J. B., Bubenick, O., et al. Delayed hypersensitivity: Indicator of acquired failure of host defenses in sepsis and trauma. *Ann. Surg.* 186:241, 1977.
39. Meguid, M. M., Debonis, D., Meguid, V., Hill, L. R., and Terz, J. J. Complications of abdominal operations for malignant disease. *Am. J. Surg.* 156:341, 1988.
40. Meguid, M. M., Stabile, B. E., Shizgal, H. M., and Cerra, F. B. Aggressive preoperative nu-

tritional support in the major surgery patient. *Contemp. Surg.* 20:115, 1982.

41. Moghissi, K., Hornshaw, J., Teasdale, P. R., and Dawes, E. A. Parenteral nutrition in carcinoma of the oesophagus treated by surgery: Nitrogen balance and clinical studies. *Br. J. Surg.* 64:125, 1977.

42. Moore, F. D., and Boyden, C. M. Body cell mass and limits of hydration of the fat-free body: Their relation to estimated skeletal weight. *Ann. N.Y. Acad. Sci.* 110:62, 1963.

43. Moore, F. D., Olesen, K. H., McMurrey, J. D., Parker, H. V., Ball, M. R., and Boyden, C. M. *The Body Cell Mass and Its Supporting Environment.* Philadelphia: W. B. Saunders, 1963.

44. Mullen, J. L., Buzby, G. P., Matthews, D. C., Smale, B. F., and Rosato, E. F. Reduction of operative morbidity and mortality by combined preoperative and postoperative support. *Ann. Surg.* 192:604, 1980.

45. Mullen, J. L., Buzby, G. P., Waldman, T. G., Gertner, M. H., Hobbs, C. L., and Rosato, E. F. Prediction of operative morbidity and mortality by preoperative nutritional assessment. *Surg. Forum* 30:80, 1979.

46. Mullen, J. L., Gertner, M. H., Buzby, G. P., Goodhart, G. L., and Rosato, E. F. Implications of malnutrition in the surgical patient. *Arch. Surg.* 114:121, 1979.

47. Müller, J. M., Brenner, U., Dienst, C., and Pichlmaier, H. Preoperative parenteral feeding in patients with gastrointestinal carcinoma. *Lancet* 1:68, 1982.

48. Müller, J. M., Keller, H. W., Brenner, U., Walter, M., and Holzmeller, W. Indications and effects of preoperative parenteral nutrition. *World J. Surg.* 10:53, 1986.

49. Pinchcofsky-Devin, G., Kaminski, M. V., and Bailey, A. Correlation between serum albumin levels, length of hospitalization and mortality. *J. Am. Coll. Nutr.* 4:363, 1985.

50. Reinhardt, G. F., Myscofski, J. W., Wilkens, D. B., Dobrin, P. B., Mangan, J. E., and Stannard, R. T. Incidence and mortality of hypoalbuminemic patients in hospitalized veterans. *J. Parenter. Enter. Nutr.* 4:357, 1980.

51. Rhoads, J. E., and Alexander, C. E. Nutritional problems of surgical patients. *Ann. N.Y. Acad. Sci.* 63:268, 1955.

52. Rhoads, J. E., Fliegelman, M. T., and Panzer, L. M. The mechanisms of delayed wound healing in the presence of hypoproteinemia. *J.A.M.A.* 118:21, 1942.

53. Rickard, K. A., Grosfeld, J. L., Kirksey, A., Ballantine, T. V. N., and Baehner, R. L. Reversal of protein-energy malnutrition in children during treatment of advanced neoplastic disease. *Ann. Surg.* 190:771, 1979.

54. Roza, A. M., Tuitt, D., and Shizgal, H. M.
Transferrin: A poor measure of nutritional status. *J. Parenter. Enter. Nutr.* 8:523, 1984.

55. Schildt, B., Groth, O., Larsson, J., Sjodahl, R., Symreng, T., and Wetterfors, J. Failure of preoperative TPN to improve nutritional status in gastric carcinoma. (Abstract) *J. Parenter. Enter. Nutr.* 5:360, 1981.

56. Seltzer, M. H., Fletcher, H. S., Slocum, B. A., and Engler, P. E. Instant nutritional assessment in the intensive care unit. *J. Parenter. Enter. Nutr.* 5:70, 1981.

57. Seltzer, M. H., Slocum, B. A., Cataldi-Belcher, E. L., Fileti, C., and Gerson, N. Instant nutritional assessment: Absolute weight loss and surgical mortality. *J. Parenter. Enter. Nutr.* 6:218, 1982.

58. Shizgal, H. M. Body composition and nutritional support. *Surg. Clin. North Am.* 61:729, 1981.

59. Shizgal, H. M. Body composition of patients with malnutrition and cancer: Summary of methods of assessment. *Cancer* 55:250, 1985.

60. Shizgal, H. M., Spanier, A. H., and Kurtz, R. S. The effect of parenteral nutrition on body composition in the critically ill. *Am. J. Surg.* 131:156, 1976.

61. Simms, J. M., Oliver, E., and Smith, J. A. R. A study of total parenteral nutrition (TPN) in major gastric and esophageal resection for neoplasia. *J. Parenter. Enter. Nutr.* 4:422, 1980.

62. Simms, J. M., Smith, J., and Weeds, H. F. A modified prognostic index based upon nutritional measurements. *Clin. Nutr.* 1:71, 1982.

63. Smale, B. F., Mullen, J. L., Buzby, G. P., and Rosato, E. F. The efficacy of nutritional assessment and support in cancer surgery. *Cancer* 47:2375, 1981.

64. Smale, B. F., Mullen, J. L., Hobbs, C. L., Buzby, G. B., and Rosato, E. F. Serum protein response to acute dietary manipulation. *J. Surg. Res.* 28:379, 1980.

65. Smith, R. C., and Hartemink, R. Improvement of nutritional measures during preoperative parenteral nutrition in patients selected by the prognostic nutritional index: A randomized control trial. *J. Parenter. Enter. Nutr.* 12:587, 1988.

66. Spanier, A. H., Pietsch, J. B., Meakins, J. L., MacLean, L. S., and Shizgal, H. M. The relationship between immune competence and nutrition. *Surg. Forum* 27:332, 1976.

67. Starker, P. M., LaSala, P. A., Askanazi, J., Todd, G., Hensle, T. W., and Kinney, J. M. The influence of preoperative total parenteral nutrition upon morbidity and mortality. *Surg. Gynecol. Obstet.* 162:569, 1986.

68. Studley, H. O. Percentage of weight loss: A basic indicator of surgical risk in patients with chronic peptic ulcer. *J.A.M.A.* 106:458, 1936.

69. Thompson, W. D., Ravdin, I. S., and Frank, I. L. Effect of hypoproteinemia on wound disruption. *Arch. Surg.* 36:500, 1938.

70. Tuten. M. B., Wogt, S., Dasse, F., and Leider, Z. Utilization of prealbumin as a nutritional parameter. *J. Parenter. Enter. Nutr.* 9:709, 1985.

71. Twomey, P., Ziegler, D., and Rombeau, J. Utility of skin testing in nutritional assessment: A critical review. *J. Parenter. Enter. Nutr.* 6:50, 1982.

72. Woolfson, A. M. F., and Smith, J. A. R. Elective nutritional support after major surgery: A prospective randomized trial. *Clin. Nutr.* 8:15, 1989.

Inflammatory Bowel Disease

Josef E. Fischer

Inflammatory bowel disease in the Western world generally consists of two forms—Crohn's disease (or granulomatous inflammatory bowel disease [GIBD]) and ulcerative colitis. There are less common forms of inflammatory bowel disease that enter but little in the discussion of nutritional support. Clindamycin-associated colitis is not strictly an inflammatory bowel disease, but does occasionally confuse the issue, and total parenteral nutrition (TPN) has on occasion been utilized to tide the patient over the associated diarrhea. Cholera is not, strictly speaking, an "inflammatory bowel disease" in this frame of reference, but again TPN may be used with profit in patients with severe cholera. Diverticulitis is, of course, a common form of inflammation, but is not, in this connotation, an inflammatory bowel disease. Patients are treated with parenteral nutrition when fistulas supervene or following severe complications of operation for diverticulitis such as fistulas, abscesses, and intestinal obstruction. Amoebic colitis, tuberculous enteritis, and

schistosomiasis are situations in which parenteral nutrition might potentially be useful, but will not enter this discussion further.

GIBD was probably first described by a Scottish surgeon, Sir Kennedy Dalziel, in 1913 [13]. The article was remarkable in a number of ways. Nine patients with what was probably regional enteritis were described and operated on successfully, with no mortality, and with no recurrence reported, a remarkable feat considering the primitive state of surgery at that time. Another noteworthy feature of that article was the identification of atypical mycobacteria in the specimens, etiologic agents that are still under investigation. The article was forgotten, however, and the entity was confused with tuberculous enteritis, at least in the United States, for the next 20 years. It was not until Crohn et al.'s classic description in 1932 [12] that regional enteritis ("Crohn's disease" or GIBD) was separated from tuberculous enteritis. It is important to note that acute forms of enteritis exist. It is not clear that those cases described in Gump et al.'s classic paper [26] of acute ileitis, for which most patients underwent resection and almost all did not have a recurrence in long-term follow-up, were due to *Yersinia*, other infective agents, or an acute form of enteritis amenable to surgery that is not chronic and recurrent.

Until the late 1950s, it all seemed very simple: Crohn's disease or regional enteritis infected the small bowel, and all large-bowel disease was ulcerative colitis. However, by 1960 it was clear that there were at least two different forms of inflammatory bowel disease affecting the colon. For the sake of simplicity, and especially from a surgical point of view, the mucosal disease generally known as ulcerative colitis is limited to the colon, affects the mucosa, and usually presents with bleeding and toxicity. The rectum is almost never spared, even if the disease is mild, and the disease tends to be confluent. Perirectal abscesses and fistulas are rare. There is small-bowel involvement, the so-called "backwash ileitis," but in 20 years of extensive experience in patients with ulcerative colitis, I have never found backwash ileitis, whatever its etiology, to be of much surgical or prognostic significance.

GIBD is transmural, not confluent, and associated with rectal sparing and the small-bowel disease is significant. Its presentation is somewhat different, with bleeding and megacolon playing a less prominent role, and toxicity, perforation, and internal and external fistulas more prominent. It is important for surgeons to be able to differentiate the two, but this is not always possible. In my own experience with total proctocolectomies and ileoanal pull-throughs and pouches (Soave procedures) for ulcerative colitis [36, 37], the one diagnostic criterion that will lead me not to do an operation for ulcerative colitis is the presence of chronic rectal fistulas. In the few instances in which patients have had rectal fistulas, and I allowed myself to be persuaded that they had ulcerative colitis, I was usually sorry: The diagnosis was GIBD. Between 10 to 15% of patients, however, have indeterminant colitis; that is, even after the pathologic specimen has been in the

hands of the pathologist, the diagnosis is not clear—Crohn's disease of the colon or ulcerative colitis. Such patients do not appear to have a different prognosis than those patients with clear-cut ulcerative colitis.

MALNUTRITION IN GRANULOMATOUS INFLAMMATORY BOWEL DISEASE

In GIBD the causes of malnutrition are various, but most occur as a result of the disease. Patients may voluntarily limit intake because of the associated pain and cramps of partial intestinal obstruction, learning from experience that if they voluntarily avoid intake, their pain and obstructive symptoms as well as cramps and mucous diarrhea are avoided. Thus, they voluntarily skip meals, often losing weight in the process.

Protein Loss

Protein loss in GIBD may be substantial, up to 80 to 90 g/24 hr. There is a normal loss of brush border, desquamated enterocytes, and epithelium, as well as digestive enzymes. Normally, these products undergo digestion, are reabsorbed, and enter the portal circulation, with a normal stool nitrogen level of less than 1 g/24 hr. In inflammatory bowel disease, this process may not proceed to completion. First, there may be losses of protein with inflammatory exudates. Second, there may be a substantial amount of bleeding or mucus production with GIBD. Third, there may be denudation of substantial mucosal areas of either the small or large bowel. If denudation of the small-bowel mucosa is substantial, absorption will be interfered with. Fourth, there may be areas of partial obstruction in which the bowel becomes massively distended, losing its absorptive ability. Fifth, there may be short bowel complicating the disease, particularly following repeated resections for Crohn's disease. For all of these reasons, the loss of protein may be very substantial and may contribute to the malnutrition.

Malabsorption

There are many reasons for malabsorption of specific nutrients in GIBD:

1. **Rapid transit.** Rapid transit appears to be part and parcel of the irritation that certainly the small bowel experiences with GIBD. This prevents nutrients from being sufficiently in contact with the gut mucosa so that absorption can take place.

2. **Denudation of mucosa.** While Crohn's disease mostly affects the distal ileum, and it is rare to find patients with excessively long segments of denuded mucosa, there are patients in whom the Crohn's disease is so prevalent throughout the small bowel that absorption is interfered with. Indeed, a prevalent concept of Crohn's disease is that the entire enteral tract from mouth to anus is affected, a suggestion that bears some credence with the presence of microscopic oral lesions in patients with Crohn's disease.

3. **Short-bowel syndrome.** Repeated resections for Crohn's disease and/or bypasses, internal fistulas, and so on, result in short-bowel syndrome and an inability to absorb nutrients.

4. **Blind loops and bacterial overgrowths.** While bypass for GIBD has become much less fashionable as surgical techniques have improved and mortality for resection decreased, and the association between small-bowel bypass and adenocarcinoma complicating Crohn's disease becomes better known, an occasional patient will have a blind loop with bacterial overgrowth, which leads to local consumption of vitamins and nutrients as well as the lack of absorption of others. A more common cause of bacterial overgrowth is partial intestinal obstruction, which provides large reservoirs of bacteria that may prevent absorption. Other reasons for bacterial overgrowth include frequent use of histamine H_2 antagonists or other inhibitors of gastric acid secretion, thus doing away with an important mechanism for keeping the small bowel free of bacteria. Anastomoses between the small bowel and the colon, which resect the ileocecal valve (the most common resection in Crohn's disease), may also be responsible for the colonization of the small bowel with bacteria.

5. **Poor mixing of intestinal contents and normal digestive enzymes.** Surgery in Crohn's disease, particularly that involving bypass of the Crohn's disease–affected duodenum, or perhaps other rearrangements of normal small-bowel anatomy, leads to the poor mixing of food with bile and pancreatic secretions. Proper mixing is particularly important for the digestion of fat. It is thought that protein is adequately digested and absorbed if there is 120 cm of normal small bowel, and there is great reserve capacity with respect to most forms of carbohydrates with the exception, of course, of lactose and secondary lactase insufficiency. There is not a great deal of reserve with respect to fat absorption, in which adequate mixing of bile and pancreatic juices is essential for normal digestion. In addition, increased length of the resected part of the ileum leads to poor bile-salt absorption, bile-salt diarrhea, as well as a decrease in enterohepatic absorption of bile leading to a decreased bile-salt pool, which in turn results in decreased fat absorption.

6. **Mechanical interference.** Edema, chronic fibrosis, and thickening may lead to anatomic disruption of lymphatic absorption channels and normal capillary and venous absorptive channels.

Specific Malabsorption

Resection of the ileum often leads to impairment of vitamin B_{12} absorption. In my own experience, even with massive resections of the ileum, some patients adapt and have normal findings on the Schilling test. However, if the entire ileum is resected, it is well to supplement vitamin B_{12}, 1 mg monthly. If the duodenum is resected or bypassed, there may be malabsorption of calcium and iron, which are normally absorbed in the duodenum. Some medications may interfere with the metabolism and/or absorption of various nutrients; an example is sulfasalazine (Azulfidine) and its supposed effect on the absorption of folic acid.

Medications

Certain medications, such as steroids, are thought to contribute to the proteolysis and catabolism so common in GIBD. Steroids probably stimulate proteolysis, and in concert with catabolic cytokines (candidates such as interleukin-1 and/or tumor necrosis factor, or cachectin), proteolysis continues. Azathioprine and other antiinflammatory or antineoplastic agents not only are associated with proteolysis, but also may provoke certain complications such as pancreatitis (in conjunction with steroids). Sulfasalazine (Azulfidine), in addition to causing gastric upset that may result in decreased oral intake, sometimes interferes with absorption of nutrients.

Proteolysis and Catabolism

Obviously, when systemic illness and toxicity supervene, proteolysis, lack of protein synthesis, and other complications of inflammation complicate the patients' course.

NUTRITION AND THE GUT

Specific Effects of Total Parenteral Nutrition on the Gut

Since publication of the last edition of this book, much more has been learned about the effects of TPN on the gut. Although it has been known since 1972 that the use of TPN decreases villous height and perhaps decreases gut thickness, sufficient attention was not paid to this early in the history of parenteral nutrition. More recently, it has become appreciated that there are specific fuels for enterocytes [42, 47], and that these specific fuels may be more important for enterocytes at one level of the gut than at others. Much recent attention has focused on the requirement for glutamine for certain enterocytes

[47] and the short-chain fatty acids (SCFAs) for others [42] (see Chaps. 11 and 26). Since much of this work is in flux and relatively new, and its full significance is not yet appreciated, I summarize my concept of the current research in enterocyte fuels:

Glutamine

Glutamine is thought to be a preferred fuel of at least some of the small-bowel enterocytes. Much work has been done with respect to the jejunum [47, 53], yet recent work appears to favor ileal enterocytes as a point where glutamine appears maximally effective [52]. The cell where such fuel is effective appears to be the enterocyte itself, rather than the lymphocytes. Administration of oral glutamine, at least in the experimental animal, is associated with increased villous height, gut protein, and DNA content. The results of the current work have often been inconsistent, and the effects of intravenously administered glutamine have been considerably less than, for example, those of epidermal growth factor. The relationship between glutamine and human nutrition has been investigated in only a preliminary manner [48]. Thus, although a recent study [48] using a glutamine peptide showed decreased negative nitrogen balance following a standard operation in a relatively small group of patients, it is unlikely that the difference reported would improve outcome. A much more profound difference in nitrogen balance and nutritional outcome would be essential, in my opinion, to improve outcome.

Specific Enterocyte Fuels— Short-Chain Fatty Acids

Another class of fuels that appear to be specific are the SCFAs acetate, proprionate, and butyrate, in which there has been considerable interest over the past number of years [42]. Proprionate and butyrate are (at least in the gut) largely products of bacterial fermentation of soluble fiber such as pectin, present in the Western diet largely in the form of solid material from citrus and other fruits. Fermentation of pectin by the bacteria in the colon may be stoichiometrically expressed by the following formulas [46]:

$35\ C_6H_{10}O_5 \rightarrow 48$ acetic acid
$\quad + 11$ proprionic acid $+ 5$ butyric acid
$\qquad + 24\ CH_4 + 34\ CO_2 + 10\ H_2O$

$34.4\ C_6H_{12}O_6 \rightarrow G4\ SCFA + 23.75\ CH_4$
$\qquad + 37.23\ CO_2 + 10.5\ H_2O$

Once fermented, the fate of the SCFAs varies. As a group, the SCFAs are utilized only 10% and the remainder is exported to the portal circulation, where it is taken up by the liver and metabolized. However, among the three components, there are remarkable differences. Whereas only 10% of acetate is utilized by the enterocytes, with 90% being absorbed into the portal vein, this increases to 50% in the case of proprionate and to 80% with respect to butyrate. Butyrate appears to have a specific local effect on gut mucosa, including increasing villous height, gut wall thickness, gut protein, and presumably DNA content (although data to confirm this point are not yet available), as well as an endocrine-type effect from within the circulation on the ileum [33]. Again, there has been less work utilizing parenteral formulations incorporating the SCFAs, but this is a fertile field.

Growth Factors

There are a number of identified growth factors that have an effect on gut wall thickness, villous height, and protein and DNA content. Presumably, these also translate into increased defense of the gut barrier against translocation of bacteria and/or absorption of bacterial products. When compared with the effects of glutamine, for example, the growth factors seem to have a much more profound effect, with greater gut thickness, protein and DNA content, and villous height, thus presumably providing additional protection [53].

None of the above three nutritional factors have been applied to nutritional support in the case of GIBD. It is conceivable, for example, that GIBD may be the result of a shortage of such nutritional material, and that supplying such substrates and/or growth factors may help support, in either a specific or a nonspecific way, the regrowth of gut mucosa

to the extent of improved healing. Clearly, this area requires investigation.

Enteral Nutriton and Immunology

With the increased interest in enteral nutrition for nutritional support, as well as a number of studies that purport to show long-term success with the administration of enteral diets, some review of the possible effects of enteral nutrition on gut function and immunology is appropriate. It would be simplistic to say that stimulation of the gut by food increases thickness of the gut wall and reverses the atrophy that accompanies parenteral nutrition. The specific effect of enteral nutrition in the elicitation of various hormones such as enteroglucagon and gastrin, which may or may not be trophic to certain portions of the gut [32], is probably important. Probably more important is the elicitation of certain hepatic secreted proteins, such as IgA [4], which are probably important in the immunology of the gut. With increased recognition of the importance of gut lymphocytes and a gut role in secreting various immunologic proteins, it is clear that the gut is an important immunologic organ. Presumably, although this has been more difficult to show, malfunction of the gut in its function as an immunologic organ results in disease.

Translocation

One of the more active areas of investigation over the past several years has been the translocation of gut bacteria. Translocation appears to be a natural process by which bacteria are engulfed by macrophages and perhaps other cells, carried across the gut wall, and lodge in lymph nodes. The process itself is probably not as important as absorption of various gut bacterial products such as endotoxin. Indeed, to my knowledge, despite the level of interest in translocation, no one has yet identified endotoxin within the portal vein, even utilizing the more sensitive chromogenic assay, except in patients with burns. The presumption underlying the various studies is that whenever various host defenses are decreased, either because of intrinsic disease, decreased gut wall thickness, and/or dissolution of the tight junctions, translocation of bacteria that have been engulfed, but presumably not killed by various gut macrophages, increases. These bacteria then become liberated in the lymph nodes and enter the body, thus increasing nosocomial infections. Indeed, a leading hypothesis concerning multiple-organ failure syndrome, or in patients who are so terribly depleted that they cannot muster the defenses against such endogenous invaders, is that the nonseptic patient without a definable source of infection does, in fact, have nosocomial infections that arise in the gut. Translocation and/or the absorption of enteral products is thought to be important in burns [30, 31], shock [5, 24], and a number of other human pathologic conditions, and at least in one of these (i.e., burns) it is now clear that some of the hypermetabolism that accompanies a burn may be obviated by early gut feedings [1], findings confirmed both in guinea pigs and in humans, but apparently not in the rat [54].

Translocation appears to depend on both the nature and the concentration of various gut bacteria and is increased by the usual total parenteral nutrition formulas given either parenterally or enterally [3]. This has not been confirmed independently. Starvation itself does not appear to trigger translocation [15]. Diminished IgA secretion may contribute to translocation when protein-depleted animals are repleted by TPN.

Although much of the work is suggestive, few studies have confirmed that changes from TPN to enteral nutrition result in differences in outcome, except perhaps in burned patients [2].

ENTERAL NUTRITION IN GRANULOMATOUS INFLAMMATORY BOWEL DISEASE

A logical outgrowth of all of the above work with translocation, nosocomial infection, and so on, has been to suggest that enteral nutrition may be more efficacious than parenteral nutrition. Not surprisingly, this has been subjected to a variety of randomized, prospective trials. The results have been disappointing. Postoperative studies utilizing enteral versus parenteral nutrition reveal little difference in ultimate nitrogen balance, although TPN appears to restore patients to positive nitrogen balance more quickly [7]. This is probably true even when the efficacy of TPN as far as restoring patients to nitrogen balance is made slightly more efficacious by the addition of glutamine in the form of esters and/or growth hormone. No one has yet argued that the addition of such components will result in improved outcome.

In postoperative patients, the achievement of positive nitrogen balance is marginally better with TPN as opposed to enteral nutrition, but the difference is minor [7]. Most investigators have focused on expense in that enteral nutrition seems to be less expensive. Other investigators have focused on the immunologic consequences. Kudsk et al. [34] demonstrated in protein-depleted rats that nutritional repletion using TPN did not protect as well against hemoglobin adjuvant peritonitis as did enteral nutrition. Studies in patients, particularly those patients at risk, vary according to disease state. It seems reasonably well established from a variety of studies, including a number carried out at the University of Cincinnati, that patients who are able to receive a greater amount of their nutrition by gut seem to have a lower incidence of infection and a higher survival rate following burns that those who did not [2]. Whether they were able to take more of their nutritional support because of other variables that were not detected is not clear. Additional studies utilizing a variety of diets, which are presented separately in this volume (see Chap. 26), suggest that various components may make it possible for enteral diets to be more efficacious. In critical care patients, however, there do not appear to be, at least in a relatively small group, any clearly definable differences in outcome [10, 11].

USE OF ENTERAL NUTRITION IN GRANULOMATOUS INFLAMMATORY BOWEL DISEASE

As stated above, there has been increased interest in the use of enteral nutrition in patients with inflammatory bowel disease. This may take two forms. First, there may be prolonged treatment of patients with GIBD with chemically defined diets. These may be sufficient to induce and maintain remission in some patients. An additional use of enteral diets in patients with GIBD has been to utilize chemically defined diets once a remission has been induced with TPN. This is clearly necessary, since the long-term results of patients who have gone into remission utilizing TPN suggest that the long-term outcome is not as hopeful. In a recent review by Shiloni et al. [44], 45% of patients went into early remission, but at the end of 15 months all but 20% required operation. Whether or not maintenance on a chemically defined diet of enteral nutrition, once such patients had gone into remission with TPN, would have prolonged remission is not clear.

USES OF TOTAL PARENTERAL NUTRITION IN PATIENTS WITH INFLAMMATORY BOWEL DISEASE

Granulomatous Inflammatory Bowel Disease

Patients with GIBD are theoretically good candidates for the use of TPN. Because they voluntarily limit their intake because of pain and malabsorb because of short-bowel syndrome, diarrhea, and excessive losses of protein and/or blood, the use of an alternative form of nutrition seems logical. In my own experience, the following indications for parenteral nutrition in GIBD have proved useful:

1. To induce remission in patients in whom other forms of medical therapy have failed
2. To taper steroids while preventing flare of disease
3. To treat rapid recurrence following surgery or other therapy
4. In the preoperative period, to prepare patients for operation
5. To close fistulas
6. When the extent of disease is so extensive that it is not possible to perform resection

These are discussed in turn.

Inducing Remission

The initial indication for TPN was in a group of patients with GIBD in whom we attempted to induce remission. With rare exception, these were patients in whom other forms of medical therapy had failed [22]. Our initial experience suggested that the prognosis depended on the location of the disease [22], a finding that has not been corroborated by all. In our own experience, in that group of patients who had extensive small-bowel disease, but did not have colon involvement, remission could be induced in approximately 75%. We have been unsuccessful however, in defining the characteristics allowing us to predict which of the patients would go into remission. Patients with granulomatous colitis had a much lower rate of remission, approximately 50%. The main problem, which has remained so, has been the maintenance of such remission. In Table 16-1 are data from studies on attempts to catalogue those patients with GIBD who were treated with TPN. One can see that although the rate of initial remission is relatively high, with a singular exception the late remissions are comparatively low.

Various procedures can be used in an attempt to increase the duration of maintenance of remission. In our own studies [22, 41], we found that a low dose of steroids (e.g., 5 mg/day of prednisone) prevented the flare-up of GIBD when TPN was discontinued. Other suggestions include the use of enteral nutrition to promote a long-term remission. The cessation of such remissions were quite sudden; one patient who had gone into complete remission flared within 24 hours after TPN was discontinued. The basis for such remission is not clear. Clearly,

Table 16-1. Results of Total Parenteral Nutrition (TPN) and Bowel Rest in Patients with Granulomatous Inflammatory Bowel Disease

Study	Year	No. of Patients	Duration of TPN (d)	Nutritional Response (%)	Hospital Remission (%)	Late Remission (%)
Fischer et al. [22]	1973	—	—	—	67	—
Vogel et al. [50]	1974	14	9–50	78	100	50
Eisenberg et al. [19]	1974	46	5–46	—	—	—
Reilly et al. [41]	1976	23	29–36	74	61	—
Fazio et al. [21]	1976	67	20	—	77	—
Greenberg et al. [25]	1976	43	25	—	77	67
Dudrick et al. [18]	1976	52	—	—	54	—
Dean et al. [14]	1976	16	—	—	43	—
Harford et al. [27]	1978	—	—	—	—	21
Mullen et al. [38]	1978	50	26–37	—	38	—
Driscoll and Rosenberg [17]	1978	16	—	100	75	50
Elson et al. [20]	1980	20	36	100	65	25
Dickinson et al. [16]	1980	9	18–24	—	66	16
Bos and Weterman [6]	1980	115	41	—	41	—
Holm [29]	1981	6	60–98	—	86	86
Shiloni and Freund [45]	1983	19	21–150	100	56	37.5
Müller et al. [39]	1983	30	84	—	83	43
Ostro et al. [40]	1985	100	25	—	77	—
Kushner et al. [35]	1986	10	124	—	—	60
Shiloni et al. [44]	1989	49	30	—	45	23

there are alterations in gut hormones [23], some of which may have specific effects on the bowel. As stated earlier, specific nutrients for the bowel have not been tested as yet.

Tapering Steroids

Long-term steroid therapy for patients with Crohn's disease can be almost as debilitating as the disease. Thus, it is occasionally useful to utilize TPN to reduce the dosage of steroids. This is a useful aspect of TPN that is not often utilized, but should be kept in mind.

Treating Rapidly Appearing Recurrences

Whereas recurrence following surgery generally occurs comparatively late in the course, especially if an adequate resection is done, an occasional patient will flare in the immediate

postoperative period. It seems inappropriate to reoperate on such a patient; the use of parenteral nutrition is a valid alternative. In my experience, this usually results in remission and the patient can be discharged.

Perioperative Parenteral Nutrition

It has now been clearly established that there is a group of patients who have lost a great deal of weight, probably have immunologic defects, and are at increased risk for surgery. There has been difficulty in identifying this group, although much progress has been made. Studies by both Christou in Montreal and Mullen's group in Philadelphia attempted to define a perioperative nutritional index. In Christou's studies (see Chap. 8),

$$P|death| = 1/\{1 + e^{(-3.45 + 1.75*(albumin) + 0.3*(ln[DTH\ score])}\}$$

where P is probability and DTH is delayed-type hypersensitivity; while in studies by Mullin's group [9],

$$PNI = 158 - 16.6 \, (ALB) - 0.78 \, (TSF) \\ - 0.20 \, (TFN) - 5.8 \, (DH)$$

where PNI is Prognostic Nutritional Index, ALB is serum albumin level, TSF is triceps skinfold, TFN is serum transferrin level, and DH is delayed hypersensitivity. It is of interest that in both of the prognostic indices, albumin figures prominently. A more recent interpretation of this feature suggests that when patients are either malnourished, anergic, or both, but have an immunologic defect, short-turnover, acute-phase reactant hepatic protein synthesis may be increased, but albumin synthesis is down-regulated [51]. The decreased serum concentration of albumin may reflect an increased percentage of extravascular albumin secondary to the increased extracellular water accompanying starvation. This in turn increases the degradation of albumin.

Several recent studies attempted to elucidate whether nutritional depletion in patients with inflammatory bowel disease is associated with identifiable increased risk. Higgens et al. [28] operated on a series of 127 patients, most of whom had GIBD, and found no correlation between the degree of weight loss, serum albumin level, or a series of other relatively basic nutritional parameters, and outcome with respect to either mortality and/or major or minor infection. Of interest was that 90 days after the operation was completed, the weight gain of the group that was very depleted (i.e., that had lost 10 to 20% or even greater than 20% of their body weight) was more rapid than that of the group that was not very depleted, so their percentage of ideal body weight was identical. In a randomized, prospective multicenter trial, Buzby [8] demonstrated in the severely malnourished group (by their definition) that perioperative parenteral nutrition for between 10 and 14 days preoperatively successfully decreased the incidence of perioperative complications. However, in the mildly to moderately depleted perioperative group,

any decrease in perioperative complications was offset by an increase in non–catheter-related infections. That patients with interference with their immune mechanisms may have an increased incidence of either catheter- or non–catheter-related infections has also been seen in patients with pancreatitis, in two independent studies [24, 43].

Thus, although one can make an argument that in severely malnourished individuals, a period of perioperative TPN may decrease the incidence of complications, it has been difficult to establish. If one does intend to prevent perioperative complications in severely malnourished individuals, it is suggested that a period of perioperative TPN in patients with benign disease extend for between 10 and 14 days.

Fistulas
Fistulas are a common complication of GIBD, and certainly TPN usually results in the closure of fistulas. In my experience, such fistulas almost always reopen, and therefore I personally utilize TPN to close the fistula and decrease the abdominal wall sepsis. When the abdominal wall sepsis is quiescent, I operate on these patients under the cover of TPN. Resection and end-to-end anastomosis are carried out. If the fistula is from the colon and/or colonic anastomosis is required and/or there is an internal fistula between the ileum, for example, and the sigmoid colon (Fig. 16-1), a sleeve resection of sigmoid and reanastomosis are carried out. A gastrostomy is then placed and the anastomosis not tested with food for approximately 7 to 10 days postoperatively while the patient is kept nourished by TPN. Other authorities utilizing either steroids, metronidazole, or azathioprine, have claimed good long-term success with some fistulas in GIBD, but this has not been my experience.

Extensive Small-Bowel Disease
Occasionally one sees patients in whom the extent of inflammatory bowel disease throughout the small and large bowel is so great that resection cannot be contemplated. These patients may respond to a relatively

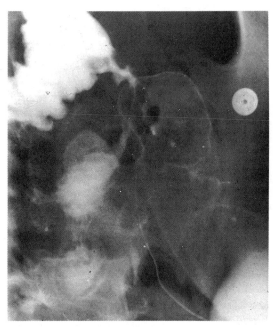

Figure 16-1. Crohn's disease with a cecal-sigmoid fistula. The fistula emerged on the umbilicus. The fistulas, cecum, and sigmoid were resected. The patient did well.

short course of TPN. More often, however, they require long-term home TPN.

Recurrence

Recurrence of disease remains a problem in patients with GIBD. As stated above, the period of remission induced by TPN can be as short as 24 hours. However, the mean time of recurrence is approximately 11 months. Once recurrence occurs, it is possible to undergo a period of additional TPN, although the chances for inducing remission under these circumstances are considerably less. In the recent experience of Shiloni et al. [44], although 45% of the patients originally avoided surgery, at the end of 15 months, recurrence had claimed all but 20%, and surgery was necessary.

ULCERATIVE COLITIS

Early experience with ulcerative colitis suggested that patients with fulminant ulcerative colitis that was out of medical control were not candidates for TPN. A few reports in the interim suggested that long-term home TPN may quiet ulcerative colitis, but I fail to see what purpose this serves, since patients with extensive and debilitating ulcerative colitis can now undergo a curative procedure in which permanent ileostomy is not the outcome [36, 37]. My own extensive experience with the Soave procedure or ileoanal pull-through with a pouch reservoir (my own preference is for the S-pouch) suggests that it is almost never worthwhile to treat such a patient with home TPN for ulcerative colitis. Indeed, with the increased incidence of carcinoma in patients with 10 years' activity of ulcerative colitis, treatment of ulcerative colitis patients with home TPN is rare.

More recent experience suggests one situation in which in-hospital TPN may be useful for patients with ulcerative colitis: those who are about to undergo rectal mucosal stripping and ileoanal pull-through with reservoir for ulcerative colitis, but in whom it is difficult to obtain quiescence of the rectal segment; the quiescent segment need be no more than approximately 10 cm of the rectum. In my own experience, hospitalization of such patients, treatment with short-term TPN for 2 to 6 weeks (2 weeks is often sufficient) plus rectal steroid suppositories and intravenous chloramphenicol (Chloromycetin) or metronidazole has been sufficient to render these patients quiescent enough to undergo operation.

HOME TPN

Crohn's disease remains one of the principal indications for the use of home TPN, often in three circumstances: (1) repeated small-bowel resections or the short-gut syndrome, (2) Crohn's disease that is so extensive that resection cannot be contemplated, and (3) fistulas that are recurrent and remain open despite repeated surgical interventions.

The success rate of restoration to function with home TPN is very high. Most of the patients are extraordinarily well motivated and, in my experience, approximately 90% return to their previous occupations. Several home

TPN patients run medium-size companies, care for households of growing children unaided, and so on. The average duration of catheter life has now been extended to approximately 6 years with the proper care.

The organization of home TPN will depend on local custom, intelligence of the patient, and the ability to obtain reimbursement (see Chap. 23). My own preference remains for pharmacy manufacture of solutions utilizing either glucose amino acids in one bottle and fat in another bottle or, more recently, a "three-in-one" mixture. Following manufacture, the solutions are delivered at weekly intervals and kept refrigerated. The patient is trained extensively in the hospital, utilizing tape recordings and books, and by special home TPN nurses. The patient must be trained to care for every conceivable complication of home TPN. There is always someone on call to make house visits or care for patients in case of problems in the middle of the night.

Utilizing such an approach, we have been successful in restoring our patients to function within society.

Home TPN in Children

A common indication for home TPN is in the pediatric group, when stunting of growth will scar the individual for life. To my knowledge, there are no clear-cut indications for when such an individual should be placed on home TPN except that it has been a general rule that when a child falls below the 10th percentile on a growth curve, home TPN should be undertaken. My own experience suggests that a period of approximately 3 to 4 weeks of in-hospital TPN will be followed by a 6-month growth spurt. Such a growth spurt can be made more or less permanent by the use of home TPN [49]. In addition, home TPN will have the salutory effect of reducing the activity of GIBD.

SUMMARY

Parenteral nutrition continues to play an active role in the therapy of inflammatory bowel disease. Most of the salutary effect occurs in patients with GIBD, with the role of TPN in ulcerative colitis largely limited to preparation of patients for operation and in therapy of the complications of ulcerative colitis. Enteral nutrition with chemically defined diets has received much more prominence recently, and reasonable success rates are being reported. In children, the use of home TPN in an effort to prevent growth stunting proves to be an excellent adjunct to therapy and can result in a more normal life. If other therapy fails as a result of repeated resections or short-gut syndrome, home TPN is a useful adjunct in the treatment of such patients.

REFERENCES

1. Alexander, J. W. Nutrition and infection: New perspectives for an old problem. *Arch. Surg.* 121:966, 1986.
2. Alexander, J. W., MacMillan, B. G., Stinnett, J. D., et al. Beneficial effects of aggressive protein feeding in severely burned children. *Ann. Surg.* 192:505, 1980.
3. Alverdy, J. C., Aoys, E., and Moss, G. S. Total parenteral nutrition promotes bacterial translocation from the gut. *Surgery* 104:185, 1988.
4. Alverdy, J., Chi, H. S., and Sheldon, G. F. The effect of parenteral nutrition on gastrointestinal immunity: The importance of enteral stimulation. *Ann. Surg.* 202:681, 1986.
5. Baker, J. W., Deitch, E. A., Berg, R., and Ma, L. Hemorrhagic shock impairs the mucosal barrier, resulting in bacterial translocation from the gut and sepsis. *Surg. Forum* 38:73, 1987.
6. Bos, L. P., and Weterman, I. T. TPN in Crohn's disease. *World J. Surg.* 4:163, 1980.
7. Bower, R. H., Talamini, M. A., Sax, H. C., Hamilton, F., and Fischer, J. E. Postoperative enteral versus parenteral nutrition: A randomized, controlled trial. *Arch. Surg.* 121:1040, 1986.
8. Buzby, G. P. The case for preoperative nutritional support. Presented at American College of Surgeons 1981 Clinical Congress Postgraduate Course on Pre- and Postoperative Care: Metabolism and Nutrition, Chicago, IL, October 25–28, 1988.
9. Buzby, G. P., Mullen, J. L., Matthews, D. C., Hobbs, C. L., and Rosato, E. F. Prognostic nutritional index in gastrointestinal surgery. *Am. J. Surg.* 139:160, 1980.
10. Cerra, F. B., McPherson, J. P., Konstantinides, F. N., Konstantinides, N. N., and Teas-

ley, K. M. Enteral nutrition does not prevent multiple organ failure syndrome (MOFS) after sepsis. *Surgery* 104:727, 1988.

11. Cerra, F. B., Shronts, E. P., Konstantinides, N. N., et al. Enteral feeding in sepsis: A prospective, randomized, double-blind trial. *Surgery* 98:632, 1985.

12. Crohn, B. B., Ginzburg, L., and Oppenheimer, G. D. Regional ileitis: A pathologic and clinical entity. *J.A.M.A.* 99:1323, 1932.

13. Dalziel, T. K. Chronic interstitial enteritis. *Br. Med. J.* 2:1068, 1913.

14. Dean, R. F., Campos, M. M., and Barrett, B. Hyperalimentation in the management of chronic inflammatory intestinal disease. *Dis. Colon Rectum* 19:601, 1976.

15. Deitch, E. A., Berg, R., and Specian, R. Endotoxin promotes the translocation of bacteria from the gut. *Arch. Surg.* 122:185, 1987.

16. Dickinson, R. J., Ashton, M. G., Axon, A. T. E., Smith, R. C., Yeung, C. K., and Hill, G. L. Controlled trial of intravenous hyperalimentation and total bowel rest as an adjunct to the routine therapy of acute colitis. *Gastroenterology* 79:1199, 1980.

17. Driscoll, R. H., and Rosenberg, I. H. Total parenteral nutrition in inflammatory bowel disease. *Med. Clin. North Am.* 62:185, 1978.

18. Dudrick, S. J., MacFadyen, B. V., and Daly, J. M. Management of inflammatory bowel disease with parenteral hyperalimentation. In H. R. Clearfield and V. P. Dinoso (eds.), *Gastrointestinal Emergencies.* New York: Grune & Stratton, 1976. P. 193.

19. Eisenberg, H. W., Turnbull, R. B., and Weakley, F. L. Hyperalimentation as preparation for surgery in transmural colitis (Crohn's disease). *Dis. Colon Rectum* 17:469, 1974.

20. Elson, C. O., Layden, T. J., Nemchausky, B. A., Rosenberg, J. L., and Rosenberg, I. H. An evaluation of total parenteral nutrition in the management of inflammatory bowel disease. *Dig. Dis. Sci.* 25:42, 1980.

21. Fazio, V. W., Kodner, I., Jagelman, D. G., Turnball, R. B., and Weakley, F. L. Inflammatory disease of the bowel: Nutrition as primary or adjunctive treatment. *Dis. Colon Rectum* 19:574, 1976.

22. Fischer, J. E., Foster, G. S., Abel, R. M., Abbott, W. M., and Ryan, J. A. Hyperalimentation as primary therapy for inflammatory bowel disease. *Am. J. Surg.* 125:165, 1973.

23. Gimmon, Z., Murphy, R. F., Chen, M. H., Nachbauer, C. A., Fischer, J. E., and Joffe, S. N. The effect of parenteral and enteral nutrition on portal and systemic immunoreactivities of gastrin, glucagon and vasoactive intestinal polypeptide (VIP). *Ann. Surg.* 196:571, 1982.

24. Goodgame, J. T., and Fischer, J. E. Parenteral nutrition in the treatment of acute pancreatitis: Effect on complications and mortality. *Ann. Surg.* 186:651, 1977.

25. Greenberg, G. R., Haber, G. B., and Jeejeebhoy, K. N. Total parenteral nutrition and bowel rest in the management of Crohn's disease. *Gut* 17:828, 1976.

26. Gump, F. E., Lepore, M., and Barker, H. G. A revised concept of acute regional enteritis. *Ann. Surg.* 166:942, 1967.

27. Harford, F. J., and Fazio, V. W. Total parenteral nutrition as primary therapy for inflammatory disease of the bowel. *Dis. Colon Rectum* 21:555, 1978.

28. Higgens, C. S., Keighley, M. R. B., and Allan, R. N. Impact of preoperative weight loss and body composition changes on postoperative outcome in surgery for inflammatory bowel disease. *Gut* 25:732, 1984.

29. Holm, L. Benefits of total parenteral nutrition in the treatment of Crohn's disease and ulcerative colitis. *Acta Chir. Scand.* 147:271, 1981.

30. Inoue, S., Epstein, M. D., Alexander, J. W., Trocki, O., Jacobs, P., and Gura, P. Prevention of yeast translocation across the gut by a single enteral feeding after burn injury. *J. Parenter. Enter. Nutr.* 13:565, 1989.

31. Inoue, S., Wirman, J. A., Alexander, J. W., Trocki, O., and Cardell, R. R. *Candida albicans* translocation across the gut mucosa following burn injury. *J. Surg. Res.* 44:479, 1988.

32. Johnson, L. R., Lichtenberger, L. M., Copeland, E. M., Dudrick, S. J., and Castro, G. A. Action of gastrin on gastrointestinal structure and function. *Gastroenterology* 68:1184, 1975.

33. Kripke, S. A., Fox, A. D., Berman, J. M., De Paula, J. A., Rombeau, J. L., and Settle, R. G. Inhibition of TPN-associated colonic atrophy with beta-hydroxybutyrate. *Surg. Forum* 39:48, 1988.

34. Kudsk, K. A., Carpenter, G., Petersen, S., and Sheldon, G. F. Effect of enteral and parenteral feeding in malnourished rats with *E. coli* hemoglobin adjuvant peritonitis. *J. Surg. Res.* 31:105, 1981.

35. Kushner, R. F., Shapir, J., and Sitrin, M. D. Endoscopic, radiographic, and clinical response to prolonged bowel rest and home parenteral nutrition in Crohn's disease. *J. Parenter. Enter. Nutr.* 10:568, 1986.

36. Martin, L. W., and Fischer, J. E. Preservation of anorectal continence following total colectomy. *Ann. Surg.* 196:700, 1982.

37. Martin, L. W., Fischer, J. E., Sayers, H. J., Alexander, F., and Torres, M. A. Anal continence following Soave procedure: Analysis of results in 100 patients. *Ann. Surg.* 203:525, 1986.

38. Mullen J. L., Hargrove, W. C., Dudrick, S. J., Fitts, W. T., and Rosato, E. F. Ten years' experience with intravenous hyperalimentation and inflammatory bowel disease. *Ann. Surg.* 187:523, 1978.
39. Müller, J. M., Keller, H. W., Erasmi, H., and Pichlmaier, H. Total parenteral nutrition as the sole therapy in Crohn's disease: A prospective study. *Br. J. Surg.* 70:40, 1983.
40. Ostro, M. J., Greenberg, G. R., and Jeejeebhoy, K. N. Total parenteral nutrition and complete bowel rest in the management of Crohn's disease. *J. Parenter. Enter. Nutr.* 9:280, 1985.
41. Reilly, J., Ryan, J. A., Strole, W., and Fischer, J. E. Hyperalimentation in inflammatory bowel disease. *Am. J. Surg.* 131:192, 1976.
42. Roediger, W. E. W. Utilization of nutrients by isolated epithelial cells of the rat colon. *Gastroenterology* 83:424, 1982.
43. Sax, H. C., Warner, B. W., Talamini, M. A., et al. Early total parenteral nutrition in acute pancreatitis: Lack of beneficial effects. *Am. J. Surg.* 153:117, 1987.
44. Shiloni, E., Coronado, E., and Freund, H. R. The role of total parenteral nutrition in the treatment of Crohn's disease. *Am. J. Surg.* 157:180, 1989.
45. Shiloni, E., and Freund, H. R. Total parenteral nutrition in Crohn's disease: Is it primary or supportive mode of therapy? *Dis. Colon Rectum* 26:275, 1983.
46. Soergel, K. H. Absorption of fermentation products from the colon. In H. Caspar and H. Goebell (eds.), *Colon and Nutrition*. Lancaster, PA: MTP Press, 1982.
47. Souba, W. W., and Wilmore, D. W. Gut-liver interaction during accelerated gluconeogenesis. *Arch. Surg.* 120:66, 1985.
48. Stehle, P., Zander, J., Mertes, N., et al. Effect of parenteral glutamine peptide supplements on muscle glutamine loss and nitrogen balance after major surgery. *Lancet* 1:231, 1989.
49. Strobel, C. T., Byrne, W. J., and Ament, M. E. Home parenteral nutrition in children with Crohn's disease: Effective management alternative. *Gastroenterology* 77:272, 1979.
50. Vogel, C. M., Corwin, T. R., and Baue, A. E. Intravenous hyperalimentation in the treatment of inflammatory diseases of the bowel. *Arch. Surg.* 108:460, 1974.
51. Von Allmen, D., Hasselgren, P. O., Li, S., and Fischer, J. E. Effect of ischemia on protein synthesis in septic liver. Presented at the 9th Annual Meeting of the Surgical Infection Society, Denver, CO, April 13–14, 1989.
52. Wang, X., Jacobs, D. O., O'Dwyer, S. T., Smith, R. J., and Wilmore, D. W. Glutamine-enriched parenteral nutrition prevents mucosal atrophy following massive small bowel resection. *Surg. Forum* 39:44, 1988.
53. Smith, R. J., and Wilmore, D. W. Glutamine nutrition and requirements. *J. Parenter. Enter. Nutr.* 14(Suppl.): 945, 1990.
54. Wood, R. H., and Caldwell, F. J. Effect of early feeding on post-burn metabolism. *Surg. Forum* 37:111, 1986.

Fistulas

Daniel W. Benson
Josef E. Fischer

Many factors important to the management of gastrointestinal fistulas have been clearly defined and yet fistulas remain a potentially catastrophic complication associated with high morbidity and mortality, lengthy hospitalizations, and excessive health care costs. Fluid and electrolyte imbalances, malnutrition, and sepsis are among the myriad of problems that must be dealt with in order to avoid the downward spiralling course of multiorgan system failure and death. To the physician, the treatment of enterocutaneous fistulas can be a humbling and sometimes demoralizing experience, while to the patient it may result in major depression and a loss of confidence in the health care team. This chapter reviews the management of gastrointestinal fistulas, with emphasis on the role of nutritional support, particularly the role of parenteral nutrition.

PATHOPHYSIOLOGY

A basic understanding of the pathophysiology behind the changes that occur with enterocutaneous fistulas is important for a successful outcome. The three factors most associated with mortality are fluid and electrolyte imbalance, malnutrition, and sepsis.

Fluid and Electrolyte Imbalance

Fluid and electrolyte imbalance is primarily associated with high-output fistulas, defined as those with outputs greater than 500 ml daily. The amount of fistula drainage will depend in part on the proximity to the ligament of Treitz and may comprise the majority of gastrointestinal secretions. For example, the total diversion of gastrointestinal secretions at the ligament of Treitz may drain up to 4 liters/day, approximately 2 liters of which originates from the stomach and saliva, and an additional 2 liters from pancreatic or biliary secretions. These losses are composed of a highly complicated solution, rich in protein, electrolytes, and other components. It is not difficult to imagine how the continued loss of this fluid might quickly wreak havoc with total body fluid economy. A critical feature is that these pancreatic and biliary losses are hypertonic to plasma, particularly in regard to sodium (Na^+), bicarbonate (HCO_2), and potassium (K^+). A significant amount of energy is expended to maintain this gradient.

The replacement of these losses in the past posed another problem due to the lack of suitable hypertonic parenteral solutions. With the advent of hyperalimentation and experience with total parenteral nutrition (TPN), one can now meet most of the needs of electrolyte losses utilizing hyperalimentation alone without utilizing supplemental electrolyte infusions.

Malnutrition

Even with aggressive nutritional support, malnutrition remains a major problem in patients with enterocutaneous fistulas. There are three main contributing factors: (1) the lack of adequate food intake; (2) the hypercatabolism of the associated sepsis; and (3) the loss of protein-rich, energy-requiring secretion from the fistula.

The inability to take in adequate nourishment is self-explanatory. Furthermore, ingestion of food into the gut has been shown to increase the output of small-bowel fistulas. Parenteral nutrition now provides a method of delivering nutrients irrespective of the state of the gastrointestinal tract.

The hypermetabolism of sepsis results in a rapid breakdown of lean body mass. This autocannibalization serves as a form of internal nutritional support and, while initially adaptive, leads to multiorgan system failure and death if it is unchecked.

Under normal circumstances, almost all of the protein content of small-bowel secretions is reabsorbed as free amino acids and, in the presence of sufficient energy, enters the free amino acid pool to be reutilized in protein synthesis. Obviously, in a high-output fistula, much of this protein-rich material is lost.

Sepsis

Sepsis is the most common cause of death in patients with enterocutaneous fistulas. This

is not surprising, given the nature of the insult. That is, postsurgical disruption, abscess formation, and necrotic devitalized tissue all play a role in providing a suitable culture medium for bacterial growth. The most common organisms tend to be those of bowel origin (i.e., coliforms, bacteroides, and enterococci). *Staphylococcus* also plays a role in intrabdominal abscesses. Sepsis remains the most frequent indication for operation.

ETIOLOGY

In general, enterocutaneous fistulas result from one of four conditions: (1) the extension of bowel disease to surrounding structures, (2) the extension of disease in the surrounding viscera into the bowel, (3) unrecognized trauma to the bowel, and (4) breakdown of an intestinal anastomosis.

The first two conditions predispose to nonoperative causes of fistulas and occur most commonly with inflammatory bowel disease, irradiation, benign and malignant neoplasms, and vascular diseases. These have been increasing in frequency and now constitute approximately 25% of spontaneous fistulas.

The latter two conditions, however, still account for the majority of enterocutaneous fistulas. These are usually the result of an operative misadventure such as direct injury to the small bowel during lysis of adhesions, disruption of an anastomosis, or a perianastomotic abscess.

Finally, the prevailing cause of enterocutaneous fistulas at a given institution varies, to some extent depending on areas of general interest and referral patterns.

DEFINITION AND CATEGORIZATION OF FISTULAS

Gastrointestinal fistulas represent an abnormal communication between the bowel and another organ. They have been categorized in a variety of ways, including anatomic location, the amount of drainage, and whether they are internal or external, to name but a few. These descriptive classifications are helpful in predicting the likelihood of spontaneous closure, and later in formulating a management plan. In this chapter, we primarily discuss the management of external fistulas arising from the small bowel, with outputs greater than 200 ml daily for at least 48 hours' duration.

ROLE OF NUTRITIONAL SUPPORT

The management of enterocutaneous fistulas has evolved significantly over the last three decades, and although it has been a point of contention, nutritional support has gained a prominent role in their management. Critical evaluation of the impact of nutritional support is difficult, owing to the nature of the disease. Enterocutaneous fistulas are relatively rare, with a varied presentation, and consequently much of the literature is composed of anecdotal reports or poorly controlled, retrospective series collected over many years. Unfortunately, this has not prevented some authors from drawing sweeping conclusions, further complicating interpretation of the literature. It is unlikely, however, that a prospective randomized series comparing types of nutritional support will ever be done, owing to the length of time such a study would require. A careful review of the literature, nevertheless, can still be helpful in gaining an appreciation for the role of nutritional support in the management of enterocutaneous fistulas.

In their classic article in 1960, Edmunds et al. [4] for the first time called attention to the serious nature of and the high mortality related to enterocutaneous fistulas, in part owing to their association with electrolyte imbalance, malnutrition, and sepsis. They reported an overall mortality rate of 43% in 157 patients with fistulas from 1945 to 1959 at the Massachusetts General Hospital. The mortality rate increased to 61% in patients with malnutrition. These authors advocated early surgical intervention in an attempt to restore bowel continuity, to institute "refunc-

tionalization," to provide for nutritional intake, and hopefully to avoid malnutrition and its attendant complications.

These findings were later confirmed in a study from the same institution on 119 patients from 1960 to 1970 [10]. In patients with severe malnutrition, moderate malnutrition, or no malnutrition, the mortality rates were 28%, 10%, and 7%, respectively.

In 1964, Chapman et al. [2], at the University of California, took the concept one step further by emphasizing that one of the keys to successful management was to maintain adequate nutritional support from the very beginning. They studied the effect of nutritional support and reported an increased fistula closure rate and decreased mortality rate (14%) in those patients treated with more than 1600 kcal/day, using a combination of peripheral nutritional support and tube feedings. In contrast to Edmunds et al. [4], they recommended conservative surgical management, with surgery reserved only for those patients who failed to respond to nutritional support.

In 1971, Sheldon et al. [9] reported on 51 patients with fistulas who were treated using the management principles established by Chapman. In patients who received greater than 3000 kcal/day, they reported a 76% spontaneous closure rate and a 12% mortality rate.

The studies discussed above used enteral means of nutritional support. This necessarily led to the exclusion of many patients with high-output jejunal fistulas, intraabdominal sepsis, bowel obstruction, inflammatory bowel disease, radiation enteritis, and gastrointestinal malignancy. The potential for bias and erroneous conclusions is obvious. Valid conclusions on the impact of nutritional support on outcome in patients with fistulas could not be drawn until it became possible to nourish all patients, regardless of the status of their gastrointestinal tracts. It was with the introduction and standardization of parenteral nutrition that this became possible.

In 1973, McPhayden and Dudrick [6], at the University of Pennsylvania, reported on 62 patients with internal and external gastrointestinal fistulas treated with hyperalimentation. They achieved a spontaneous closure rate of 70.5% and an overall mortality rate of 6.45%. Reports such as these led most surgeons during the early 1970s to come to rely on TPN in the belief that it would afford both a high rate of spontaneous closure and a low mortality.

This concept was challenged by Aguirre et al. [1] who reported on a series of patients with gastrointestinal-cutaneous fistulas that did not close spontaneously with TPN and required operation. Their findings, when presented to the American Surgical Association, were controversial, but found strong support in two studies in the late 1970s that also questioned the role of TPN alone, without surgery, in patients with fistulas. The first study, by Reber et al. [8] in 1978, reported on 186 patients with enteric fistulas from 1968 to 1977. They divided their experience into an early group from 1968 to 1971 (82 patients) and a later group from 1972 to 1977 (104 patients). In the first group, 35% of the patients received TPN, compared to 71% in the second group. The majority of patients who did not receive TPN were treated with enteral nutrition. The fistula-related mortality rate for the entire 10-year period was 11%, with no difference between the earlier (13%) and later (10%) years. Likewise, there was no statistically significant difference in spontaneous closure rates for the earlier (26%) and later (35%) years. When patients who were adequately nourished by tube feeding were compared to those treated with TPN, neither mortality (7 versus 14%) nor spontaneous closure rates (22 versus 37%) of the fistulas were significantly different. Reber et al. concluded that the principal impact of TPN was to simplify management rather than to alter the outcome.

The second study, by Soeters et al. [10], updated the earlier report by Edmunds et al. [4]. Soeters et al. [10] reported on 404 patients with fistulas who were grouped into three chronologic eras: 1945 to 1960, 1960 to 1970, and 1970 to 1975. The mortality rates were 43%, 15%, and 21%, respectively. The authors pointed out that the decrease in mortality occurred in the 1960 to 1970 era, prior to

the introduction of TPN, and was probably the result of improved intensive care monitoring. Furthermore, the addition of TPN did not lead to further improvements in outcome. They ascribed the decrease in mortality to advances in parasurgical care. However, they did find that spontaneous closure rates improved, with the introduction of TPN, from 10 to 32%.

In contrast to these two reports, three other series compared the pre- and post-TPN eras. Investigators found both a decrease in mortality rate and an increased spontaneous closure rate when using TPN [3, 5, 11].

In the final analysis, when evaluating the beneficial effects of TPN on the treatment of gastrointestinal fistulas, the following factors need to be considered: (1) mortality rate, (2) spontaneous closure rate, (3) efficacy of nutritional support, and (4) preparation for corrective surgery.

Although not all studies reported a decrease in mortality, they have found increased spontaneous closure rates with TPN. Both means of nutritional support are effective, with acceptable rates of spontaneous closure; however, enteral nutrition usually takes several days to achieve full nutritional support. TPN would appear to be a more expedient method of nutritional support. Finally, even in patients whose fistulas do not close spontaneously, they will be much better prepared to tolerate a major operation after 4 to 6 weeks of TPN.

RECOGNITION

The recognition of an external gastrointestinal fistula is rarely a problem, due to the nature of the drainage. The finding of greenish digestive juices or brownish material if the fistula is colonic in origin, discovered on the wound dressing, or draining through an abdominal wound, through a drain tract, or spontaneously after drainage of an intraabdominal abscess all too clearly signals to the surgeon what has happened. A fairly common story is a patient not doing well and running a fever of 101 to 102°F (38.3–

38.9°C). On the sixth postoperative day, a wound infection is drained and purulent material is obtained. Twenty-four hours later, bowel contents drain from the wound.

PHASES OF MANAGEMENT

Management of these fistulas requires a systematic and rational approach. It is helpful to divide the management of enterocutaneous fistulas into five sequential but overlapping phases: (1) stabilization, (2) investigation, (3) decision, (4) definitive therapy, and (5) healing.

Stabilization

Minimize Fistula Output
On recognition of the fistula, the patient should be put at complete bowel rest and started on anticholinergics or histamine H_2 blockers, or both, to reduce fistula output. More recently, the naturally occurring peptide somatostatin has been used to decrease fistula output in cases refractory to standard treatment. Somatostatin has a wide range of inhibitory effects on gut endocrine, secretory, and motor function. The exact role of somatostatin in the management of enterocutaneous fistulas is yet to be defined [7]. If indwelling tubes such as a gastrostomy or jejunostomy are already in place, they should be opened and placed to gravity drainage. The placement of a decompressive tube, either nasogastric or long gastrointestinal, should be avoided unless severe ileus or intestinal obstruction is present. Several series have been unable to demonstrate any improvement in outcome from the use of decompressive tubes. Furthermore, the presence of an indwelling nasogastric tube for a prolonged period of time not only is uncomfortable to the patient, but also may contribute to the development of impaired cough, aspiration pneumonia, serous otitis media, pharyngitis, or acid reflux esophagitis that may ultimately lead to late esophageal stricture formation. If long-term decompression is necessary, a gastrostomy tube should be placed; this can be done under local anesthesia, if necessary, or

by the more recently popularized percutaneous endoscopic technique.

Restoration of Fluid and Electrolytes
Restoration of fluid volume, electrolytes, and acid-base balance must be achieved next. These patients' blood volume is often depleted and should be rapidly restored with albumin, plasma, and packed cells so that a hematocrit of at least 35% and an albumin level of at least 3.5 g/dl are achieved. As previously noted, the drainage from enterocutaneous fistulas tends to be hypertonic to plasma with high sodium, potassium, and bicarbonate content; the crystalloid fluids used for replacement should reflect this. Deficits of calcium, magnesium, and phosphorus also need to be corrected. Following the initial resuscitation, it should be possible in most patients to meet maintenance fluid and electrolyte needs with TPN.

Drainage of Abscesses
As previously noted, uncontrolled sepsis remains the major cause of mortality in these patients. Therefore, the presence of abscesses must be aggressively looked for and, when found, promptly drained. With today's technology, it should not be necessary to perform exploratory laparotomy to diagnose an intraabdominal abscess. Using CT scan or ultrasonography, the diagnosis can usually be made and drainage can often be carried out percutaneously by the invasive radiologist.

Patients receive, on the average, seven to nine different antibiotics during the course of treatment. Antibiotics should therefore be reserved for specific instances when sepsis cannot be controlled by other means, and then only after adequate cultures and sensitivity studies have been done, if possible. It is to be stressed, however, that the primary treatment is surgical drainage and not antibiotic therapy.

Skin Care and Sump Drainage
Local control of the fistula and care of the skin surrounding the fistula are accomplished by sump drainage of the fistula and the application of various protective sub-

stances and appliances to the skin. The importance of this cannot be overemphasized. Surgical therapy may be delayed or made more difficult if maceration, digestion, cellulitis, and cutaneous necrosis around the fistula have occurred. Sump drainage can be accomplished by inserting a soft, brown latex nephrostomy tube through which a 14-gauge Intracath is placed down the center, as an air vent, to end near the tip of the larger tube. The nephrostomy tube is then connected for continuous suction. The 14-gauge Intracath can be irrigated with antibiotic solution to break the suction if needed. Various sizes of nephrostomy tubes are available, and the choice should be based on the consistency of the intestinal contents being drained. In addition to protecting the skin, placement of a sump is helpful in quantitating fistula losses. When drainage is decreasing, the sump can be replaced by a well-fitting appliance that will provide greater freedom in movement for the patient.

A variety of protective substances are available, and include karaya powder, ion exchange resin, Stomadhesive, as well as other local favorites. Our preference, when suitable, is Stomadhesive. If available, specialist nurse/enterostomal therapists should be involved, as excellent skin care is often the product of cooperation between the physician and these experts.

Institution of Nutritional Support

Nutritional support is essential for these patients and should not be unnecessarily delayed. As previously noted, satisfactory rates of spontaneous closure have been achieved using either parenteral or enteral nutritional support. However, parenteral nutrition is usually the easiest and most expedient method in the majority of cases. Even if enteral support is considered, it will take 4 or 5 days to achieve caloric balance. Therefore, parenteral nutrition should be initiated at the outset.

Parenteral Nutrition

The institution of parenteral nutrition should be delayed only to allow time for adequate hydration so that central-line placement is easier and safer, and for the treatment of frank bacteremia that has an easily identifiable source. The techniques of catheter insertion have been described elsewhere. Caloric requirements for these patients can be estimated from the Harris-Benedict equation and verified by indirect calorimetry. This will approximate 35 kcal/day. A calorie-nitrogen ratio of between 125 and 160 nonprotein calories to 1 g of nitrogen is usually acceptable. Of the nonprotein calories, 15 to 20% should be derived from fat, both to prevent essential fatty acid deficiency and to maximize hepatic protein synthesis. Infusions are generally begun at 40 ml/hr, utilizing D25W solutions with approximately 50 g of protein per liter. The infusions are increased by 20 ml/hr every 24 to 48 hours, with careful monitoring of urinary and blood glucose levels. Insulin may be added as required to maintain glucose levels below 200 mg/dl. In patients with glucose intolerance, fat may be used as a caloric source supplying up to 30% of nonprotein calories.

Although trace elements and vitamins are now routinely administered with parenteral nutrition solutions, one should be constantly alert to the possibility of deficiencies developing in these patients. Water-soluble vitamins are given daily and the fat-soluble vitamins, on at least a weekly basis. B and C vitamins should be provided at two to five times the minimal daily requirement. Anemia is frequently seen in these patients even in the presence of normal amounts of vitamin B_{12}, folate, and iron. Some believe that this may be due to a copper deficiency. Finally, supplementation with zinc is necessary in these patients.

Enteral Nutrition

Our primary reliance is on parenteral nutrition, with the use of enteral nutrition by chemically defined formulas reserved for low-output ileal and colonic fistulas. It is our belief that although elemental formulas are a low-residue means of providing adequate nutrition, they do not give complete bowel rest and have been associated in some cases with an increase in fistula drainage after insti-

tution as well as in the reopening of fistulas that had previously closed.

If enteral nutrition is to be used, at least 122 cm (4 ft) of small bowel is required. The enteral diet should be administered preferably through a soft, small-bore feeding tube that has been passed nasally into the stomach or small bowel, or through a gastrostomy or jejunostomy tube if one is present. Endoscopic or fluoroscopic guidance may be helpful in some cases. Placement of feeding tubes should always be confirmed by x-ray before institution of enteral therapy. The solution is begun in an iso-osmotic form at a slow rate of infusion (25 ml/hr), which is best controlled by a pump. If this is tolerated, the diet may be slowly increased first in osmolality and then in volume if the infusion is into the stomach. If gut access is by way of the small bowel, the volume and then concentration should be increased, owing to the poor tolerance of hypertonic solutions by the small bowel.

Morale and Ambulation

Loss of morale may be a major cause of morbidity and mortality in the patient with an enterocutaneous fistula. As it is anticipated that most fistulas will heal spontaneously, it is important from the outset to maintain good morale and start these patients on ambulation as quickly as possible. This is all the more reason to remove sutures, drains, and tubes as soon as possible.

Investigation

Sinography

If the appropriate measures have been taken, and after 48 hours patients have stabilized, definition of the fistula can begin, although we frequently will delay this for 7 to 10 days to allow the fistula tract to mature. Radiologic investigations are usually the most important step in defining the anatomy of the fistula. These, however, should be undertaken after the patient has stabilized. Sinography, using contrast medium (either 60% Renograffin or Hypaque) infused with a No. 5 French pediatric feeding tube through the fistula, is the easiest means of delineation of the anatomy. This should be a collaborative effort with both a senior surgeon and a radiologist in attendance, since the manner in which the dye runs into the various fistula tracts is often as important as the appearance of these tracts on the still radiographs. The surgeon hopes to answer several questions through these investigations. Is the bowel in continuity? As a corollary: Is the fistula a sinus from the lateral wall of the bowel or is it an end fistula? What is the nature of the surrounding area? Is there a large adjacent abscess cavity? What is the nature of the bowel immediately adjacent to the fistula? Is it of normal caliber or narrowed and strictured? Is it inflamed, boggy, or edematous? Is the mucosa normal or ulcerated? Finally, is there distal obstruction?

We rarely perform classic gastrointestinal tract radiologic studies, as they are not often helpful and often do not define the fistula in a manner to be helpful.

Decision

Following a thorough investigation, two questions need to be answered. First, is surgery required? If so, when should it be performed? In answering the first question, it is usually possible to predict which fistulas require operative intervention based on the following criteria. First are the nature and behavior of the drainage. Usually, fistula output decreases in response to TPN. If it does not decrease, operation is probably required. Duration of drainage is also important. If after 4 to 5 weeks of sepsis-free adequate parenteral nutrition, the fistula output is not decreasing, the fistula is unlikely to close.

Next, the nature of the fistula, including the site and its anatomic and radiographic characteristics, must be taken into account. Ileal fistulas close spontaneously less than 50% of the time. Other areas that are difficult to heal include the ligament of Treitz and gastric fistula. In contrast, esophageal, lateral duodenal, and jejunal fistulas as well as pancreatic and biliary fistulas tend to close spontaneously. Anatomic and radiographic characteristics adverse to spontaneous closure include: (1) loss of bowel continuity, (2) adjacent small bowel that is severely abnormal, (3) unremitting distal obstruction, (4) a large adjacent abscess into which the fistula drains, (5) short fistula (< 2 cm) with epithelialization of the tract down to the opening into the bowel, (6) the presence of a foreign body, and (7) an opening in the bowel greater than 1 cm². Finally, in specific disease states such as cancer, radiation, and inflammatory bowel disease, fistulas may close, only to reopen after a diet is resumed.

Regardless of how these questions are answered, a period of TPN is usually indicated to allow for healing of the skin surrounding the fistula and for restoration of nutritional balance, and because most fistulas meet criteria favorable for healing. In deciding the exact timing of therapy, we have found it helpful to follow the short-turnover proteins. Patients whose serum retinol-binding protein, thyroxin-binding prealbumin, and transferrin levels are increasing usually withstand an operation. However, global assessment of the patient's condition is often as accurate an index of timing of operation as any measurement.

Definitive Therapy

Nonoperative Therapy

If the nature of the fistula suggests that closure is likely, it is appropriate to allow a trial of bowel rest and parenteral nutrition. As long as the patient is continuing to improve metabolically, it is reasonable to continue with the conservative form of therapy. As previously noted, even if spontaneous closure does not occur, a period of 3 to 6 weeks of TPN is often invaluable in improving the patient's condition prior to operation, allowing for restoration of positive nitrogen balance, lean body mass, immunologic competence, and healing capacity. Furthermore, following many major operations, especially when the bowel wall has fistulated, there is a dense peritoneal reaction that is maximal from 10 to 21 days and lasts about 6 to 8 weeks before beginning resolution. Total resolution may take months and is unpredictable. If the abdomen is opened during this

period, a form of obliterative peritonitis may be encountered and may render dissection almost impossible. Premature operations at this time are ill-advised.

Operative Therapy

Prevention
Given that the major cause of fistulas is iatrogenic, the foremost principle in management is prevention. This can be accomplished by following exact operative technique, with adherence to rigid surgical principles in performing intestinal anastomosis, including: (1) watertight anastomoses without tension, (2) preservation of uncompromised blood supply, (3) avoidance of anastomoses in the presence of sepsis, (4) release of distal obstruction, (5) proximal decompression when indicated, and (6) careful closure of abdominal incisions.

Salvage Procedure
Sometimes early surgical intervention is necessary, using procedures that have been referred to by various names, including: (1) salvage or rescue procedure, (2) indirect therapy, or (3) conservative surgical therapy. These are temporizing measures when uncontrolled sepsis or fistula output makes early surgical intervention urgent but the patient's general condition prohibits a major surgical procedure, and include drainage of abscesses, exteriorization of the bowel, or proximal diversion of the bowel.

Definitive Procedure
Major indications for operation are persistent drainage, sepsis, or abscess. Operations for fistulas should not be undertaken lightly, and one should be prepared to devote the entire day to the procedure. The patient should be well prepared both mentally and physically. All orifices should be cultured, sensitivities obtained, and appropriate antibiotics given in adequate dosages preoperatively. If available, an infectious disease team of the institution should be consulted. Adequate amounts of blood should be reserved, as the intraoperative transfusion of large volumes of blood is often necessary.

If possible, the operative approach should take place through a new incision or an extension of the old incision that is away from the area of sepsis, and placed in such a way that the abscess cavity can be drained at a distance from the incision through a separate stab wound. After the skin is incised, wound towels or wound barrier drapes should be placed to protect the skin, subcutaneous tissue, and muscles from septic abdominal contents. Great care must be taken to avoid injury to the underlying bowel, which is invariably adherent to the abdominal wall. The entire bowel and fistula must then be freed up. Next, the fistulous tract and surrounding skin should be completely resected. The anastomosis itself should be carried out in a clean field, using healthy bowel that is not inflamed. Meticulous technique and hemostasis are absolutely essential to prevent further abscess or fistula formation and further anastomotic breakdown. Any rent in the serosa, even if not associated with rents in the mucosa, should be closed with Lembert sutures of nonabsorbable material to prevent further fistulization. All abscesses are drained and extensive abdominal irrigation with antibiotic solution is used both during and after the procedure.

It is clear that the best results are obtained with resection of the fistula with end-to-end anastomoses [10]. We use a two-layer silk interrupted anastomosis. In situations where excision is judged too precarious, exclusion of the fistula from the mainstream of the gastrointestinal tract may be appropriate. A blind loop should be avoided and at least one end brought out as a mucous fistula. Direct suture closure of the fistula without resection is an undesirable alternative, as it is usually followed by breakdown. Others have advocated Roux-en-Y bypass or serosal patching of fistulas in certain difficult cases; however, it is our opinion that if the fistula can be sufficiently mobilized for one of these procedures, it can be resected, and the success rate from these compromised procedures is usually less than that from resection and end-to-end anastomosis [10]. Following the repair, intestinal decompression should be provided by gastrostomy tube for comfort and the pro-longed drainage during the ileus that may follow.

The final element of successful operation is secure closure of the abdominal wall. In the case of large abdominal wall defects, a repair utilizing muscle flaps may be required for adequate closure. For this reason, on completion of a long and tedious operation, we believe strongly about the use of a fresh plastic and reconstructive surgery team to reconstruct difficult abdominal wall closures.

Postoperative Care
Antibiotics should be continued for at least 72 hours after the procedure, unless an obvious abscess cavity or cellulitis is present, in which case antibiotics are therapeutic, not prophylactic, and should be used longer. It is our practice not to stress the bowel with oral intake until at least a week postoperatively, regardless of how quickly bowel function returns. Drains should always be of a soft latex, sump-type in a closed system, and are left in place for at least 1 week postoperatively until a tract is well established or, if drainage is profuse, until drainage ceases. The drain is then slowly advanced so that the tract can be established and drainage can continue after the foreign body is removed. "Two-way" drains are only used for abscess cavities. For drainage of noninfected areas, for example, raw and bleeding areas, closed-suction drains are used. We also use gastrostomy tubes liberally, to avoid rushing in removing nasogastric tubes prematurely.

Healing

Nutritional management and continued support, as outlined in the stabilization phase, must be maintained during the final healing phase. The cornerstone to this phase of management is to provide patients with sufficient caloric intake during this crucial transitional phase, since otherwise newly laid-down protein and collagen may be catabolized as an energy source and refistulization may occur if nutritional support is withdrawn too soon. If all has gone well, 10 to 14 days after surgery a patient will be ready to make the transition to a regular diet. A patient receiving parenteral nutrition for several weeks, however, may not have an appetite and it may be necessary to discontinue the parenteral nutrition, run normal saline solution through the line, and in some cases ask the family to bring in food the patient wants. When the patient is able to take in at least two-thirds of his or her estimated caloric needs by mouth, the line can be removed.

RESULTS

Historically, the principal causes of mortality have been electrolyte imbalance, malnutrition, and sepsis. To a certain extent, all of these remain problems, particularly in high-output fistulas. Advances in patient monitoring and surgical intensive care have reduced, but not eliminated, electrolyte imbalance, while nutritional support has blunted malnutrition. Uncontrolled sepsis remains the major cause of mortality today. Other causes include the primary disease, as in cancer, or gastrointestinal bleeding. Most contemporary studies of fistulas still report mortality rates between 6 and 20%. In general, mortality decreases as one moves away from the ligament of Treitz. Following the control of sepsis, one can expect a spontaneous closure rate of 25 to 80%, although here again location, cause, and associated clinical conditions play an important role. Of those fistulas that are going to close, 80 to 90% do so within 4 to 6 weeks of the control of sepsis.

SUMMARY

The infamous reputation of enterocutaneous fistulas is well deserved. Although mortality has been significantly reduced, it remains an undeniable reality in the management of these patients. The successful management of enterocutaneous fistulas hinges on a carefully orchestrated, multidisciplinary approach that utilizes nonoperative and operative strategies in a complementary fashion. Early and aggressive nutritional support plays a significant role in the overall scheme. The primary goal of therapy should be an attempt at spontaneous closure, which is aided by good skin care through sump drainage of fistulas, parenteral nutritional support, aggressive control of intraabdominal sepsis, and careful radiologic definition of the fistula. When it is judged that spontaneous closure is unlikely, a carefully timed operation is called for, usually after 3 to 6 weeks of conservative therapy. Ideally, resection of the involved bowel with end-to-end anastomosis is carried out. Finally, we stress the importance of secure closure of the abdominal wall and the use of a fresh plastic and reconstructive surgery team in difficult cases.

REFERENCES

1. Aguirre, A., Fischer, J. E., and Welch, C. E. The role of surgery and hyperalimentation in therapy of gastrointestinal-cutaneous fistulae. *Ann. Surg.* 180:393, 1974.
2. Chapman, R., Foran, R., and Dunphy, J. E. Management of intestinal fistulas. *Am. J. Surg.* 108:157, 1964.
3. Deitel, M. Nutritional management of external gastrointestinal fistulas. *Can. J. Surg.* 19:505, 1976.
4. Edmunds, L. H., Williams, G. H., and Welch, C. E. External fistulas arising from the gastrointestinal tract. *Ann. Surg.* 152:445, 1960.
5. Himal, H. S., Allard, J. R., Nadeau, J. E., Freeman, J. B., and MacLean, L. D. The importance of adequate nutrition in closure of small intestinal fistulas. *Br. J. Surg.* 61:724, 1974.
6. McPhayden, V. B., Jr., and Dudrick, S. J. Management for gastrointestinal fistulas with parenteral hyperalimentation. *Surgery* 74:100, 1973.
7. Mulvihill, S., Pappas, T. N., Passaro, E., Jr., and Debas, H. T. The use of somatostatin and its analogs in the treatment of surgical disorders. *Surgery* 100:467, 1986.
8. Reber, M. A., Roberts, C., Way, L. W., and Dunphy, J. E. Management of external gastrointestinal fistulas. *Ann. Surg.* 188:460, 1978.
9. Sheldon, G. F., Gardiner, B. N., Way, L. W., and Dunphy, J. E. Management of gastrointestinal fistulas. *Surg. Gynecol. Obstet.* 133:385, 1971.
10. Soeters, P. B., Ebeid, A. M., and Fischer, J.E. Review of 404 patients with gastrointestinal fistulas: Impact of parenteral nutrition. *Ann. Surg.* 190:189, 1979.
11. Thomas, R. J. S., and Rosalion, A. The use of parenteral nutrition in the management of external gastrointestinal tract fistulas. *Aust. N.Z. J. Surg.* 48:535, 1978.

Nutritional Support in Hepatic Failure: The Current Role of Disease-Specific Therapy

Darryl T. Hiyama
Josef E. Fischer

As the field of nutritional support continues to develop, its role in the management of specific disease states also continues to be defined shaped by the critical review of indications for, and the demonstrable efficacy of its use. Nutrition is recognized as an important adjunct in the management of hepatic failure, yet controversy exists as to what role nutritional support currently serves, particularly in relation to the problem of hepatic encephalopathy. The complication of hepatic encephalopathy is an integral aspect of hepatic failure, and imposes severe restrictions on necessary protein administration. In the corresponding chapter in the first edition of this book, it was proposed that the use of branched-chain amino acids (BCAA)-enriched formulations could provide adequate nutritional supplementation in patients with hepatic failure and possibly be useful as a form of therapy in the treatment of hepatic encephalopathy. At that time, only data from animal studies were available. In the decade that has passed, several clinical trials concerning the use of BCAA-enriched formulations in both enteral and parenteral nutritional support have been reported. This chapter focuses on the current status of nutritional support in the management of hepatic failure, with emphasis on the review of the relevant clinical studies.

HEPATIC FAILURE

In humans, the presence of clinical evidence of liver failure represents the loss of 70% of the functional hepatocyte mass. This loss of function may result from one of three disease processes: (1) massive hepatocellular necrosis; (2) portal-systemic shunting of blood and chronic deprivation of substrate; or, more rarely, (3) ultrastructural changes without significant cellular necrosis. The causes of hepatic failure are varied and are discussed in later sections. It is sufficient to note that the common deficit that results from any of the above-mentioned disease processes is a reduction in the number of functioning hepatocytes due to physical destruction, metabolic impairment, or ischemia. In any of the above-mentioned situations, recovery from hepatic failure is dependent on the restoration of cellular function, whether by repletion of hepatocyte mass or via the repair of demaged cellular organelles. Recovery of structural and functional integrity requires adequate calories, protein, and micronutrients. The need for nutritional support becomes evident when these factors cannot be obtained via an oral diet.

From a clinical standpoint, and for the purposes of this discussion, the types of hepatic failure are distinguished by the acuity of the disease. This segregation has significance in terms of the underlying disease process, the incidence and severity of complicating hepatic encephalopathy, and the relative efficacy of nutritional support. There are three variants of hepatic failure in which nutritional support has been applied: (1) acute hepatic failure, (2) chronic hepatic failure, and (3) chronic hepatic failure complicated by acute exacerbation.

ACUTE HEPATIC FAILURE

In the majority of cases, the underlying disease process is one of widespread hepatocellular necrosis. In most instances, the cause is fulminant viral hepatitis; however, several drugs and toxins are known to produce this degree of liver damage (Table 18-1). An alternative form of this disease occurs in Reye's syndrome, acute fatty liver of pregnancy, and acute fatty liver following tetracycline toxicity, in which the clinical presentation is similar but the major histologic change is intracellular fatty infiltration and minimal hepatocyte necrosis [47].

Fulminent hepatic failure is much less common than chronic liver failure, but the clinical course is often dramatic, characterized by an acute onset and rapid deterioration in liver function. Although the affected patients are frequently younger individuals without preexisting liver disease, malnutrition, or com-

Table 18-1. Precipitating Causes of Acute Hepatic Failure

Viral hepatitis
Isoniazid
Para-aminosalicylic acid
Rifampin
Monoamine oxidase inhibitors
Methyldopa
Halothane
Amanita phalloides mushroom toxicity
Chloroform
Carbon tetrachloride
Acetaminophen toxicity
Tetracycline toxicity

comitant medical problems, the prognosis for survival often is guarded.

Several complications can develop and must be considered in the application of nutritional support. From a technical standpoint, coagulation abnormalities may preclude the percutaneous placement of central venous catheters for parenteral nutrition unless exogenous coagulation factors are given to correct deficiencies. Hypervolemia, as evidenced by ascites, and peripheral edema may require judicious fluid management as well as sodium restriction. The development of cerebral edema may also mandate fluid restriction. Hypoglycemia, occasionally heralded by hypothermia (in about 5% of patients) [47], can develop, requiring adequate glucose administration.

The most severe complication of acute hepatic failure is hepatic encephalopathy, and the maximal degree of encephalopathy can be correlated with overall survival [9]. The encephalopathy that accompanies acute failure is rapid in onset, with a brief prodrome. The progression from drowsiness, delirium, and convulsions to deep coma can occur over a short period. Cerebral edema is more likely to develop, and death may result from tentorial herniation. Once coma is present, the prognosis for survival becomes poor. Awakening from coma has been reported, occurring both spontaneously and following therapy [22, 51], but there is little evidence of effective therapy for the coma complicating acute fulminant hepatitis.

Characteristically, the serum amino acid profile (amino-acid-gram) of patients with fulminant hepatic failure reveals a pronounced, generalized elevation, presumably secondary to diffuse cellular destruction [56]. An exception to this trend are the BCAAs, which are not elevated and may be slightly decreased. However, the severity of the hyperaminoacidemia in fulminant hepatic failure precludes the effective use of infusion techniques alone, directed toward the correction of amino acid abnormalities. Normalization of the amino acid profile requires the adjunct use of perfusion or filtration techniques utilizing a polyacrylonitrile membrane or charcoal filter or hemodialysis. Unfortunately, none of these techniques as yet has shown sufficient promise to be adopted for widespread application. Thus, the role of nutritional support in acute (fulminant) hepatic failure is very limited. It may be useful as adjunctive therapy to perfusion and filtration techniques.

CHRONIC HEPATIC FAILURE

Chronic hepatic failure is characterized by the progressive development of hepatic insufficiency. In the United States, this most commonly develops following a long history of ethanol abuse, although it can also develop following viral hepatitis, primary biliary cirrhosis, and a variety of other less common diseases [47]. The classic anatomic correlation for this condition is cirrhosis, and the well-known syndrome of jaundice, ascites, edema, and cachexia is often present. Acute episodes of hepatic failure can be superimposed on a state of chronic hepatic insufficiency. Often these episodes are precipitated by specific, reversible causes: gastrointestinal bleeding, sepsis, or dehydration [16].

The natural history in these patients is often marked by episodes of hepatic encephalopathy, which coincide with acute exacerbations of failure ("acute-on-chronic"

encephalopathy). Milder episodes of encephalopathy and even subclinical episodes are also recognized in "stable" patients with chronic hepatic failure [61]. It is in this area that the majority of clinical experience concerning nutritional support and hepatic failure is currently available.

Pathophysiology of Chronic Hepatic Failure

Under normal circumstances the portal vein provides approximately 80% of the total hepatic blood flow, which is relatively rich in nutrients but somewhat depleted in oxygen. In contrast, the remaining 20% of hepatic blood flow, supplied by the hepatic artery, is rich in oxygen and poor in nutrients. Within the hepatic lobule, flow originates at the periphery, within the portal triad, with blood admixture (portal and systemic) occurring at the level of the hepatic sinusoids. The "composite" blood flows toward the central venule in a centripetal direction, perfusing radially arranged "plates of hepatocytes" (which are a single hepatocyte in thickness) in sequential progression. At the central venule, deoxygenated, nutrient-poor blood is collected and eventually carried to the hepatic veins. It has been suggested that within a given hepatic lobule, there exists a spectrum of metabolic activity. A progression of diminishing activity may be found within a given plate as flow moves centripetally. This would coincide with the perfusion of central hepatocytes with partially deoxygenated and nutrient-depleted blood.

The natural evolution of chronic liver disease (cirrhosis) is marked by a pattern of repeated physiologic insults, cell death followed by regeneration and repair. Distortions in lobular architecture result from the formation of nodules of regenerated hepatocytes surrounded by fibrous scar tissue. These nodules aberrantly derive their blood supply from hepatic arterioles and thus become exquisitely sensitive to changes in hepatic artery blood flow. Dehydration, shock, sepsis, or general anesthesia can rapidly lead to sudden decreases in hepatic artery blood flow and a reduction in hepatic function. The situation forms the basis of the common episodes of acute deterioration of hepatic function observed in cirrhotic patients ("acute-on-chronic" failure) following gastrointestinal bleeding, sepsis, or surgery.

The subsequent development of portal hypertension following cirrhosis may initially be considered a "homeostatic" response to altered lobular perfusion. The perfusion pressure of portal vein blood is gradually elevated to maintain a "normalized" perfusion pattern, to compensate for the increased vascular resistance within the altered hepatic lobule. Eventually, although not inevitably, portal venous pressure exceeds systemic venous pressure, leading to portal-systemic venous shunting through various collaterals whose vascular resistance is less than the scarred liver. This diversion of portal blood flow causes decreased transport of substrate, as well as substances that require metabolism or degradation, to the hepatic parenchyma. Portal-systemic shunting also leads to variceal changes in the esophagogastric and hemorrhoidal venous plexuses, with esophageal varices extremely sensitive to spontaneous rupture and bleeding, especially when large.

The anatomic distortion may also lead to ascites. In cirrhosis, with increased vascular resistance, hepatic lymphatic flow increases, presumably to provide easier egress of plasma rather than through the distorted pathway through the central veins. As hepatic architectural distortion increases secondary to either fibrosis and scarring (chronic cirrhosis) or swelling (fatty infiltration, alcoholic hepatitis), the ability of the liver to export lymph is exceeded by its production and ascites results, usually by the lymph escaping from the surface of the liver into the peritoneal cavity. The accumulation of serum protein, fluid, and electrolytes within the peritoneal cavity decreases intravascular volume, aggravates portal hypertension, and complicates fluid management in these patients.

Malnutrition is commonly found in patients with chronic hepatic failure. While the cachexia associated with cirrhosis obviously contributes to the nutritional status, the pathophysiologic mechanism behind the anorexia has not been defined. The dietary habits of chronic alcoholics have been well documented; they often consist of low protein and a high proportion of carbohydrate (alcohol) calories with deficiencies in macronutrients (zinc, vitamin A, B-complex vitamins, folate, and magnesium) [34].

Metabolic Alterations in Chronic Hepatic Failure

Accelerated catabolism characterizes the net metabolic effect in chronic liver failure. Glucagon levels are probably elevated as a result of release of gluconeogenic amino acids and ammonia, portal-systemic shunting, and impaired degradation [62]. Increased concentrations of ammonia and aromatic amino acids have been demonstrated to stimulate glucagon secretion [69]. In contrast to the hormonal milieu following acute injury, insulin levels are also elevated [65, 66]. However, peripheral insulin resistance is present and effectively reduces the influence of insulin. Thus, it appears that the effective insulin to glucagon ratio is decreased, resulting in net hyperglucagonemia. Contributing to the catabolic state are elevated circulating levels of epinephrine and cortisol [13], probably again due to impaired hepatic deactivation of circulating hormones.

Hepatic and skeletal muscle carbohydrate stores are depleted by accelerated glycogenolysis and inadequate glycogenesis. In response to hyperglucagonemia, hepatic, renal, and intestinal gluconeogenesis is also accelerated. Increased glucose production, in combination with decreased insulin-dependent peripheral cellular uptake of glucose and the decreased insulin-dependent hepatic glycolysis, results in fasting and postprandial hyperglycemia.

Alternative energy sources are recruited to support the catabolic state. Hepatic lipolysis of triglycerides yielding glycerol and free fatty acids is increased. Under normal circumstances, fat, a major energy source, accounts for 75 to 80% of the resting energy expenditure during starvation. However, impaired hepatic metabolism of long-chain free fatty acids to ketone bodies results in the accumulation of short-chain free fatty acids and the reduction in ketone bodies, an important alternative energy source. The impaired utilization of fat limits the provision of exogenous lipid calories in hypercatabolic patients with glucose intolerance. Alterations in fat absorption also occur in up to 50% of cirrhotics, also limiting the enteral administration of fat [24].

Under normal circumstances, following a large protein meal, the BCAAs are largely cleared by the liver. Approximately 60 to 100% of the splanchnic clearance of amino acids is the form of BCAAs. Similarly, under the conditions of nitrogen equilibrium, 60 to 100% of the peripheral nitrogen exchange is in the form of BCAAs, which undergo direct oxidation in cardiac and skeletal muscle or are utilized for protein synthesis [72]. The peripheral utilization (skeletal muscle) of BCAAs accounts for 6 to 7% of energy needs in the healthy individual. Under conditions of stress, BCAA metabolism may theoretically contribute as much as 25 to 30% of energy requirements, and the increased oxidation of these amino acids leads to a significant reduction in the plasma BCAA levels [21, 48, 63]. In addition, in conditions of increased insulin resistance and catabolism, BCAAs may play a regulatory role in the efflux of other amino acids across the myocyte membrane [1, 19, 30]. Decreases in plasma BCAA concentrations may thus lead to impaired protein synthesis (in skeletal muscle) and, as will be subsequently detailed, also contribute to the development of hepatic encephalopathy.

Alterations in nitrogen metabolism are probably the most prominent biochemical changes in chronic hepatic failure. Hyperammonemia is common and probably results from several causes: (1) active amino acid deamination and gluconeogenesis in intestine and muscle, (2) intraluminal bacterial degradation of protein and absorption of ammonia in gut, (3) impaired or inadequate ureagenesis, and (4) inadequate delivery to the liver

due to portal-systemic shunting. While hyperamonemia is a prominent metabolic finding, its significance as the sole cause of hepatic encephalopathy is doubtful (see Hepatic Encephalopathy below).

The aromatic amino acids (AAAs)—phenylalanine, tyrosine, and free tryptophan—are notably elevated in cirrhosis [1, 19, 30, 32, 33, 64, 74]. In part, this can be attributed to increased release into the circulation by muscle proteolysis and decreased incorporation into synthesized proteins. However, it is most likely that the major cause is a decreased clearance of ammonia by the liver. Under normal circumstances, the AAAs, methionine, glutamine, asparagine, and histidine all undergo 80 to 100% first-pass hepatic clearance. In contrast, other amino acids, such as alanine, lysine, proline, and arginine, undergo 20 to 40% hepatic clearance. It would seem logical that those amino acids subject to high clearance would be most affected by portal-systemic shunting.

Tryptophan, in contrast to the other AAAs, is unique in being albumin-bound [4]. In hepatic failure, a normal plasma concentration of tryptophan may not truly reflect the elevation of free tryptophan, which is most available for transport into the brain and which is the significant fraction in terms of hepatic encephalopathy [10, 50, 59]. Several factors that may contribute to elevations in the free fraction include hypoalbuminemia, competitive displacement by nonesterified (free) fatty acids, and hyperbilirubinemia [50].

The amino acid disturbances in chronic hepatic failure are thus characterized by elevated levels of phenylalanine, tyrosine, free (but not necessarily total) tryptophan, methionine, glutamine, as well as asparagine and histidine, and by lowered levels of BCAAs. Clinically, it is useful to describe this relationship in terms of plasma molar ratios of BCAAs to AAAs: [(valine) + (leucine) + (isoleucine)] / [(phenylalanine) + (tyrosine)]; some have included tryptophan. Characteristic amino acid patterns have been described (Table 18-2). In hepatic failure, a BCAA/AAA molar ratio of 1.4 to 2.0 usually represents significant liver disease, and a ratio of 1.0 or

Table 18-2.   Characteristic Plasma Amino Acid Alterations in Selected Disease and Metabolic Conditions

| Condition | Plasma Amino Acid Profile | |
	Increased	Decreased
Hepatic failure	Phenylalanine,[a] tyrosine,[a] tryptophan,[a] methionine, glutamate, aspartate, histidine	Leucine,[b] isoleucine,[b] valine[b]
Malnutrition	Nonessential amino acids, tyrosine,[a] glycine	Total essential amino acids (especially leucine,[b] isoleucine,[b] valine[b]), lysine
Renal failure	—	Valine, leucine,[b] isoleucine,[b] tryptophan,[b] histidine
Sepsis	Leucine,[b] isoleucine,[b] valine[b] (late stages of sepsis)[c]	Leucine,[b] isoleucine,[b] valine[b] (early stages of sepsis)

[a] Aromatic amino acid.
[b] Branched-chain amino acid.
[c] In late sepsis with hepatic impairment, phenylalanine, tyrosine, free tryptophan, methionine cysteine, and taurine are increased. Arginine is reduced.
From Shronts, E., Teasley, K. M., Thoele, S. L., and Cerra, F. B. Nutrition support of the adult liver transplant candidate. *J. Am. Diet. Assoc.* 87:441, 1987.

less usually correlates with the presence of hepatic encephalopathy.

HEPATIC ENCEPHALOPATHY

It is well known that a variety of neurologic and behavioral disturbances can accompany liver disease and especially hepatic failure. Collectively, these syndromes have been referred to using a variety of terms such as hepatic encephalopathy, portal-systemic encephalopathy, or hepatic coma. In reality, a spectrum of syndromes exists, with some variation according to the etiology of hepatic dysfunction. In general, syndromes of portal-systemic encephalopathy can be distinguished between those that accompany acute fulminant hepatitis and those associated with chronic liver disease.

As noted above, the course of encephalopathy following fulminant hepatic failure is characterized by a short prodrome, rapid onset, and swift progression of behavioral changes from drowsiness to deep coma. Often this progression can occur within a short period of time, less than 24 hours.

In contrast, the syndrome accompanying chronic liver disease is marked by episodes of encephalopathy representing acute exacerbations often precipitated by an identifiable and reversible cause, with seeming complete recovery between episodes. In a study of 100 episodes of hepatic coma, the principal causes (in order of occurrence) were azotemia, injudicious sedation, tranquilizers, gastrointestinal hemorrhage, hypokalemia, alkalosis, and protein intoxication [16]. The progression in the severity of symptoms is much slower and often (initially) indolent. During the prodrome, euphoria or depression may be evident, along with anorexia, changes in day and night rhythm, apathy, and impairment in judgment. These subtle changes in themselves may be socially disruptive or cause endangerment to safety or property. Progressive symptomatology consists of increasing depression and impaired neurologic function. Eventually, fine-motor and then gross-motor function is lost, followed by unconsciousness [18].

Previously it was thought that during the intervals between episodes of acute-on-chronic encephalopathy, cerebral function was normal. Sophisticated psychological measurements manifest subtle alterations in function such as a lack of awareness to surroundings, decreased responsiveness to noxious stimuli, and poor reaction time [18]. It is thought that the etiology of these episodes of subclinical encephalopathy may be similar to that seen in acute-on-chronic encephalopathy.

Encephalopathy is a severe complication of hepatic failure. Impaired judgment and motor skills can place the patient at risk of self-injury or financial ruin. The effects of the progressive loss of cerebral function are obvious. Altered mental status can lead to an increased risk of gastric aspiration; immobility, atelectasis, and pneumonia may also result. While protein administration is critical for hepatocellular regeneration and support of body function, the development of protein intolerance (encephalopathy) imposes dietary restrictions. Much of current disease-specific nutritional support in this area is focused on this problem.

Etiology of Hepatic Encephalopathy

Several theories of the causation of hepatic encephalopathy have been offered. The most conventional of these indict ammonia as a direct cerebral toxin. While it is clear that patients with hepatic disease are especially sensitive to the cerebral effects of ammonia [52], it is evident that it is not the only etiologic factor. The correlation of venous ammonia levels with the degree of encephalopathy is poor, and only slightly better with arterial specimens [70]. Further, the cerebral uptake of ammonia has not been demonstrated in severe coma, and the site of ammonia toxicity within the brain does not correspond with those regions thought to be involved in hepatic encephalopathy.

Other investigators have implicated short-chain fatty acids as the etiologic factor. These are found in increased concentrations both in the blood and in the cerebrospinal fluid (CSF) of patients with hepatic encephalopathy [8, 71]. However, in another study, short-chain fatty acids were administered to patients with cirrhosis in large doses without toxic effects [43].

Zieve et al. [75, 76] proposed that a syner-gistic relationship exists between ammonia, methanethiols, and fatty acids. While coma can be produced in normal animals by infusing ammonia salts with fatty acids, the doses of ammonia are massive, much higher than those observed in most patients with encephalopathy. The major problems with this hypothesis are the poor correlation of methanethiol levels with the degree of cerebral dysfunction, and the methodology used to measure these substances.

A more recent hypothesis proposes that gamma-aminobutyric acid (GABA), an inhibitory neurotransmitter, is responsible for the symptomatology of hepatic coma [60]. However, the concentrations of GABA in the brains of rats [3] and dogs [53] with hepatic coma or after ammonia intoxication [60] were not increased, nor is there any difference in CSF concentrations of GABA in patients with or without hepatic coma [44]. More recent work has hypothesized an up-regulation of $GABA_A$ receptors, but these are normal in hepatic coma [5].

The amino acid and neurotransmitter theory and, later, the unified theory of hepatic encephalopathy were developed in an attempt to integrate the various findings in cirrhotic patients with encephalopathy. An in-depth discussion of these concepts is beyond the scope of this chapter, and the interested reader is referred to the references. The following is a brief review.

Amino Acid and Neurotransmitter Hypothesis

Under the conditions of chronic hepatic failure, characterized by catabolism and energy deficiency (as discussed above), there is a significant breakdown of lean body mass. The BCAAs released are utilized as a peripheral energy source. Plasma levels of AAAs along with ammonia further stimulate glucagon secretion, perpetuating the cycle. Both BCAAs and AAAs share a common pathway (system L) across the blood-brain barrier and compete for transport into the CNS. Since plasma levels of BCAAs are reduced, the AAAs are preferentially transported and accumulate in the brain. Increased free-tryptophan levels in the plasma also lead to increased transport into the brain. Ammonia indirectly increases this process by crossing the blood-brain barrier and, with glutamic acid, being synthesized into glutamine, probably largely in the glia. Glutamine, in turn, is exchanged across the blood-brain barrier for the large neutral amino acid group, which by plasma concentrations are more likely to include AAAs than under normal circumstances. Studies in both animals and humans have shown elevated CNS concentrations of AAAs and their aminergic products as well as glutamine, methionine, and histidine. In addition, there is good correlation between CSF levels of octopamine, a weak or "false" neurotransmitter product of phenylalanine and tyrosine, and CSF glutamine levels and the degree of encephalopathy [36, 39, 46, 57].

Increased CNS levels of phenylalanine and tyrosine can result in the formation of weak or "false" neurotransmitters, normally occurring transmitters whose actions are weaker or different than the catecholamines, norepinephrine and dopamine, normally present in much greater abundance, and these weak or false neurotransmitters are thought to compete with normal neurotransmitters for binding sites. Tryptophan gives rise to 5-hydroxytryptamine (serotonin), a true transmitter, whose actions are thought to increase sleep or lethargy, or be inhibitory. Increased free (unbound) tryptophan increases CNS levels of tryptophan and thereby serotonin. Excess tyrosine is converted to tyramine and then to octopamine. Phenylalanine is converted into phenylethylamine and then to phenylethanolamine. All agree that brain norepinephrine levels are decreased in hepatic coma. This may occur in two ways: Phenylalanine and tyrosine may block formation of dopamine and norepinephrine by competing for enzyme activity, or octopamine may inhibit dopamine B-oxidase. Alternatively, tyramine, octopamine, phenylethanolamine, and so on are good releasers of norepinephrine. Tryptophan is converted to serotonin, an inhibitory neurotransmitter. The general effect of these substances is to impair excitatory stimulation of various brain regions, increase inhibitory influences, and impair normal neurotransmission [36, 39, 46, 57].

BASIS FOR THEORY

Based on the above information, it appeared logical that the manipulation of the plasma and hence brain amino acid concentrations would serve as primary treatment for hepatic encephalopathy. With normal hepatic function, plasma concentrations of AAAs are regulated independent of exogenous intake [55]. Under conditions of impaired hepatic function, however, exogenous intake (parenteral or enteral) influences plasma levels of AAAs, as the liver can no longer do so [55]. This suggests that one method of manipulation would be the regulation of exogenous intake.

Another observation made in rats following portacaval shunting showed that plasma and brain AAA concentrations and brain octopamine levels varied inversely with the presence or absence of positive nitrogen balance. In animals converted to anabolism, plasma phenylalanine and tyrosine and brain tyrosine and octopamine levels were decreased [55]. It was suggested that the AAAs are reduced by incorporation into intracellular protein synthesis. It has been noted that even modest protein intake (20–40 g/day) is preferable to the traditional absolute protein restriction [2], as there is less endogeneous protein breakdown. Total restriction of protein intake is in reality a high protein diet.

The third influence on the plasma and brain levels of AAAs is the plasma concentration of BCAA. The administration of small doses of equimolar concentrations of the BCAA to rats with portacaval shunts decreased both plasma and brain tyrosine levels. This was interpreted as showing that BCAAs may decrease skeletal muscle breakdown and decrease the release of AAAs, as well as decreasing brain AAA levels by increased competition for transport [15].

Based on the above and other information, BCAA-enriched formulations were developed to allow adequate protein and caloric supplementation to induce anabolism while simultaneously ameliorating or eliminating hepatic encephalopathy. There are several theoretic advantages to the use of such formulations in patients with liver disease:

1. BCAAs are a useful energy source. Patients with hepatic encephalopathy begin with decreased stores of glycogen and fat reserves. They are highly catabolic and glucose intolerant, and ketogenesis and the utilization of fatty acids are probably decreased because of impairment of the hepatic mechanism by which ketone bodies are produced from fatty acids. Although under normal circumstances, the BCAAs comprise only about 6 to 7% of the energy needs, on a theoretic basis, in hepatic failure the BCAAs could conceivably supply over 30% of the energy needs since the BCAAs may be utilized directly by muscle, heart, liver, and brain.
2. BCAAs decrease the efflux of other amino acids through the myocyte membrane, thus decreasing the AAAs in the circulation.
3. In humans, leucine decreases muscle proteolysis and increases muscle protein synthesis. The effect on proteolysis is probably a characteristic of alpha-keto-isocaproate, the keto derivative of leucine.
4. Hepatic protein synthesis is apparently increased by all amino acids in humans. There is some evidence in humans that leucine is more capable of sustaining plasma levels of hepatic proteins [4].
5. Administration of BCAAs normalizes the plasma amino acid pattern secondary to: (a) decreased muscle breakdown; and (b) increased protein synthesis, thus utilizing the AAAs. A caloric source of glucose appears to be better in this particular regard than fat, perhaps because of the influence of insulin [23].
6. The large neutral amino acids including the AAAs phenylalanine, tyrosine, methionine, histidine, and to some extent tryptophan, and the BCAAs all compete for entry through system L across the blood-brain barrier. Under normal circumstances, the BCAAs represent the bulk of the competition. Thus, increasing the BCAAs in the plasma, in addition to lowering plasma AAA levels, prevents their penetration across the brain by direct competition for the neutral amino acids via system L.
7. In hepatectomized animals, the administration of BCAAs increases reduced brain norepinephrine levels in three out of the seven regions [28].
8. On a theoretic basis, peripheral plasma catecholamine synthesis will be normalized by having a more normal precursor amino acid pool.
9. BCAAs increase the metabolism of ammonia by muscle. The BCAAs probably donate the amino group for glutamine synthesis.

Furthermore, there is some evidence suggesting that BCAA-enriched amino acid solutions are more supportive of hepatic protein synthesis than are standard solutions. The factors that may contribute to control of hepatic regeneration are given in Figure 18-1. Many of these factors are permissive. Nutrition is the one factor physicians can influence rather easily. Thus, on this basis alone, a BCAA-enriched amino acid solution might be more useful [54].

CLINICAL STUDIES

It must be noted that a significant amount of controversy still exists concerning the etiology of hepatic encephalopathy. However, BCAA-enriched formulations, developed on the basis of one of these hypotheses, has been shown to be at least as efficacious as standard therapy directed toward a reduction in blood ammonia level, according to the ammonia hypothesis, a classic toxic hypothesis.

A number of uncontrolled anecdotal studies were performed using BCAA-enriched solutions and hypertonic dextrose in patients with liver disease [6, 11, 20, 37, 49, 68]. The conclusions drawn from these studies were:

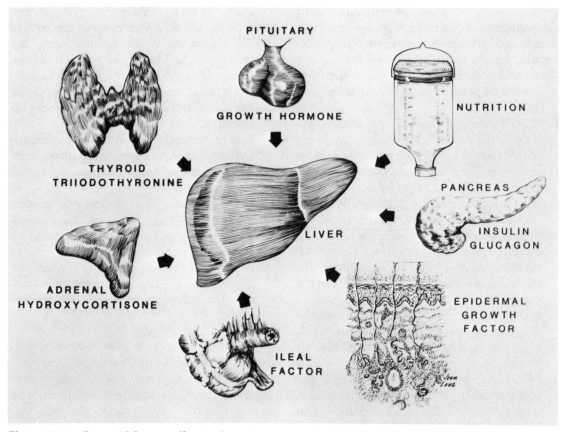

Figure 18-1.   Potential factors affecting hepatic regeneration, including the unknown ileal factor.

1. In patients intolerant of standard solutions, infusions of up to 125 g/day of BCAA-enriched solution are well tolerated.
2. In many if not most instances, arousal from hepatic encephalopathy accompanies the infusion.
3. In patients with cirrhosis and acute-on-chronic encephalopathy, the use of 80 g/day of a 35% BCAA-enriched mixture is associated with both arousal and nitrogen equilibrium as well as normalization of the plasma amino acid pattern.

These initial studies stimulated a significant volume of clinical research into the use of mixtures containing increased proportions of BCAAs and relative deficiencies of AAAs. An analysis of the results is facilitated by considering the type of encephalopathy being treated: (1) subclinical (latent) encepha-

lopathy, (2) chronic encephalopathy, and (3) acute hepatic encephalopathy (with cirrhosis).

Subclinical Encephalopathy

Only one clinical trial has been performed in this area to date. Egberts et al. [12], in a double-blind crossover study, examined a group of 22 patients with cirrhosis but without previous history of encephalopathy (grade 0). The presence of subclinical encephalopathy was diagnosed by extensive psychometric testing. A diet of 35 kcal/kg/day containing 1 g of protein/kg/day was provided. BCAAs (leucine 43%, valine 28.5%, isoleucine 28.5%) or casein in a dose of 0.25 g/kg/day were subsequently given in crossover fashion. Nitrogen balance was positive for both groups, although a larger increase was noted in those patients receiving BCAAs.

Further, during BCAA treatment, serum ammonia concentration tended to decrease, and significant improvements in psychomotor function, attention, and practical intelligence were noted. These studies may have more than theoretic significance, as patients with latent subclinical encephalopathy may be unable to drive because of poor reaction times, and so on. Treatment with BCAAs may improve patients' psychometric testing sufficiently to enable them to drive safely.

Chronic Encephalopathy

Eriksson et al. [14] performed a double-blind, randomized, crossover trial with seven patients with cirrhosis and encephalopathy (grade 1–2) on entry. Only four of seven patients were receiving protein restriction on entrance into the study. A defined diet of 40 to 100 g/day of dietary protein was provided. The test group received supplemental 30 g of mixed BCAAs, while the control group received a placebo. In addition, four patients in the control group also received lactulose. After 14 days of treatment, no improvement in encephalopathy was reported, although a careful examination of the results showed improvement in practical intelligence in the test group receiving BCAAs, and 30 g of protein equivalent was tolerated, thus improving nutritional status.

McGhee et al. [40], in a similar study with four patients, compared a casein diet with 50 g of protein to a study diet containing 20 g of casein and 30 g of BCAAs (HepaticAid). While positive nitrogen balance was achieved, no significant improvement in encephalopathy was reported.

Both these studies are glaring examples of a statistical type II error, that is, with too few patients to achieve a valid distinction *even if it were present*. The fact that the two groups were no different does not mean they were the same. A valid difference may not have been detected given the miniscule number of patients.

In contrast, Horst et al. [31], in a double-blind randomized study followed 37 patients with encephalopathy (grade 0–1) for 4 weeks in a more carefully controlled study. Both the control and the test groups were initiated on a 20-g protein diet during the first week. At 1-week intervals dietary protein was increased by 20 g, with the test group receiving the additional protein as BCAAs (HepaticAid). By week 4, both groups were receiving 80 g/day of protein and were in positive nitrogen balance. The frequency of encephalopathy was found to be significantly higher in the control group than in the test group.

If the results from the studies performed by Horst et al. [31] and Egberts et al. [12] are confirmed, then BCAA-enriched formulations may also be utilized, in addition to primary therapy for encephalopathy, as a safer means of improving the long-term nutritional status in patients with cirrhosis. Marchesini et al. published a carefully done long-term study in which 3.6 g BCAA/10 kg/day were randomized against chronic encephalopathy patients receiving isonitrogenous casein. There was a statistically significant improvement in the BCAA group as compared with the casein group.

Acute Encephalopathy (With Cirrhosis)

Despite a number of clinical trials studying the efficacy of parenterally administered BCAA-enriched solutions, only seven have been performed in an appropriate prospective and randomized fashion.

Rossi-Fanelli et al. [58] reported a multicenter trial in which 40 patients with acute encephalopathy or chronic recurrent encephalopathy (grade 3–4) were randomized to receive either hypertonic 20% dextrose and lactulose or 57 g of BCAAs in an isocaloric amount of hypertonic dextrose. Three patients failed to complete the trial and there was no difference in survival between the two groups. After 2 days of treatment, arousal from encephalopathy was noted in 70% of the test patients versus 49% of the control subjects. This difference was close to, but did not achieve, statistical significance.

Fiaccadori et al. [17], in an Italian trial, divided patients into three groups. The control group received lactulose alone, while the second group received a BCAA-enriched formulation (HepatAmine) and hypertonic dextrose. The third group received both forms of therapy. Arousal was significantly higher in both groups receiving BCAA-enriched formulations compared to the group receiving lactulose alone. More important, there were no deaths in the group receiving both forms of therapy, one death in the group receiving the BCAA-enriched mixture and dextrose, and five deaths in the group treated with lactulose alone. These results were statistically significant.

The largest group studied to date was in the U.S. Multicenter Trial reported by Cerra et al. [7]. Eighty patients from eight centers with grade 2 to 4 encephalopathy by clinical and EEG criteria were entered into the study following unresponsiveness to conventional therapy. Patients were randomized to receive either a 35% solution enriched with BCAAs and deficient in AAAs and hypertonic dextrose (25 kcal/kg/day) or neomycin and an isocaloric amount of hypertonic dextrose. The treatment period was 4 to 14 days, and the rate of arousal from encephalopathy was followed. A significantly more rapid rate of arousal was noted in the BCAA-treated group (77%) versus controls (45%) for days 1 and 2 of the study. In addition, a significant improvement in nitrogen balance was noted in the BCAA-treated group. Most striking is the difference in survival: The overall survival rate was 65% in the BCAA-treated group, significantly better than the 37% in controls, and for those patients completing the study was 83% in the BCAA-treated group versus 45% in the control group.

Another study using HepatAmine was performed by Strauss et al. [67] in a Brazilian multicenter trial. Thirty-two patients were enrolled and received either HepatAmine and hypertonic dextrose, or neomycin and isocaloric dextrose. While arousal appeared more rapid (not statistically significant) in the BCAA-treated group, no difference in survival rates was noted. Gluud et al. [25] con-

ducted a similar multicenter trial in Denmark, with similar results.

Wahren et al. [73], in a multicenter trial in Sweden and France, studied 50 patients with encephalopathy (grade 2–4) who were previously treated with conventional therapy. The duration of previous treatment was 23.5 ± 35 hours for the test group and 25.5 ± 30 hours for the control group, the wide variation suggesting long periods of prior therapy for some patients. The test group received a BCAA-enriched formulation containing 70% leucine, 20% valine, and 11% isoleucine, a lethal combination that depressed other plasma amino acids below a safe level to support protein synthesis. Both groups received isocaloric amounts (30 kcal/kg/day) of glucose and fat mixtures (50% fat). The control group did not receive lactulose. No statistically significant difference in arousal was reported. Mortality at 5 days of treatment was 40% in the BCAA-treated group and 20% in controls, but 20% in both groups if patients who died of gastrointestinal bleeding (which was supposedly excluded) are eliminated, and 70% in both groups at 25 days. Both differences were not statistically significant. The control group was significantly younger (52 years versus 59 years) despite randomization.

Michel et al. [42] compared a standard amino acid formulation containing 20% BCAAs and a high concentration of arginine and a formulation containing 35% BCAAs. Both groups received approximately 67% of calories as fat, and neither group received additional conventional therapy. No difference in arousal between the two groups was noted. Nitrogen balance was not reported.

It is somewhat difficult to make an appropriate analysis of the data, since there are marked differences between studies in terms of type of BCAA formulation used, type and number of nonprotein calories administered, and the use of cathartics. At best, what can be concluded is that the use of BCAAs in hepatic encephalopathy, when used with hypertonic dextrose as the energy source, can result in clinical improvement at least equal to that obtained using conventional therapy. This is true even in patients resistant to standard therapy. In addition, there is a possibility that overall patient survival can also be improved, although this remains to be confirmed. Naylor et al. [45], by the techniques of meta-analysis, reached these same conclusions.

Acute Fulminant Hepatitis

There are fewer data on acute fulminant hepatitis. A few anecdotal studies reported improvement in encephalopathy in patients treated with amino acid solutions enriched with BCAAs and deficient in AAAs.

ALTERNATIVE FORMS OF NUTRITIONAL THERAPY

In a series of patients with chronic hepatic encephalopathy, protein tolerance was increased for long periods of time when patients were fed a mixture of the keto-analogues of five essential amino acids and four nonessential amino acids [38]. Resolution of encephalopathy was observed in some patients in an unpredictable fashion. While it was thought that ammonia may have been reduced by amination of the keto-acid to form the amino acid, glutamine appears to be the nitrogen donor [38]. An alternative beneficial effect may be reduced muscle catabolism. A subsequent study by Herlong et al. [29] compared the effects of administration of the ornithine salts of the keto-analogues of the BCAAs with a small dose of BCAAs. While both groups were improved, greater improvement in encephalopathy was noted in the group receiving the ornithine salts, possibly due to a reduction in blood ammonia levels. Further work in this area is needed.

Recent clinical trials suggested that vegetable protein may be better tolerated (fewer episodes of encephalopathy) in patients with cirrhosis [26, 27, 35]. The mechanism of action is not clear, since neither ammonia nor plasma amino acid levels are markedly altered, and few data are available concerning the CSF levels of ammonia, amino acids, and glutamine. In a study involving five patients,

plasma levels of tyrosine decreased in patients receiving a vegetable protein diet compared to a group fed a meat diet [35]. Flatulence appears to be a major problem with this diet, as is long-term compliance due to the monotony of the diet.

SUMMARY

Hepatic failure remains a challenging clinical problem, where therapy is largely limited to supportive measures while awaiting regeneration and recovery of function. Nutritional support plays a key role in management of this disease. The most progress has been achieved in the treatment of patients with chronic liver disease. Nutritional support in this area is disease specific and directed toward the provision of adequate calories and protein to support anabolism and intracellular protein synthesis, while preventing or eliminating development of hepatic encephalopathy. The use of oral BCAA supplements in preventing and treating chronic encephalopathy is promising. The clinical experience of similar formulations for parenteral use in treating acute-on-chronic encephalopathy has demonstrated efficacy, comparable to standard therapy, and may improve chance of survival. The clinical use of nutritional support in hepatic failure should be in conjunction with standard forms of therapy.

REFERENCES

1. Aguirre, A., Yoshimura, N., Westman, T., and Fischer, J. E. Plasma amino acids in dogs with two experimental forms of liver damage. *J. Surg. Res.* 16:339, 1974.
2. Anonymous. Diet and hepatic encephalopathy. (Editorial) *Lancet* 1:625, 1983.
3. Biebuyck, J., Funovics, J., Dedrick, D. F., Scherer, Y. D., and Fischer, J. E. Neurochemistry of hepatic coma: Alterations in putative neurotransmitter amino acids. In R. Williams and I. M. Murray-Lyon (eds.), *Artificial Liver Support*. London: Pitman Medical, 1975, P. 51.
4. Bower, R. H., and Fischer, J. E. Hepatic indications for parenteral nutrition. In J. L. Rombeau and M. D. Caldwell (eds.), *Clinical Nutrition*. Vol. 2: Parenteral Nutrition. Philadelphia: W. B. Saunders, 1986, P. 602.
5. Butterworth, R. F., Lavoie, J., Giguere, J. F., and Pomier-Layrargues, G. Affinities and den-

sities of high-affinity [³H]muscimol (GABA-A) binding sites and of central benzodiazepine receptors are unchanged in autopsied brain tissue from cirrhotic patients with hepatic encephalopathy. *Hepatology* 8:1084, 1988.

6. Capocaccia, L., Calcaterra, V., Cangiano, C., et al. Therapeutic effect of branched chain amino acids in hepatic encephalopathy: A preliminary study. In M. J. Orloff, S. Stippa, and V. Ziparo (eds.), *Medical and Surgical Problems of Portal Hypertension.* New York: Academic Press, 1979. P. 239.

7. Cerra, F. B., Cheung, N. K., Fischer, J. E., et al. Disease-specific amino acid infusion (FO80) in hepatic encephalopathy: A prospective, randomized, double-blind, controlled trial. *J. Parenter. Enter. Nutr.* 9:288, 1985.

8. Chen, S., Mahadevan, V., and Zieve, L. Volatile fatty acids in the breath of patients with cirrhosis of the liver. *J. Lab. Clin. Med.* 75:622, 1970.

9. Conn, H. O. Cirrhosis. In L. Schiff and E. R. Schiff (eds.), *Diseases of the Liver.* Philadelphia: J. B. Lippincott, 1982, P. 947.

10. Cummings, M. G., James, J. H., Soeters, P. B., Keane, J. M., Foster, J., and Fischer, J. E. Regional brain study of indoleamine metabolism in the rat in acute hepatic failure. *J. Neurochem.* 27:741, 1976.

11. Delafosse, B., Bouletreau, P., and Motin, J. Variation des acides amines plasmatiques au cours des hèpatites graves avec encephalopathie. *Nouv. Presse Med.* 6:1207, 1977.

12. Egberts, E. H., Schomerus, H., Hamster, W., and Jurgens, P. Effective treatment of latent porto-systemic encephalopathy with oral branched chain amino acids. In L. Capococcia, J. E. Fischer, and F. Rossi-Fanelli (eds.), *Hepatic Encephalopathy in Chronic Liver Failure.* New York: Plenum Press, 1984. P. 351.

13. Eigler, N., Sacca, L., and Sherwin, R. S. Synergistic interactions of physiologic increments of glucagon, epinephrine, and cortisol in the dog: A model for stress-induced hyperglycemia. *J. Clin. Invest.* 63:114, 1979.

14. Eriksson, L. S., Persson, A., and Wahren, J. Branched chain amino acids in the treatment of chronic hepatic encephalopathy. *Gut* 23:801, 1982.

15. Escourrou, J., James, J. H., Hodgman, J. M., and Fischer, J. E. Effect of branched chain amino acids on plasma and brain amino acids and brain neurotransmitters. *Gastroenterology* 71:904, 1976.

16. Fessel, J. M., and Conn, H. O. An analysis of the causes and prevention of hepatic coma. *Gastroenterology* 62:191, 1972.

17. Fiaccadori, F., Ghinelli, F., Pedretti G., et al. Branched chain amino acid enriched solutions in the treatment of hepatic encephalopathy: A

controlled trial. In L. Capocaccia, J. E. Fischer, and F. Rossi-Fanelli (eds.), *Hepatic Encephalopathy in Chronic Liver Failure.* New York: Plenum Press, 1984. P. 323.

18. Fischer, J. E. Portal systemic encephalopathy. In R. Wright, G. H. Millward-Sadler, K. G. M. M. Alberti, and S. Karran (eds.), *Liver and Biliary Disease* (2nd ed.). London: W. B. Saunders, 1985. P. 1245.

19. Fischer, J. E., Yoshimura, N., James, J. H., Cummings, M. G., Abel, R. M., and Deindoerfer, F. Plasma amino acids in patients with hepatic encephalopathy: Effects of amino acid infusions. *Am. J. Surg.* 127:40, 1974.

20. Freund, H. R., Dienstag, J., Lehrich, F., et al. Infusion of BCAA solution in patients with hepatic encephalopathy. *Ann. Surg.* 196:209, 1982.

21. Fulkes, R. M., Li, J. B., and Goldberg, A. L. Effect of insulin, glucose and amino acids on protein turnover in rat diaphragm. *J. Biol. Chem.* 250:280, 1975.

22. Gazzard, B. G., Portmann, B., Weston, M. J., et al. Charcoal hemoperfusion in the treatment of fulminant hepatic failure. *Lancet* 1:1301, 1974.

23. Gelfand, R. A., Hendler, R. G., and Sherwin, R. S. Dietary carbohydrate and metabolism of ingested protein. *Lancet* 1:65, 1979.

24. Gitlin, N., and Heyman, M. B. Nutritional support in advanced liver disease. *Nutr. Supp. Serv.* 4:14, 1984.

25. Gluud, C., Dejgaard, A., Hardt, F., et al., and the Copenhagen Coma Group. Preliminary results of treatment with balanced amino acid infusion in patients with hepatic encephalopathy. *Scand. J. Gastroenterol. Suppl.* 18:19, 1983.

26. Greenberger, N. J., Carley, J. E., and Schenker, S. Diet therapy of chronic hepatic encephalopathy (CHE): Role of vegetable protein and carbohydrate loading. *Gastroenterology* 69:825, 1976.

27. Greenberger, N. J., Carley, J. E., Schenker, S., Bettinger, I., Stamnes, C., and Beyer, P. Effects of vegetable and animal protein diets in chronic hepatic encephalopathy. *Am. J. Dig. Dis.* 22:845, 1977.

28. Herlin, P. M., James, J. H., Nachbauer, C. A., and Fischer, J. E. Effect of total hepatectomy and administration of branched chain amino acids on regional norepinephrine, dopamine, and amino acids in rat brain. *Ann. Surg.* 198:172, 1983.

29. Herlong, H. F., Maddrey, W. C., and Walser, M. Ornithine salts of branched chain ketoacids in portal systemic encephalopathy. *Ann. Intern. Med.* 93:545, 1980.

30. Higashi, T., Watanabe, A., Hayashi, S., Obata, T., Tanei, N., and Nagashima, H. Effect of branched chain acid infusion on alter-

ations in CSF neutral amino acids and their transport across the blood-brain barrier in hepatic encephalopathy. In M. Walser and R. Williamson (eds.), *Metabolism and Clinical Implications of Branched Chain and Ketoacids*. New York: Elsevier North-Holland, 1981. P. 465.

31. Horst, D., Grace, N., Conn, H. O., et al. Comparison of dietary protein with an oral branched chain-enriched amino acid supplement in chronic portal-systemic encephalopathy: A randomized controlled trial. *Hepatology* 4:279, 1984.

32. Iber, F. L., Rosen, H., Levenson, S. M., and Chalmers, T. C. The plasma amino acids in patients with liver failure. *J. Lab. Clin. Med.* 50:417, 1957.

33. Iob, V., Mattson, W. J., Jr., Sloan, M., Coon, W. W., Turcotte, J. G., and Child, C. G. Alterations in plasma-free amino acids in dogs with hepatic insufficiency. *Surg. Gynecol. Obstet.* 130:794, 1970.

34. Isselbacher, K. J. Disturbances of bilirubin metabolism. In K. J. Isselbacher, R. D. Adams, E. Braunwald, R. G. Petersdorf, and J. D. Wilson (eds.), *Harrison's Principles of Internal Medicine* (9th ed.). New York: McGraw-Hill, 1980. P. 1454.

35. Jeppsson, B., Kjallman, A., Aslund, U., Alwmark, A., Gullstrand, P., and Joelsson, B. Effect of vegan and meat protein diets in mild chronic portal systemic encephalopathy. In L. Capococcia, J. E. Fischer, and F. Rossi-Fanelli (eds.), *Hepatic Encephalopathy in Chronic Liver Failure*. New York: Plenum Press, 1984. P. 359.

36. Lam, K. C., Tall, A. R., Goldstein, G. B., and Mistilis, S. P. Role of a false neurotransmitter, octopamine, in the pathogenesis of hepatic and renal encephalopathy. *Scand. J. Gastroenterol.* 8:465, 1973.

37. Leon, I. M., Martinez, J. L., Martin, P. M., Dorado-Pombo, M. S., Leon, P. B., and Perez, A. S. Parenteral nutrition in patients with hepatic encephalopathy: Preliminary considerations in 10 treated cases. *Rev. Clin. Esp.* 151:129, 1978.

38. Maddrey, W. C., Weber, F. L., Coulter, A. W., and Walser, M. Effects of ketoanalogues of essential amino acids in portal systemic encephalopathy. *Gastroenterology* 71:190, 1976.

39. Manghani, K. K., Lunzer, M. R., Billing, B. H., and Sherlock, S. Urinary and serum octopamine in patients with portal systemic encephalopathy. *Gastroenterology* 71:190, 1975.

40. McGhee, A., Henderson, J. M., Millikan, W. J., et al. Comparison of the effects of Hepatic-Aid and a casein modular diet on encephalopathy, plasma amino acids, and nitrogen balance in cirrhotic patients. *Ann. Surg.* 197:288, 1983.

41. McMenamy, R. H., and Oncley, J. L. The specific binding of L-tryptophan to serum albumin. *J. Biol. Chem.* 233:1436, 1958.

42. Michel, H., Pomier-Layrargues, G., Duhamel, O., Lacombe, B., Cuilleret, G., and Bellet, H. Intravenous infusion of ordinary and modified amino acid solutions in the management of hepatic encephalopathy (controlled study, 30 patients). *Gastroenterology* 79:1038, 1980.

43. Morgan, M. Y., Bolton, C. H., Morris, J. S., and Read, E. A. Medium chain triglycerides and hepatic encephalopathy, *Gut* 15:180, 1974.

44. Moroni, F., Riggio, O., Carla, V., et al. Hepatic encephalopathy: Lack of changes of gamma-aminobutyric acid content in plasma and cerebrospinal fluid. *Hepatology* 7:816, 1987.

45. Naylor, C. D., O'Rourke, K., Detsky, A. S., and Baker, J. P. Parenteral nutrition with branched-chain amino acids in hepatic encephalopathy: A meta-analysis, *Gastroenterology* 97:1033, 1989.

46. Nespoli, A., Bevilacqua, G., Staudacher, C., Rossi, N., Salerno, E., and Castelli, M. R. Pathogenesis of hepatic encephalopathy and hyperdynamic syndrome in cirrhosis: Role of false neurotransmitters. *Arch. Surg.* 116:1129, 1981.

47. O'Brien, M. J., and Gottlieb, L. S. The liver and the biliary tract. In S. L. Robbins and R. S. Cotran (eds.), *Pathologic Basis of Disease* (2nd ed.). Philadelphia: W. B. Saunders, 1979. P. 1009.

48. Oddessey, R., and Goldberg, A. L. Oxidation of leucine by rat skeletal muscle. *Am. J. Physiol.* 223:1376, 1972.

49. Okada, A., Kamata, S., Kim, C. W., and Kawashima, Y. Treatment of hepatic encephalopathy with BCAA-rich amino acid mixture. In M. Walser and R. Williamson (eds.), *Metabolism and Clinical Implications of Branched Chain Amino and Ketoacids*. New York: Elsevier North-Holland, 1981. P. 447.

50. Ono, J., Hutson, D. G., Dombro, R. S., Levi, J. U., Livingstone, A., and Zeppa, R. Tryptophan and hepatic coma. *Gastroenterology* 74: 196, 1978.

51. Opolon, P., Rapian, J. R., Huguet, C., et al. Hepatic failure coma treated by polyacrylonitrile membrane hemodialysis. *Trans. Am. Soc. Artif. Organs* 22:701, 1976.

52. Phillips, G. B., Schwartz, R., Gabuzda, G. J., and Davidson, C. S. The syndrome of impending hepatic coma in patients with cirrhosis of liver given nitrogenous substances. *N. Engl. J. Med.* 247:239, 1952.

53. Pomier-Layrargues, G., Bories, P., Mirouze, D., et al. Brain gamma aminobutyric acid in acute hepatic encephalopathy in dogs following hepatectomy with or without abdominal

evisceration. In L. Copocaccia, J. E. Fischer and F. Rossi-Fanelli (eds.), *Hepatic Encephalopathy in Chronic Liver Failure.* New York: Plenum Press, 1984. P. 127.

54. Rigotti, P., Peters, J. C., Tranberg, K. G., and Fischer, J. E. Effects of amino acid infusions on liver regeneration after partial hepatectomy in the rat. *J. Parenter. Enter. Nutr.* 10:17, 1986.

55. Rosen, H. M., Soeters, P. B., James, J. H., Hodgman, J., and Fischer, J. E. Influences of exogenous intake and nitrogen balance on plasma and brain aromatic amino acid concentrations. *Metabolism* 27:393, 1978.

56. Rosen, H. M., Yoshimura, N., Hodgman, J., and Fischer, J. E. Plasma amino acid patterns in hepatic encephalopathy of differing etiology. *Gastroenterology* 72:483, 1977.

57. Rossi-Fanelli, F., Cangiano, C., Attili, A., et al. Octopamine plasma levels and hepatic encephalopathy: A reappraisal of the problem. *Clin. Chem. Acta* 67:255, 1976.

58. Rossi-Fanelli, F., Riggio, O., Cangiano, C., et al. Branched-chain amino acids vs. lactulose in the treatment of hepatic coma: A controlled study. *Dig. Dis. Sci.* 27:929, 1982.

59. Salerno, F., Dioguardi, F. S., and Abbiati, R. Tryptophan and hepatic coma. (Letter) *Gastroenterology* 75:769, 1978.

60. Schafer, D. F., and Jones, E. A. Potential neural mechanisms in the pathogenesis of hepatic encephalopathy. In H. Popper and F. Schaffner (eds.), *Progress in Liver Disease.* New York: Grune & Stratton, 1982. P. 615.

61. Schomerus, H., Hamster, W., Blunck, H., Reinhard, U., Mayer, K., and Dolle, W. Latent portal systemic therapy. I. Nature of cerebral functional defects and their effects on fitness to drive. *Dig. Dis. Sci.* 26:622, 1981.

62. Sherwin, R., Joshi, P., Hendler, R., Felig, P., and Conn, H. O. Hyperglycagonemia in Laennec's cirrhosis. *N. Engl. J. Med.* 290:239, 1974.

63. Sherwin, R. S. Effect of starvation on the turnover and metabolic response to leucine. *J. Clin. Invest.* 21:1471, 1978.

64. Smith, A. R., Rossi-Fanelli, F., Ziparo, V., James, J. H., Perelle, B. A., and Fischer, J. E. Alterations in plasma and CSF amino acids, amines and metabolites in hepatic coma. *Ann. Surg.* 187:343, 1978.

65. Soeters, P. B., and Fischer, J. E. Insulin, glucagon, amino acid imbalance and hepatic encephalopathy. *Lancet* 2:880, 1976.

66. Soeters, P. B., Weir, G. C., Ebeid, A. M., and Fischer, J. E. Insulin, glucagon, portal systemic shunting, and hepatic failure in the dog. *J. Surg. Res.* 23:183, 1977.

67. Strauss, E., Santos, W. R., DaSilva, E. C., Lacet, C. M., Capacci, M. L. L., and Bernardini, A. P. A randomized controlled clinical trial for the evaluation of the efficacy of an enriched branched chain amino acid solution compared to neomycin in hepatic encephalopathy. *Hepatology* 3:862, 1983.

68. Streibel, J., Holm, E., Lutz, M., and Storz, L. W. Parenteral nutrition and coma therapy with amino acids in hepatic failure. *J. Parenter. Enter. Nutr.* 3:240, 1979.

69. Strombeck, D. R., Roger, Q., and Stern, J. S. Effects of intravenous ammonia infusion on plasma levels of amino acids, glucagon and insulin in dogs. *Gastroenterology* 74:1165, 1978.

70. Summerskill, W. H. J., and Wolfe, S. J. The metabolism of ammonia and alpha-keto acids in liver disease and hepatic coma. *J. Clin. Invest.* 36:361, 1957.

71. Takahashi, Y. Serum lipids in liver disease: Liver disease and the relationship of serum lipids and hepatic coma. *Jpn. J. Gastroenterol.* 60:571, 1963.

72. Wahren, J., Felig, P., and Hagenfeldt, L. Effect of protein ingestion on splanchnic and leg metabolism in normal man and in patients with diabetes mellitus. *J. Clin. Invest.* 57:987, 1976.

73. Wahren, J. J., Denis, J., Desurmont, P., et al. Is intravenous administration of branched chain amino acids effective in the treatment of hepatic encephalopathy? A multicenter study. *Hepatology* 4:475, 1983.

74. Watanabe, A., Tanesue, A., Higashi, T., and Nagashima, N. Serum amino acids in hepatic encephalopathy: Effects of branched chain amino acid infusion on serum aminogram. *Acta Hepato-Gastroenterol.* 26:346, 1979.

75. Zieve, F. J., Zieve, L., Doizaki, W. M., and Gilsdorf, R. B. Synergism between ammonia and fatty acids in the production of coma: Implications for hepatic coma. *J. Pharmacol. Exp. Ther.* 191:10, 1974.

76. Zieve, L., Doizaki, W. M., and Zieve, F. J. Synergism between mercaptans and ammonia or fatty acids in the production of coma: A possible role for mercaptans in the pathogenesis of hepatic coma. *J. Lab. Clin. Med.* 83:16, 1974.

19

Parenteral Nutrition in the Burned Patient

Michele M. Gottschlich
Glenn D. Warden

Nutritional support of the burned patient represents a special challenge because of the complex interactions of injury, organ function, wound healing, and immunocompetence. Nutrition is an important effector of each of these events. Inefficient diet therapy will exacerbate metabolic abnormalities and catabolic sequelae such as erosion of lean body mass and deterioration of blood proteins as well as disturb cellular and organ function [46, 48, 73, 123, 130]. For example, active transport of sodium and potassium across the cell membrane is inhibited in both erythrocytes and muscle if sufficient calories are not delivered [46, 48]. Loss of respiratory musculature, impaired ventilatory effort, and secondary pulmonary infection are additional morbid consequences of inadequate or improper nutrient provision [14, 28]. Wound healing deteriorates [20, 21, 23, 75, 80, 125, 139]. Intestinal villi may be degraded for energy, hence impairing digestion and absorption [73, 150]. It is also well known that the predisposition to infection is greatly influenced by nutritional status [21, 25, 26, 44, 63, 66, 153]. Evidence that malnutrition can increase susceptibility to infection represents a major problem for burned patients [32, 40, 54, 148, 163] as sepsis is the most frequent cause of morbidity and mortality in these patients.

With nutritional needs of burned patients nearly double that required prior to injury, the clinician is faced with serious decisions regarding what and how to feed them. A thorough understanding of the pathophysiologic changes associated with burn injury is necessary to plan and provide an optimal diet therapy program. This chapter outlines the impact of acute thermal injury on energy and nutrient metabolism, describes the hormonal environment that directs these changes, and examines methods of nutritional support that may expedite recovery, with particular emphasis on total parenteral nutrition (TPN). Indications and guidelines for the proper use of intravenous nutritional support in burn care are provided.

METABOLIC CONSEQUENCES OF THERMAL INJURY

There is no physiologic insult greater than an extensive thermal injury. The burn wound either directly or indirectly initiates significant alterations in hormonal milieu and metabolism, which has been characterized as having two distinct phases: the "ebb" and "flow" responses. The initial or ebb phase is manifested by decreased oxygen consumption, inadequate circulation, fluid imbalance, and cellular shock. This period of depressed metabolism provides a protective environment, but only for a short time. Within days, the patient enters a severely catabolic state. During the acute phase of the flow response, the sympathoadrenal axis is activated with elevations in the counterregulatory hormones, namely glucagon [88, 121, 142, 163, 172], catecholamines [1, 164, 169], and glucocorticoids [18, 57, 155]. Insulin levels are normal or elevated. Nevertheless, insulin is low in relation to glucagon. The change in endocrine relationships heightens metabolic rate and accelerates protein breakdown, lipolysis, and gluconeogenesis [158]. Although the flow phase is initially a catabolic, hypermetabolic period, the transition to anabolism must be made if the patient is to survive [49]. The metabolic and hormonal alterations in terms of energy and nutrient requirements have important implications in the design of parenteral feeding regimens for the burned patient.

Hypermetabolism

Energy requirements increase following thermal injury, and the magnitude of hypermetabolism is virtually unsurpassed by any other form of trauma or critical illness. Metabolic rate is directly related to burn size, rising in linear proportion to a maximum level approximately twice normal, with burns over 50% of the total body surface area [164]. The heat production of patients with burns exceeding 50% of the surface area appears to reach a plateau. This has led to the concept of a "ceiling" to metabolic rate which patients cannot exceed.

Metabolic rate also varies with time after injury. Wilmore et al.'s [164] classic study showed that following the shock phase, oxygen consumption increases dramatically, peaking between the sixth and tenth day after injury. Thereafter, metabolic rate slowly returns to normal as coverage of the burn wound is achieved [158]. Reactivation of hypermetabolism can occur with complications such as infection or organ failure.

Several factors are responsible for the heightened metabolic response. Loss of cutaneous integrity results in a large evaporative fluid loss with significant surface cooling. This evaporation requires energy. For many years, the tremendous evaporative loss from the wound was considered to be the major causative factor for the hypermetabolic state [41, 42, 119, 128], until Zawacki et al. demonstrated that blocking evaporation by application of impermeable dressings to the burn wound produced only a modest reduction in metabolic rate [175].

Ambient temperature is another factor that influences metabolic rate in burned patients. Burn care conducted in a higher environmental temperature minimizes the hypermetabolic response [27, 36, 53, 164, 165]. Metabolic expenditure appears to be temperature sensitive but not temperature specific, as environmental heating does not totally abolish hypemetabolism.

Catecholamines are the major mediators augmenting energy expenditure. Increased levels of catecholamines in plasma and the rate of urinary catecholamine excretion in burned patients are markedly elevated and correlate with burn size, fever, and metabolic rate [1, 31, 79, 164, 169]. Supporting this concept is the fact that beta-adrenergic blockade has been shown to partially block hypermetabolism in burned patients, and epinephrine infused into normal humans significantly increased their metabolic rate [164].

Alterations in Carbohydrate Metabolism

An important pathophysiologic phenomenon of thermal injury is the radical derangement in carbohydrate metabolism manifested by hyperglycemia and glycosuria [10, 17, 151, 159, 172]. There is a marked rise in serum glucose level during burn shock, which is probably due to a temporary decrease in peripheral utilization because of impaired tissue perfusion. Following resuscitation, increased blood glucose flow is directed to the wound, as reparative cells in the burn wound rely almost exclusively on glucose for energy via anaerobic glycolytic pathways. Glucose consumption in burned tissue is significantly greater than that in normal tissue [158, 160]. However, in spite of the wound's high requirement for glucose, hyperglycemia often persists during the acute-phase response. Previously, the syndrome of burn-induced pseudodiabetes was thought to be due to impaired glucose utilization. That glucose intolerance might be due to the inability of the burned patient to oxidize glucose has since been disproved [104, 142, 166, 167, 171]. Glucose is oxidized at a normal or even enhanced rate [104]. An altered glucoregulatory hormonal environment, having the effect of accelerating hepatic glucose production, accounts for the continued state of hyperglycemia [88, 104, 162, 172]. Specific hormonal changes that exacerbate gluconeogenesis include elevations in the catecholamines [1, 164, 169] and glucocorticoids [18, 57, 155], and reversal in the normal insulin-glucagon ratio [163, 172]. As a consequence, gluconeogenic amino acids tend to be unavailable for protein synthesis. Instead, large amounts of the gluconeogenic precursors are supplied to the liver from peripheral tissues such as muscle. The result is muscle wasting.

Protein Considerations

Protein nutriture is severely compromised by thermal injury. Several factors are involved. The burn wound is a significant source of nitrogen loss. The daily decrement may average 2 to 3 g of protein/day for each percent of body surface area burn [120]. This aspect of protein loss can be lessened by early excision and grafting of the burn wound.

Another significant source of nitrogen loss is the endogenous hypercatabolism mediated by the altered hormonal balance. Protein catabolism allows for nitrogen mobilization to support the formation of nonessential amino acids for wound healing and the synthesis of vital acute-phase proteins associated with host defense. Protein breakdown also serves the increased energy needs of the host through the deamination of amino acids, particularly alanine and glutamine, in the generation of carbon skeletons for glucose [15, 37, 62, 162, 170, 172]. Alanine is the major gluconeogenic precursor to be cycled to the liver, and the glucose that is produced is sent to glucose-dependent tissues such as the healing wound. Glutamine, on the other hand, serves as a significant gluconeogenic substrate for the gut. The major reservoir of these priority amino acids and carbon fragments is the skeletel muscle. Their production is paralleled by enhanced urea formation, the urinary excretion of which can be used as an index of the severity of injury and the nitrogen needs of the patient [92]. In summary, accelerated wound and urinary nitrogen losses together with a progressive reduction in somatic protein status following burns reflect a serious state of protein malnutrition.

Although an increase in protein synthesis likewise exists, anabolism is inefficient in the presence of hormonal disturbances and suboptimal nutritional support. One goal in the prescription of a parenteral feeding program is the selection of an appropriate amino acid mixture and total quantity that will maximize viscera and wound anabolism while overshadowing the coincident carcass breakdown that occurs with stress (Fig. 19-1). Over the years, the effects of improved protein intake on outcome in burns has been the subject of extensive research. It is undisputed that the burned patient has high protein requirements [4, 81, 92, 140, 146, 174]. Alexander et al. [4] demonstrated that severely burned children receiving a high protein diet containing approximately 25% of calories as protein (calorie-protein ratio of 100:1) had higher levels of total protein, transferrin, C_3, IgG, and opsonic index, compared to patients

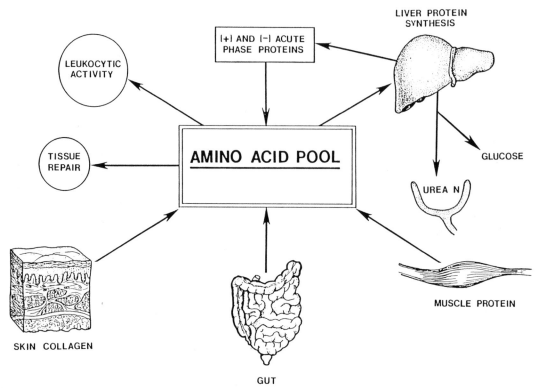

Figure 19-1. Alterations in protein metabolism following injury create a function redistribution of protein to aid increased synthetic activity of the viscera and healing of wounds. (Adapted from Benotti, P., Blackburn, G. L., et al. *Crit. Care Med.* 7:520, 1979.)

supplied 16% of calories as protein (calorie-protein ratio of 150:1). In addition, the high protein group had an improved survival rate and a decreased incidence of bacteremia.

Fat Metabolism

Another physiologic sequela of the acute phase of burn injury is the pronounced change in lipid metabolism. Serum cholesterol levels fall dramatically [29, 30, 36, 45, 77], coincident with a drop in low-density lipoprotein (LDL) [30, 35]. The burn wound is a significant route of loss of LDL and cholesterol [30].

Burn-mediated increases in catecholamines and glucagon stimulate lipolysis, producing a marked elevation in serum levels of triglycerides [6, 29, 45, 78, 143], free fatty acids [6, 35, 36, 77, 78, 164], and glycerol [78]. Whether this increase in lipolysis is beneficial

to thermally injured patients in a manner similar to normal humans during starvation or exercise is debatable. Wilmore [158] demonstrated that burned tissues preferentially utilize glucose, and fat stores cannot meet this need. Even though patients with minimal stress do equally well with either high fat or high glucose calories, lipid appears to represent an inefficient source of calories for the maintenance of nitrogen equilibrium and lean body mass following major injury [64, 105, 141, 147]. Long et al. [105] evaluated parenteral support containing various glucose-fat ratios and demonstrated intravenous fat emulsions to be less effective in nitrogen sparing than carbohydrate in the burned patients. In studies of stressed animals, Freund et al. [64] and Souba et al. [147] also found glucose to be superior to fat as an intravenous calorie substrate for nitrogen balance. Goodenough and Wolfe [67] demonstrated the energy contribution from the oxidation of intravenous lipid to be insignificant in a study of six burned patients. Rather, most of the fat oxidized was from endogenous fat stores. It is likely that burned patients do not benefit from a high fat intake due to the apparent limitations in fatty acid oxidation in the presence of ongoing stimulation of endogenous fat mobilization.

METHODS OF NUTRITIONAL SUPPORT

Patients with burns over more than 25% of the total body surface area require some form of specialized nutritional therapy. In most cases, no absolute contraindication to enteral feeding exists following burns. In smaller-size burns, meals supplemented with protein-rich beverages suffice, but more often a nonvolitional means of nutritional support is required.

Alert patients with a functional gastrointestinal tract generally do quite well with gastrointestinal tube feedings, if proper attention is given to methodology. Constant drip infusions are recommended, with hourly monitoring of gastric residual. Since burned patients usually have normal digestive and absorptive capabilities (unless the gastrointestinal tract was traumatized), there are no contraindications to utilizing intact enteral formulations. Most tube-feeding products can be started at full strength. The initial hourly infusion rate should begin at approximately half of the final desired volume and be increased by 5 ml/hr in the child and by 10 ml/hr in the adult as tolerated until the final hourly rate is achieved.

In the past, nutritional intake (e.g., oral or nasogastric) was limited by posttraumatic gastrointestinal ileus. This often meant that the most critically ill burn patients could not be fed. During the last part of the 1960s, it became possible to provide caloric support to virtually any patient with the application of parenteral hyperalimentation [58]. This feeding technique has subsequently been employed in the nutritional support of burned children [56, 122, 124, 168] and adults [84, 86, 108, 144, 161, 168], with many clinicians favorably regarding the ability to deliver caloric-dense intravenous substrates as a solution to the starvation syndrome and high mortality associated with extensive burns.

More recently, with the development of fairly sophisticated tube-feeding tools (e.g., soft, radiopaque, weighted enteric feeding tubes; stylets to aid in placement; tube-feeding pumps; and portable fluoroscopy), enteral support has resurfaced as a viable option. Indeed, most patients with even large thermal injuries can be successfully fed enterally [3, 70, 90, 95, 96, 107]. During periods of gastroparesis, duodenal tube feeding is possible since the small intestine usually maintains its functional capabilities. Fluoroscopically or endoscopically guiding the feeding tube distal to the pylorus lessens the chances of gastroesophageal reflux, tracheobronchial aspiration, and tube displacement [95]. Enteral nutritional support is therefore possible, even during critical periods such as resuscitation, surgery, ketamine-induced anesthesia for major dressing changes, or septic ileus.

ENTERAL VERSUS PARENTERAL SUPPORT

Because it is now possible to provide diets enterally or parenterally, it is important to examine whether the route of nutrient administration makes a difference. In an animal model, atrophy of the small-bowel mucosa was observed following burn injury, but this finding could be improved or prevented by gavage feeding [113, 134]. Saito et al. [134] also demonstrated that preservation of mucosal mass was associated with a reduction in the posttraumatic secretion of catabolic hormones (assessed by urinary VMA excretion, plasma cortisol, and plasma glucagon), suggesting that enteral regimens may be preferable to parenteral feeding systems.

It is now widely appreciated that a functioning alimentary tract is the preferred route of nutritional support in the thermally injured patient. TPN offers no advantage except in atypical cases of prolonged alimentary tract dysfunction due to concomitant gastrointestinal disease or injury. In fact, parenteral feeding is associated with more frequent positive blood cultures, lower helper-suppressor cell ratios, impaired neutrophil function, and lower secretory IgA, compared to enteral hyperalimentation [7, 84, 98, 133].

Herndon et al. [84] randomly assigned 28 patients with burns over more than 50% of the total body surface area to receive TPN (25% dextrose, 4.25% crystalline amino acid solution) or no TPN (5% dextrose) during the first 10 days after the burn. TPN supplementation demonstrated no apparent clinical benefit and was associated with significantly increased T suppressor-helper cell ratios. Since no clear advantage could be demonstrated with TPN, the routine use of TPN early in the burn course should be avoided.

Enteral feedings, on the other hand, increase gut blood flow, preserve gastrointestinal function, and maintain gut mucosal integrity [3, 7, 73, 101, 133, 134], thus decreasing the absorption of endotoxin or the direct translocation of bacteria across the gastrointestinal tract [3, 54, 55, 93, 114, 134]. These observations support the concept that optimal nutritional support for victims of burns is via the alimentary tract. Efforts to maintain small-bowel integrity offer immunologic, gastrointestinal, and metabolic benefits.

INDICATIONS FOR TOTAL PARENTERAL NUTRITION

While enteral alimentation is the preferred route to provide nutrients to the burned patient, under certain circumstances intravenous feeding can become a necessary and even life-saving part of burn management. For example, if the gastrointestinal tract cannot be used because of concurrent abdominal trauma or preburn pathologic conditions, parenteral nutrition assumes a major role. Gastrointestinal complications associated with large burns that are definite indications

for intravenous feeding include stress ulceration of the stomach or duodenum (Curling's ulcer) [52], severe pancreatitis [68], septic ileus, or pseudo-obstruction of the colon [100]. Occasionally, superior mesenteric artery syndrome [32, 99, 124] is observed in burned patients following a period of rapid weight loss, necessitating the use of TPN. Another important indication for intravenous hyperalimentation is as an adjunct to enteral support. Frequently, the enormous caloric demands cannot be met entirely by enteral support. The development of vomiting, abdominal distention, or intractable diarrhea limits the number of calories that can be delivered by the enteral route. In situations such as these, the use of TPN is extremely beneficial in making up the enteral caloric deficit.

CALORIC GOAL

The first objective of any intravenous diet therapy program is to satisfy caloric requirements. The burned patient is unable to direct nutrients toward tissue repair if the regimen is deficient in calories. Instead the body oxidizes important endogenous fuel stores for energy. Accurate identification of caloric needs is likewise necessary to avoid overfeeding. Administering inordinate numbers of calories has been associated with increased metabolic rate, hyperglycemia, hypernatremia secondary to solute diuresis, liver abnormalities, and increased carbon dioxide production. Importantly, tailoring caloric delivery to the patient is cost-effective in avoiding the use of costly hyperalimentation solutions.

Establishing an individualized caloric goal in the field of burns can be accomplished in one of several ways. Many mathematic derivations exist for calculating daily energy requirements. Traditional formulas do not account for the severity of injury [116]. The two formulas used most frequently were introduced by Curreri et al. [47] and Long and colleagues [102, 103]. Curreri et al. accounted for extent of burn in their formula [47]:

Caloric needs = (25 kcal/kg of body weight)
+ (40 kcal/% burn).

Long et al.'s formula [102, 103] is a modification of the Harris-Benedict equation [76]. It predicts energy expenditure on the basis of age, sex, height, and weight, and then applies a factor for burn injury:

Caloric needs (male) =
$(66.473 + 13.75W + 5.0H - 6.76A)$
$\times$ (activity factor) $\times$ (injury factor)

Caloric needs (female) =
$(655.1 + 9.56W + 1.85H - 4.68A)$
$\times$ (activity factor) $\times$ (injury factor)

where W is weight (kg), H is height (cm), A is age (years), activity factor is 1.2 (confined to bed) or 1.3 (out of bed), and injury factor is 2.0 to 2.5 (burns).

In independent studies using indirect calorimetry, the clinical validity of these equations was challenged [87, 132, 154]. Indeed, no formula provides for the great variation observed in individual patients. Predicting energy needs is complicated by room temperature, humidity, dressing changes, anesthesia, medications, surgery, fever, infection, pain, anxiety, nutrient intake, activity level, and other factors. As with most other nutritional assessment procedures, the more severely ill the patient, the less accurate the index. With the advent of portable indirect calorimetry, resting energy expenditure can be routinely determined from the measurement of oxygen consumption and carbon dioxide production. It is recommended that compensation be made for clinical conditions that heighten energy needs beyond those measured at rest. The burned patient's caloric goal should be calculated at 120 to 130% of the measured resting energy expenditure [71, 132] in an effort to adjust for physical therapy, stress, temperature spikes, dressing changes, and other effectors of metabolic rate. Since postburn hypermetabolism tends to fluctuate during the clinical course and gradually decreases with convalescence, indirect calorimetry should be conducted at least twice weekly for proper adjustment of the hyperalimentation regimen.

INTRAVENOUS CARBOHYDRATE INTAKE

Parenteral carbohydrate delivery exerts several benefits to the burn victim. First, it can be directly oxidized as an energy-providing nutrient [171]. In addition, carbohydrate stimulates insulin release, a key hormonal signal that suppresses gluconeogenesis [159]. Both of these effects promote protein sparing in burns [105, 108]. In severely hypermetabolic burned patients receiving isonitrogenous regimens, intravenous carbohydrate decreases nitrogen excretion whereas equicaloric doses of fat fail to evoke a similar effect [105]. Carbohydrate also helps restore normal sodium and potassium cell pump activity following burns [48]. Thus, carbohydrate is an important component of a parenteral feeding program for burned patients; however, a limit exists to its effectiveness as an intravenous substrate [105]. This is an important consideration because of the ease with which large amounts of dextrose can be delivered using central venous hyperalimentation techniques. Glucose oxidation accelerates with increases in glucose up to about 5 mg/kg/min (504 g/70 kg/day) in injured patients, but little additional glucose is oxidized at higher rates [40, 105]. Burke et al. [40] documented increases in the respiratory quotient above 1.0, increased respiratory work, and fat deposition in the livers of burned patients dying after intravenous glucose infusions of 9.3 to 17 mg/kg/min, which suggests a disadvantage of carbohydrate loads in excess of caloric needs. Askanazi et al. [12, 13] also demonstrated increased carbon dioxide production that may influence weaning from ventilators at high levels of intravenous glucose infusion in depleted septic patients.

Admixed central venous hyperalimentation solutions containing a final concentration of dextrose ranging from 5 to 35% have been administered to burned patients. Standard regimens for this patient population usually consist of a final concentration of 25% dextrose; however, more concentrated solutions may be indicated in the presence of renal failure and less concentrated formulations may be used during cases of carbon dioxide retention or severe hyperglycemia unresponsive to insulin therapy.

Dextrose-rich solutions may aggravate burn-induced hyperglycemia and glycosuria. If the renal threshold for glucose is exceeded, calories are lost in the urine. Osmotic diuresis secondary to glucose also results in excessive loss of water. Glucosuria thus results not only in calorie depletion but also in dehydration. By frequently measuring blood and urine glucose concentration and administering insulin as indicated, a large glucose load can usually be infused while maintaining serum glucose levels between 100 and 200 mg/dl. If a relatively constant glucose load has been tolerated by the patient for several days without hyperglycemia, the appearance of an elevated blood sugar may indicate the presence of sepsis. Should the patient be unresponsive to insulin, excessive caloric or carbohydrate infusion should be ruled out or adjusted accordingly.

AMINO ACIDS

Instead of the recommended daily allowance of protein devised for normal, healthy people, a more appropriate protein allowance for burned patients approximates 20 to 25% of their total energy needs [4, 174]. In order to meet these requirements, intravenous hyperalimentation solutions composed of a final concentration of 5% crystalline amino acids are necessary. When fluid intake is not restricted and kidney function is normal, burned patients tolerate such protein loads extremely well. It is vital to concurrently provide sufficient energy for efficient protein utilization.

Particular care must be taken when high protein feedings are administered to children under 1 year old, as excessive amounts can have adverse effects on immature or compromised kidneys. Fluid status and serum electrolytes, BUN, and serum creatinine levels must be monitored on all patients receiving high protein parenteral regimens. In addi-

tion, protein status should be periodically evaluated using nitrogen balance studies along with selected plasma proteins to ensure that appropriate nutritional support is taking place [33, 92, 115, 116].

When deciding on a crystalline amino acid product, attention should be given to commercial differences in nitrogen concentration, amino acid profiles, and electrolyte content. Amino acid distribution is as important a consideration as the amount of nitrogen being delivered because an inadequacy of one amino acid can be a significant limiting factor for protein synthesis. There are different amino acid requirements following burns, and it appears that many reparative and immunologic functions are dependent on the availability of specific amino acids. Such changes in amino acid metabolism are evidenced by the altered levels of the plasma amino acids observed in the thermally injured patient [4, 15, 16, 50, 51, 74, 85, 145, 148, 173]. The combination of enhanced skeletal muscle catabolism, essentiality of certain amino acids for wound healing and gluconeogenesis, possible changes in enzyme activity, and wound tissue debris all contribute to alterations in plasma amino acid concentration.

The amino acid solution must contain all of the essential and sufficient nonessential amino acids. Furthermore, an adequate ratio must be maintained between the essential and nonessential amino acids. Incorrect administration of amino acids may result in imbalances leading to hyperchloremic metabolic acidosis, hyperammonemia, and elevation of BUN. Manipulation of crystalline amino acids may be of value. For example, phenylalanine is usually elevated in the plasma of severely burned individuals [15, 50, 74, 85, 145, 148], with a positive correlation to eventual mortality [85, 148]. Consequently, the hyperalimentation solution should contain reduced phenylalanine.

Branched-chain amino acid–enriched hyperalimentation solutions may be useful in the burned [43, 122] or septic [39, 137] patient in terms of hepatic protein synthesis and improved nitrogen retention, even though enteral branched-chain amino acid supplementation has not proved beneficial [71, 112, 137]. In addition, the amino acid formulation should contain arginine despite the fact that it is not considered to be an essential dietary constituent for normal humans [129]. In both animals and humans, plasma arginine levels drop following burn injury [148, 173], suggestive of a relative deficiency. Low plasma levels of arginine are significantly associated with weight loss [148]. Regarding the therapeutic effects of arginine supplementation, Heird et al. [82] documented hyperammonemia in three infants receiving a parenteral alimentation solution practically devoid of arginine. The syndrome was corrected by administering 2 mmol/kg of arginine glutamate, or 3 mmol/kg of arginine HCl to the infusate. [*Editor's Note:* Since that report, no more patients with hyperammonemia have been observed and reported.] Likewise, Najarian and Harper [118] infused 15 patients who had hyperammonemia with 25 to 30 g/day of arginine HCl and observed improved mental status and reduced blood ammonia concentrations. Clearly, arginine is an important urea cycle intermediate for the removal of excess ammonia. Arginine supplementation also represents a nutritional means of enhancing nitrogen retention [25, 111, 126], accelerating wound healing [20, 21, 23, 71, 138], and augmenting insulin and human growth hormone secretion [25, 109, 117]. Furthermore, it has immunostimulatory capabilities [21, 22, 24–26, 72, 136]. Saito et al. [136] demonstrated that 2% arginine supplementation in guinea pigs with burns over 30% of the body surface area had a beneficial effect in restoring immunocompetence.

USE OF FAT EMULSION

The optimal amount and composition of intravenous fat for burned patients are still largely a matter of speculation. Saito et al. [135] demonstrated in a 30% burned guinea pig model that animals receiving fish oil had better preservation of lean tissue mass and improved response to dinitrofluorobenzene (DNFB) skin tests compared to animals receiving safflower oil, a rich source of linoleic acid. Arachidonic acid metabolites may be responsible for the adverse effects observed from an overabundance of linoleic acid following burns [5, 69, 135]. Linoleic acid is a precursor of arachidonate. Arachidonic acid is metabolized primarily by oxygenation to numerous biologically active compounds, including the 2- series of prostaglandins. The dienoic prostaglandins have been found to be major immunosuppressive substances [5, 11, 59, 153]. Prostaglandins of the 2- series have also been associated with enhanced protein breakdown [19, 127]. Further research is needed to determine the optimal balance of fatty acids such as linoleic acid and perhaps the beneficial effects of omega-3 fatty acids as modulators of prostaglandin synthesis.

Additional undesirable effects of fat in general and intravenous fat in particular include cholestasis, hepatomegaly, overloading syndrome, and impaired clotting. It is also noteworthy that parenteral lipids have been reported to depress the immune response [30, 61, 63, 89, 149]. For these reasons conservative utilization of fat emulsion in total parenteral regimens for burned patients is recommended. Nevertheless, several desirable features of lipid as an intravenous substrate, including isotonicity, concentrated calorie source, and infusion into peripheral veins tend to encourage overzealous use of fat emulsions.

The main purpose of including intravenous fat in a diet therapy program is to prevent the onset of essential fatty acid deficiency (EFAD). EFAD, manifested as dermatitis, hemolytic anemia, thrombocytopenia, impaired wound healing, and a triene-to-tetraene ratio greater than 0.4, is uncommon in burned humans or animals unless fat-free parenteral alimentation represented the only source of nutrients for a prolonged period of time [77, 83, 110, 168]. [*Editor's Note:* Other studies suggested that EFAD may result from fat-free parenteral nutrition for as short as 1 week in relatively unstressed patients.] All fat emulsions contain significant amounts of linoleic acid. It is estimated that 1 to 2% of total caloric intake should be derived from linoleic acid. When glucose and amino acids provide 100% of energy needs, 500 ml of 10% lipid emulsion infused two to three times weekly suffices in meeting most patients' essential fatty acid requirement. Peripheral vessels are frequently not available in the burned patient. "Piggybacking" the fat emulsion's tubing into the tubing of the water-based glucose and amino acid solution is a safe alternative. [*Editor's Note*: a 3-in-1 mixture containing all three components—amino acids, fat, and carbohydrates—is being increasingly utilized.]

FLUID AND ELECTROLYTES

The management of fluid and electrolyte status is mandatory prior to commencing TPN, and requires daily reassessment while providing parenteral alimentation. Proper fluid balance is essential to maintain adequate tissue perfusion and electrolyte concentration. Over- or underhydration, in addition to altering end-organ function, may result in ionic disequilibrium of cellular constituents. Central hyperalimentation, with its requisite high osmotic load, can significantly affect cell function by altering fluid and electrolyte concentrations. Concentrated dextrose solution in the presence of an impaired insulin response can precipitate osmotic diuresis, leading to decreased intravascular fluid volume with resultant hypernatremia and dehydration. Hyperchloremic metabolic acidosis, frequently associated with the delivery of excessive chloride on crystalline amino acids, represents another example of the detrimental effects for early parenteral nutrition replenishment. Therefore, it is imperative first to correct any fluid or electrolyte imbalance prior to initiating TPN.

Following burn shock resuscitation, the parenteral feeding formulation should be designed to deliver nutritional needs in a fluid volume appropriate for the burned patient's cardiovascular and renal status. The heightened water requirements needed to replace the evaporative fluid losses of patients with extensive burns [157] facilitate the administration of a high calorie, high protein regimen. The coincident fluid volume and energy requirements of most severely burned patients result in a nutrient solution containing approximately 1 cal/ml.

Electrolytes and minerals that are added to the parenteral diet include sodium, potassium, chloride, phosphate, magnesium, and calcium. Potassium losses are generally large, and potassium supplementation is usually required in generous amounts. The requirements of phosphorus, calcium, and magnesium are also increased in burned patients. If the patient has acid-base alterations, or if there is hyperchloremic acidosis, acetate may be added instead of chloride. Frequent monitoring of serum sodium, potassium, chloride, calcium, magnesium, and phosphorus levels along with arterial blood gases is the best clinical guide to determining individual requirements of these constituents.

MICRONUTRIENTS

In addition to tailoring parenteral fluids, macronutrients, and electrolyte intake based on the unique needs of burn patients, appropriate vitamins and trace elements must be added daily to meet heightened requirements without excessive wastage or toxicity. Macronutrients will not be efficiently processed if intake of these vital cofactors and coenzymes is inadequate. Metabolic functions, assessment techniques, and the basis for supplementation of vitamins and trace minerals during burn care recently were reviewed elsewhere [70, 72]; however, our understanding of the micronutrient requirements for burned patients is rudimentary. The appropriate parenteral micronutrient provision to the thermally injured patient is largely a matter of conjecture, as current data available regarding guidelines for intake center around the normal individual or enterally fed burned patient. Patients dependent on intravenous nutritional support are usually prescribed the standard dosage for vitamins [8] and trace elements [9] recommended by the Nutrition Advisory Group of the American Medical Association (AMA), unless symptoms of deficiency occur. It seems prudent, however, to supplement the AMA guidelines with ascorbic acid (250–500 mg daily) and zinc (2–5 mg/day) in view of their important roles in wound repair [65, 75, 94, 139] and immunocompetence [44, 152], combined with frequent reports of deficiencies of these two micronutrients in burns [75, 97, 106, 125].

CATHETER ACCESS AND CARE

When parenteral feeding represents the sole source of nutrients, the infusion of very hypertonic solutions becomes necessary to meet the supranormal needs of the burn victim. Hyperalimentation infusions must be delivered into a vessel with a high blood flow where rapid dilution occurs, to minimize the risk of phlebitis, sclerosis, and thrombosis. Therefore, venous catheters for TPN are commonly placed into the superior caval system through unburned skin whenever possible. The most popular access site is the subclavian vein, although the catheter can also be introduced safely through the internal and external jugular veins. The small diameter of the external jugular vein, however, predisposes it to a higher incidence of thrombosis. The external jugular vein is therefore primarily used as a short-term means of central venous feeding, and then only when no other access is present. It should be used only as a last resort.

In addition to the superior vena caval route, catheters can be inserted into the inferior vena cava by way of venipuncture at the groin. Cannulation of the femoral vein provides an additional access site when upper veins are unavailable and when frequent changes of cannula are mandated; however,

this approach is associated with a high incidence of infection and thrombosis [156]. These patients must also be carefully monitored for the development of phlebitis and pulmonary embolism.

It is not surprising that the placement of catheters through burn wounds is associated with a higher infection rate. Studies from the 1970s reported an extremely high incidence of sepsis ranging from 50 to 88% in burned patients receiving TPN [56, 124, 161]. Popp et al. [124] observed no serious complications with the placement of central lines through unburned skin; however, the authors reported a 50% incidence of sepsis, diagnosed by the presence of positive blood cultures, in patients cannulated through the burn wound. Although the high risk of catheter-related infection in burns is not questioned, its diagnosis is problematic. Incidence may be inflated if one uses the criterion of a positive culture of material from the catheter or blood as the only index of catheter-related infection. Sadowski et al. [131] recently showed that demonstrating the origin of positive culture material from the catheter tip may be difficult in thermally injured patients, as the same organism is frequently matched to simultaneous cultures from the wound and blood. Resolution of clinical sepsis on removal of the hyperalimentation line, with a positive culture of material from the catheter tip, is much more diagnostic of catheter-seeded infection.

The importance of aseptic technique during central-line placement and catheter care to the ultimate success of the TPN program is especially true in the thermally injured patient, already heavily colonized with bacteria and thus very susceptible to infection. Proper skin preparation for catheter placement requires that the area be cleansed with an antiseptic soap followed by an iodine solution. In addition, the rotation of catheter sites at 48 to 72 hours is imperative. Development and adherence to strict protocols for care of central lines and infection control (see Chap. 7) are directly responsible for the decline in catheter-related complications.

COMPLICATIONS

The use of TPN in burns presents several special problems, which may be divided into three general categories: mechanical, metabolic, and infectious. Insertion and utilization of an indwelling central venous catheter impose significant risks including pneumothorax, microbial contamination of the catheter, phlebitis, venous thrombosis, air embolism, pulmonary or hepatic dysfunction, and nutrient imbalances. Most of these complications can be minimized or prevented by the use of rigorous implementation protocols, meticulous catheter care, experienced personnel, and finally, an ongoing monitoring system. Early recognition is the key to successful management of any complication.

PERIPHERAL PARENTERAL NUTRITION

Peripheral parenteral nutrition (PPN) is a technique in which near isotonic mixtures of glucose, amino acids, fat, vitamins, minerals, and/or electrolytes are administered through a peripheral vein. Although the risk of sepsis is reduced during PPN by the fact that the needle or peripheral catheter is usually changed more often than the central catheter, strict aseptic technique and care in the delivery of PPN remain important components of patient care. Another issue is the possibility of causing local tissue damage from infiltration of the infusion. A third concern during peripheral feeding is the risk of thrombophlebitis. Osmolarity and potassium content of PPN are directly related to its development. Feeding a patient by the peripheral venous route is different from TPN through a central venous catheter, in that blood flow through a peripheral vein is lower and the solution's osmotic density is less. Thus, the glucose concentration of the solutions given peripherally should not exceed 10%.

Peripheral intravenous alimentation is rarely useful in burns. The ability to feed burned patients successfully with peripheral venous solutions is limited by the availability of peripheral veins, osmolarity of the substrate, and the existing caloric deficit. It is impossible to provide the seriously injured burn patient sufficient energy by peripheral vein infusions alone [108]. Instead, PPN should be viewed as a temporizing measure when short delays are anticipated prior to obtaining central venous access. Peripheral intravenous nutritional support may also be effective in burns when it is used to supplement a marginally inadequate enteral intake due to gastrointestinal intolerance of large volumes of tube feedings.

Peripheral parenteral feeding regimens have been shown to be safe and useful as the sole source of nutrition support in various patient populations whose caloric requirements are not exceedingly high [34, 38, 60]. On the other hand, Morath et al. [115] described a case where a similar program consisting of an admixture of 4.25% crystalline amino acids and 10% dextrose was used in a 50-year-old man with a 42% total body surface area, 32% full-thickness burn injury. PPN was employed as a temporary means of minimizing negative nitrogen balance during a period when both central-line and gastrointestinal feedings were contraindicated. A marked elevation in BUN to 122 mg/dl and serum creatinine to 3.4 mg/dl ensued (Table 19-1), but cleared rapidly following the removal of the intravenous amino acids. The etiology of the azotemia remains unclear; however, it might be speculated that excessive nitrogen was being released from deamination of exogenous and endogenous amino acids relative to the patient's excretion or utilization capabilities, with carbon chains derived from the gluconeogenic amino acids serving as a significant source of oxidative fuel in the presence of grossly inadequate caloric support. Analysis of the aforementioned clinical chain of events leads one to believe that PPN may not be appropriate as the sole means of alimentation in intensely hypermetabolic burn patients. The major problem with such regimens is the extremely low final caloric density of the solution. While peripheral infusions are often considered to be "safer" than central venous systems, this case highlights the serious na-

Table 19-1.   Nutritional Assessment of a Burn Patient Receiving Various Nutrition Support Modalities

	Admission	*Week 2*	*Week 3*	*Week 4*	*Week 5*	*Week 13*	*Discharge*
% Kcal needs met	43%	42%	23%	60%	74%	80%	100%
% Protein needs met	37%	36%	30%	58%	64%	80%	100%
BUN (mg/dl)	48	28	122	44	21	16	18
Serum creatinine (mg/dl)	3.6	1.5	3.4	1.8	1.2	1.0	1.3
Mode of feeding	D5W	TPN	PPN	TPN	TPN	PO	PO
Weight (lb)	205	186	172	160	153	195	192
Albumin (g/dl)	3.4	2.6	2.4	3.2	3.9	4.4	4.0
Skin tests	0/4	0/4	0/4	0/4	0/4	2/4	2/4
(positive reaction/total tests administered)							

D5W = 5% dextrose solution; TPN = central venous hyperalimentation; PPN = peripheral parenteral nutrition; PO = oral diet.

ture of PPN. Although the mechanism for the impairment of nitrogen utilization or excretion is equivocal, its tendency to cause azotemia should be kept in mind.

MONITORING

The high incidence of associated dangerous complications with TPN or PPN necessitates frequent monitoring of the burned patient's response to parenteral nutrition, and the regimen should be altered as indicated. Variables that should be evaluated include the patient's temperature, blood pressure, fluid balance, and urinary glucose and acetone levels every 8 hours. Serum electrolyte, BUN, creatinine, and glucose levels and blood gases are determined daily until levels stabilize within normal ranges, and then every 2 to 3 days thereafter. Weekly measurements of serum calcium, phosphorus, magnesium, SGOT, SGPT, and alkaline phosphatase should be performed to ensure adequate mineral replacement and monitoring of liver function. The best measures of assessing the nutritional adequacy of the parenteral regimen involve biweekly indirect calorimetry, nitrogen balance, serum albumin, serum transferrin, body weight, and calculation of energy and protein intake from all sources (e.g., oral, tube feeding, and intravenous). Interpretation of these data has been exten-

sively reviewed elsewhere [33, 91, 92, 116, 132].

CONCLUSIONS

An extensive burn injury introduces a complex nutritional challenge that is closely related to the ultimate survival of the patient. The application of parenteral nutrition has undoubtedly contributed to improved outcome in burned patients unable to be supported enterally. No longer does the thermally injured patient need to deteriorate when enteral feeding is insufficient or contraindicated; however, the metabolic and mechanical complications of parenteral hyperalimentation and the markedly increased susceptibility to infection of the burned patient speak for reserving TPN for those whose nutritional needs cannot be met by the enteral route. Adherence to strict protocols of infection control, along with individual balancing and continuous monitoring, will most often promote a successful intravenous feeding program.

Although exciting advances have been made in this field during the past two decades, there are still many considerations that are far from clear. Our knowledge regarding the precise nutrient needs of the burn victim is incomplete. Many of the guidelines for nutrient intake in burns are based on enteral studies, and it is likely that there are some differences in nutrient requirements, depending on the route of administration. Future efforts should be directed toward improving the composition of parenteral formulations, delivery systems, and clinical monitors in an effort to maximize nutritional rehabilitation while minimizing complications.

Acknowledgment

Supported in part by a grant from the Shriners of North America.

The authors wish to express their appreciation for the contribution of Marilyn Jenkins, R.N., M.B.A., Al Waldbillig, R.N., Mary McErlane, and Joanne Orr to this manuscript.

REFERENCES

1. Aikawa, N., Caufield, J. B., Thomas, R. J. S., and Burke, J. F. Postburn hypermetabolism: Relation to evaporative heat loss and catecholamine level. *Surg. Forum* 26:74, 1975.
2. Alexander, J. W. Nutrition and infection: New perspectives for an old problem. *Arch. Surg.* 121:966, 1986.
3. Alexander, J. W. Nutrition and metabolic response to injury. In *Proceedings of the International Society for Burn Injuries.* Istanbul, Turkey, 1988. P. 109.
4. Alexander, J. W., MacMillan, B. G., Stinnett, J. P., et al. Beneficial effects of aggressive protein feeding in severely burned children. *Ann. Surg.* 192:505, 1980.
5. Alexander, J. W., Saito, H., Ogle, C. K., and Trocki, O. The importance of lipid type in the diet after burn injury. *Ann. Surg.* 204:1, 1986.
6. Allison, S. P., Hinton, P., and Chamberlain, M. J. Intravenous glucose tolerance, insulin and free fatty acid levels in burned patients. *Lancet* 2:1113, 1968.
7. Alverdy, J., Chi, H. S., and Sheldon, G. F. The effect of parenteral nutrition on gastrointestinal immunity: The importance of enteral stimulation. *Ann. Surg.* 202:681, 1985.
8. American Medical Association Department of Foods and Nutrition. Multivitamin preparations for parenteral use: A statement by the Nutrition Advisory Group. *J. Parenter. Enter. Nutr.* 3:258, 1979.
9. American Medical Association Department of Foods and Nutrition. Guidelines for essential trace element preparations for parenteral use. *J.A.M.A.* 241:2051, 1979.
10. Arney, G. K., Pearson, E., and Sutherland, A. B. Burn stress pseudodiabetes. *Ann. Surg.* 152:77, 1960.
11. Arturson, M. G., Arachidonic acid metabolism and prostaglandin activity following burn injury. In J. L. Ninnemann (ed.), *Traumatic Injury: Infection and Other Immunologic Sequela.* Baltimore: University Park Press, 1983. P. 57.
12. Askanazi, J., Elwyn, D. H., Silverberg, P. A., Rosenbaum, S. H., and Kinney, J. M. Respiratory distress secondary to high carbohydrate load. *Surgery* 87:596, 1980.
13. Askanazi, J., Rosenbaum, S. H., Hyman, A. I., Silverberg, P. A., Milic-Emili, J., and Kinney, J. M. Respiratory changes induced by large glucose loads of total parenteral nutrition. *J.A.M.A.* 243:1444, 1980.
14. Askanazi, J., Weissman, C., Rosenbaum, S. H., Hyman, A. I., Milic-Emili, J., and Kinney, J. M. Nutrition and the respiratory system. *Crit. Care Med.* 10:163, 1982.
15. Aulick, L. H., and Wilmore, D. W. Increased peripheral amino acid release following burn injury. *Surgery* 85:560, 1979.
16. Aussel, C., Cynober, L., Lioret, N., et al. Plasma branched-chain keto acids in burn patients. *Am. J. Clin. Nutr.* 44:825, 1986.
17. Bailey, B. N. Hyperglycemia in burns. *Br. Med. J.* 2:1783, 1960.
18. Bane, J. W., McCaa, R. E., and McCaa, C. S. The pattern of aldosterone and cortisone blood levels in thermal burn patients. *J. Trauma* 14:605, 1974.
19. Baracos, V., Rodemann, H. P., Dinarello, C. A., and Goldberg, A. L. Stimulation of muscle protein degradation and prostaglandin E$_2$ release by leukocytic pyrogen (interleukin-1): A mechanism for the increased degradation of muscle proteins during fever. *N. Engl. J. Med.* 308:553, 1983.
20. Barbul, A., Fishel, R. S., Shimaz, S., et al. Intravenous hyperalimentation with high arginine levels improves wound healing and immune function. *J. Surg. Res.* 38:328, 1985.
21. Barbul, A., Rettura, G., Levenson, S. M., and Seifter, E. Arginine: A thymotrophic and wound-healing promoting agent. *Surg. Forum* 28:101, 1977.
22. Barbul, A., Rettura, G., Levenson, S. M., and Seifter, E. Thymotrophic actions of arginine, ornithine and growth hormone. *Fed. Proc.* 37:264, 1978.
23. Barbul, A., Rettura, G., Levenson, S. M., and Seifter, E. Wound healing and thymotrophic effects of arginine: A pituitary mechanism of action. *Am. J. Clin. Nutr.* 37:786, 1983.
24. Barbul, A., Sisto, D. A., Wasserkrug, H. L., and Efron, G. Arginine stimulates lymphocyte immune response in healthy human beings. *Surgery* 90:244, 1981.

25. Barbul, A., Sisto, D. A., Wasserkrug, H. L., Yoshimura, N., and Efron, G. Nitrogen-sparing and immune mechanisms of arginine: Differential dose-dependent responses during post-injury intravenous hyperalimentation. *Curr. Surg.* 40:114, 1983.

26. Barbul, A., Wasserkrug, H. L., Sisto, D. A., et al. Thymic stimulatory actions of arginine. *J. Parenter. Enter. Nutr.* 4:446, 1980.

27. Barr, P. O., Birke, G., Liljidahl, S. O., and Plantin, L. O. Oxygen consumption and water loss during treatment of burns with warm dry air. *Lancet* 1:164, 1968.

28. Barrocas, A., Tretola, R., and Alonso, A. Nutrition and the critically ill pulmonary patient. *Respir. Care* 28:50, 1983.

29. Batstone, G. F., Alberti, K. G., and Hinks. L. Metabolic studies in subjects following thermal injury. *Burns* 2:207, 1976.

30. Baxter, C. R., Roberts, C., Germany, B., Heck, E., Ireton, C., and Dobke, M. Effect of Intralipid on polymorphological function. *Proc. Am. Burn. Assoc.*, Vol. 17, 1985.

31. Becker, R. A., Vaughn, G. M., Goodwin, C. W., et al. Interactions of thyroid hormones and catecholamine in severely burned patients. *Rev. Infect. Dis.* 5:S908, 1983.

32. Beckler, J. M., Bruck, H. M., Munster, A. M., Curreri, P. W., and Pruitt, B. A. Superior mesenteric artery syndrome as a consequence of burn injury. *J. Trauma* 12:979, 1972.

33. Bell, S. J., Molnar, J. A., Krasker, W. S., and Burke, J. F. Prediction of total urinary nitrogen from urea nitrogen for burned patients. *J. Am. Diet. Assoc.* 85:1100, 1985.

34. Berman, M. L., Hamrell, C. E., Lagasse, L. D., et al. Parenteral nutrition by peripheral vein in the management of gynecologic oncology patients. *Gynecol. Oncol.* 7:318, 1979.

35. Birke, G., Carlson, L. A., and Liljedahl, S. O. Lipid metabolism and trauma. III. Plasma lipids and lipoproteins in burns. *Acta Med. Scand.* 178:337, 1965.

36. Birke, G., Carlson, L. A., Von Euler, U. S., Liljedahl, S. O., and Plantin, L. C. Lipid metabolism, catecholamine excretion, basal metabolic rate and water loss during treatment of burns with dry air. *Acta Chir. Scand.* 138:321, 1972.

37. Birkhahn, R. H., and Border, J. R. Alternate or supplemental energy sources. *J. Parenter. Enter. Nutr.* 5:24, 1981.

38. Blackburn, G. L., Flatt, J. P., Clowes, G. H., and O'Donnell, T. E. Peripheral intravenous feeding with isotonic amino acid solutions. *Am. J. Surg.* 125:447, 1973.

39. Bower, R. H., Muggia-Sullam, M., Vallgren, S., et al. Branched chain amino acid–enriched solutions in the septic patient: A randomized, prospective trial. *Ann. Surg.* 203:13, 1986.

40. Burke, J. F., Wolfe, R. R., Mullany, C. J., Mathews, D. E., and Bier, D. M. Glucose requirements following burn injury: Parameters of optimal glucose infusion and possible hepatic and respiratory abnormalities following excessive glucose intake. *Ann. Surg.* 190:274, 1979.

41. Caldwell, F. T. Energy metabolism following thermal burns. *Arch. Surg.* 111:181, 1976.

42. Caldwell, F. T., Bowser, B. H., and Crabtree, J. H. The effect of occlusive dressings on the energy metabolism of severely burned children. *Ann. Surg.* 193:579, 1981.

43. Cerra, F., Hirsch, J., Mullen, K., Blackburn, G., and Luther, W. The effect of stress level, amino acid formula, and nitrogen dose on nitrogen retention in traumatic and septic stress. *Ann. Surg.* 205:282, 1987.

44. Chandra, R. K., and Au, B. Single nutrient deficiency and cell-mediated immune responses. I. Zinc. *Am. J. Clin. Nutr.* 33:736, 1980.

45. Coombes, E. J., Shakespeare, P. G., and Batstone, G. F. Lipoprotein changes after burn injury in man. *J. Trauma* 20:971, 1980.

46. Curreri, P. W., Hicks, J. E., Aronoff, R. J., and Baxter, C. R. Inhibition of active sodium transport in erythrocytes from burn patients. *Surg. Gynecol. Obstet.* 139:538, 1974.

47. Curreri, P. W., Richmond, D., Marvin, J., and Baxter, C. R. Dietary requirements of patients with major burns. *J. Am. Diet. Assoc.* 65:415, 1974.

48. Curreri, P. W., Wilmore, D. W., Mason, A. D., Newsome, T. W., Asch, M. J., and Pruitt, B. A. Intracellular cation alterations following major trauma: Effect of supranormal caloric intake. *J. Trauma* 11:390, 1971.

49. Cuthbertson, D. P. Post-shock metabolic response. *Lancet* 1:433, 1942.

50. Cynober, L., Nguyen Dinh, F., Blonde, F., Saizy, R., and Giboudeau, J. Plasma and urinary amino acid pattern in severe burn patients: Evolution throughout the healing period. *Am. J. Clin. Nutr.* 36:416, 1982.

51. Cynober, L., Nguyen Dinh, F., Saizy, R., Blonde, F., and Giboudeau, J. Plasma amino acid levels in the first few days after burn injury and their predictive value. *Intens. Care Med.* 9:325, 1983.

52. Czaja, A. J., McAlhany, J. C., and Pruitt, B. A. Gastric acid secretion and acute gastroduodenal disease after burns. *Arch. Surg.* 111:243, 1976.

53. Danielsson, U., Arturson, G., and Wennberg, L. Variations of metabolic rate in burned patients as a result of the injury and the care. *Burns* 5:169, 1978.

54. Deitch, E. A., Maejima, K., and Berg, R. Effect of oral antibiotics and bacterial overgrowth on the translocation of the gastrointestinal tract microflora in burned rats. *J. Trauma* 25:385, 1985.

55. Dietch, E. A., Winterton, J., and Berg, R. Thermal injury promotes bacterial translocation from the gastrointestinal tract in mice with impaired T cell-mediated immunity. *Arch. Surg.* 121:97, 1986.

56. Derganc, M. Parenteral nutrition in severely burned children. *Scand. J. Plast. Reconstr. Surg.* 13:195, 1979.

57. Dolocek, R., Adamkova, M., and Sotornikova, T. Endocrine response after burn. *Scand. J. Plast. Reconstr. Surg.* 13:9, 1979.

58. Dudrick, S., Wilmore, D., Vars H., and Rhoads, J. E. Can intravenous feeding as the sole means of nutrition support growth in the child and restore weight loss in an adult? *Ann. Surg.* 169:974, 1969.

59. Ellner, J. J. Suppressor cells of man. *Clin. Immunol. Rev.* 1:119, 1981.

60. Elwyn, D. H., Gump, F. E., Iles, M., Long, C. L., and Kinney, J. M. Protein and energy sparing of glucose added in hypocaloric amounts to peripheral infusions of amino acids. *Metabolism* 27:325, 1978.

61. English, D., Roloff, J. S., Lukens, J. N., Parker, P., Greene, H. L., and Ghishan, F. K. Intravenous lipid emulsions and human neutrophil function. *J. Pediatr.* 99:913, 1981.

62. Felig, P. The glucose-alanine cycle. *Metabolism* 22:179, 1973.

63. Fischer, S. W., Hunter, K. W., Wilson, S. R., and Mease, A. D. Diminished bacterial defenses with Intralipid. *Lancet* 2:819, 1980.

64. Freund, H. R., Yoshimura, N., and Fischer, J. E. Does intravenous fat spare nitrogen in the injured rat? *Am. J. Surg.* 140:377, 1980.

65. Gang, R. K. Adhesive zinc tape in burns: Results of a clinical trial. *Burns* 7:322, 1981.

66. Garre, M. A., Boles, J. M., and Youinou, P. Y. Current concepts in immune derangement due to undernutrition. *J. Parenter. Enter. Nutr.* 11:309, 1987.

67. Goodenough, R. D., and Wolfe, R. R. Effect of total parenteral nutrition on free fatty acid metabolism in burned patients. *J. Parenter. Enter. Nutr.* 8:357, 1984.

68. Goodwin, C. W., and Pruitt, B. A. Increased incidence of pancreatitis in thermally injured patients: A prospective study. *Proc. Am. Assoc. Surg. Trauma* 13:106. 1981.

69. Gottschlich, M. M., and Alexander, J. W. Fat kinetics and recommended dietary intake in burns. *J. Parenter. Enter. Nutr.* 11:80, 1987.

70. Gottschlich, M. M. Acute thermal injury. In C. E. Lang (ed.), *Nutritional Support in Critical Care.* Rockville, MD: Aspen, 1987. Pp. 159–181.

71. Gottschlich, M. M., Jenkins, M., Warden, G. D., et al. Differential effects of three enteral feeding regimens on selected outcome variables in burn patients. *J. Parenter. Enter. Nutr.* 14:225, 1990.

72. Gottschlich, M. M. Micronutrients. In A. Skipper (ed.), *The Dietitian's Handbook of Enteral and Parenteral Nutrition.* Rockville, MD: Aspen, 1989. Pp. 163–203.

73. Gottschlich, M. M., Warden, G. D., Michel, M. A., et al. Diarrhea in tube-fed burn patients: Incidence, etiology, nutritional impact, and prevention. *J. Parenter. Enter. Nutr.* 12:338, 1988.

74. Groves, A. C., Moore, J. P., Woolf, L. I., and Duff, J. H. Arterial plasma amino acids in patients with severe burns. *Surgery* 83:138, 1978.

75. Henzel, J. W., DeWeese, M. S., and Lichit, E. L., Zinc concentrations within healing wounds. *Arch. Surg.* 100:349, 1970.

76. Harris, J. A., and Benedict, F. G. *Biometric Studies of Basal Metabolism In Man.* Publication no. 279. Carnegie Institute of Washington, 1919.

77. Harris, R. L., Cottam, G. L., Johnston, J. M., and Baxter, C. R. The pathogenesis of abnormal erythrocyte morphology in burns. *J. Trauma* 21:13, 1981.

78. Harris, R. L., Frenkel, R. A., Cottam, G. L., and Baxter, C. R., Lipid mobilization and metabolism after thermal trauma. *J. Trauma* 22:194, 1982.

79. Harrison, T. S., Seaton, J. F., and Feller, I. Relationship of increased oxygen consumption to catecholamine excretion in thermal burns. *Ann. Surg.* 165:169, 1967.

80. Haydock, D. A., and Hill, G. L. Improved wound healing response in surgical patients receiving intravenous nutrition. *Br. J. Surg.* 74:320, 1987.

81. Hebiert, J. M., and Botens, J. Protein requirements in the burned patient: Controlled interaction of injury, protein and calories. *J. Parenter. Enter. Nutr.* 8:87, 1984.

82. Heird, W. C., Nicholson, J. F., Driscoll, J. M., Schullinger, J. N., and Winters, R. W. Hyperammonemia resulting from intravenous alimentation using a mixture of synthetic L-amino acids: A preliminary report. *J. Pediatr.* 81:162, 1972.

83. Helmkamp, G. M., Wilmore, D. W., Johnson, A. A., and Pruitt, B. A., Essential fatty acid deficiency in red cells after thermal injury: Correction with intravenous fat therapy. *Am. J. Clin. Nutr.* 26:1331, 1973.

84. Herndon, D. N., Stein, M. D., Rutan, T. C., Abston, S., and Linares, H. Failure of TPN

supplementation to improve liver function, immunity, and mortality in thermally injured patients. *J. Trauma* 27:195, 1987.

85. Herndon, D. N., Wilmore, D. W., Mason, A. D., and Pruitt, B. A. Abnormalities in phenylalanine and tyrosine kinetics: Significance in septic and nonseptic burned patients. *Arch. Surg.* 113:133, 1978.

86. Hunt, D. R., Lane, H. W., Beesinger, D., et al. Selenium depletion in burn patients. *Parenter. Enter. Nutr.* 8:695, 1984.

87. Ireton, C. S., Turner, W. W., Hunt, J. L., and Liepa, G. U. Evaluation of energy expenditures in burn patients. *J. A-M. Diet. Assoc.* 86:331, 1986.

88. Jahoor. F., Herndon, D. H., and Wolfe, R. R. Role of insulin and glucagon in the response of glucose and alanine kinetics in burn-injured patients. *J. Clin. Invest.* 78:807, 1986.

89. Jarstrand, C., Berghem, L., and Lahnborg, G. Human granulocytes and reticuloendothelial system function during Intralipid infusion. *J. Parenter. Enter. Nutr.* 2:663, 1978.

90. Jenkins, M., Gottschlich, M. M., Waymack, J. P., Alexander, J. W., and Warden, G. D. An evaluation of the effect of immediate enteral feeding on the hypermetabolic response following severe burn injury. *Proc. Am. Burn Assoc.* 20: 1988.

91. Jensen, T. G. Determination of nutritional status in critical care. *J. Am. Diet. Assoc.* 84:1345, 1984.

92. Kagan, R. J., Matsuda, T., Hanumadass, M., Castillo, B., and Jonasson, O. The effect of burn wound size on ureagenesis and nitrogen balance. *Ann. Surg.* 195:70, 1982.

93. Keller, G. A., West, M. A., Cerra, F. B., and Simmons, R. L. Multiple systems organ failure: Modulation of hepatocyte protein synthesis by endotoxin activated Kupffer cells. *Ann. Surg.* 201:87, 1985.

94. Kramer, G. M., Dillios, L. C., and Bowler, E. C. Ascorbic acid treatment on early collagen production and wound healing in the guinea pig. *J. Peridontol.* 50:189, 1979.

95. Kravitz, M., Woodruff, J., Petersen, S., and Warden, G. D. The use of the Dobhoff tube to provide additional nutritional support in thermally injured patients. *J. Burn Care Rehabil.* 3:226, 1982.

96. Larkin, J. M., and Moylan, J. A. Complete enteral support of thermally injured patients. *Am. J. Surg.* 131:722, 1976.

97. Larson, D. L., Maxwell, R., Abston, S., and Dobrokovsky, M. Zinc deficiency in burned children. *Plast. Reconstr. Surg.* 46:13, 1970.

98. Lennard, E. S., Alexander, J. W., Craycraft, T., and MacMillan, B. G. Association in burn patients of improved antibacterial defense with nutritional support by the oral route. *Burns* 1:98, 1974.

99. Lescher, T. J., Sirinek, K. R., and Pruitt, B. A. Superior mesenteric artery syndrome in thermally injured patients. *J. Trauma* 19:567, 1979.

100. Lescher, T. J., Teejarden, D. K., and Pruitt, B. A. Acute pseudo-obstruction of the colon in thermally injured patients. *Dis. Colon Rectum* 21:618, 1978.

101. Levine, G., Deren, J., Steiger, E., and Zinno, R. Role of oral intake in maintenance of gut mass and disaccharide activity. *Gastroenterology* 67:975, 1974.

102. Long, C. L. Energy expenditure of major burns. *J. Trauma* 19:904, 1979.

103. Long, C. L., Schaffel, N., Geiger, J. W., Schiller, W. R., and Blakemore, W. S. Metabolic response to injury and illness: Estimation of energy and protein needs from indirect calorimetry and nitrogen balance. *J. Parenter. Enter. Nutr.* 3:452, 1979.

104. Long, C. L., Spencer, J. L., Kinney, J. M., and Geiger, J. W. Carbohydrate metabolism in man: Effect on elective operations and major injury. *J. Appl. Physiol.* 31:110, 1971.

105. Long, J. M., Wilmore, D. W., Mason, A. D., and Pruitt, B. A. Effect of carbohydrate and fat intake on nitrogen excretion during total intravenous feeding. *Ann. Surg.* 185:417, 1977.

106. Lund, C. C., Levenson, S. M., and Green, R. W. Ascorbic acid, thiamine, riboflavin and nicotinic acid in relation to acute burns in man. *Arch. Surg.* 55:557, 1947.

107. McArdle, A. H., Palmason, C., Brown, R. A., Brown, H. C., and Williams, H. B. Early enteral feeding of patients with major burns: Prevention of catabolism. *Ann. Plast. Surg.* 13:396, 1984.

108. McDougal, W. S., Wilmore, D. W., and Pruitt, B. A. Effects of intravenous near isosmotic nutrient infusions and nitrogen balance in critically ill injured patients. *Surg. Gynecol. Obstet.* 145:408, 1977.

109. Merimee, T. J., Lillicrap, D. A., and Rabinowitz, D. Effect of arginine on serum levels of human growth hormone. *Lancet* 2:668, 1965.

110. Meurling, S., and Roos, K. A. Liver changes in rats on continuous and intermittent parenteral nutrition with and without fat (Intralipid 20%). *Acta Chir. Scand.* 147:475, 1981.

111. Minuskin, M. L., Lavine, M. E., Ulman, E. A., and Fisher, H. Nitrogen retention, muscle creatinine and orotic acid excretion in traumatized rats fed arginine and glycine enriched diets. *J. Nutr.* 111:1265, 1981.

112. Mochizuki, H., Trocki, O., Dominioni, L.,

and Alexander, J. W. Effect of a diet rich in branched chain amino acids on severely burned guinea pigs. *J. Trauma* 26:1077, 1986.

113. Mochizuki, H., Trocki, O., Dominioni, L., Brackett, K., Joffe, S. N., and Alexander, J. W. Mechanism of prevention of post-burn hypermetabolism and catabolism by early enteral feeding. *Ann. Surg.* 200:297, 1984.

114. Moore, E. E., and Jones, T. Benefits of immediate jejunostomy feeding after major abdominal trauma: A prospective randomized study. *J. Trauma* 26:874, 1986.

115. Morath, M. A., Miller, S. F., and Finley, R. K. Use and abuse of peripheral parenteral nutrition: A case study. In *Proceedings of the International Society for Burn Injuries.* San Francisco, 1982. P. 67.

116. Morath, M. A., Miller, S. F., Finley, R. K., and Jones, L. M. Interpretation of nutritional parameters in burn patients. *J. Burn Care Rehabil.* 4:361, 1983.

117. Mulloy, A. L., Kari, F. W., and Visek, W. J. Dietary arginine, insulin secretion, glucose tolerance and liver lipids during repletion of protein-depleted rats. *Horm. Metab. Res.* 14:471, 1982.

118. Najarian, J. S., and Harper, H. A. A clinical study of the effect of arginine on blood ammonia. *Am. J. Med.* 21:832, 1956.

119. Neely, W. A., Petro, A. B., Holloman, G. H., Rushton, F. W., Turner, M. D., and Hardy, J. D. Reseaches on the cause of burn hypermetabolism. *Ann. Surg.* 179:291, 1974.

120. Nylen, B., and Wallenius, G. The protein loss via exudation from burns and granulating wound surfaces. *Acta Chir. Scand.* 122:97, 1961.

121. Orton, C. I., Segal, A. W., Bloom, S. R., and Clarke, J. Hypersecretion of glucagon and gastrin in severely burnt patients. *Br. Med. J.* 2:170, 1975.

122. Pachl, J., Kruf, M., Zabrodsky, V., et al. Total parenteral nutrition in severe paediatric burns. *Acta Chir. Plast.* 25:194, 1983.

123. Pine, R. W., Wertz, W. J., Lennard, E. S., Dellinger, E. P., Carrico, C. J., and Minshew, B. H. Determinants of organ malfunction or death in patients with intra-abdominal sepsis: A discriminant analysis. *Arch. Surg.* 118:242, 1983.

124. Popp, M. B., Law, E. J., and MacMillan, B. G. Parenteral nutrition in the burned child: A study of twenty-six patients. *Ann Surg.* 179:219, 1974.

125. Pories, W. J., Henzel, J. H., Rob, C. G., and Strain, W. H. Acceleration of wound healing in man with zinc sulfate given by mouth. *Lancet* 1:121, 1967.

126. Pui, Y. M. L., and Fisher, H. Factorial supplementation with arginine and glycine on nitrogen retention and body weight gain in the traumatized rat. *J. Nutr.* 109:240. 1979.

127. Rodemann, H. P., and Goldberg, A. L. Arachidonic acid, prostaglandin E_2 and F_2 influence rates of protein turnover in skeletal and cardiac muscle. *J. Biol. Chem.* 257:1632, 1982.

128. Roe, C. F., Kinney, J. M., and Blau, C. Water and heat exchange in third degree burns. *Surgery* 56:212, 1964.

129. Rose, W. C. The amino acid requirements of adult man. *Nutr. Abstr. Rev.* 27:631, 1957.

130. Royle, G. T., and Kettlewell, M. G. W. Liver function tests in surgical infection and malnutrition. *Ann. Surg.* 192:192, 1981.

131. Sadowski, D. A., Harrell, D. A., Maley, M. P., and Warden, G. D. The value of culturing central-line catheter tips in burn patients. *J. Burn Care Rehabil.* 9:66, 1988.

132. Saffle, J. R., Medina, E., Raymond, J., Westenskow, D., Kravitz, M., and Warden, G. D. Use of indirect calorimetry in the nutritional management of burned patients. *J. Trauma* 25:32, 1985.

133. Saito, H., Trocki, O., and Alexander, J. W. Comparison of immediate postburn enteral versus parenteral nutrition. *J. Parenter. Enter. Nutr.* 9:115, 1985.

134. Saito, H., Trocki, O., Alexander, J. W., Kopcha, R., Heyd, T., and Joffe, S. N. The effect of route of nutrient administration on the nutritional state, catabolic hormone secretion, and gut mucosal integrity after burn injury. *J. Parenter. Enter. Nutr.* 11:1, 1987.

135. Saito, H., Trocki, O., Heyd, T., and Alexander, J. W. Effect of dietary unsaturated fatty acids and indomethacin on metabolism and survival after burn. *Proc. Am. Burn Assoc.* 17:1985.

136. Saito, H., Trocki, O., Wang, S., Gonce, S. J., Joffe, S. N., and Alexander, J. W. Metabolic and immune effects of dietary arginine supplementation after burn. *Arch. Surg.* 122:784, 1987.

137. Sax, H. C., Talamini, M. A., and Fischer, J. E. Clinical use of branched chain amino acids in liver disease, sepsis, trauma and burns. *Arch. Surg.* 121:358, 1986.

138. Seifter, E., Rettura, G., Barbul, A., and Levenson, S. M. Arginine: An essential amino acid for injured rats. *Surgery* 84:224, 1978.

139. Sengupta, K. P., and Deb, S. K. Role of vitamin C in collagen synthesis. *Indian J. Exp. Biol.* 16:1061, 1978.

140. Serog, P., Baigts, F., Apfelbaum, M., Guilbaud, J., Chauvin, B., and Pecquer, M. L. Energy and nitrogen balances in 24 severely burned patients receiving 4 isocaloric diets of about 10 MJ/m²/day (2392 Kcalories/m²/day). *Burns* 9:422, 1983.

141. Shizgal, H. M., and Forse, R. A. Protein and caloric requirements with total parenteral nutrition. *Ann. Surg.* 192:562, 1980.

142. Shuck, J. M., Eaton, R. P., Shuck, L. W., Wachtel, T. L., and Schade, D. S. Dynamics of insulin and glucagon secretion in severely burned patients. *J. Trauma* 17:706, 1977.

143. Schumer, W. Consensus summary on metabolism. *J. Trauma* 19:910, 1979.

144. Smith, R. C., Hartemink, R. J., and Duggan, D. Prolonged multipurpose venous access in burned patients: Three years experience with Hickman right atrial catheters. *J. Trauma* 25:634, 1985.

145. Snelling, C. F. T., Woolf, L. I., Groves, A. C., Moore, J. P., and Duff, J. H. Amino acid metabolism in patients with severe burns. *Surgery* 91:474, 1982.

146. Soroff, H. S., Pearson, E., and Artz, C. P. An estimation of nitrogen requirements for equilibrium in burned patients. *Surg. Gynecol. Obstet.* 112:159, 1961.

147. Souba, W. W., Long, J. M., and Dudrick, S. J. Energy intake and stress as determinants of nitrogen excretion in rats. *Surg. Forum* 29:76, 1978.

148. Stinnett, J., Alexander, J. W., Watanabe, C., et al. Plasma and skeletal muscle amino acids following severe burn injury in patients and experimental animals. *Ann. Surg.* 195:75, 1982.

149. Strunk, R. C., Kunke, K. S., Kolski, G. B., and Revsin, B. K. Intralipid alters macrophage membrane fatty acid composition and inhibits complement (C_2) synthesis. *Lipids* 18:493, 1983.

150. Suskind, R. Gastrointestinal changes in the malnourished child. *Pediatr. Clin. North Am.* 22:873, 1975.

151. Taylor, F. H. L., Levenson, S., Adams, M. A. Abnormal carbohydrate metabolism in human thermal burns. *N. Engl. J. Med.* 231:437, 1944.

152. Thomas, W. R., and Holt, P. G. Vitamin C and immunity: An assessment of the evidence. *Clin. Exp. Immunol.* 32:370, 1978.

153. Trocki, O., Heyd, T. J., Waymack, J. P., and Alexander, J. W. Effects of fish oil on postburn metabolism and immunity. *J. Parenter. Enter. Nutr.* 11:521, 1987.

154. Turner, W. W., Ireton, C. S., Hunt, J. C., and Baxter, C. R. Predicting energy expenditures in burned patients. *J. Trauma* 25:11, 1985.

155. Vaughn, G. M., Becker, R. A., Allen, J. P., Goodwin, C. W., Pruitt, B. A., and Mason, A. D. Cortisol and corticotrophin in burned patients. *J. Trauma* 22:263, 1982.

156. Warden, G. D., Wilmore, D. W., and Pruitt, B. A. Central venous thrombosis: A hazard of medical progress. *J. Trauma* 13:620, 1973.

157. Warden, G. D., Wilmore, D. W., Rogers, P. W., Mason, A. D., and Pruitt, B. A. Hypernatremic state in hypermetabolic burn patients. *Arch. Surg.* 106:420, 1973.

158. Wilmore, D. W. Nutrition and metabolism following thermal injury. *Clin. Plast. Surg.* 1:603, 1974.

159. Wilmore, D. W. Glucose metabolism following severe injury. *J. Trauma* 21:705, 1981.

160. Wilmore, D. W., Aulick, L. H., Mason, A. D., and Pruitt, B. A. Influence of the burn wound on local and systemic responses to injury. *Ann. Surg.*, 186:444, 1977.

161. Wilmore, D. W., Curreri, P. W., Spitzer, K. W., Spitzer, M. E., and Pruitt, B. A. Supranormal dietary intake in thermally injured hypermetabolic patients. *Surg. Gynecol. Obstet.* 132:881, 1971.

162. Wilmore, D. W., Goodwin, C. W., Aulick, L. H., Powanda, M. C., Mason, A. D., and Pruitt, B. A. Effect of injury and infection on visceral metabolism and circulation. *Ann. Surg.* 192:491, 1980.

163. Wilmore, D. W., Lindsey, C. A., Moylan, J. A., Faloona, G. R., Pruitt, B. A., and Unger, R. H. Hyperglucagonemia after burns. *Lancet* 1:73, 1974.

164. Wilmore, D. W., Long, J. M., Skreen, R., Mason, A. D., and Pruitt, B. A. Catecholamines: Mediator of the hypermetabolic response following thermal injury. *Ann. Surg.* 180:653, 1974.

165. Wilmore, D. W., Mason, A. D., Johnson, D. W., and Pruitt, B. A. Effect of ambient temperature on heat production and heat loss in burn patients. *J. Appl. Physiol.* 38:593, 1975.

166. Wilmore, D. W., Mason, A. D., and Pruitt, B. A. Alterations in glucose kinetics following thermal injury. *Surg. Forum* 26:81, 1975.

167. Wilmore, D. W., Mason, A. D., and Pruitt, B. A. Insulin response to glucose in hypermetabolic burn patients. *Ann. Surg.* 183:314, 1976.

168. Wilmore, D. W., Moylan, J. A., Helmkamp, G. M., and Pruitt, B. A. Clinical evaluation of a 10% fat emulsion for parenteral nutrition in thermally injured patients. *Ann. Surg.* 178:503, 1973.

169. Wilmore, D. W., Orcutt, T., Mason, A. D., and Pruitt, B. A. Alterations in hypothalamic function following thermal injury. *J. Trauma* 15:697, 1975.

170. Wilmore, D. W., and Aulick, L. Systemic responses to injury and the healing wound. *J. Parenter. Enter. Nutr.* 4:147, 1980.

171. Wolfe, R. R., and Burke, J. F. Effect of burn trauma on glucose turnover, oxidation and recycling in guinea pigs. *Am. J. Physiol.* 233:E80, 1977.

172. Wolfe, R. R., Durkot, M. J., Allsop, J. R., and Burke, J. F. Glucose metabolism in severely burned patients. *Metabolism* 28:1031, 1979.

173. Xiao-jun, C., Chih-chun, Y., Wei-shia, H., Wei-tsung, H., and Tsi-siang, S. Changes of serum amino acids in severely burned patients. *Burns* 10:109, 1983.

174. Young, V. R., Motil, K. J., and Burke, J. F. Energy and protein metabolism in relation to requirements of the burned pediatric patient. In R. M. Suskind (ed.), *Textbook of Pediatric Nutrition*. New York: Raven Press, 1981. P. 309.

175. Zawacki, B. E., Spitzer, K. W., Mason, A. D., and Johns, L. A. Does increased evaporative water loss cause hypermetabolism in burn patients? *Ann. Surg.* 171:236, 1970.

Parenteral Nutrition in the Pediatric Patient

Brad W. Warner

When compared with that for adults, nutritional support of the pediatric population is unique, since early in life, growth consumes a major component of the calories and substrate administered. The degree of growth is dependent on age and is greatest during the 2- to 12-week interval of extrauterine life. Roughly 40% of total energy utilized by the 2-week-old infant is delegated to growth, and this percentage falls off rapidly over the ensuing 10 weeks (Fig. 20-1) [6]. Even during the adolescent growth spurt, growth rarely accounts for greater than 2 to 3% of total energy utilized. In special situations, such as very-low-birth- weight infants (< 1200 g), approximately 60% of total metabolizable energy intake is accounted for by growth alone [100].

An appreciation of the changes in body composition that occur during growth is important as it relates to caloric reserve during periods of starvation and the composition of body weight gain during growth. One of the most remarkable changes noted to occur during late fetal development is in the rapid deposition of body fat (Fig. 20-2) [67]. The relative paucity of body fat present in the premature infant is deleterious, since the relatively poor insulation allows for greater susceptibility to cold stress–induced hypermetabolism. Further, since fat is a major source of energy during periods of starvation, one can appreciate the relatively dismal reserve present in a 1000-g infant when compared with a 3500-g term infant, and even a 70-kg adult (Table 20-1) [138]. While the 70-kg adult has a fat reserve of roughly 141,000 kcal, the term infant (assuming 15% of body weight as adipose tissue) has a fat reserve of 4800 kcal. In contrast, the 1000-g premature infant has only 200 kcal of fat reserve. If one accepts that these infants require roughly 120 kcal/kg/day, it would not be difficult to understand why complete starvation for more than a day or two is poorly tolerated [65].

If it is assumed that the estimated energy cost of depositing protein is 8.66 kcal/g and of fat is 12.0 kcal/g [46], the energy cost of

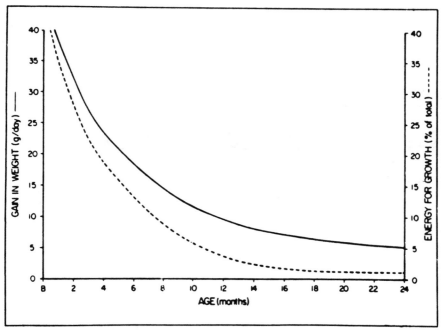

Figure 20-1. Daily gain in body weight and percentage of energy intake utilized for growth at 2 weeks to 2 years old. Solid line = weight gain (g/day); dashed line = energy for growth (%). (From Anderson, T. A. Birth through 24 months. In Rudolph, A. M. (ed.), *Pediatrics* (18th ed.). Norwalk, CT: Appleton & Lange, 1987. P. 158.)

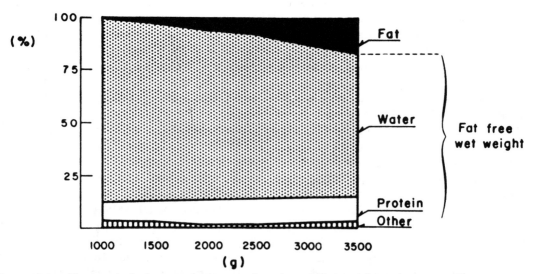

Figure 20-2. Changes in body composition as a function of fetal weight and gestational age. (From Heird, W. C., and Winters, R. W. Total parenteral nutrition: The state of the art. *J. Pediatr.* 86:2, 1975.)

Table 20-1. Endogenous Fuel Composition of Humans

	Body Weight (kg)		
	70.0	3.5	1.0
Fat (adipose triglyceride)			
Kg	15.0 (21%)*	0.53 (15%)*	0.023 (2.3%)*
Kcal	141,000	4800	200
Protein (mainly muscle)			
Kg	6.0	0.45	0.085
Kcal	24,000	1800	340
Glycogen (muscle)			
Kg	0.15	—	—
Kcal	600	—	—
Glycogen (liver)			
Kg	0.75	—	—
Kcal	300	—	—

*Percent of body weight.
From Zlotkin, S. H., Stallings, V. A., and Pencharz, P. B. Total parenteral nutrition in children. *Surg. Clin. North Am.* 32:381, 1985.

weight gain can be calculated from knowledge of body compositional changes during growth. The composition of body weight gain during growth appears to change most dramatically during the first 4 months of life (Table 20-2) [44], when a fairly rapid deposition of body fat is noted to occur. Thus, energy requirements per gram of weight appear to rise and fall in concert with the proportion of fat synthesized and deposited during late fetal development and early infancy [46].

INDICATIONS

With a few notable exceptions, the indications for parenteral nutrition in the pediatric population are similar to those for adults. Enteral nutrition is usually preferred since it is more physiologic, less expensive, and associated with fewer technical complications. There exist several circumstances in infants and children, however, whereby use of the gut is either contraindicated or not feasible.

Pediatric surgical disorders in which parenteral nutrition is commonly used include congenital anomalies that prevent the use of the gastrointestinal tract. Examples of these include gastroschisis, omphalocele,

tracheoesophageal fistula, intestinal atresia, meconium ileus, neonatal necrotizing enterocolitis, and the enterocolitis associated with Hirschsprung's disease. The role of parenteral nutrition in these situations is primarily for nutritional support until surgical correction of the anomaly allows for resumption of enteral intake. While there are no known controlled studies on the efficacy of parenteral nutrition in infants requiring gastrointestinal surgery, the available data overwhelmingly argue in favor of its continued use [31, 41, 59, 67, 116]. Such trials comparing parenteral nutrition versus the only alternative, starvation, are not likely to be generated due to obvious ethical considerations.

The short-bowel syndrome results from massive intestinal resection and mandates the parenteral route of nutrition administration. The minimum length of intact small bowel without an ileocecal valve required for survival without parenteral nutrition was reported by Wilmore to be 40 cm [129]. In that study, a survival rate of 50% was noted in patients with 15 to 38 cm of small bowel with an intact ileocecal valve, and no survivors were reported to have less than 15 cm of small bowel. With the use of parenteral nutrition, survival in patients with less than 15 cm of small bowel has been reported [75]. More recently, Grosfeld et al. [60] suggested that 20 cm of small intestine may be the minimum length required for survival. Zlotkin et al. [138] indicated that although the potential for survival after massive intestinal resection has dramatically improved since the advent of total parenteral nutrition (TPN), data as to the effect of this therapy on ultimate outcome are purely testimonial.

Intractable diarrhea of infancy is historically associated with a 40% mortality rate and has been reduced to essentially nil with parenteral nutritional support during the period of gut regeneration [61, 72].

Another situation whereby parenteral nutritional support has become increasingly important is in premature infants with necrotizing enterocolitis (NEC). Although the actual cause of this entity is still not known, enteral

Table 20-2. Body Composition of Reference Children

| | | | Fat | | | | Water | | | Minerals | | |
| | | | | | | | | | | | | |
Age	Length (cm)	Weight (gm)	g	%	Fat-Free Body Mass	Protein	Total Body Water	Extra-cellular Water	Cellular Water	Osseous	Non-osseous	Carbo-hydrate
Boys												
Birth	51.6	3545	486	13.7	3059	12.9	69.6	42.5	27.0	2.6	0.6	0.5
1 mo	54.8	4452	671	15.1	3781	12.9	68.4	41.1	27.3	2.6	0.6	0.5
2 mo	58.2	5509	1095	19.9	4414	12.3	64.3	38.0	26.3	2.4	0.6	0.5
3 mo	61.5	6435	1495	23.2	4940	12.0	61.4	35.7	25.8	2.3	0.6	0.5
4 mo	63.9	7060	1743	24.7	5317	11.9	60.1	34.5	25.7	2.3	0.5	0.4
5 mo	65.9	7575	1913	25.3	5662	11.9	59.6	33.8	25.8	2.3	0.5	0.4
6 mo	67.6	8030	2037	25.4	5993	12.0	59.4	33.4	26.0	2.3	0.5	0.4
9 mo	72.3	9180	2199	24.0	6981	12.4	60.3	33.0	27.2	2.3	0.6	0.5
12 mo	76.1	10150	2287	22.5	7863	12.9	61.2	32.9	28.3	2.3	0.6	0.5
18 mo	82.4	11470	2382	20.8	9088	13.5	62.2	32.3	29.9	2.5	0.6	0.5
24 mo	87.2	12590	2456	19.5	10134	14.0	62.9	31.9	31.0	2.6	0.6	0.5
3 yr	95.3	14675	2576	17.5	12099	14.7	63.9	31.1	32.8	2.8	0.6	0.5
4 yr	102.9	16690	2656	15.9	14034	15.3	64.8	30.5	34.2	2.9	0.6	0.5
5 yr	109.9	18670	2720	14.6	15950	15.8	65.4	30.0	35.4	3.1	0.6	0.5
6 yr	116.1	20690	2795	13.5	17895	16.2	66.0	29.6	36.4	3.2	0.6	0.5
7 yr	121.7	22850	2931	12.8	19919	16.5	66.2	29.1	37.1	3.3	0.6	0.5
8 yr	127.0	25300	3293	13.0	22007	16.6	65.8	28.3	37.5	3.4	0.6	0.5
9 yr	132.2	28130	3724	13.2	24406	16.8	65.4	27.6	37.8	3.5	0.6	0.5
10 yr	137.5	31440	4318	13.7	27122	16.8	64.8	26.7	38.0	3.5	0.6	0.5

Components of Fat-Free Body Mass (% of Body Wt)

Components of Fat-Free Body Mass (% of Body Wt)

Age	Length (cm)	Weight (gm)	Fat g	Fat %	Fat-Free Body Mass	Protein	Water Total Body Water	Water Extra-cellular Water	Water Cellular Water	Minerals Osseous	Minerals Non-osseous	Carbo-hydrate
Girls												
Birth	50.5	3325	495	14.9	2830	12.8	68.6	42.0	26.7	2.6	0.6	0.5
1 mo	53.4	4131	668	16.2	3463	12.7	67.5	40.5	26.9	2.5	0.6	0.5
2 mo	56.7	4989	1053	21.1	3936	12.2	63.2	37.1	26.1	2.4	0.6	0.5
3 mo	59.6	5743	1366	23.8	4377	12.0	60.9	35.1	25.8	2.3	0.6	0.5
4 mo	61.9	6300	1585	25.2	4715	11.9	59.6	33.8	25.8	2.3	0.5	0.4
5 mo	63.9	6800	1769	26.0	5031	11.9	58.8	33.0	25.9	2.2	0.5	0.4
6 mo	65.8	7250	1915	26.4	5335	12.0	58.4	32.4	26.0	2.2	0.5	0.4
9 mo	70.4	8270	2066	25.0	6204	12.5	59.3	32.0	27.3	2.3	0.5	0.4
12 mo	74.3	9180	2175	23.7	7005	12.9	60.1	31.8	28.3	2.3	0.5	0.5
18 mo	80.2	10780	2346	21.8	8434	13.5	61.3	31.4	29.8	2.4	0.6	0.5
24 mo	85.5	11910	2433	20.4	9477	13.9	62.2	31.5	30.8	2.4	0.6	0.5
3 yr	94.1	14100	2606	18.5	11494	14.4	63.5	31.3	32.2	2.5	0.6	0.5
4 yr	101.6	15960	2757	17.3	13203	14.8	64.3	31.2	33.1	2.5	0.6	0.5
5 yr	108.4	17660	2949	16.7	14711	15.0	64.6	31.0	33.6	2.5	0.6	0.5
6 yr	114.6	19520	3208	16.4	16312	15.2	64.7	30.8	34.0	2.6	0.6	0.5
7 yr	120.6	21840	3662	16.8	18178	15.2	64.4	30.3	34.1	2.5	0.6	0.5
8 yr	126.4	24840	4319	17.4	20521	15.2	63.8	29.6	34.2	2.5	0.6	0.5
9 yr	132.2	28460	5207	18.3	23253	15.1	63.0	28.9	34.1	2.5	0.6	0.5
10 yr	138.3	32550	6318	19.4	26232	15.0	62.0	28.1	33.9	2.5	0.6	0.5

From Foman, S. J., Haschke, F., Ziegler, E. E., and Nelson, S. E. Body composition of reference children from birth to age 10 years. *Am. J. Clin. Nutr.* 35:1169, 1982.

feeding early in life has been postulated to be an important associated factor [78, 81]. Parenteral nutrition during this vulnerable period may contribute to an attenuated risk for the development of NEC in high-risk infants. Evidence for this is provided by a study whereby 17 very-low-birth-weight infants were randomized to receive parenteral nutrition or enteral feeding of milk. Four patients in the control group developed NEC as compared with none of the parenterally fed infants [133]. Parenteral nutrition becomes even more important when the infant actually develops NEC, as the gut cannot be used for prolonged periods either during conservative management or after intestinal resection.

Very-low-birth-weight infants (< 1200 g) are often limited in their ability to ingest, tolerate, and absorb nutrients. As previously discussed, energy stores in the premature infant are scant, and nutritional supplementation must begin early. The most concentrated period of brain growth occurs during the thirteenth week of gestation to the fifth month of extrauterine life [27]. Irreversible reduced brain growth during malnutrition at this critical interval has been reported in laboratory animals [30, 130, 131]. The sole reliance on enteral nutrition is often impossible in these infants due to such factors as incompetence of the lower esophageal sphincter, uncoordinated gastrointestinal motility, and delayed gastric emptying. Intravenous nutrition is therefore a needed supplement while the immature intestinal tract gradually adapts to extrauterine life.

REQUIREMENTS

Energy

Energy requirements from birth through childhood are partitioned into maintenance of existing body tissues, provision for growth, and energy expended during activity. The importance of this latter consideration is illustrated in Table 20-3, as energy requirements decline from birth to the middle of the first year of life, and likely reflect re-

Table 20-3. Average Energy Requirement by Age

Age (mo)	Average Energy Requirement* (kcal/kg/d)
0–1	124
1–2	116
2–3	109
3–4	103
4–5	99
5–6	96.5
6–7	95
7–8	94.5
8–9	95
9–10	99
10–11	100
11–12	104.5

*Based on measured intakes.
From Beaton, G. H. Nutritional needs during the first year of life: Some concepts and perspectives. *Pediatr. Clin. North Am.* 32:275, 1985.

duced rates of growth. The rise in requirements during the latter half of the first year probably represents increased physical activity [13].

In considering low-birth-weight and premature infants, the Committee on Nutrition of the American Academy of Pediatrics [3] stated that the goal of feeding should be to obtain prompt resumption of growth at a rate approximating intrauterine growth. Using continuous, open-circuit indirect calorimetry, Reichman et al. [100] were able to determine energy requirements in 13 very-low-birth-weight infants (Fig. 20-3). Maintenance requirements were noted to be approximately 51 kcal/kg/day. To achieve the equivalent expected rate of intrauterine weight gain, it was determined that an additional 60 kcal/kg/day be provided. These calculations were based on enterally fed infants and must therefore allocate losses for unabsorbed nutrients, due primarily to fat malabsorption.

Fewer calories are required when nutrition is administered intravenously, and adequate growth in neonates has been documented with parenteral intakes in the range of 88 to 90 kcal/kg/day [19, 23]. In a study of 22 premature, parenterally fed infants, significant

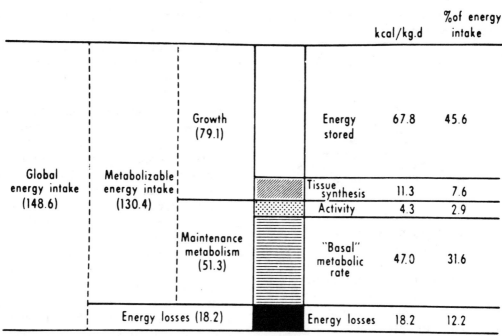

Figure 20-3. Partition of energy utilization from 22 metabolic and nutritional balance studies in 13 very-low-birth-weight, formula-fed infants under thermoneutral conditions. Results are expressed as mean kilocalories per kilogram per day and percent of gross energy intake. (From Reichman, B. L., Chessex, P., Putet, G., et al. Partition of energy metabolism and energy cost of growth in the very low-birth-weight infant. *Pediatrics* 69:446, 1982.)

increases in nitrogen retention and weight gain were reported when a constant nitrogen intake was administered and energy intake was increased from 50 to 80 nonprotein kcal/kg/day [137]. Beyond an energy intake of 70 kcal/kg/day, further increases in energy intake had only minimal effect on nitrogen retention, thus suggesting that basal metabolic needs were probably met at this level. Intrauterine nitrogen accretion rates were duplicated when energy intake was greater than 70 kcal/kg/day and nitrogen was provided at a rate of 2.7 to 3.5 g of protein/kg/day.

In a controlled trial, Anderson et al. [5] evaluated two isocaloric parenteral feeding regimens in 14 premature infants. Each regimen provided 60 kcal/kg/day, with one providing glucose alone and the other providing glucose plus amino acids at a rate of 2.5 g/kg/day. Not surprisingly, positive nitrogen balance was documented with the latter regimen. Of interest was the development of essential fatty acid deficiency in infants receiving amino acids, but not in those receiving glucose alone. Since equivalent nitrogen retention has been demonstrated with glucose versus combined glucose and lipid as the nonprotein energy source [101], the latter regimen is preferred since the development of essential fatty acid deficiency is prevented.

Caloric requirements for older pediatric patients are depicted in Table 20-4 [73] and notably decline with age. It must be stressed that these figures represent mean values derived from studying populations of children and that a great deal of variation is possible with each individual child. Indirect calorimetry may therefore play an important role in the determination of energy requirements of individual patients.

Glucose

Glucose represents an important source of nonprotein calories. Rates of administration and concentration in solution are often limiting factors in the parenteral nutrition of small infants. The maintenance of blood

Table 20-4. Caloric Requirements on Total Parenteral Nutrition

Age (yr)	Caloric Requirement (cal/kg/d)
0–1	90–120
1–7	75–90
7–12	60–75
12–18	30–60

From Kerner, J. A., Jr. Fat requirements. In J. A. Kerner, Jr. (ed.), *Manual of Pediatric Parenteral Nutrition.* New York: John Wiley and Sons, 1983. P. 65.

glucose levels to within a narrow window is extremely important, since hypoglycemia (blood glucose levels < 40 mg/dl) is associated with seizures and resultant brain damage. Hyperglycemia (blood glucose levels > 125 mg/dl) and varying serum osmolality may result in brain cell dehydration, capillary dilatation, and intracranial hemorrhage [43]. Further, significant hyperglycemia produces glycosuria with an attendant osmotic diuresis and dehydration.

Glucose metabolism in small, premature infants is very fragile during the first few days of life. Hyperglycemia was demonstrated to occur frequently in infants with birth weights of 1100 g or less when parenteral glucose infusion rates exceeded 6 mg/kg/min [34]. In general practice, glucose infusion is started at a rate less than 6 mg/kg/min and gradually increased as endogenous insulin production is stimulated to a target rate of 11 to 12 mg/kg/min. This rate of infusion is usually tolerated after 5 to 7 days.

If hyperglycemia prevents sufficient caloric intake, insulin may be added to the parenteral solution. A word of caution with regard to insulin is in order, since blood glucose levels may vary greatly in the low-birth-weight infant and hypoglycemia may result. Another factor that may act to augment levels of blood glucose is parenteral lipids via the effects of serum free fatty acids on glucose and insulin metabolism [125].

Fat

The advantages of lipid administration to very-low-birth-weight infants include its high caloric content as well as the fact that it is isotonic and can be administered by a peripheral vein. Intralipid (derived from soybean oil and stabilized with egg phospholipid) and Liposyn (derived from safflower oil) are the two primary lipid sources available.

The beneficial effects of lipid administration include the prevention of essential fatty acid deficiency. The requirements for essential fatty acids are quite high in the neonate due to rapid growth and relatively low tissue stores. The clinical findings of essential fatty acid deficiency in infants may appear as early as 1 week following administration of fat-free parenteral nutrition [28, 48] and include scaly dermatitis, sparse hair growth, increased susceptibility to infection, failure to thrive, and thrombocytopenia [95, 99].

Another benefit of lipid administration in infants is more optimal nitrogen retention. Nose et al. [90] noted lower basal metabolic rates, lower respiratory quotients, and higher nitrogen retention rates in infants and children receiving nonprotein calories as glucose plus lipid when compared with glucose alone. Other investigators confirmed higher metabolic rates and higher respiratory quotients in infants receiving glucose alone as the source of nonprotein calories [103, 123]. Clearance of infused lipid is inversely related to the gestational age of the infant, as tolerance improves with maturation [7, 109]. Further, small-for-gestational-age infants tolerate intravenous lipid less well than infants who are of appropriate size for gestational age [7]. Premature infants under 27 weeks' gestation have been found to have less than one-third of the lipase reserves of infants older than 27 weeks [28]. The above findings suggest that a critical mass of adipose tissue must be present to adequately metabolize circulating triglycerides. This is further suggested by the finding of a significant correlation between lipolytic activity of the serum after heparin administration, and body weight and body fat [64].

The administration of heparin has been suggested to aid the clearance of intravenous fat in infants and children, due to its ability to stimulate the release of lipoprotein lipase

[25]. Total lipid levels and turbidity were reduced when heparin was given as a single injection of 50 to 100 IU/kg to infants who were small for their gestational age [62]. Despite these observations, Coran et al. [25] were unable to demonstrate any significant effect of heparin on clearance of intravenously administered fat from the bloodstream in infants receiving 150 IU/kg/day of heparin. Currently, heparin is not routinely administered to enhance clearance of intravenous lipid.

Despite the fact that plasma concentrations of carnitine are higher in premature infants than in term infants, their ability to synthesize carnitine is reduced and plasma levels fall during the first 3 days of life without supplemental carnitine [91]. Carnitine, present in both human and cow's milk, is absent from intravenous nutrient solutions and facilitates transfer of free fatty acids across the mitochondrial membrane for beta oxidation. A deficiency of carnitine may therefore contribute to the premature infant's inability to metabolize administered fatty acids. Indeed, infants fed carnitine-free parenteral nutrition were found to have lower plasma carnitine levels and lower urinary carnitine excretion when compared with a group of orally fed infants of similar gestational age [104]. Further, postmortem analysis of liver, heart, and skeletal muscle tissue from infants who received intravenous nutrition for more than 15 days revealed very low carnitine levels, with levels in the heart tissue in the range reported for systemic carnitine deficiency [96]. As yet, there are no recognized clinical problems associated with the lack of carnitine in parenteral nutrition formulations. The degree to which this deficiency contributes to relative intolerance to lipids in the neonate is at present only speculative and deserves further consideration.

The use of intravenous lipids should be restricted in the presence of hyperlipemia, since hyperlipemia following Intralipid infusion may interfere with pulmonary diffusing capacity [56] or induce pulmonary fat embolism [11]. Another situation whereby intravenous lipids may be harmful is in the infant with jaundice. Free fatty acids released during the hydrolysis of intravenous lipid are capable of displacing bilirubin from albumin, producing free (unbound) bilirubin, which may increase the risk of kernicterus [14, 115, 121]. Fatty acids do not begin to displace bilirubin until the fatty acid to serum albumin molar ratio is greater than 6 in vivo [8]. This ratio may be conveniently monitored in these infants during the course of parenteral nutrition and rates of lipid infusion adjusted accordingly [15].

To prevent the development of ketonemia, no more than 60% of nonprotein calories are administered as lipid [74] and it has been recommended to limit the rate of infusion of lipid to 3.0 g/kg/day [2]. Lipid is infused in infants continuously over a 24-hour interval, as Brans et al. [16] demonstrated wide fluctuations and higher concentrations of plasma lipid fractions in infants administered lipids intermittently versus continuously. Additionally, these investigators were able to demonstrate that the occurrence of gross hyperlipemia was related to the hourly infusion rate, regardless of the duration of infusion. In general, lipid infusions are started at 0.5 g/kg/day in premature infants or 1.0 g/kg/day in term infants and progressed in daily increments of 0.25–0.5 g/kg/day until a maximum of 3.0 g/kg/day is reached.

If the rate of intravenous fat administration exceeds the rate of clearance, then visible lactescence and hyperlipidemia occur. Unfortunately, visual inspection of plasma for turbidity is unreliable for monitoring patients receiving intravenous fat [105]. Further, while nephelometric determinations have an excellent correlation with plasma turbidity, nephelometry does not reliably predict elevated triglyceride or cholesterol levels or free fatty acid–albumin molar ratio [29]. Lipid intolerance is defined by Zlotkin et al. [137] as a lipid emulsion–triglyceride ratio greater than 100 mg/100 g. The American Academy of Pediatrics [2] recommended that serum triglyceride levels be maintained below 150 mg/dl. By whatever method utilized, it is important that infants are monitored carefully during administration of fat. An excellent review of the subject of lipid administration in infants was written by Stahl et al. [114].

Protein

Protein may be administered via the parenteral route as either protein hydrolysates of fibrin or casein, or as various mixtures of crystalline amino acids. Due to more optimal nitrogen utilization [32], greater ability to vary individual amino acid concentrations, and lower preformed ammonia load, crystalline amino acids are currently preferred.

The quantity and concentration of amino acids required are varied given the age of the patient and metabolic state of the patient (i.e., during sepsis or stress). Although the ideal composition of amino acids for the premature infant is not presently known, it intuitively seems unwise to administer the same amino acid formulation to a premature, septic infant as one would give to an adult recovering from trauma. Although several specialized amino acid formulations have been proposed for preterm infants [50, 112], superiority over standard formulations has not been sufficiently established.

Several amino acids are suggested to be uniquely essential in the parenteral nutritional support of premature infants. Due to low activity of cystathionase (the enzyme that converts methionine to cysteine) in hepatic tissue of newborns, cysteine is considered essential. Further, cysteine is not currently available in amino acid solutions because of the relatively poor solubility of cystine, the oxidized form of cysteine. Despite this, Zlotkin et al. [136] were unable to demonstrate any benefit of cysteine supplementation of a cysteine-free parenteral nutrition solution when administered to a group of premature and term newborns. Taurine must also be considered essential, since it is synthesized from cysteine.

Other amino acids of concern to infants include methionine, phenylalanine, and glycine. Those amino acid formulations with higher methionine or phenylalanine concentrations result in abnormally high plasma levels of these amino acids [5, 138]. Solutions containing high amounts of gylcine should be used with caution, since hyperglycemia and hyperammonemia may result [5, 67].

From a practical standpoint, amino acid solutions are begun at a dose of 0.5 g of protein/kg/day and increased in increments of 0.5 g/kg/day to a generally accepted maximum dose. The generally accepted maximum dose for a given age of a patient is fairly controversial. In premature infants, Zlotkin et al. [137] were able to duplicate in utero nitrogen accretion rates at a protein intake of 2.7 to 3.5 g/kg/day when nonprotein energy was provided at a level greater than 70 kcal/kg/day. Provisions of this higher amount of protein may result in acidosis, hyperammonemia, azotemia, and cholestatic jaundice in some infants [74, 126]. A more appropriate maximum level of protein for premature infants may well be in the range of 2.5 to 3.0 g/kg/day. When comparing this to healthy infants fed human milk, Zlotkin [135] was able to duplicate nitrogen retention and weight gain in a group of full-term infants undergoing surgery, with protein intakes of 2.3 to 2.7 g/kg/day. A protein intake of 2.0 to 3.0 g/kg/day is considered acceptable for older infants and children [74].

In one study, hyperammonemia during the parenteral nutrition of infants was reported to occur up to 75% of the time [106]. Elevated levels of ammonia are usually associated with overinfusion of protein and occur more commonly in the premature, but may also be noted in full-term infants. Clinical signs of hyperammonemia include lethargy, which proceeds to muscle twitching and, ultimately, grand mal seizures. Treatment is withdrawal of the parenteral nutrition, and resolution of clinical symptoms should follow [66]. Azotemia usually precedes hyperammonemia and, thus, BUN levels should be serially followed.

Although hyperammonemia was observed in infants receiving protein hydrolysates as the nitrogen source [70], it has also been reported during infusion of crystalline amino acids [66, 122]. Other factors that may cause or contribute to hyperammonemia in the infant should be considered and include de-

Table 20-5. Normal Plasma Amino Acid Values in Neonates and Infants*

Amino Acid	Premature First Day	Newborn before First Feeding	16 D– 4 Mo	9 Mo– 2 Yr
Taurine	105–255	101–181	—	14–91
OH-Proline	0–80	0	—	—
Aspartic	0–20	4–12	17–21	0–9
Threonine	155–275	196–238	141–213	33–128
Serine	195–345	129–197	104–158	24–172
Aspartate and Glutate	655–1155	623–895	—	46–290
Proline	155–305	155–305	141–245	51–185
Glutamic	30–100	27–77	—	—
Glycine	185–735	274–412	178–248	56–308
Alanine	325–425	274–384	239–345	99–313
Valine	80–180	97–175	123–199	57–262
Cysteine ½	55–75	49–75	33–51	—
Methionine	30–40	21–37	15–21	3–29
Isoleucine	20–60	31–47	31–47	26–94
Leucine	45–95	55–89	56–98	45–155
Tyrosine	20–220	53–85	33–75	11–122
Phenylalanine	70–110	64–92	45–65	23–69
Ornithine	70–110	66–116	37–61	10–107
Lysine	130–250	154–246	117–163	45–144
Histidine	30–70	61–93	64–92	24–112
Arginine	30–70	37–71	53–71	11–65
Tryptophan	15–45	15–45	—	—
Citrulline	8.5–23.7	10.8–21.1	—	—
Ethanolamine	13.4–105	32.7–72	—	—
α-Amino-n-butyric	0–29	8.7–20.4	—	—
Methylhistidine	—	—	—	—

*Values are in μmol/liter; range for ± 1 standard deviation from the mean.
From Cox, J. H. High risk neonates and infants. In C. E. Lang (ed.), *Nutritional Support in Critical Care*. Rockville, MD: Aspen, 1987. P. 19.

ranged hepatic function, perinatal asphyxia [51], and sepsis [121], or they may occur transiently in preterm infants from undetermined causes [10, 36]. No established guidelines exist as to what maximum blood level of ammonia should mandate a reduction in protein intake, although Seashore [106] suggested this level to be 250 μg/dl.

In addition to monitoring levels of blood ammonia during parenteral nutrition, following plasma amino acid levels may be important both to uncover inborn errors of metabolism and to follow the development of significantly deranged patterns. Normal plasma amino acid values for premature infants and toddlers are depicted in Table 20-5

[83]. Although none of the currently available amino acid formulations result in "normal" plasma amino acid patterns when administered to pediatric patients, data derived from serial amino acid profiles may allow for the development of more appropriate formulas.

Vitamins, Minerals, and Trace Elements

Vitamins

The need for separate adult and pediatric formulations for multivitamin supplements to parenteral nutrition solutions was first suggested in 1979 by the Nutrition Advisory Group of the American Medical Association

Table 20-6. Suggested Intakes of Parenteral Vitamins in Infants and Children

Vitamin	Term Infants and Children (dose/d)	Preterm Infants* Current Suggestions (dose/kg body weight)	Preterm Infants* Best Estimate for New Formulation (dose/kg body weight)
Lipid soluble			
A (μg)	700	280	500
E (mg)	7	2.8	2.8
K (μg)	200	80	80
D (μg)	10	4	4
(IU)	400	160	160
Water soluble			
Ascorbic acid (mg)	80	32.0	25
Thiamin (mg)	1.2	0.48	0.35
Riboflavin (mg)	1.4	0.56	0.15
Pyridoxine (mg)	1.0	0.4	0.18
Niacin (mg)	17	6.8	6.8
Pantothenate (mg)	5	2.0	2.0
Biotin (μg)	20	8.0	6.0
Folate (μg)	140	56	56.0
Vitamin B_{12} (μg)	1.0	0.4	0.3

*Maximum not to exceed term infant dose.
From Greene, H. L., Hambidge, K. M., Schanler, R., and Tsang, R. C. Guidelines for the use of vitamins, trace elements, calcium, magnesium, and phosphorus in infants and children receiving total parenteral nutrition. *Am. J. Clin. Nutr.* 48:1324, 1988.

[4]. Although the United States Food and Drug Administration approved the adult formulation in 1979, the pediatric formulation was not accepted until 1981. More recently, a subcommittee of the American Society for Clinical Nutrition reviewed existing data on the use of multivitamin preparations in pediatric patients and proposed new guidelines [55]. A summary of these suggested modifications is reproduced in Table 20-6.

The fat-soluble vitamins (A, D, E, and K) differ in several ways from the water-soluble vitamins in the pediatric population. Requirements for fat-soluble vitamins are more dependent on age and degree of maturation, and since these vitamins are stored in body tissues, the potential for overdosage and toxicity exists. In contrast, body tissue stores of water-soluble vitamins are very limited, primarily due to efficient renal excretion, and toxicity occurs very rarely.

Vitamin A
Normal adult hepatic stores of vitamin A may prevent the development of clinical defi-

ciency for roughly 1 year. Due to much more limited hepatic reserve, the risk of vitamin A deficiency is greater in growing children [92] and greatest in preterm infants, whose hepatic stores of vitamin A are virtually absent [86]. Low plasma retinol levels have been associated with the development of bronchopulmonary dysplasia in preterm infants [69] and one randomized, blinded trial confirmed higher plasma retinol levels and a significant reduction in the incidence of bronchopulmonary dysplasia in vitamin A–supplemented infants [108]. Toxicity of vitamin A is represented clinically by dermatitis, irritability, chelosis, and gingivitis. Radiographically, thick periosteal new bone formation and dense metaphyses of long bones have been described [107].

Vitamin E
Vitamin E functions primarily as a biologic antioxidant protecting membrane phospholipids from peroxidation. Deficiency of vitamin E may result in increased red cell hemolysis [94], progressive neuronal damage [88,

119], and skeletal muscle degeneration [93]. A relative state of vitamin E deficiency exists in infants, as total body content is roughly 20 mg in a 3-kg infant. In low-birth-weight infants, the total body content is much less and is approximately 3 mg in a 1-kg infant. Deficiency of vitamin E in patients receiving the currently recommended dose in parenteral nutrition formulations has not been described. Low-birth-weight and preterm infants appears to be more susceptible to potential toxicity of vitamin E, which is manifested as coagulopathy with progressive liver disease and ultimate liver failure [71, 82]. For this reason, the recommended daily dose in these infants is less.

Vitamin K

Although vitamin K is not present in adult formulations of multivitamins, the pediatric multivitamin solutions contain the lipid-soluble phylloquinone form of vitamin K. Vitamin K is administered prophylactically in the newborn period, since the neonate has no intestinal flora to produce vitamin K. Toxicity to parenterally administered vitamin K in newborns is clinically apparent as hemolysis, hyperbilirubinemia, and occasionally, kernicterus. Toxicity appears to be dose dependent, occurring rarely at dosages less than 1 mg/day.

Vitamin D

Vitamin D is required for normal metabolism of calcium, phosphorus, and magnesium. While a lack of vitamin D in adults is represented by osteomalacia, vitamin D deficiency in infants and children is characterized by rickets, which includes the rachitic rib rosary, craniotabes, bowed legs, and muscle weakness [113]. The importance of maintaining adequate blood levels of vitamin D during development is underscored by recent implications of its role in normal cell differentiation of bone marrow cultures [20, 37]. No reported instances of vitamin D toxicity (e.g., hypercalcemia, vomiting, constipation, growth retardation) have been reported to date with the current recommended dosages as outlined in Table 20-6 [73].

Vitamin C (Ascorbic Acid)

Vitamin C is a necessary cofactor in several hydroxylation reactions, including the metabolism of tyrosine, phenylalanine, dopamine, carnitine, and collagen. Hepatic tyrosine transaminase activity is low in premature infants, and vitamin C supplementation allows for the normal metabolism of tyrosine and phenylalanine [120]. Toxicity of parenterally administered vitamin C is extremely rare, since it is cleared rapidly by the kidneys. This factor must be considered in the clinical context of renal failure.

Thiamin

Thiamin functions as a cofactor in oxidative decarboxylation reactions involving carbohydrates and, thus, needs are directly proportional to carbohydrate intake. Deficiency of thiamin results in beriberi and may present clinically as lactic acidosis and high-output congestive heart failure. Erythrocyte transketolase activity is a useful marker of thiamin deficiency, although whole-blood thiamin levels are becoming available.

Riboflavin

Although riboflavin is inactivated by indirect sunlight and phototherapy light [49], deficiency of riboflavin has not been reported in children receiving parenteral nutrition. Current recommendations for dosages of riboflavin in premature infants may be excessive, since blood levels are markedly elevated [54] and excess riboflavin may induce photohemolysis [17].

Vitamin B₆ (Pyridoxine)

A deficiency of this vitamin is rare and characterized by hypochromic microcytic anemia, gastrointestinal disturbances, failure to thrive, irritability, and seizures. No reported instances of deficiency have been reported in parenterally fed infants. Current recommended dosages may be excessive in premature infants, since blood levels achieved were greater than 10-fold over cord blood and maternal levels when the recommended dose was administered to eight premature infants [54].

Niacin

Pellagra is the resultant syndrome of niacin deficiency and has not been reported in parenterally fed infants or children receiving the recommended supplements.

Pantothenic Acid

Because of the ubiquitous nature of this vitamin, deficiency states do not occur naturally. Requirements of this vitamin during parenteral nutrition have been reported only in small numbers of children [87].

Biotin

Until recently, parenteral vitamin preparations in the United States did not contain biotin. Biotin deficiency is rare, owing to the ubiquitous nature of biotin in food and the fact that it is synthesized by intestinal bacteria. The clinical syndrome of biotin deficiency has been reported in a child with short-bowel syndrome receiving parenteral nutrition and consisted of an exfoliative dermatitis, alopecia, pallor, irritability, and lethargy [85]. The deficiency state in infants likely results from a combination of impaired intestinal absorption as well as impaired bacterial synthesis due to antibiotic administration. No reports of toxicity exist for biotin administration in children.

Folic Acid

Folate deficiency is one of the most common nutritional vitamin deficiencies in humans, with low serum levels occurring after 3 weeks and hypersegmentation of polymorphonuclear leukocytes after 7 weeks [52]. No toxic conditions have been reported for folate, and no deficiency states have been reported in children receiving parenteral folate supplementation.

Vitamin B₁₂

No specific deficiency or toxicity has been reported to occur in children receiving parenteral nutrition supplementation.

Electrolytes and Minerals

General guidelines for electrolyte and mineral requirements in infants and children are

Table 20-7. Recommended Daily Intake of Electrolytes and Minerals for Parenteral Nutrition Solutions

Element	Daily Amount
Sodium	2–4 mEq/kg
Potassium	2–3 mEq/kg
Chloride	2–3 mEq/kg
Magnesium	0.25–0.50 mEq/kg
Calcium gluconate*	100–500 mg/kg
Phosphorus	1–2 mmol/kg

*Gluconate is the recommended calcium salt for use in parenteral nutrition solutions.
From Poole, R. L. Electrolyte and mineral requirements. In J. A. Kerner (ed.), *Manual of Pediatric Parenteral Nutrition*. New York: John Wiley & Sons, 1983. P. 130.

depicted in Table 20-7 [98]. Actual requirements for each individual must be considered and are dependent on such factors as diuretic administration, increased electrolyte losses in gastrointestinal fluids (nasogastric tubes, diarrhea, various fistulas), renal function, and degree of hydration.

Calcium is the most abundant mineral in the body. A relatively high content of this mineral plus phosphorus in parenteral nutrition is desirable in early infancy [57]. Because these requirements may not be as high in older pediatric patients, it has been suggested that age-related guidelines rather than one pediatric recommendation may be indicated [55]. During periods of fluid restriction, it is important not to inadvertently increase the concentration of calcium and phosphorus in the parenteral solution, since this may result in precipitation. This becomes an important issue when using very small tubing that is sometimes utilized to deliver parenteral nutrition to very small infants. Factors that act to reduce solubility of calcium and phosphorus in parenteral solutions include low amino acid or glucose content, high pH, and prolonged exposure of intravenous tubing to the high temperature of infant incubators [124].

Trace Elements

The problem of trace element deficiency is especially important in infants and children

Table 20-8.   Recommended Intravenous Intakes of Trace Elements[a]

| Element | Infants | | Children |
	Preterm[b]	Term	
	$g \cdot kg^{-1} \cdot d^{-1}$		$g \cdot kg^{-1} \cdot d^{-1}$ [maximum g/d]
Zinc	400	250 < 3 mo	50 [5000]
		100 > 3 mo	
Copper[c]	20	20	20 [300]
Selenium[d]	2.0	2.0	2.0 [30]
Chromium[d]	0.20	0.20	0.20 [5.0]
Manganese[c]	1.0	1.0	1.0 [5.0]
Molybdenum[d]	0.25	0.25	0.25 [5.0]
Iodide	1.0	1.0	1.0 [1.0]

[a]When total parenteral nutrition is only supplemental or limited to < 4 wk, only zinc need be added. Thereafter, addition of the remaining elements is advisable.
[b]Available concentrations of manganese and molybdenum are such that dilution of the manufacturer's product may be necessary.
[c]Omit in patients with obstructive jaundice.
[d]Omit in patients with renal dysfunction.
From Greene, H. L., Hambidge, K. M., Schanler, R., and Tsang, R. C. Guidelines for the use of vitamins, trace elements, calcium, magnesium, and phosphorus in infants and children receiving total parenteral nutrition. *Am. J. Clin. Nutr.* 48:1324, 1988.

since normal growth and development are dependent on sufficient amounts in the diet. Recommended intakes of the various trace elements for the pediatric population are shown in Table 20-8 [55].

Zinc is one example of a trace element whose requirements are determined primarily by growth in early infancy [77]. Zinc is an essential component of multiple enzyme reactions, and the earliest sign of deficiency in the infant is a decline in growth velocity. With more severe depletion, the infant is irritable, lethargic, or both, and a characteristic acro-orificial rash develops with diarrhea and alopecia. Other contributing factors in the development of zinc deficiency include increased losses, as in persistent diarrhea or excessive gastrointestinal losses from fistulas or ostomies [102, 132].

The term neonate has substantial hepatic stores of copper despite relatively low serum levels. Limited synthesis of ceruloplasmin is thought to account for the lower serum copper levels. Clinical characteristics of copper deficiency include osteoporosis, neutropenia, and microcytic anemia. Preterm infants may develop neurologic abnormalities, failure to thrive, and hepatomegaly. Since 80% of absorbed copper is excreted by the biliary system [63], one of the main considerations in intravenous copper replacement is hepatic function. Copper deficiency may develop when there are excessive losses of copper-containing biliary secretions [111]. Conversely, copper toxicity may occur in situations whereby biliary excretion is impaired (including TPN-associated cholestasis); thus, caution should be exercised in the administration of copper in these situations. For the same reasons, manganese is another trace element that should be withheld in patients with cholestasis.

It has been suggested by Greene et al. [55] that zinc is the only needed trace element when parenteral nutrition is administered for only 1 to 2 weeks. The other trace elements (as cited in Table 20-8) are considered essential if parenteral nutrition continues for greater than 4 weeks [55].

TECHNIQUE

Primarily because of body size and degree of physical activity, the ability to safely secure and maintain reliable venous access in infants and children poses many unique challenges. One major issue in the pediatric population is whether parenteral nutrition should be administered via the central or peripheral venous route. Risks of anesthesia, technical and infectious complications, and limited venous accessibility have all been cited as deterrents in the use of central veins. On the other hand, inability to reliably cannulate and maintain access for prolonged periods as well as delivery of solutions restricted in caloric density argues against the use of peripheral veins.

In addressing this issue, Ziegler et al. [134] reviewed the records of 585 children who received parenteral nutrition by either the central or the peripheral venous route. In that study, central administration of parenteral nutrition resulted in a greater daily caloric intake (128 versus 63 kcal/kg) for longer periods (33.7 versus 11.4 mean days) and more weight gain (82.5 versus 63%). Although infectious and metabolic complications were encountered more frequently in the group receiving central administration, technical complications were documented more often in the group receiving peripheral administration and consisted primarily of soft tissue sloughs. When these data were analyzed per day of therapy, no significant differences in complication rates between the two routes of administration were noted. Based on these results, it was recommended that the primary factor in deciding the method of therapy should be the caloric needs of the individual patient. Peripheral alimentation is suggested for nonstressed infants for brief courses of maintenance therapy when full growth and development are not the primary goal.

Several methods exist for central venous access in the pediatric patient. One of the more common techniques involves the use of a Broviac catheter inserted through a relatively large, surgically exposed vein, with the catheter tip residing in the superior vena cava. Available sites for central venous access in infants are illustrated in Figure 20-4 [76]. The catheter is tunneled subcutaneously to exit at an area separate from the original inci-

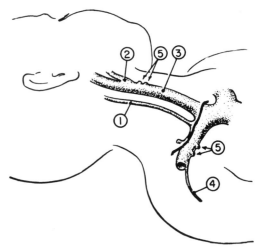

Figure 20-4. Sites for central venous access in infants, in order of preference. *1* = external jugular vein; *2* = facial vein; *3* = internal jugular vein; *4* = cephalic vein; *5* = tributaries of subclavian and internal jugular veins. (From Kosloske, A. M., and Klein, M. D. Techniques of central venous access for long term parenteral nutrition in infants. *Surg. Gynecol. Obstet.* 154:395, 1982.)

sion and is usually on the posterior part of the scalp or anterior part of the chest. The inferior vena cava may also be used via a saphenous vein cutdown (Fig. 20-5) as advocated by Fonkalsrud et al. [45]. Although not universally accepted, this technique was found to be technically easier and associated with fewer complications when compared with use of the superior vena cava for central venous access [89].

Broviac catheters in the pediatric population are associated with an incidence of catheter-related sepsis in the range of 6 to 9.8% and mechanical complications requiring removal of the catheter in 5 to 11.5% [21, 128]. Warner et al. [127] reported the multiple-purpose use of these catheters for parenteral nutrition, replacement fluids, and medication administration in a group of 20 premature infants weighing less than 1000 g. The rates of catheter-associated sepsis and mechanical complications in this high-risk group were 9 and 18%, respectively.

Percutaneous subclavian vein catheterization is another method of central venous access and offers the advantages of repeated

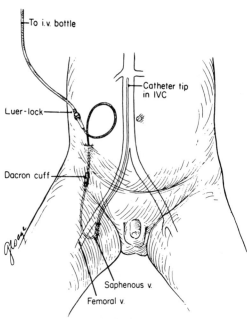

Figure 20-5. A catheter is inserted into the inferior vena cava (IVC), with the tip placed at the level of the renal veins by saphenous venorrhapy. The Dacron cuff on the catheter is placed in the subcutaneous tunnel at least 1 cm inferior to the catheter exit site on the abdominal wall. *i.v.* = intravenous; *v.* = vein. (From Fonkalsrud, E. W., Berquist, W., Burke, M., and Ament. M. E. Long term hyperalimentation in children through saphenous central venous catheterization. *Am. J. Surg.* 143:209, 1982.)

catheterization of the same vessel, with the avoidance of surgical exposure and vessel ligation. The incidence of catheter-related sepsis with this technique is in the range of 2.5 to 15.9% and mechanical complications, in the range of 12 to 31.8% [42, 58]. This method has not become widespread, since significant morbidity [35] and mortality [58] have been reported. A significant learning curve is involved and requires the participation of a surgeon highly experienced in this technique.

A more recently described method involves the threading of silicone elastomer tubing from a peripheral to a central position [26, 33, 80, 110]. The attractiveness of this method lies in the fact that no transportation to the operating room is required, no anesthesia is needed, and central venous access can be obtained by nonsurgical physicians.

The overall incidence of sepsis and mechanical complications (including the inability to thread the catheter into a central position) is similar to that for other described methods.

COMPLICATIONS

Complications related to parenteral nutrition in the pediatric population are not unlike those encountered in adults, and are discussed in detail elsewhere in this volume. The types of complications are generally categorized as either metabolic, technical (as related to placement and maintenance of the catheter), or septic.

Metabolic complications are generally related to disorders of either glucose metabolism (hyperglycemia or hypoglycemia) or specific deficiencies or toxicities of various components of the infused solution. These have been mentioned already in the discussion regarding requirements of each component.

One of the more common metabolic complications encountered in pediatric parenteral nutrition is the development of hepatobiliary dysfunction. This entity is second only to technical problems with the catheter, being the most common complication requiring discontinuation of therapy in infants and children [38]. In adults, parenteral nutrition–related hepatic abnormalities consist primarily of steatosis with elevations of alkaline phosphatase and transaminases. In contrast, a pattern of cholestasis is noted in children with conjugated hyperbilirubinemia and lesser elevations of other hepatocellular enzymes.

Several factors have been implicated in the pathogenesis of hepatobiliary dysfunction, but no single causal factor has been identified. Gestational age is important, since gestational age was shown to be inversely related to peak serum bilirubin levels in parenterally fed infants [97]. Further, the incidence of cholestasis was reported to be 50%, 18%, and 7% in infants with birth weights less than 1000 g, 1000 to 1500 g, and 1500 to 2000 g, respectively [12]. Another important factor seems to be the duration of parenteral therapy [97]. The incidence is fairly low in infants receiving therapy for less than 2 weeks, but rises to 80% if parenteral therapy is continued for more than 60 days [12].

Since degree of prematurity and duration of therapy are main factors in the development of liver abnormalities, immaturity of the hepatobiliary system has been suggested to be an important underlying factor. Implicating this factor is difficult since severe prematurity, prolonged parenteral therapy, extended periods of enteral fasting, and exposure to many potential hepatotoxins (drugs, blood component transfusions, and so on) often coexist. Immature organisms have a decreased bile salt pool, reduced hepatic uptake of bile salts, and diminished terminal ileal salvage of conjugated bile acids [9]. Further, biotransformation of bile acids by conjugation and sulfation is reduced and associated with low specific enzyme activity [117, 118].

Enteral feeding promotes secretion of multiple gastrointestinal hormones, several of which influence production and flow of bile. Lack of enteral feeding, which frequently occurs in the setting of parenteral nutrition, may attenuate hormone-stimulated bile flow and thus contribute to cholestasis. Another phenomenon associated with enteral starvation is reduced villus height and atrophy with reduced intraluminal levels of secretory IgA. It has been suggested that these factors allow for translocation of bacteria and/or endotoxin from the gut into the portal blood, thus affecting the liver [1]. Further evidence for the role of intestinal bacteria is provided by the attenuation of liver function derangements by administration of metronidazole during parenteral therapy [47, 79]. [*Editor's Note:* It is probably bacterial products, not bacteria, that do the damage. We and others have had extraordinary difficulty in identifying endotoxin in portal blood.]

In contrast to adults, steatosis due to overfeeding is uncommon in neonates with parenteral nutrition–associated cholestasis [68]. Since cholestasis has been reported in infants receiving glucose-only parenteral solutions as well as glucose-plus-fat solutions, administration of intravenous fat has not been implicated in the pathogenesis of cholestasis.

Amino acids are known to have cholestatic potential. However, the incidence of cholestasis was not found to be significantly greater in a prospective trial of infants fed higher levels of protein [126]. Further, cholestasis may occur in the face of inadequate protein supplementation. The notion that specific amino acids may be toxic to the liver was suggested in a report by Grant et al. [53] that documented fatty changes of the liver of rats infused with solutions containing tryptophan that were exposed to light. [*Editor's Note:* This apparently requires the presence of bisulfite, previously added as a preservative. It is no longer added; thus this mechanism is unlikely.] These observations were extended by Merritt et al. [84] who injected suckling rat pups with individual amino acids found in standard hyperalimentation solutions. Only tryptophan was cholestatic in a dose-dependent fashion, and only in rats of 12 days old or less.

Deficiency of certain amino acids—particularly taurine—may also play a role, since current amino acid solutions do not contain taurine. This amino acid is considered to be essential in the neonate, owing to reduced synthetic ability. In a controlled trial, however, taurine supplementation did not alter biochemical tests of hepatic toxicity [22].

From a clinical standpoint, the onset of hyperbilirubinemia is usually 3 to 4 weeks after the start of parenteral nutrition, and the first detectable biochemical abnormality is an increase in the concentration of serum bile acids [39, 40]. Serum levels of alkaline phosphatase are not helpful, since these levels are normally quite high in the newborn period. Hepatic synthetic function is usually normal [97].

The diagnosis of parenteral nutrition–induced cholestasis in the infant is one of exclusion, since the differential diagnosis of hyperbilirubinemia is quite extensive. Sepsis (from any cause) must be ruled out, and non-invasive imaging of the hepatobiliary system should be performed to exclude structural abnormalities. Deficiency of α_1-antitrypsin is one of the leading causes of neonatal cholestasis and should be considered. Other diseases associated with hepatic dysfunction include cystic fibrosis, viral infections, and inborn errors of metabolism such as galactosemia or tyrosinemia. In a study of 47 patients referred for evaluation of presumed parenteral nutrition–associated cholestasis, Farrell and Balistreri [38] were able to make a definitive diagnosis of other disorders in 10% of the patients.

Once the diagnosis of parenteral nutrition–associated cholestasis has been established, the physician caring for the patient is faced with a dilemma. Discontinuation of parenteral nutrition and institution of enteral feeding are therapeutic. However, this is often impossible to do since enteral feeding is usually poorly tolerated or contraindicated by virtue of the patient's underlying disease. Suggestions for continued parenteral nutrition in these patients include decreasing the amount of protein infused to the minimum amount required and reducing abnormally high calorie-nitrogen ratios (> 200–250 kcal/g of nitrogen) [38]. There appear to be no indications to limit the use of intravenous fat or to administer the parenteral solution in a cyclic fashion.

REFERENCES

1. Alverdy, J. C., Aoys, E., and Moss, G. S. Total parenteral nutrition promotes bacterial translocation from the gut. *Surgery* 104:185, 1988.
2. American Academy of Pediatrics. Use of intravenous fat emulsions in pediatric patients. *Pediatrics* 68:738, 1981.
3. American Academy of Pediatrics Committee on Nutrition. Nutritional needs of low-birth-weight infants. *Pediatrics* 75:976, 1985.
4. American Medical Association Department of Foods and Nutrition. Multivitamin preparations for parenteral use: A statement by the Nutrition Advisory Group, 1975. *J. Parenter. Enter. Nutr.* 3:258, 1979.
5. Anderson, G. H., Bryan, H., Jeejeebhoy, K. N., and Corey, P. Dose-response relationships between amino acid intake and blood levels in newborn infants. *Am. J. Clin. Nutr.* 30:1110, 1977.
6. Anderson, T. A. Birth through 24 months. In A. M. Rudolph (ed.), *Pediatrics* (18th ed.). Norwalk, CT: Appleton & Lange, 1987.
7. Andrew, G., Chan, G., and Schiff, D. Lipid metabolism in the neonate. I. The effects of Intralipid infusion on plasma triglyceride and free fatty acid concentrations in the neonate. *J. Pediatr.* 88:273, 1976.
8. Andrew, G., Chan, G., and Schiff, D. Lipid metabolism in the neonate. II. The effect of Intralipid on bilirubin binding in vitro and in vivo. *J. Pediatr.* 88:279, 1976.
9. Balistreri, W. F., Heubi, J. E., and Suchy, F. J. Immaturity of the enterohepatic circulation in early life: Factors predisposing to "physiologic" maldigestion and cholestasis. *J. Pediatr. Gastroenterol. Nutr.* 2:346, 1983.
10. Ballard, R. A., Vinocur, B., Reynolds, J. W., et al. Transient hyperammonemia of the preterm infant. *N. Engl. J. Med.* 299:920, 1978.
11. Barson, A. J., Chiswick, M. L., and Doig, C. M. Fat embolism in infancy after intravenous fat infusions. *Arch. Dis. Child.* 53:218, 1978.
12. Beale, E. F., Nelson, R. M., Bucciarelli, R. L., Donnelly, W. H., and Eitzman, D. V. Intrahepatic cholestasis associated with parenteral nutrition in premature infants. *Pediatrics* 64:342, 1979.
13. Beaton, G. H. Nutritional needs during the first year of life: Some concepts and perspectives. *Pediatr. Clin. North Am.* 32:275, 1985.
14. Berde, C., Rasmussen, F., Benitz, W., Kerner, J., Johnson, J., and Wennberg, R. Binding of bilirubin and fatty acids in the sera of neonates. (Abstract) *Clin. Res.* 27:134A, 1979.
15. Berde, C. B., Kerner, J. A., and Johnson, J. D. Use of the conjugated polyene fatty acid, parinaric acid, in assaying fatty acids in serum or plasma. *Clin. Chem.* 26:1173, 1980.
16. Brans, Y. W., Andrew, D. S., Carrillo, D. W., Dutton, E. P., Menchaca, E. M., and Puleo-Scheppke, B. A. Tolerance of fat emulsions in very-low-birth-weight neonates. *Am. J. Dis. Child.* 142:145, 1988.
17. Brown, M. C., and Roe, D. A. Role of riboflavin in drug-induced photohemolysis. *Clin. Res.* 36:755, 1988.
18. Caldwell, M. D., Jonsson, H. T., and Othersen, H. B. Essential fatty acid deficiency in an infant receiving prolonged parenteral alimentation. *J. Pediatr.* 81:894, 1972.
19. Cashore, W. J., Sedaghatian, M. R., and Usher, R. H. Nutritional supplements with intravenously administered lipid, protein hydrolysate, and glucose in small premature infants. *Pediatrics* 56:88, 1975.
20. Chaplinski, T. J., and Bennett, T. E. Induction of insulin receptor expression of human

leukemic cells by 1-alpha, 25-dihydroxyvi-tamin D_3. *Leuk. Res.* 11:37, 1987.

21. Colombani, P. M., Dudgeon, D. L., Buck, J. R., et al. Multipurpose central venous access in the immunocompromised pediatric patient. *J. Parenter. Enter. Nutr.* 9:38, 1985.

22. Cooke, R. J., Whitington, P. F., and Kelts, D. Effect of taurine supplementation on hepatic function during short-term parenteral nutrition in the premature infant. *J. Pediatr. Gastroenterol. Nutr.* 3:234, 1984.

23. Coran, A. G. The long-term total intravenous feeding of infants using peripheral veins. *J. Pediatr. Surg.* 8:801, 1973.

24. Coran, A. G. Total intravenous feeding of infants and children without the use of a central venous catheter. *Ann. Surg.* 179:445, 1974.

25. Coran, A. G., Edwards, B., and Zaleska, R. The value of heparin in the hyperalimentation of infants and children with a fat emulsion. *J. Pediatr. Surg.* 9:725, 1974.

26. Dalcourt, J. L., and Bose, C. L. Percutaneous insertion of Silastic central venous catheters in newborn infants. *Pediatrics* 70:484, 1982.

27. Denson, S. E. Nutritional considerations of IV support of the neonate. In A. G. Coran, S. E. Denson, A. B. Fletcher (eds.), *The Compromised Neonate*. New York: Pro Clinica, 1980. P. 10.

28. Dhanireddy, R., Hamosh, M., Sivasubramanian, K. N., Chowdhry, P., Scanlon, J. W., and Hamosh, P. Postheparin lipolytic activity and Intralipid clearance in very low-birth-weight infants. *J. Pediatr.* 98:617, 1981.

29. D'Harlingue, A., Hopper, A. O., Stevenson, D. K., Shahin, S. M., and Kerner, J. A., Jr. Limited value of nephelometry in monitoring the administration of intravenous fat in neonates. *J. Parenter. Enter. Nutr.* 7:55, 1983.

30. Dickerson, J. W. T., Dobbing, J., and McCance, R. A. The effect of undernutrition on the postnatal development of the brain and cord in pigs. *Proc. R. Soc. Lond. (Biol.)* 166:396, 1966–67.

31. Dudrick, S. J., Copeland, E. M., and Mac Fadyen, B. V. Long-term parenteral nutrition: Its current status. *Hosp. Pract.* 10:47, 1975.

32. Duffy, B., Gunn, T., Collinge, J., and Pencharz, P. The effect of varying protein quality and energy intake on the nitrogen metabolism of parenterally fed very low birthweight (<1600 g) infants. *Pediatr. Res.* 15:1040, 1981.

33. Durand, M., Ramananthan, R., Martinelli, B., and Tolentino, M. Prospective evaluation of percutaneous central venous Silastic catheters in newborn infants with birth weights of 510 to 3,920 grams. *Pediatrics* 78:245, 1986.

34. Dweck, H. S., and Cassady, G. Glucose intol-erance in infants of very low birth weight. I. Incidence of hyperglycemia in infants of birth weights 1,100 grams or less. *Pediatrics* 53:189, 1974.

35. Eichelberger, M. R., Rous, P. G., Hoelzer, D. J., Garcia, V. F., and Koop, C. E. Percutaneous subclavian venous catheters in neonates and children. *J. Pediatr. Surg.* 16:547, 1981.

36. Ellison, P. H., and Cowger, M. L. Transient hyperammonemia in the preterm infant: Neurologic aspects. *Neurology* 31:767, 1981.

37. Fabian, I., Kletter, Y., and Bleiberg, I. The effect of 1,25-dihydroxy-vitamin D_3 on hematopoiesis in long-term human bone marrow cultures. *Proc. Soc. Exp. Biol. Med.* 185:434, 1987.

38. Farrell, M. K., and Balistreri, W. F. Parenteral nutrition and hepatobiliary dysfunction. *Clin. Perinatol.* 13:197, 1986.

39. Farrell, M. K., Balistreri, W. F., and Suchy, F. J. Serum sulfate lithocholate as an indicator of cholestasis during parenteral nutrition in infants and children. *J. Parenter. Enter. Nutr.* 6:30, 1982.

40. Farrell, M. K., Gilster, S., and Balistreri, W. F. Serum bile acids: An early indicator of parenteral nutrition–associated liver disease. *Gastroenterology* 86:1074, 1984.

41. Filler, R. M., Eraklis, A. J., Das, J. B., and Schuster, S. R. Total intravenous nutrition: An adjunct to the management of infants with a ruptured omphalocele. *Am. J. Surg.* 121:454, 1971.

42. Filston, H. C., and Grant, J. P. A safer system for percutaneous subclavian venous catheterization in newborn infants. *J. Pediatr. Surg.* 14:564, 1979.

43. Finberg, L. Dangers to infants caused by changes in osmolal concentration. *Pediatrics* 40:1031, 1967.

44. Foman, S. J., Haschke, F., Ziegler, E. E., and Nelson, S. E. Body composition of reference children from birth to age 10 years. *Am. J. Clin. Nutr.* 35:1169, 1982.

45. Fonkalsrud, E. W., Berquist, W., Berke, M., and Ament, M. E. Long term hyperalimentation in children through saphenous central venous catheterization. *Am. J. Surg.* 143:209, 1982.

46. Forbes, G. B. Fetal growth and body composition: Implications for the premature infant. *J. Pediatr. Gastroenterol. Nutr.* 2(Suppl. 1):S52, 1983.

47. Freund, H. R., Muggia-Sullam, M., La-France, R., Enrione, E. B., Popp, M. B., and Bjornson, H. S. A possible beneficial effect of metronidazole in reducing TPN-associated liver function derangements. *J. Surg. Res.* 38:356, 1985.

48. Friedman, Z., Danon, A., Stahlman, M. T., and Oates, J. A. Rapid onset of essential fatty acid deficiency in the newborn. *Pediatrics* 58:640, 1976.

49. Fritz, I., Said, H., Harris, C., Murrell, J., and Greene, H. L. A new sensitive assay for plasma riboflavin using high performance liquid chromatography. *J. Am. Coll. Nutr.* 6: 449, 1987.

50. Ghadimi, H. Newly devised amino acid solutions for intravenous administration. In H. Ghadimi (ed.), *Total Parenteral Nutrition: Premises and Promises.* New York: Wiley, 1975. P. 393.

51. Goldberg, R. N., Cabal, L. A., Sinatra, F. R., Plajstek, C. E., and Hodgman, J. Hyperammonemia associated with perinatal asphyxia. *Pediatrics* 64:336, 1979.

52. Goldsmith, G. C. Vitamin B complex. *Prog. Food Nutr. Sci.* 1:559, 1975.

53. Grant, J. P., Cox, C. E., Kleinman, L. M., et al. Serum hepatic enzyme and bilirubin elevations during parenteral nutrition. *Surg. Gynecol. Obstet.* 145:573, 1977.

54. Greene, H., Smith, R., Murrell, J., Powers, J., and Baeckert, P. HPLC measurement of pyridoxine vitamers in infants receiving total parenteral nutrition. (Abstract) *J. Parenter. Enter. Nutr.* 13(Suppl.):5s, 1989.

55. Greene, H. L., Hambidge, K. M., Schanler, R., and Tsang, R. C. Guidelines for the use of vitamins, trace elements, calcium, magnesium, and phosphorus in infants and children receiving total parenteral nutrition: Report of the Subcommittee on Pediatric Parenteral Nutrient Requirements from the Committee on Clinical Practice Issues of the American Society for Clinical Nutrition. *Am. J. Clin. Nutr.* 48:1324, 1988.

56. Greene, H. L., Hazlett, D., and Demares, R. Relationship between Intralipid induced hyperlipemia and pulmonary function. *Am. J. Clin. Nutr.* 29:127, 1976.

57. Greer, F. R., and Tsang, R. C. Calcium, phosphorus, magnesium and vitamin D requirements for the preterm infant. In R. C. Tsang (ed.), *Vitamin and Mineral Requirements in Preterm Infants.* New York: Dekker, 1985. P. 99.

58. Groff, D. B., and Ahmed, N. Subclavian vein catheterization in the infant. *J. Pediatr. Surg.* 9:171, 1974.

59. Grosfeld, J. L. Jejunoileal atresia and stenosis. In K. J. Welch, J. G. Randolph, M. M. Ravitch, J. A. O'Neill, and M. I. Rowe (eds.), *Pediatric Surgery.* Chicago: Year Book, 1986. P. 838.

60. Grosfeld, J. L., Rescorla, F. J., and West, K. W. Short bowel syndrome in infancy and childhood: Analysis of survival in 60 patients. *Am. J. Surg.* 151:41, 1986.

61. Gunn, T., Bram, R. S., Pencharz, P., and Colle, E. Total parenteral nutrition in malnourished infants with intractable diarrhea. *Can. Med. Assoc. J.* 117:357, 1977.

62. Gustafson, A. Kjellmer, I., Olegard, R., and Victorin, L. H. Nutrition in low-birth-weight infants. II. Repeated intravenous injections of fat emulsion. *Acta Paediatr. Scand.* 63:177, 1974.

63. Hambidge, K. M. Trace elements in pediatric nutrition. *Adv. Pediatr.* 24:191, 1977.

64. Hamosh, M., Dhanireddy, R., Zaidan, H., and Hamosh, P. Total parenteral nutrition with Intralipid in the neonate: The enzymes and cofactors active in the clearing of circulating lipoprotein-triglyceride. In L. Stern, M. Xanthou, and B. Friis-Hansen (eds.), *Physiologic Foundations of Perinatal Care.* New York: Praeger, 1985. P. 176.

65. Heim, T., Putet, G., and Verellen, G. J. E. Energy cost of intravenous alimentation in the newborn infant. In L. Stern, B. Salle, and B. Friis-Hansen (eds.), *Intensive Care in the Newborn, III.* New York: Masson, 1981. P. 219.

66. Heird, W. C., Nicholson, J. F., Driscoll, J. M., Jr., Schullinger, J. N., and Winters, R. W. Hyperammonemia resulting from intravenous alimentation using a mixture of synthetic L-amino acids: A preliminary report. *J. Pediatr.* 81:162, 1972.

67. Heird, W. C., and Winters, R. W. Total parenteral nutrition: The state of the art. *J. Pediatr.* 86:2, 1975.

68. Hirai, Y., Sanada, Y., and Fujiwara, T. High calorie infusion induced hepatic impairment in infants. *J. Parenter. Enter. Nutr.* 3:146, 1979.

69. Hustead, V. A., Gutcher, G. R., Anderson, S. A., and Zachman, R. D. Relationship of vitamin A (retinol) status to lung disease in the preterm infant. *J. Pediatr.* 105:610, 1984.

70. Johnson, J. D., Albritton, W. L., and Sunshine, P. Hyperammonemia accompanying parenteral nutrition in newborn infants. *J. Pediatr.* 81:154, 1972.

71. Johnson, L., Bowen, F. W., Jr., Abbassi, S., et al. Relationship of prolonged pharmacologic serum levels of vitamin E to incidence of sepsis and necrotizing enterocolitis in infants with birth weight 1,500 grams or less. *Pediatrics* 75:619, 1985.

72. Keating, J. P., and Ternberg, J. L. Amino acid and hypertonic glucose treatment for intractable diarrhea in infants. *Am. J. Dis. Child.* 122:226, 1971.

73. Kerner, J. A., Jr. Caloric requirements. In J. A. Kerner, Jr. (ed.), *Manual of Pediatric Parenteral Nutrition.* New York: Wiley, 1983. P. 63.

74. Kerner, J. A., Jr. Fat requirements. In J. A.

Kerner, Jr. (ed.), *Manual of Pediatric Parenteral Nutrition.* New York: Wiley, 1983. P. 103.

75. Klish, W. J., and Putnam, T. C. The short gut. *Am. J. Dis. Child,* 135:1056, 1981.

76. Kosloske, A. M., and Klein, M. D. Techniques of central venous access for long term parenteral nutrition in infants. *Surg. Gynecol. Obstet.* 154:395, 1982.

77. Krebs, N. F., and Hambidge, K. M. Zinc requirements and zinc intakes of breast-fed infants. *Am. J. Clin. Nutr.* 43:288, 1986.

78. Krouskop, R. W., Brown, E. G., and Sweet, A. Y. The relationship of feeding to necrotizing enterocolitis. *Pediatr. Res.* 8:383, 1974.

79. Lambert, J. R., and Thomas, S. M. Metronidazole prevention of serum liver enzyme abnormalities during total parenteral nutrition. *J. Parenter. Enter. Nutr.* 9:501, 1985.

80. Loeff, D. S., Matlak, M. E., Black, R. E., Overall, J. C., and Dolcourt, J. L., and Johnson, D. G. Insertion of a small central venous catheter in neonates and young infants. *J. Pediatr. Surg.* 17:944, 1982.

81. Marchildron, M. B., Buck, B. E., and Abdenour, G. Necrotizing enterocolitis in the unfed infant. *J. Pediatr. Surg.* 17:620, 1982.

82. Martone, W. J., Williams, W. W., Mortensen, M. L., et al. Illness with fatalities in premature infants: Association with an intravenous vitamin E preparation, E-ferol. *Pediatrics* 78:591, 1986.

83. Meites, S. (ed.). *Pediatric Clinical Chemistry.* Washington, DC: American Association for Clinical Chemistry, 1977. P. 29.

84. Merritt, R. J., Sinatra, F. R., Henton, D., and Neustein, H. Cholestatic effect of intraperitoneal administration of tryptophan to suckling rat pups. *Pediatr. Res.* 18:904, 1984.

85. Mock, D. M., DeLorimer, A. A., Liebman, W. M., Sweetman, L., and Baker, H. Biotin deficiency: An unusual complication of parenteral alimentation. *N. Engl. J. Med.* 304:820, 1981.

86. Montreewasuwat, N., and Olson, J. A. Serum and liver concentrations of vitamin A in Thai fetuses as a function of gestational age. *Am. J. Clin. Nutr.* 32:601, 1979.

87. Moore, M. C., Greene, H. L., Phillips, B., et al. Evaluation of a pediatric multiple vitamin preparation for total parenteral nutrition in infants and children. I. Blood levels of water-soluble vitamins. *Pediatrics* 77:530, 1986.

88. Muller, D. P., Lloyd, J. K., and Wolff, D. H. Vitamin E and neurologic function: Abetalipoproteinemia and other disorders of fat absorption. *Ciba Found. Symp.* 101:106, 1983.

89. Mulvihill, S. J., and Fonkalsrud, E. W. Complications of superior versus inferior vena caval occlusion in infants receiving central total parenteral nutrition. *J. Pediatr. Surg.* 19:753, 1984.

90. Nose, O., Tipton, J. R., and Ament, M. E. Administration of lipid improves nitrogen retention in children receiving isocaloric TPN. *Pediatr. Res.* 19:228A, 1985.

91. Novak, M., Monkus, E. F., Chung, D., and Buch, M. Carnitine in the perinatal metabolism of lipids. I. Relationship between maternal and fetal plasma levels of carnitine and acylcarnitines. *Pediatrics* 67:95, 1981.

92. Olson, J. A., Gunning, D. B., and Tilton, R. A. Liver concentrations of vitamin A and carotenoids as a function of age and other parameters of American children who died of various causes. *Am. J. Clin. Nutr.* 39:903, 1984.

93. Oppenheimer, E. H. Focal necrosis of striated muscle in an infant with cystic fibrosis of the pancreas and evidence of lack of absorption of fat-soluble vitamins. *Bull. Johns Hopkins Hosp.* 98:353, 1956.

94. Oski, F. A., and Barness, L. A. Vitamin E deficiency: A previously unrecognized cause of hemolytic anemia in the premature infant. *J. Pediatr.* 70:211, 1967.

95. Paulsrud, J. R., Pensler, L., Whitten, C. F., Stewart, S., and Holman, R. T. Essential fatty acid deficiency in infants caused by fat-free intravenous feeding. *Am. J. Clin. Nutr.* 25:897, 1972.

96. Penn, D., Schmidt-Sommerfeld, E., and Pascu, F. Decreased tissue carnitine concentrations in newborn infants receiving total parenteral nutrition. *J. Pediatr.* 98:976, 1981.

97. Pereira, G. R., Sherman, M. S., DiGiacomo, J., Ziegler, M., Roth, K., and Jacobowski, D. Hyperalimentation-induced cholestasis: Increased incidence and severity in premature infants. *Am. J. Dis. Child.* 135:842, 1981.

98. Poole, R. L. Electrolyte and mineral requirements. In J. A. Kerner, Jr. (ed.), *Manual of Pediatric Parenteral Nutrition.* New York: Wiley, 1983. P. 129.

99. Postuma, R., Pease, P. W. B., Watts, R., Taylor, S., and McEvoy, F. A. Essential fatty acid deficiency in infants receiving parenteral nutrition. *J. Pediatr. Surg.* 13:393, 1978.

100. Reichman, B. L., Chessex, P., Putet, G., et al. Partition of energy metabolism and energy cost of growth in the very low-birthweight infant. *Pediatrics* 69:446, 1982.

101. Rubecz, I., Mestyan, J., Varga, P., and Klujber, L. Energy metabolism, substrate utilization, and nitrogen balance in parenterally fed postoperative neonates and infants. *J. Pediatr.* 98:42, 1981.

102. Ruz, M., and Solomons, N. Fecal zinc excre-

tion during oral rehydration therapy for acute infectious diarrhea. *Fed. Proc.* 46:748, 1987.

103. Sauer, P., Van Aerde, J., Smith, J., Pencharz, P., and Swyer, P. Substrate utilization of newborn infants fed intravenously with or without a fat emulsion. (Abstract) *Pediatr. Res.* 18:804, 1984.

104. Schiff, D., Chan, D., Seccombe, D., and Hahn, P. Plasma carnitine levels during intravenous feeding of the neonate. *J. Pediatr.* 95:1043, 1979.

105. Schriener, R. L., Glick, M. R., and Nordschow, C. D. An evaluation of methods to monitor infants receiving intravenous lipids. *J. Pediatr.* 94:197, 1979.

106. Seashore, J. H. Metabolic complications of parenteral nutrition in infants and children. *Surg. Clin. North Am.* 60:1239, 1980.

107. Seibert, J. J., Byrne, W. J., and Golladay, E. S. Development of hypervitaminosis A in a patient on long-term parenteral hyperalimentation. *Pediatr. Radiol.* 10:173, 1981.

108. Shenai, J. P., Kennedy, K. A., Chytil, F., and Stahlman, M. T. Clinical trial of vitamin A supplementation in infants susceptible to bronchopulmonary dysplasia. *J. Pediatr.* 111:269, 1987.

109. Shennan, A. T., Bryan, M. H., and Angel, A. The effect of gestational age on Intralipid tolerance in newborn infants. *J. Pediatr.* 91:134, 1977.

110. Sherman, M. P., Vitale, D. E., McLaughlin, G. W., and Goetzman, B. W. Percutaneous and surgical placement of fine silicone elastomer central catheters in high-risk newborns. *J. Parenter. Enter. Nutr.* 7:75, 1983.

111. Shike, M., Roulet, M., Kurian, R., Whitwell, J., Stewart, S., and Jeejeebhoy, K. N. Copper metabolism and requirements in total parenteral nutrition. *Gastroenterology* 81:290, 1981.

112. Snyderman, S. E. Recommendations for parenteral amino acid requirements. In R. W. Winters and E. G. Hasselmeyer (eds.), *Intravenous Nutrition in the High Risk Infant.* New York: Wiley, 1975. P. 422.

113. Specker, B. L., Greer, F., and Tsang, R. C. Vitamin D. In R. C. Tsang and B. F. Nichols (eds.), *Nutrition in Infancy.* Philadelphia: Hanley & Belfus, 1988. P. 175.

114. Stahl, G. E., Spear, M. L., and Hamosh, M. Intravenous administration of lipid emulsions to premature infants. *Clin. Perinatol.* 13:133, 1986.

115. Starinsky, R., and Shafrir, E. Displacement of albumin-bound bilirubin by free fatty acids: Implications for neonatal hyperbilirubinemia. *Clin. Chim. Acta* 29:311, 1970.

116. Stothert, J. C., Jr., McBride, L., Lewis, J. E.,

Danis, R. K., and Barner, H. B. Esophageal atresia and tracheoesophageal fistula: Preoperative assessment and reduced mortality. *Ann. Thorac. Surg.* 28:54, 1979.

117. Suchy, F. J., Courchene, S. M., and Balistreri, W. F. The development of hepatic bile acid conjugation in the rat. *Pediatr. Res.* 17:202, 1983.

118. Suchy, F. J., Courchene, S. M., and Balistreri, W. F. Ontogeny of hepatic bile acid conjugation in the rat. *Pediatr. Res.* 19:97, 1985.

119. Sung, J. H., Park, S. H., Mastri, A. R., and Warwick, W. J. Axonal dystrophy in the gracile nucleus in congenital biliary atresia and cystic fibrosis (mucoviscidosis): Beneficial effect of vitamin E therapy. *J. Neuropathol. Exp. Neurol.* 39:584, 1980.

120. Sunshine, P. Nutrition of the low birthweight infant. In E. J. Quilligan and N. Kretchmer (eds.), *Fetal and Maternal Medicine.* New York: Wiley, 1980. P. 637.

121. Thiessen, H., Jacobsen, J., and Brodersen, R. Displacement of albumin bound bilirubin in fatty acids. *Acta Paediatr. Scand.* 61:285, 1972.

122. Thomas, D. W., Sinatra, F. R., Hack, S. L., Smith, T. S., Platzker, A. C. G., and Merritt, R. J. Hyperammonemia in neonates receiving intravenous nutrition. *J. Parenter. Enter. Nutr.* 6:503, 1982.

123. Van Aerde, J., Sauer, P., Smith, J., Wesson, D., Swyer, P., and Pencharz, P. Contribution of glucose and fat to the energy expenditure of parenterally fed neonates. (Abstract) *Pediatr. Res.* 19:322A, 1985.

124. Venkateraman, P. S., Brissie, E. O., and Tasng, R. C. Stability of calcium and phosphorus in neonatal parenteral nutrition solutions. *J. Pediatr. Gastroenterol. Nutr.*, 2:640, 1983.

125. Vileisis, F. A., Cowett, R. M., and Oh, W. Glycemic response to lipid infusion in the premature neonate. *J. Pediatr.* 100:108, 1982.

126. Vileisis, R. A., Inwood, R. J., and Hunt, C. E. Prospective controlled study of parenteral nutrition–associated cholestatic jaundice: Effect of protein intake. *J. Pediatr.* 96:893, 1980.

127. Warner, B. W., Gorgone, P., Schilling, S., Farrell, M., and Ghory, M. J. Multiple purpose central venous access in infants less than 1000 grams. *J. Pediatr. Surg.* 22:820, 1987.

128. Weber, T. R., West, K. W., and Grosfeld, J. L. Broviac central venous catheterization in infants and children. *Am. J. Surg.* 145:202, 1983.

129. Wilmore, D. W. Factors correlating with a successful outcome following extensive intes-

tinal resection in newborn infants. *J. Pediatr.* 80:88, 1972.

130. Winick, M., and Noble, A. Cellular response in rats during malnutrition at various ages. *J. Nutr.* 89:300, 1966.

131. Winick, M., and Rosso, P. The effect of severe early malnutrition on cellular growth of human brain. *Pediatr. Res.* 3:181, 1969.

132. Wolman, S. L., Anderson, G. H., Marliss, E. B., and Jeejeebhoy, K. N. Zinc in total parenteral nutrition: Requirements and metabolic effects. *Gastroenterology* 76:458, 1979.

133. Yu, V. Y. H., Joseph, R., Bajuk, B. F., Orgill, A., and Astbury, J. Necrotizing enterocolitis in very low birthweight infants: A four-year experience. *Aust. Paediatr. J.* 20:29, 1983.

134. Ziegler, M., Jakobowski, D., Hoelzer, D., Eichelberger, M., and Koop, C. E. Route of pediatric parenteral nutrition: Proposed criteria revision. *J. Pediatr. Surg.* 15:472, 1980.

135. Zlotkin, S. H. Intravenous nitrogen intake requirements in full-term newborns undergoing surgery. *Pediatrics* 73:493, 1984.

136. Zlotkin, S. H., Bryan, M. H., and Anderson, G. H. Cysteine supplementation to cysteine-free intravenous feeding regimens in newborn infants. *Am. J. Clin. Nutr.* 34:914, 1981.

137. Zlotkin, S. H., Bryan, M. H., and Anderson, G. H. Intravenous nitrogen and energy intakes required to duplicate in utero nitrogen accretion in prematurely born human infants. *J. Pediatr.* 99:115, 1981.

138. Zlotkin, S. H., Stallings, V. A., and Pencharz, P. B. Total parenteral nutrition in children. *Surg. Clin. North Am.* 32:381, 1985.

Nutritional Support in the Cancer Patient

Lisa M. Sclafani
Murray F. Brennan

The cancer patient commonly presents with significant nutritional deficits that are potentially deleterious to treatment and outcome. In an effort to better design nutritional support modalities, careful documentation of those deficits and an understanding of the etiology of the malnutrition is essential. When nutritional support is indicated and offered, it must be performed with low morbidity and serious attempts to evaluate efficacy must be documented.

NUTRITIONAL DEFICITS IN THE CANCER PATIENT

Incidence

Hospitalized cancer patients are commonly malnourished. The prevalence of malnutrition varies according to the parameters measured, the type and stage of cancer, and treatment modality [10, 71, 100]. Tables 21-1 and 21-2 document the prevalence of malnutrition in hospitalized cancer patients according to whether anthropometric measurements or serum deficiencies are used to indicate malnutrition. Weight loss is common in patients with gastrointestinal malignancy, especially esophageal and gastric cancer, which often presents with weight loss [12]. In contrast, patients with early-stage small-cell lung cancer may have less significant weight loss [30]. Clearly with advanced stage, the degree of weight loss is markedly increased.

Bozetti et al. [10] studied 280 cancer patients and noted body weight, cutaneous delayed hypersensitivity, and serum albumin level as the most commonly altered parameters. They noted that patients with resectable carcinoma of the colon, rectum, or head, neck cancer, oat-cell carcinoma, lymphoma, or carcinoma of unknown primary had no significant alteration of nutritional status. Patients with carcinoma of the esophagus or stomach showed significant depletion of weight, triceps skinfold thickness, and total protein, albumin, and cholinesterase levels. Nixon et al. [71] reviewed 54 consecutive pa-

Table 21-1. Incidence of Malnutrition in Cancer Patients Measured by Anthropometric Parameters

Parameter	Study	Patient Population	Weight Loss	% of Patients
Weight loss	DeWys et al. [25]	Protocol chemotherapy patients before treatment	Yes > 10%	54% 15%
	Shike et al. [95]	Small-cell lung carcinoma pretreatment	5.6% average	—
	Shils and Coiso [97]	All admissions to a cancer hospital	> 10% > 20%	25% 17.5%
		Outpatient chemotherapy patients	> 5%	25%
	Burke et al. [14]	Gastrointestinal malignancies	Yes	75%
Triceps skinfold thickness	Nixon et al. [71]	Hospitalized medical oncology patients	< 80%	42%
	Bistrian et al. [8]	Hospitalized medical oncology patients	< 60%	60%
Arm muscle circumference	Bistrian et al. [8]	Hospitalized medical oncology patients	< 90%	70%
Creatinine-height index	Nixon et al. [71]	Hospitalized medical oncology patients	< 80%	85%

tients admitted to a medical oncology ward and found that 42% had triceps skinfolds of less than 80% of standard. Creatinine-height ratios were less than 80% of standard values in 85% of cancer patients. Serum albumin level and midarm muscle circumference was also low in 23 to 31% of cancer patients. In a large study including 3047 patients entering chemotherapy protocols, DeWys et al. [24] reported that 54% of patients showed weight loss. In 15%, the weight loss was greater than 10%. The incidence of weight loss was dependent on diagnosis, with the highest incidence in gastric and pancreatic tumors (87%)

Table 21-2. Deficits in Serum Components in the Cancer Patient

Component	Study	Patient Population	Results
Albumin	Nixon et al. [71]	Hospitalized medical oncology patients	31% patients < 80% standard
	Bozzetti et al. [10]	Patients with unresectable gastric-esophageal cancer	Mean = 87% of controls
	Rombeau et al. [82]	Preop. colon & rectal cancer patients	16% < controls ($p < 0.01$)
Vitamins	Inculet et al. [42]	Hospitalized oncology patients	40% had low niacin levels; 15% had low B_{12} levels
Transferrin	Shike et al. [95]	Hospitalized oncology patients undergoing chemotherapy	25% decrease during chemotherapy
	Rombeau et al. [82]	Preop. colon & rectal cancer patients	17% < controls ($p < 0.05$)
Cholinesterase	Bozzetti et al. [9]	Advanced malnourished cancer patients	Mean = 1.37 U/ml; normal = 1.90–3.80 U/ml
Retinol-binding protein	Bozzetti et al. [9]	Advanced malnourished cancer patients	Mean = 2.0 mg/dl; normal = 3–6 mg/dl

Body Composition

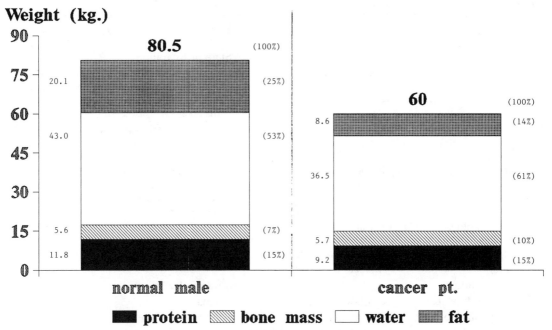

Figure 21-1. Body composition in a normal middle-age male, and a weight-losing cancer patient. The cancer patient has lost 25% of his total body weight: 57% of body fat, 22% of body protein, and 15% of body water. The numbers in parentheses represent percent of total body weight that each compartment represents. (Data from Cohn, S. H., Ellis, K. J., Vartsky, D., et al. Comparison of methods of estimating body fat in normal subjects and cancer patients. *Am. J. Clin. Nutr.* 34:2839, 1981.)

and lowest in patients with breast cancer (36%) and sarcoma (40%).

Body Composition

A knowledge of body composition is necessary for understanding, measuring, and treating nutritional deficits. Body composition in normals is dependent on gender and age, but can be divided into four components: body fat, body water, bone mineral mass, and protein [20]. The composition of body weight is illustrated in Figure 21-1 in a normal middle-age male and a weight-losing cancer patient. Bone mineral mass is constant for an individual and is measured by neutron activation of calcium. Body fat is anhydrous and not a major site of metabolism. It can be measured indirectly by densitometry or tri-

ceps skinfold thickness. Body weight less body fat equals the lean body mass, which can be divided into intracellular and extracellular components. The extracellular component can be measured by electric impedance methods and is most affected by changes in hydration status. When fat and the extracellular fluid is subtracted from the total body mass, the body cell mass, which includes the protein and water compartments of muscle and viscera, is obtained. It is responsible for the majority of metabolism and is a reflection of the actively metabolizing cells in the human body. The body cell mass is proportional to oxygen consumption, caloric requirement, and basal metabolic expenditure as described by Moore et al. in 1963 [68]. The maintenance of the body cell mass is the aim of nutritional support.

Table 21-3. Body Compartment Measurements and Sources of Error

Method	Compartment Measured	Source of Error	Ease of Measurement
Weight/height	All	Body frame, state of hydration	+ + +
% Weight loss	All	State of hydration	+ + +
Creatinine-height index	Muscle mass	Dietary intake of creatinine, variability creatinine excretion, renal disease	+ + +
Densitometry	Fat mass	Age and nutrition-related changes in density	+ +
Anthropomorphics			
Arm muscle circumference	Muscle mass	Depends on age, sex, race, and site of measurement; observer-dependent	+ + +
Triceps skinfold thickness	Fat mass		
K_{40}—Whole-body counter	Body cell mass; Skeletal muscle plus viscera	Intracellular hypokalemia	+
K_e—Isotope dilution		Intracellular hypokalemia	+ +
D_2O—Total body water	Lean body mass	Edema	+ +
Na_e—Isotope dilution	Extracellular mass— indirectly body cell mass	State of hydration	+ +
Neutron activation— Analysis of total body nitrogen	Total body protein	Differences in size and shape of patients	+
Electric impedance	Extracellular fluid volume and total body water	Electrolyte changes	+ +
CT scan	Fat content	Severe malnutrition, fatty infiltration of muscle, limited area of study	+ +
MRI	Fat and muscle mass	Limited area of study	+ +

K_{40} = potassium 40; K_e = exchangeable potassium; Na_e = exchangeable sodium; + + + = suitable for routine in-hospital use; + + = requires skilled personnel and research equipment; + = research facility necessary.

Methods of Measurement

Methods of measuring body compartments range from simple anthropometric measurements to sophisticated radioactive labeling methods and are summarized in Table 21-3. Anthropometric measurements include body weight, weight-height ratio, triceps skinfold thickness, and midarm muscle circumference. Triceps skinfold thickness is measured midway between the olecranon and acromion using Lange calipers. Arm circumference is measured at the same point, and tri-

ceps skinfold thickness is subtracted from this value to derive midarm muscle circumference. These measurements are compared to historical standards and used as indirect estimates of fat and muscle depletion. While easy and inexpensive to perform, these measurements are dependent on the experience of the observer and on the age, sex, and race of the patient. Comparison with standard controls is valid only within the same population group [49].

In a comparison of CT scan and anthropometric measurements of midarm composition, Heymsfield et al. pointed out that several assumptions in measuring midarm muscle circumference are incorrect [38]. First, the arm is rarely circular but more often elliptical, the muscle compartment is "cloverleaf" in configuration, and fat is distributed asymmetrically. The bone area, not taken into account, varies according to body build and patient population and is not influenced by malnutrition. Muscle area is then underestimated in undernourished subjects. In subjects with greater than 15% ideal body weight, estimates of midarm fat area and muscle area differed from radiographic values by more than 50%. Despite these limitations, anthropometric measurements are still used for nutritional assessment because of their low cost and availability.

Muscle mass may be estimated by determining creatinine-height index. This is calculated by dividing the 24-hour creatinine excretion rate by the standard creatinine excretion rate expected for a person of the same height. While this was noted to be the most sensitive indicator of malnutrition in a large series of cancer patients studied by Nixon et al., its reliability is limited by the variability of dietary intake and renal function, as well as the daily variability of creatinine excretion seen in the same patient [71].

The measurement of changes in body compartment ratios seen in cancer patients has been facilitated by the use of radioactive labeled compounds [20]. Potassium 40 is the naturally occurring isotope of potassium, representing 0.012% of all naturally occurring potassium in the human body. Using a whole-body counter, the total body potassium is directly measured, a technique that is expensive and cumbersome. The development of radioactive isotopes of potassium, such as potassium 42, enables the total body potassium to be measured indirectly using isotope dilution methods. A measured amount of radioactive compound is injected and distributes throughout the body, and after equilibration, the amount in a blood sample is counted. By this method, indirect measurements of total body exchangeable potassium (TBK_e) can be made. Since 98% of potassium is intracellular, total body potassium is a function of the body cell mass. The body cell mass represents the actively metabolizing compartment of the body and is the most important indicator of nutritional status [68].

The total exchangeable body water (TBW_e) and total exchangeable body sodium ($TBNa_e$) can also be measured by isotope dilution methods, using tritiated water, deuterium oxide, or sodium 122. Since fat is anhydrous, the total body water is proportional to the lean body mass. Sodium, in contrast to potassium, is almost entirely extracellular and the total body sodium is a measure of the extracellular mass. Both TBK_e and $TBNa_e$ vary with body size, but are best corrected when expressed as a function of total body water. With malnutrition, the body cell mass decreases and the extracellular mass increases, with an increase in the ratio of Na_e/K_e. This Na_e/K_e ratio is used to assess nutritional state. Shizgal measured Na_e/K_e in a group of catabolic patients and demonstrated marked contraction of the body cell mass with expansion of the extracellular component, with a Na_e/K_e of 2.05 compared to 1.0 for 18 normal volunteers. A similar increase in the Na_e/K_e ratio was seen in postoperative patients but the increase was prevented by the administration of parenteral alimentation [98]. In a group of 98 hospitalized patients in Madrid, the Na_e/K_e ratio proved to correlate best with mortality in a high-risk group (28% mortality), when the ratio was compared to measurements of serum albumin, transferrin, percentage of recent weight loss, and triceps skinfold thickness [103].

Neutron activation analysis allows direct measurement of total body nitrogen using a small dose of neutrons and measuring the gamma radiation produced by activated nitrogen nuclei [64]. Total body nitrogen is converted to total body protein by multiplying by 6.25. Other radionuclides produced by the neutron activation can be used to determine total body calcium, aluminum, sodium, and chlorine. This technique is quite accurate and noninvasive, and exposes the patient to minimum radiation. The technology is expensive,

Table 21-4. Methods of Nutritional Assessment

Serum Measurements	Measures	Sources of Error
Albumin	Visceral protein	Long half-life, liver disease, hydration, exogenous sources
Transferrin	Visceral protein	Liver disease, acute-phase reactant, dependent on iron stores
Complement	Visceral protein	Infection, liver disease, head and neck cancers, acute-phase reactant
Prealbumin	Visceral protein	Liver disease, reduced in vitamin A and zinc deficiencies
Immunoglobulin	Humoral immunity	Infection, myeloma, hematologic malignancies
Total lymphocyte count	Cellular immunity	Infection, leukemia

however, and not commonly available except in the research setting. In combination with measurement of potassium 40 and total body water, these parameters can be used for quick, easy, body compartment measurements, which can be followed over a course of treatment [20–22, 39].

In comparing measurements of body fat obtained indirectly from potassium 40, total body nitrogen, total body water, and triceps skinfold thickness, there was little difference in young, healthy volunteers. However, in wasting diseases, total body potassium is quite variable and total body nitrogen is thought to be the most accurate for measuring body fat indirectly [20].

Bioelectric impedance entails determination of resistance and reactance using a four-terminal impedance plethysmograph. Electrodes are positioned on the hands and feet in the supine patient. A current is applied and the voltage drop measured. Impedance correlates inversely with the fat-free mass, which contains the body fluids and electrolytes. This method then is used to determine lean body mass and indirectly body fat. When compared with anthropometric methods, it is found to be more accurate [60, 75, 87].

Serum protein levels are easily measured but are affected by nutritional and nonnutritional factors (Table 21-4). Serum albumin level, one of the most common parameters used in nutritional assessment, is dependent on normal liver function for production and is influenced by the patient's state of hydration. The long half-life of albumin, as well as the maintenance of normal levels in the marasmic state, prompted the measurement of more sensitive indicators of malnutrition [63]. These include transferrin (measured as a function of iron-binding capacity or directly by immunodiffusion), retinol-binding protein, and prealbumin, all of which have significantly shorter half-lives than albumin (8 days, 10 hours, 24 hours, and 20 days, respectively). All are synthesized by the liver and are influenced by liver disease and hydration. The shorter half-lives make them more useful for monitoring the acute effects of therapy.

Both CT and MRI enable a more accurate assessment of the muscle and fat compartments in an extremity. As previously mentioned, using the CT scan, Heymsfield et al. pointed out several erroneous assumptions on which anthropometric measurements are based [38]. The CT scan, however, takes into account the area of the bone and distribution of the muscle within the forearm. Limitations include a limited area of study, high cost, limited availability, and the occurrence of fatty infiltration of the muscle in severe malnutrition.

MRI provides even more striking contrast in the soft tissues [65]. Differences in proton relaxation times (T1 and T2) correlate with differences in tissue composition, hard tissues (e.g., bone, tendons), fat, cellular tissue (muscle, viscera), hemorrhage, and blood flow, allowing for a very precise analysis of body composition. MRI is also limited, however, by high cost, limited field of study, and availability.

Ease of Measurement

Many of the above-described methods are cumbersome and impractical in the average clinical setting. They are primarily research tools used to document effects of therapy and deficits in various disease states. In a more practical sense, Baker et al. [3] found that a good history, with emphasis on weight loss, dietary patterns, and gastrointestinal symptomatology, in combination with a thorough physical examination noting muscle wasting, loss of fat, and body weight, may be just as effective in identifying the malnourished patient at risk.

Specific Deficits in the Cancer Patient

Cancer patients represent a heterogeneous group of patients, making it difficult to generalize about specific deficits. Figure 22-1 illustrates the changes in body composition seen in the cancer patient. In this example of severe weight loss, normal body mass is represented as 25% fat, 53% water, 7% bone, and 15% protein. After a 25% reduction in weight, these proportions change to 14% fat, 61% water, 9.5% bone, and 15% protein. Protein is lost proportionately (22%), fat losses are greatest (57%), and the 15% water loss actually leads to an overhydrated patient [20]. Tables 21-1 and 21-2 outline various nutritional parameters that have been measured in cancer patients. Specific deficits have been noted in fat, protein, vitamins, minerals, and immunity. These deficits may be due to treatment, malnutrition, or the cancer itself, making it difficult to distinguish the cause.

Specific deficits of skeletal protein with sparing of visceral protein were seen by Cohn et al. when total body nitrogen and potassium were measured [20–22]. This was confirmed by Shike et al., who demonstrated that albumin and transferrin levels were well maintained in weight-losing cancer patients despite progressive loss of all components of body composition [95]. Creatinine-height index has been shown by several investigators [61, 71, 72, 95] to more accurately reflect weight loss and depletion of total body nitrogen in cancer patients, when compared to albumin and total serum protein measurements, probably because of this visceral sparing effect. Only in severely wasted patients with progressive disease is a decrease in serum albumin level seen [63]. Plasma amino acid levels are maintained despite cancer in mild nutrition. With marked weight loss, a decrease in total plasma amino acids has been seen [95].

Significant loss of the fat compartment was also seen by several investigators [21, 95, 114]. Watson and Sammon demonstrated higher total body fat loss in malnourished cancer patients compared to malnourished patients with nonmalignant disease [117]. Specific decreases in plasma free fatty acid (FFA) [56] and glycerol turnover [28, 56] are seen in weight-losing cancer patients, while triglyceride levels may be maintained, indicating an increase in whole-body lipolysis. Measuring water-soluble vitamin levels, Inculet et al. [42] found low levels of B_1, B_2, B_6 and niacin in 4 to 40% of cancer patients receiving total parenteral nutrition (TPN). No patients developed clinical evidence of vitamin deficiencies in this study.

Immune Deficits

Immunocompetence is impaired in patients with solid tumors and lymphoreticular cancers. The extent and quality of the immune deficit are influenced by the type and stage of the cancer, the patient's nutritional status, and the treatment the patient has received [5, 29, 76, 83].

Among the hematologic malignancies, patients with Hodgkin's disease demonstrate impairment of T cell–mediated functions, while in chronic lymphocytic leukemia and multiple myeloma, humoral (B-cell) immu-

Table 21-5. Immune Deficits in Patients with a Solid Tumor

Parameter	Study	Type of Malignancy	Stage	Cancer Patients	Controls
Delayed hypersensitivity to DNCB	Pinsky et al. [76]	Head and neck	Localized	42%	95%
		Not head and neck	Localized	83%	95%
		Not head and neck	Regional metastases	67%	95%
		Not head and neck	Distant metastases	41%	95%
		Melanoma	Distant metastases	74%	95%
		Sarcoma	Distant metastases	73%	95%
	Eilber and Morton [29]	All types	All stages	60%	95%
Response to common skin	Eilber and Morton [29]	All types	Localized	39%	90%
Antigens	Pinsky et al. [76]	All types	All stages	50%	90%
Total lymphocyte count	Haffejee and Angorn [35]	Esophagus	Unresectable	83%	100%
IgA levels (μ/dl)	Veltri et al. [112]	Head and neck	Localized Pretreatment Posttreatment	310 ($p = 0.001$) 290 ($p = 0.05$)	220
Serum complement levels (U/dl)	Veltri et al. [112]	Head and neck	Localized Pretreatment Posttreatment	150 ($p = 0.05$) 125	130 —

DNCB = dinitrochlorobenzene.

nity is affected to a greater degree. Hypogammaglobulinemia is common in patients with chronic lymphocytic leukemia. Patients with myeloma have an excess of monoclonal antibody; however, their functioning polyclonal immunoglobulin level is low. Patients with acute myelogenous leukemia and chronic myelogenous leukemia generally maintain immunocompetence until treatment is begun or blast crisis occurs.

In patients with solid tumors, immune deficits are commonly seen in disseminated disease or after treatment has occurred (Table 21-5). Certain solid tumors (e.g., cancer of the head and neck) are more likely to elicit deficits even in their early stage. Dinitrochlorobenzene (DNCB) elicits a positive de-

layed hypersensitivity reaction from 95% of control patients. Pinsky et al. showed that 83% of cancer patients with no evidence of metastases had a positive delayed reaction to DNCB, whereas only 41% of patients with distant metastases reacted to DNCB [76]. For patients with localized head and neck cancer, however, only 42% reacted to DNCB. In generalized metastatic melanoma and sarcoma, 73% maintained a positive reaction to DNCB. A positive reaction to DNCB has also been correlated with a good prognosis. Eilber and Morton tested patients with clinically early cancers preoperatively and followed them for 6 months postoperatively [29]. Ninety-three percent of patients with a negative response to DNCB were inoperable or had an early recurrence; 92% of patients with a positive recall to DNCB were free of disease for the 6-month period. Overall, 60% of these cancer patients had a positive response to DNCB, compared to 95% of normal control subjects. Common skin antigen testing in these same groups demonstrated that 90% of control subjects would respond to at least one of six antigens, whereas only 39% of cancer patients reacted to one or more antigens.

The contribution of malnutrition to the impaired immune response is often difficult to separate from the effect of the cancer itself. Haffejee and Angorn studied 20 patients with unresectable cancer of the esophagus before and after palliation with tube intubation of the esophagus [35]. All patients showed evidence of malnutrition initially. However, 3 weeks after intubation, all patients were in positive nitrogen balance, with rises in serum albumin, iron-binding capacity, and body weight, and an increase in skinfold thickness. Total lymphocyte counts, initially depressed 17% below control values, rose to normal after restoration of nitrogen balance. Transformation of lymphocytes by phytohemagglutinin (PHA) (a measure of T-cell function), initially depressed, approached normal with treatment; however, no improvement in the 0% reactivity to DNCB in cancer patients was seen after nitrogen balance was achieved.

Immune deficits present before and even after successful treatment have been attributed to circulating immune complexes. Veltri et al. demonstrated increased IgA levels and circulating serum immune complexes before and after successful treatment for head and neck cancers. These serum immune complexes are implicated in in vitro immune deficits seen in these patients [112].

Once treatment is initiated in the cancer patient, further deficits in the immune response are seen. Both T and B cells are sensitive to radiation, and defects in circulating lymphocyte counts can be documented following localized radiation, but are more common after total nodal irradiation. This is also reflected in depressed T-cell function while immunoglobulin levels are usually maintained. Bone narrow depression secondary to

radiation contributes to depressed neutrophil counts and the resultant impaired inflammatory response [5].

Surgery, with its concomitant anesthesia, also affects immune function. Roth et al. measured lymphocyte function parameters pre- and postoperatively in cancer patients and demonstrated no overall significant changes [83]. However, certain groups were identified to have significant depression of lymphocyte function, and included those undergoing intraabdominal or intrathoracic procedures, those receiving blood transfusions, and those having operations longer than 2 hours. The type of tumor also influenced the postoperative immune response, with carcinoma patients having a significantly depressed response compared to patients with melanoma or sarcoma. All of these effects were normalized by 4 weeks postoperatively.

Virtually all chemotherapeutic agents have an effect on the immune system. These effects are dependent on dose, schedule of treatment, underlying disease, parameter measured, and type of chemotherapy. By their myelosuppressive action in the bone marrow, the nonspecific inflammatory reaction is diminished, especially with absolute neutrophil counts less than 1000. Cell cycle–specific drugs and alkylating agents, especially cyclophosphamide, also affect lymphocytes to a high degree.

MECHANISMS FOR NUTRITIONAL DEFICITS

The etiology of the nutritional deficits seen in cancer patients includes decreased intake, impaired absorption and digestion, abnormal losses, altered metabolism, and increased requirements [13, 71].

Impaired Intake and Digestion

Several factors have been implicated in the anorexia of cancer patients [13, 24]. Defects of olfactory and gustatory sensations have been documented. Altered thresholds for sweet, sour, and salt are noted. Generalized debility

**Table 21-6.   Gastrointestinal
Complications of Tumors and
Their Treatment**

Tumor-related
  Gastric outlet obstruction
  Dysphagia, odynophagia
  Fistulas
  Malabsorption
  Infections
  Small- and large-bowel obstruction
  Esophageal obstruction
  Bleeding diarrhea
  Ulcerations
Chemotherapy-related
  Nausea and vomiting
  Oropharyngeal ulcerations/infections
  Anorexia
  Esophagitis
  Gastrointestinal motility disorders
  Colitis
  Anosmia
  Diarrhea
Radiation-related
  Enteritis, acute or chronic
  Mucositis
  Xerostomia
  Colitis
  Fistulas
  Malabsorption
Surgery-related
  Prolonged ileus
  Gastric atony
  Fistulas
  Malabsorption
  Short-bowel syndrome
  Bowel obstruction
  Postgastrectomy syndromes
    Dumping
    Diarrhea
    Vitamin B_{12} deficiency

and weakness impair eating, as do developed aversions to food [24]. Studies of defects in the hypothalamic appetite control center secondary to various amines have not been conclusive [13].

Table 21-6 lists the gastrointestinal effects of tumors and their treatment. Mechanical factors are most commonly seen in head and neck and upper gastrointestinal cancers [55]. In the head and neck region, pain, ulceration, obstruction, and trismus impair intake. Esophageal cancer may present with obstruc-tion, aspiration, or tracheoesophageal fistula, with patients avoiding solid food to prevent recurrent aspiration. Gastric cancers may present with early satiety even before they have become obstructing because of decreased distensibility, ulceration and pain, and extrinsic nodal or metastatic disease. Malignant obstruction of the small bowel or colon usually presents as an acute event and rarely causes chronic decreased intake and weight loss.

Impaired absorption and digestion may be secondary to loss of normal intestinal enzymes or defects in the mucosa of the gastrointestinal tract. Patients with pancreatic cancer frequently present with steatorrhea or diabetes. Obstruction of the pancreatic duct with resultant pancreatitis or atrophy of the gland accounts for these deficits in exocrine and endocrine function. Lymphoma of the small bowel may produce malabsorption. Prolonged diarrhea secondary to villous tumors of the colon and rectum can cause great losses in protein as well as fluid and electrolytes.

Obstruction of bile by common duct, duodenal, or pancreatic cancers can also cause steatorrhea. Enteric fistulas secondary to malignancy may lead to malabsorption because of the bypass of large segments of the small bowel or overgrowth of bacteria in the small bowel.

Malnutrition itself may lead to mucosal changes in the small bowel, including edema, reduced activity of mucosal enzymes, and flattening of mucosal crypts with reduced cell proliferation, contributing to impaired intestinal absorption [55]. [*Editor's Note:* Such changes may also allow translocation of intestinal bacteria, which may cause otherwise unexplained sepsis. Absorption of endotoxin into the portal circulation could also contribute to altered metabolism.]

Treatment of neoplasms, including surgery, radiation, and chemotherapy, often contributes to reduced intake and impaired absorption of nutrients [26, 66]. Major oropharyngeal resections preclude eating solid food for several weeks, and complications of fistulas, infection, and wound breakdown may prolong this. Postgastrectomy syndromes, including malabsorption of fat, and deficiencies of iron and vitamin B_{12}, dumping, and loss of the stomach reservoir with early satiety, lead to weight loss and malnutrition. Massive small-bowel resection, especially in combination with resection of the ileocecal valve, is rarely necessary for malignant disease. It can be associated with "short-bowel syndrome" resulting in diarrhea, multinutrient malabsorption, and vitamin deficiencies.

Radiation therapy has significant effects on the gastrointestinal tract, leading to nutritional deficiencies [26]. They are related to total dose, fractionation, and the volume irradiated. Head and neck radiation leads to xerostomia, mucositis, anorexia, dysosmia, and odynophagia acutely. Late sequelae include ulcers, osteoradionecrosis of the mandible, trismus, and dental caries. Radiation of the thorax commonly employed for esophageal, mediastinal, and primary lung cancers can produce dysphagia due to esophageal edema and ulceration acutely, and chronically may produce fistulas, fibrosis, and stenosis. Radiation of the abdomen commonly includes large segments of small bowel, resulting in malabsorption, diarrhea, nausea, vomiting, and loss of nutrients. Acute enteritis accompanied by shortening of villi and loss of mucosal epithelium is a predecessor of chronic radiation injury. This often presents as partial bowel obstruction, perforation, and fistulas, often requiring surgery and bowel resection, leading to further malabsorption. Chemotherapy can contribute to malnutrition in the cancer patient; frequently causing nausea and vomiting, anorexia, and generalized weakness, it restricts intake. Certain agents produce more specific insults, such as stomatitis, gastric ulcers, enteritis, diarrhea, and ileus [48, 66]. Intraperitoneal chemotherapy may cause abdominal pain and diarrhea, and intrahepatic chemotherapy induces gastric and duodenal ulceration as well as biliary sclerosis [50]. Antibiotics used to treat complications or nadir sepsis can produce diarrhea, enterocolitis, and generalized gastrointestinal upset.

Altered Metabolism

Metabolism in the cancer-bearing patient has been widely studied [7]. Defects in glucose metabolism include impaired glucose tolerance [74], increased rate of glucose oxidation and uptake, increased glucose production rates from alanine, and increased lactate production via the Cori cycle [1, 15, 36, 84]. Shaw and Wolfe [91] demonstrated increased glucose turnover in advanced tumors, with the rate of glucose oxidation proportional to tumor bulk and returning toward normal after curative resection. Protein metabolism has also been shown to be altered in the weight-losing cancer patient. We and others demonstrated increased whole-body protein turnover, synthesis, and catabolism in cancer patients compared with malnourished noncancer patients [37, 44, 47, 93].

Cancer patients have abnormal fat metabolism, with an increased rate of lipolysis, demonstrated by an increased FFA and glycerol plasma concentration and turnover [56, 92]. This has also been demonstrated in septic stressed cancer patients 57]. Measurements of the respiratory quotient (RQ) suggest a preferential fat oxidation with increased serum levels of beta-hydroxybutyrate and no significant rise in RQ with glucose infusion [84]. While some defects in metabolism are seen before the onset of weight loss and cachexia (e.g., impaired glucose tolerance), most deficits are not seen in the non–weight-losing individual with early cancer, who resembles control subjects in most instances [56, 91, 93].

The etiology of the altered metabolism is unclear. While certain deficits are seen locally, as in the tumor-bearing limb, others are demonstrable systemically [15, 74]. Circulating proteins, including tumor necrosis factor (cachectin) and interleukin, have been implicated in the altered metabolism of the cancer patient [6, 115]. Warren et al. demonstrated that the administration of tumor necrosis factor causes a net efflux of alanine and glutamine as well as a fall in the arterial amino acid concentrations, suggesting an increased uptake of amoni acids by other organs. How-

Table 21-7. Metabolic Response to Total Parenteral Nutrition (TPN) in the Malnourished Cancer Patient

	Before TPN	References	Response to TPN	References
Body weight	↓	9, 72	↑	9, 72
Caloric intake	↓	72, 84	↑	72, 84
Nitrogen balance	↓	9, 28, 72, 89	↑	9, 28, 72, 89
Protein synthesis	↑	44, 93	↑, +/−	44, 93
Protein catabolism	↑	18, 28, 44, 93	↓	18, 28, 93
Protein turnover	↑	44	↑	44
Skeletal muscle catabolism (3-methylhistidine)	↑	9, 18	↓	9, 18
Lean tissue mass	↓	16, 95	↑	16, 95
Lactate levels	↑	16, 84	↑	16, 84
Gluconeogenesis	↑	16, 107	↓	16
Alanine-glucose conversion	↑	16, 28	↓	16, 28
Glucose turnover	↑	16	↑	16
Fat synthesis	↓	84	↑	84
Fat mobilization	↑	56, 84	+/−	84
Fat oxidation	↑	84	+/−	84
Plasma free fatty acids	↑	16, 56, 84	↓, +/−	16, 84
Triceps skinfold thickness	↓	9, 28	↑, +/−	9, 28
Respiratory quotient	↓	56, 58, 84	+/−	58, 84
Resting energy expenditure	↑	84	+/−	84

+/− = unchanged.

ever, this accounts for only some of the consequences of the altered metabolism seen in cancer-bearing patients [115]. The contribution of local and systemic effects is debatable. Successful treatment of the tumor usually leads to disappearance of these metabolic abnormalities, leaving no long-term deficits [91, 100].

NUTRITIONAL SUPPORT

The presence of nutritional deficits and metabolic abnormalities in the cancer patient is not in itself justification for the use of parenteral nutrition. The study of the metabolic effects of TPN on the cancer patient provides the opportunity to investigate the etiology of the derangements present, their specificity, and the optimum use of supplemental nutri-

ents. Examination of the efficacy of nutritional support in terms of survival, treatment tolerance, and morbidity is essential. Effects of nutritional supplements on tumor growth must also be examined.

Metabolic Response to Total Parenteral Nutrition

TPN has varying abilities to reverse the metabolic deficits seen in the cancer patient (Table 21-7). In certain aspects, these patients resemble non–tumor-bearing malnourished patients, but marked differences are also noted. Malnourished cancer patients can improve their caloric intake and body weight with TPN, but there is less improvement in body weight, creatinine-height ratio, and midarm muscle circumference, compared to noncancer controls [72].

Nitrogen balance can be achieved in both cancer patients and noncancer patients. Studying protein kinetics in starved normal patients and weight-losing patients with advanced cancer or without cancer, Jeevanandam et al. were able to show a high rate of protein catabolism, synthesis, and turnover in the cancer patients, which were all decreased with TPN [44]. Finding similar protein kinetics, Shaw and Wolfe [93] demonstrated that the protein synthetic rate was increased with TPN, but a net gain of protein could not be produced despite the use of 2 g/kg/day, in marked contrast to the control patients. Jeevanandam et al. demonstrated differences in protein kinetics in response to oral supplementation versus intravenous feeding in the malnourished cancer patient. Protein synthesis was increased to a much greater degree with oral feeding compared with intravenous feeding, where no increase in protein synthesis could be demonstrated [45, 46]. Skeletal muscle catabolism, measured by urinary excretion of 3-methylhistidine, has been shown to be increased in the cancer patient but was significantly reduced by 2-week treatment with TPN. Lean tissue mass, measured by total body potassium, was also significantly increased after TPN [18].

Alterations in fat metabolism are less reliably affected by parenteral nutrition. Levinson and Russell showed that cancer patients utilize fat preferentially, as shown by a lower RQ. This was unaffected by TPN, as were the increased FFA levels and fat oxidation [57, 84]. Other workers, however, showed TPN to decrease FFA and glycerol levels and increase RQ [58]. These variations may be due to differences in cancer type, nutritional status, and supplementation. The degree of associated stress is a major factor in this response. Sauerwein et al. studied septic cancer patients and showed increased FFA turnover, which was unresponsive to glucose infusion but responsive to euglycemic hyperinsulemic clamping [86]. Most studies, however, show an increase in fat synthesis with TPN. While a 35% increase in triceps

skinfold thickness was seen by Dresler et al. in non–tumor-bearing, malnourished patients receiving TPN, no increase was seen in tumor-bearing patients receiving TPN, suggesting a decreased ability to store fat [28]. The data of Shike et al. contradicts this finding [95].

Efficacy of Total Parenteral Nutrition

Numerous attempts have been made to prove the efficacy of parenteral nutrition in improving treatment tolerance, treatment toxicity, tumor response, survival rate, and postoperative morbidity and mortality in the cancer patient (Tables 21-8, 21-9, and 21-10). Most trials are limited by the small numbers of patients, which may not allow a potential benefit to be demonstrated. Pooling of data from various studies is hazardous because of the possibility that negative trials are not being reported. Overall, however, no improvement in survival or tumor response has been shown in patients undergoing chemotherapy and receiving TPN compared with control subjects [11]. Likewise, no survival advantage and no improvement in tolerance to radiotherapy have been seen in patients undergoing radiotherapy who were randomized to receive TPN. The incidence of infectious complications seen in patients undergoing chemotherapy and receiving TPN is increased compared with controls, probably secondary to line sepsis. [Editor's Note: The increase in sepsis is probably not due to line sepsis, but other infections such as pneumonia. A number of recent studies reported an increased incidence of non–TPN-related infections, and include the Veterans Administration perioperative trial, several trials of patients with pancreatitis, and one on patients with trauma. This increased incidence is not due to hyperglycemia, but may be related to overfeeding.] It can be concluded that TPN should not routinely be used in all patients undergoing chemotherapy or radiation therapy. Individual patients, including those with significant nutritional morbidity undergoing aggressive, effective antineoplastic

Table 21-8. Randomized Trials of Total Parenteral Nutrition (TPN) in Patients Undergoing Chemotherapy

References	Cancer	No. of Patients		% of Planned Dose Given		% with Complete Response		% With Partial Response		WBC Nadir (×10³)		Mortality (%)		Median Survival (wk)	
		TPN	Control	TPN	Control	TPN	Control	TPN	Control	TPN	Control	TPN	Control	TPN	Control
78, 116	Diffuse lymphoma	17	19	88	85	—	—	—	—	2.3	2.0	—	—	—	ND
43	Lung, squamous	13	13	—	—	0	0	31	8	2.5	1.5*	—	—	—	—
54	Lung, non–oat cell	14	13	—	—	0	0	14	23	—	—	—	—	11	12
109	Lung, small cell	21	28	—	—	85	59	15	41	0	0	24	32	—	ND
88	Lung, small cell	10	9	—	—	83	80	—	—	0.6	0.8	—	—	—	—
73	Colon, metastatic	20	25	—	—	—	—	—	—	—	—	—	—	11	44
85	Testis, stage III	16	14	—	—	63	79	25	14	0.9	0.9	—	4	60	60
111	Adeno-carcinoma, lung	19	24	—	—	0	11	15	28	1.7	1.5	11	4	22	40
90	Metastatic	14	18	—	—	—	—	—	—	ND		0	27	—	—

ND = no difference at time of most recent report; WBC = white blood cell count.
*p < 0.05 versus TPN group.
Adapted from Shike, M., and Brennan, M. F. Nutritional support. In V. T. DeVita, S. Hellman, and S. Rosenberg (eds.), *Principles and Practice of Oncology* (3rd ed.). Philadelphia: J. B. Lippincott, 1989.

Table 21-9.   Randomized Trials of Total Parenteral Nutrition (TPN) in Patients Undergoing Radiation Therapy

References	Cancer	No. of Patients		% of Planned Dose Given		Median Mortality (%)		Survival (wk)	
		TPN	Control	TPN	Control	TPN	Control	TPN	Control
101	Ovarian carcinoma	42	39	—	—	—	—	39	36
110	Pelvic carcinoma	11	9	92	101	45	33	—	—
32	Pediatric ab-domon or pelvic	11	14	100	100	0	0	—	—
51	Pelvic								
	Curative	8	10	100	90	6	20	—	—
	Palliative	9	5	55	60	66	60	—	—

Adapted from Shike, M., and Brennan, M. F. Nutritional support. In V. T. DeVita, S. Hellman, and S. Rosenberg (eds.), *Principles and Practice of Oncology* (3rd ed.). Philadelphia: J. B. Lippincott, 1989.

Table 21-10.   Randomized Trials of Total Parenteral Nutrition (TPN) in Cancer Patients Undergoing Major Surgery

References	TPN in Relation to Surgery for	No. of Patients		Major Postoperative Complication		Postoperative Wound Infection		Postoperative Mortality (%)	
		TPN	Control	TPN	Control	TPN	Control	TPN	Control
	Gastrointestinal cancer								
40, 41	Pre- and post-operative	30	26	13	19	—	—	7	8
104	Variable	12	9	17	11	17	22	0	0
69	Pre- and post-operative	66	59	16	32*	21	25	5	19*
	Esophageal cancer								
67	Preoperative	10	5	—	—	0	20	—	—
27	Perioperative	10	10	40	10	30	50	10	20
	Esophageal/gastric cancer								
99	Pre- and post-operative	10	10	—	—	—	—	0	10
36	Preoperative	38	36	—	—	8	31*	16	22
70	Pre- and post-operative	58	55	8	17*	6	9	4	11

*$p = 0.05$ versus TPN group.
Adapted from Shike, M., and Brennan, M. F. Nutritional support. In V. DeVita, S. Hellman, and S. Rosenberg (eds.), *Principles and Practice of Oncology* (3rd ed.). Philadelphia: J. B. Lippincott, 1989.

therapy, may benefit but this has not been proved.

Surgical trials are difficult to interpret since patients are often not stratified to separate upper from lower gastrointestinal cancers. Underlying malnutrition, as well as operative morbidity and mortality, is clearly different in these two groups. Many studies excluded from randomization patients who were severely malnourished, when these patients were most likely to demonstrate a benefit. Likewise, the inclusion of well-nourished patients makes it difficult to prove a beneficial effect of TPN. Askanazi et al. [2] showed a significantly decreased length of stay in cystectomy patients receiving postoperative TPN. The period of preoperative nutrition also varied in these studies. In 10 surgical trials analyzed by Klein et al. [52], only one showed a statistically significant decrease in mortality in the TPN-treated group, although an additional five trials reported a nonsignificant decrease. A pooled analysis showed postoperative mortality in the TPN-treated group to be half that of control subjects. The pooled analysis of complications including eight other trials indicated a statistically significant decrease in major surgical complications in the TPN-treated group, with the odds of developing a major complication ($p = 0.01$) or a wound infection ($p = 0.05$) half that of the controls. Overall, there appears to be a benefit in providing perioperative TPN to patients with upper gastrointestinal cancers, as mortality, major complications, and wound infections decreased in some studies.

Methods of Nutritional Support

Nutritional support is indicated in the cancer patient who is malnourished or who may become malnourished during the course of proposed treatment. It may consist of dietary supplements, enteral tube feedings, or TPN. The choice is dependent on the ability of the patient to ingest and digest sufficient nutrients.

Dietary therapy is indicated if the patient can ingest the necessary number of calories by mouth. Example of special dietary regimens include postgastrectomy diets, low-fat diets for pancreatic insufficiency, low-fiber diets for radiation enteritis, and simple dietary supplements.

Enteral Nutrition
The advantages of enteral nutrition over TPN are well known and include lower cost, fewer infectious complications, and greater ease of delivery, especially for the outpatient. Enteral nutrition given via nasogastric or gastrostomy tubes is indicated if the patient has a functioning gastrointestinal tract, but is unable to ingest an adequate amount of calories. Silastic small-caliber nasogastric tubes, made specifically as feeding tubes, are preferred over Levin tubes. Their position in the distal antrum or duodenum must be ascertained, before feeding begins, to prevent aspiration from a coiled tube. For long-term feeding, a gastrostomy or jejunostomy tube, placed endoscopically or surgically, should be considered. These are considerably more comfortable for the patient, cosmetically preferred, less likely to clog, and rarely dislodge. Our recent experience [5a] with endoscopically placed gastrostomies revealed an acceptably low morbidity rate of 8.3%, making them our first choice. They can be performed on an outpatient basis and a button may be placed at the gastrostomy site, making it more comfortable and aesthetically appealing to the patient. Our limited experience with percutaneously placed jejunostomies, particularly suitable for the postgastrectomy patient, has shown the same complication rate as for percutaneous gastrostomy [96].

The availability of commercial formulas of low-osmolarity, low-fat, low-fiber, and particularly hydrolyzed enteral feeding formulas allows the clinician to choose the solution best suited to the patient. They are convenient for the outpatient, or the patient's own food may be mixed in a blender for use through the feeding tube. Commercially available enteral feeding solutions vary in their osmolarity, fat, carbohydrate, and protein ratios and in fiber content and digestion requirements. The appropriate choice should minimize diarrhea and hyperglycemia, common complications of enteral feeding.

Total Parenteral Nutrition

TPN may be indicated in the cancer patient for a variety of reasons. The presence of one or more of the gastrointestinal effects of the tumor or its treatment (see Table 21-5) may preclude adequate ingestion or digestion of nutrients, necessitating the use of TPN.

TPN is administered in the cancer patient using the same guidelines for other malnourished patients. Venous access is achieved by infraclavicular percutaneous placement of a catheter into the subclavian vein, for short-term therapy. As these patients are often receiving simultaneous chemotherapy and multiple blood products, the use of a double-lumen catheter is preferred. When placed percutaneously, these catheters have been associated with a high infection rate [62]. For more chronic therapy, a cuffed Silastic catheter, threaded into a central vein and tunneled subcutaneously on the chest wall, is used. Our preferred route, especially in the thrombocytopenic patient, is to place a Silastic catheter via a cutdown into the external jugular vein and thread the catheter centrally. X-ray confirmation of placement is essential to ensure the position of the catheter tip in the superior vena cava or right atrium and not in the internal mammary or jugular veins. Misplacement can result in thrombosis or malfunction of the catheter.

With guidelines similar to those used for other malnourished patients, TPN solutions may be used to provide calories and nutrients based on the individual patient's needs. Underlying malnutrition, specific nutrient deficits, and ongoing electrolyte and mineral losses are taken into consideration. Although special formulas have been developed for the patient with renal, hepatic, and pulmonary failure, no specific formula is used for the cancer patient [102].

The cancer patient receiving TPN initially requires close monitoring of serum chemistries, especially glucose and electrolyte levels. The development of renal or liver dysfunction, often a consequence of chemotherapy, may require adjustments in the TPN formula. Ongoing losses due to diarrhea, vomiting, and excessive urinary losses must be monitored and replaced. Specific details as to ingredients, content, volumes, and additives used in TPN are found in Chapter 5.

Effect of Nutritional Support on Tumor Growth

Because of the lack of clear uniform benefit in providing TPN to the patient with malignancy, the question of stimulation of tumor growth by TPN becomes more important [105]. Since it has been difficult to show these effects in humans, it is necessary to examine findings in animal models that have been used to study the relationship between substrate availability and tumor growth.

Although no specific difference in tumor growth could be demonstrated between rats fed standard chow and rats receiving only water 3 weeks following sarcoma implantation, starvation caused a decrease in host body and carcass weight and liver DNA activity. During starvation the tumor volume increased, while carcass weight decreased [59]. Decreased tumor growth during starvation has been shown by other investigators [23].

The effect of nutritional supplementation with TPN is clearer. Studying cachectic sarcoma-bearing rats, Kokal et al. [53] observed an increased body weight gain in rats receiving TPN, accounted for by the increased weight of the tumor. Compared to rats in which the sarcoma was resected, the tumor-bearing rats had decreased carcass protein stores and increased fat stores, indicating an impaired ability to utilize the nutrients. Popp et al. [77, 80] showed that after intravenous nutritional support, there was a direct correlation of tumor size with the amount of calories given to a group of tumor-bearing rats. With an increase in substrate infusion, increasing ratios of fat and protein accumulation were noted in the host. However, tumor growth increased to a greater extent than host lean mass with increasing caloric supplementation. Varying the rates of nitrogen infusion, Popp et al. [81] demonstrated that tumor weights increased with infused nitrogen rates. Carcass mass was maintained with TPN, without a corresponding increase in tumor growth rates, in sarcoma-bearing rats studied by Goodgame et al. although liver fat did increase [33]. Differences in tumor-bearing rats given nutritionally equivalent enteral or parenteral nutrition include similar water and protein but greater fat gain in the TPN-treated groups [79].

Because of the apparent stimulatory effects of TPN, attempts at manipulation of the diet have been made. The observation that tumors utilized glucose preferentially led to the study of diabetic rats with tumors. The early growth phase of implanted tumors is delayed in streptozocin-induced diabetic rats, as well as pair-fed control animals. The presence of insulin in the starved matched control rats was not sufficient to support tumor growth due to lack of adequate substrate. In fact, the hyperglycemic state seen in the diabetic rats had antitumor effects, perhaps due to hypoinsulinemia [113]. Hypoglycemia, induced by 3-mercaptopicolinic acid with glycerol infusion to protect brain and kidneys, was used in animals and as a phase I study in humans, with no conclusive results [17].

In another attempt to manipulate nutritional sources available to the tumor, a lipid-based TPN solution, supplying 67% of nonprotein calories as fat, was compared to an isocaloric carbohydrate-based solution supplying 5% as fat. While tumor weight was no different in these two groups, the fat-fed group accumulated more organ, tumor, and body fat [31]. Chance et al. [19] recently elicited significant increases in carcass weight and muscle savings without change in tumor growth, using the combination of TPN and insulin in the sarcoma-bearing rat. In an attempt to selectively improve host nutrient utilization while limiting tumor growth, the antimetabolite acivicin was combined with insulin and TPN. This combination stopped tumor growth, increased carcass weight, and preserved muscle mass.

Since TPN has been shown to stimulate tumor growth, several investigators attempted to exploit this response through the administration of cycle-specific chemotherapy. After a short pulse (2 hours) of TPN in tumor-bearing rats, the percentage of tumor cells in the S-phase was significantly increased. This increased the ratio of sensitive to resistant tumor cells to S-phase–specific chemotherapy [108]. Similarly, an enhanced tumoricidal effect was seen in tumor-bearing rats receiving a 48-hour course of TPN before cell cycle-specific chemotherapy with methotrexate. Final tumor volume in the TPN group was one-third that of groups fed in ad libitum diet or a protein-depleted diet preceding the methotrexate therapy. In addition, rats receiving TPN had significantly less chemotherapy-associated morbidity, compared with the protein-depleted group [107]. Similar benefits were seen with doxorubicin hydrochloride (Adriamycin) (cycle-specific) but not cyclophosphamide (Cytoxan) (non–cycle-specific) [113].

In one of the only human studies demonstrating an effect of TPN on tumor growth, Baron et al. performed flow cytometry of biopsy specimens of head and neck cancers [4]. The percentage of hyperdiploid cells increased in all eight patients after receiving TPN and in no patient not receiving TPN. No change in this ratio was seen in normal mucosa in either group. The increase in percentage of hyperdiploid cells was seen even after a short (3-day) course of TPN. While no subsequent effect on tumor growth or survival has been reported, the authors recommend that biopsy with flow cytometry during a course of TPN may be used to determine optimal time of onset for initiation of cycle-specific chemotherapy.

As yet, there are no conclusive data to answer the question of human tumor growth stimulation by TPN. Maintenance of host functional mass is seen and may account for any benefit seen clinically. TPN in humans has never been shown to promote tumor growth. Animal studies demonstrating the role of nutritional support in increased tumor size should be extrapolated to humans with caution, as these tumors often account for a large portion of the host mass and are close to killing the host. On the other hand, in advanced human cancers with no further effective therapy available, the risk-benefit ratio of TPN is minimal.

SUMMARY

Malnutrition is common in the cancer patient, but varies with disease site and stage. Studies of body composition reveal a significant loss of body fat and skeletal protein in the malnourished cancer patient. While sophisticated methods are used in the research setting to document specific deficits, standard history and physical examination identify the patients at risk for nutritional morbidity. The etiology of cancer cachexia includes impaired intake and absorption of nutrients; increased losses and requirements; and defects in carbohydrate, protein, and fat metabolism. Antitumor therapy often contributes to these factors.

TPN, given to malnourished cancer patients, can reverse negative nitrogen balance, produce weight gain, decrease protein catabolism, increase fat synthesis and storage, and restore certain immunologic parameters toward normal. However, no improvement in survival, tumor response, or tolerance to therapy has been shown in cancer patients receiving TPN while undergoing chemotherapy or radiation therapy. Increased infection rates have been associated with the administration of TPN in chemotherapy patients. Its use in malnourished surgical patients has been shown to decrease postoperative morbidity and mortality in selected studies.

TPN stimulates tumor growth in many animal models, but no evidence for this exists in humans. [Editor's Note: The caution expressed by the authors is appropriate. Decreased recurrence-free remission [89] and perhaps decreased survival rate in patients with widespread colon carcinoma [73] have raised the question in humans.] Areas for further study include the definition of subgroups of patients who may benefit from nutritional support during cancer therapy. Specific nutrient requirements and the optimal period of pre- and postoperative TPN have not been identified. Selective starvation of the tumor with maintenance of host mass is an area of active interest in animal models. Manipulation of tumor cell division to enhance cell kill by cycle-specific chemotherapy has been successful in animals but has not been proved in humans.

REFERENCES

1. Arbeit, J. M., Burt, M. E., Rubinstein, L. V., Gorschboth, C. M., and Brennan, M. F. Glucose metabolism and the percentage of glucose derived from alanine: Response to exogenous glucose infusion in tumor-bearing and non tumor-bearing rats. Cancer Res. 42:4936, 1982.
2. Askanazi, J., Hensle, T. W., Starker, P., et al. Effect of immediate postoperative nutritional support on length of hospitalization. Ann. Surg. 203:236, 1986.
3. Baker, J. P., Detsky, A. S., and Wesson, D. E. Nutritional assessment: A comparison of clinical judgement and objective measurements. N. Engl. J. Med. 306:969, 1982.
4. Baron, P. L., Lawrence, W., Chan, W. M. Y., White, F. K. H., and Banks, W. L. Effects of parenteral nutrition on cell cycle kinetics of head and neck cancer. Arch. Surg. 121:1282, 1986.
5. Bast, R. C. Effects of cancers and their treatment on host immunity. In J. P. Holland and E. Frei (eds.), Cancer Medicine. Philadelphia: Lea and Febiger, 1982.
5a. Berner, Y., Schroy, P., Herrman-Zaidans, M., et al. Long term enteral feeding with percutaneous endoscopic gastrostomy (PEG) in cancer patients (abstr.) J. Parenter. Enter. Nutr. 12(suppl.), 1988.
6. Beutler, B., and Cerami, A. Cachectin and tumor necrosis factor as two sides of the same biological coin. Nature 320:584, 1986.
7. Bistrian, B. R. Some practical and theoretic concepts in the nutritional assessment of the cancer patient. Cancer 58(Suppl.):1863, 1986.
8. Bistrian, B. R., Blackburn, G. L., Vitale, J., Cochran, D., and Naylor, J. Prevalence of malnutrition in general medical patients. J.A.M.A. 235:1567, 1976.
9. Bozzetti, F., Ammatuna, M., Migliavacca, S., et al. Total parenteral nutrition prevents further nutritional deterioration in patients with cancer cachexia. Ann. Surg. 205:138, 1987.
10. Bozzetti, F., Migliavacca, S., Scotti, A., et al. Impact of cancer type, site, stage and treatment on the nutritional status of patients. Ann. Surg. 196:170, 1982.
11. Brennan, M. F. Total parenteral nutrition in the cancer patient. N. Engl. J. Med. 305:375, 1981.

12. Brennan, M. F. Malnutrition in patients with gastrointestinal malignancy: Significance and management. *Dig. Dis. Sci.* 31(Suppl.):77S, 1986.

13. Brennan, M. F., and Elkman, L. Metabolic consequences of nutritional support of the cancer patient. *Cancer* 54:2627, 1984.

14. Burke, M., Bryson, E. I., and Kark, A. E. Dietary intakes, resting metabolic rates, and body composition in benign and malignant gastrointestinal disease. *Br. Med. J.* 280:211, 1980.

15. Burt, M. E., Aoki, T. T., Gorschboth, C. M., and Brennan, M. F. Peripheral tissue metabolism in cancer-bearing man. *Ann. Surg.* 198:685, 1983.

16. Burt, M. E., Gorschboth, C. M., and Brennan, M. F. A controlled prospective randomized trial evaluating the metabolic effects of enteral and parenteral nutrition in the cancer patient. *Cancer* 49:1092, 1982.

17. Burt, M. E., Peters, M. L., Brennan, M. F., Sato, S., Cornblath, M., and Adams, A. Hypoglycemia with glycerol infusions as antineoplastic therapy: A hypothesis. *Surgery* 97:231, 1985.

18. Burt, M. E., Stein, T. P., and Brennan, M. F. A controlled randomized trial evaluating the effects of enteral and parenteral nutrition on protein metabolism in cancer-bearing man. *J. Surg. Res.* 34:303, 1983.

19. Chance, W. T., Cao, L., and Fischer, J. E. Insulin and acivicin improve host nutrition and prevent tumor growth during total parenteral nutrition. *Ann. Surg.* 208:524, 1988.

20. Cohn, S. H., Ellis, K. J., Vartsky, D., et al. Comparisons of methods of estimating body fat in normal subjects and cancer patients. *Am. J. Clin. Nutr.* 34:2839, 1981.

21. Cohn, S. H., Gartenhaus, W., Sawitsky, A., et al. Compartmental body composition of cancer patients by measurement of total body nitrogen, potassium, and water. *Metabolism* 30:222, 1981.

22. Cohn, S. H., Gartenhaus, W., Vartsky, D., et al. Body composition and dietary intake in neoplastic disease. *Am. J. Clin. Nutr.* 34:1997, 1981.

23. Daly, J. M., Copeland, E. M., Dudrick, S. J., and Delaney, J. M. Nutritional repletion of malnourished tumor-bearing and non tumor-bearing rats: Effects on body weight, liver, muscle and tumor. *J. Surg. Res.* 28:507, 1980.

24. DeWys, W. D. Anorexia as a general effect of cancer. *Cancer* 43:2013, 1979.

25. DeWys, W. D., Begg, C., Lavin, P. T., et al., and Eastern Cooperative Oncology Group. Prognostic effect of weight loss prior to chemotherapy in cancer patients. *Am. J. Med.* 69:491, 1980.

26. Donaldson, S. S., and Lenon, R. A. Alterations of nutritional status: Impact of chemotherapy and radiation therapy. *Cancer* 43:2036, 1979.

27. Donaldson, S. S., Wesley, M. N., Ghavimi, F., Shils, M. E., Suskind, R. M., and DeWys, W. D. A prospective randomized clinical trial of total parenteral nutrition in children with cancer. *Med. Pediatr. Oncol.* 10:129, 1982.

28. Dresler, C. M., Jeevanandam, M., and Brennan, M. F. Metabolic effect of enteral feeding in malnourished cancer and noncancer patients. *Metabolism* 36:32, 1987.

29. Eilber, F. R., and Morton, D. L. Impaired immunologic reactivity and recurrence following cancer surgery. *Cancer* 25:362, 1970.

30. Enig, B., Winther, E., and Hessor, I. Energy and protein intake and nutritional status in non-surgically treated patients with small cell anaplastic carcinoma of the lung. *Acta Radiol. Oncol.* 25:19, 1986.

31. Enrione, E. B., Black, C. D., and Morre, D. M. Response of tumor-bearing rats to high-fat total parenteral nutrition. *Cancer* 56:2612, 1985.

32. Ghavimi, F., Shils, M. E., Scott, B. F., Brown, M., and Tamaroff, M. Comparison of morbidity in children requiring abdominal radiation and chemotherapy, with and without total parenteral nutrition. *J. Pediatr.* 101:530, 1982.

33. Goodgame, J. T., Lowry, S. F., and Brennan, M. F. Nutritional manipulations and tumor growth. II. The effects of intravenous feedings. *Am. J. Clin. Nutr.* 32:2285, 1979.

34. Goodgame, J. T., Pizzo, P., and Brennan, M. F. Iatrogenic lactic acidosis association with hypertonic glucose administration in patients with cancer. *Cancer* 42:800, 1978.

35. Haffejee, A. A., and Angorn, L. B. Nutritional status and the nonspecific cellular and humoral immune response in esophageal carcinoma. *Ann. Surg.* 189:475, 1979.

36. Heatley, R. V., Williams, R. H. P., and Lewis, M. H. Preoperative intravenous feeding: Controlled trial. *Postgrad. Med. J.* 55:541, 1979.

37. Heber, D., Chlebowski, R. T., Ishibashi, D. E., Herrold, J. N., and Block, J. B. Abnormalities in glucose and protein metabolism in noncachectic lung cancer patients. *Cancer Res.* 42:4815, 1982.

38. Heymsfield, S. B., Olafson, R. P., Kutner, M. H., and Nixon, D. W. A radiographic method of quantifying protein-calorie undernutrition. *Am. J. Clin. Nutr.* 32:693, 1979.

39. Hill, G. L., McCarthy, I. D., Collins, J. P., and Smith, A. H. A new method for the rapid measurement of body composition in critically ill surgical patients. *Br. J. Surg.* 65:732, 1978.

40. Holter, A. R., and Fischer, J. E. The effects of perioperative hyperalimentation on complications in patients with carcinoma and weight loss. *J. Surg. Res.* 23:31, 1977.

41. Holter, A. R., Rosen, H. M., and Fischer, J. E. The effects of hyperalimentation on major surgery in patients with malignant disease: A prospective study. *Acta Chir. Scand. (Suppl.)* 466:86, 1976.

42. Inculet, R. I., Norton, J. A., Nicholalds, G. E., Maher, M. M., White, D. E., and Brennan, M. F. Water-soluble vitamins in cancer patients on parenteral nutrition: A prospective study. *J. Parenter. Enter. Nutr.* 11:243, 1987.

43. Issell, B. F., Valdivieso, M., Zaren, H. A., et al. Protection against chemotherapy toxicity by IV hyperalimentation. *Cancer Treat. Rep.* 59:437, 1978.

44. Jeevanandam, M., Legaspi, A., Lowry, S. F., Horowitz, G. D., and Brennan, M. F. Effect of total parenteral nutrition on whole body protein kinetics in cachectic patients with benign or malignant disease. *J. Parenter. Enter. Nutr.* 12:229, 1988.

45. Jeevanandam, M., Lowry, S. F., and Brennan, M. F. Protein synthesis efficiency and the route of nutrient administration in man. *Clin. Nutr.* 6:233, 1987.

46. Jeevanandam, M., Lowry, S. F., and Brennan, M. F. Effect of the route of nutrient administration on whole body protein kinetics in man. *Metabolism* 36:968, 1987.

47. Jeevanandam, M., Lowry, S. F., Horowitz, G. D., and Brennan, M. F. Cancer cachexia and protein metabolism. *Lancet* 1:1423, 1984.

48. Jordan, W. M., Valdeviesco, M., Frankmann, C., et al. Treatment of advanced adenocarcinoma of the lung with ftorafur, doxorubicin, cyclophosphamide, and cisplatin (FACP) and intensive IV hyperalimentation. *Cancer Treat. Rep.* 65:197, 1981.

49. Kaminski, M. (ed.), *Nutritional Assessment in Hyperalimentation: A Guide for Clinicians.* New York: Marcel Dekker, 1985.

50. Kemeny, N., Daly, J., Oderman, P., et al. Hepatic artery pump infusion: Toxicity and results in patients with metastatic colorectal carcinoma. *J. Clin. Oncol.* 2:595, 1984.

51. Kinsella, T. J., Malcolm, A. W., Bothe, A., Valerio, D., and Blackburn, G. L. Prospective study of nutritional support during pelvic irradiation. *Int. J. Radiat. Oncol. Biol. Phys.* 7:543, 1981.

52. Klein, S., Simes, J., and Blackburn, G. L. Total parenteral nutrition and cancer: Clinical trials. *Cancer* 58:1378, 1986.

53. Kokal, W. A., Chan, W., Banks, W. L., and Lawrence, W. The efficacy of total parenteral nutrition in malnourished tumor bearing rats. *Cancer* 55:271, 1985.

54. Lanzotti, V., Copeland, E. M., Bhuchar, V., Wesley, M., Corriere, J., and Dudrick, S. A randomized trial of total parenteral nutrition (TPN) with chemotherapy for non-oat cell lung cancer (NOCLC). (Abstract) *Proc. Am. Assoc. Cancer Res. Am. Soc. Clin. Oncol.* 21: 377, 1980.

55. Lawrence, W. Effects of cancer on malnutrition: Impaired organ system effects. *Cancer* 43:2020, 1979.

56. Legaspi, A., Jeevanandam, M., Starnes, H. F., and Brennan, M. F. Whole body lipid and energy metabolism in the cancer patient. *Metabolism* 36:958, 1987.

57. Levinson, M. R., Groeger, J. S., Jeevanandam, M., and Brennan, M. F. Free fatty acid turnover and lipolysis in septic mechanically ventilated cancer-bearing humans. *Metabolism* 37:618, 1988.

58. Lindmark, L., Bennegard, K., Eden, E., Svaninger, G., Ternell, M., and Lundholm, K. Thermic effect and substrate oxidation in response to intravenous nutrition in cancer patients who lose weight. *Ann. Surg.* 204:628, 1986.

59. Lowry, S. F., Goodgame, J. T., Norton, J. A., Jones, D. C., and Brennan, M. F. Effect of chronic protein malnutrition on host-tumor composition and growth. *J. Surg. Res.* 26:79, 1979.

60. Lukaski, H. C., Bolonchuk, W. W., Hall, C. B., and Siders, W. A. Validation of tetrapolar bioelectrical impedance method to assess human body composition. *J. Appl. Physiol.* 60:1327, 1986.

61. Lundholm, K. G. Body composition changes in cancer patients. *Surg. Clin. North Am.* 66: 1013, 1986.

62. McCarthy, M. C., Shives, J. K., Robison, R. J., and Broadie, T. A. Prospective evaluation of single and triple lumen catheters in total parenteral nutrition. *J. Parenter. Enter. Nutr.* 11:259, 1987.

63. McCauley, R. L., and Brennan, M. F. Serum albumin levels in cancer patients receiving total parenteral nutrition. *Ann. Surg.* 197:305, 1983.

64. McNeill, G., Mernagh, J. R., Jeejeebhoy, K. N., Wolman, S. L., and Harrison, J. E. In vivo measurements of body protein based on the determination of nitrogen by prompt gamma analysis. *Am. J. Clin. Nutr.* 32:1955, 1979.

65. Mitchell, D. G., Burk, D. L., Vinitski, S., and Rifkin, M. D. The biophysical basis of tissue contrast in extracranial MR imaging. *A. J. R.* 149:831, 1987.

66. Mitchell, E. P., and Schein, P. S. Gastrointestinal toxicity of chemotherapeutic agents. *Semin. Oncol.* 9:52, 1982.

67. Moghissi, K., Hornshaw, J., Teasdale, P. R., and Dawes, E. A. Parenteral nutrition in carcinoma of the oesophagus treated by surgery: Nitrogen balance and clinical studies. *Br. J. Surg.* 64:125, 1977.

68. Moore, F. D., Olesen, K. H., McCurrey, J. D., Parker, H. V., Ball, M. R., and Boyden, C. M. *The Body Cell Mass and Its Supporting Environment: Body Composition in Health and Disease.* Philadelphia: W. B. Saunders, 1963.

69. Müller, J. M., Dienst, C., Brenner, U., and Pichlmaier, H. Preoperative parenteral feeding in patients with gastrointestinal carcinoma. *Lancet* 1:68, 1982.

70. Müller, J. M., Keller, H. W., Brenner, U., Walter, M., and Holzmüller, W. Indications and effects of preoperative parenteral nutrition. *World J. Surg.* 10:53, 1988.

71. Nixon, D. W., Heymsfield, S. B., Cohen, A. E., et al. Protein calorie undernutrition in hospitalized cancer patients. *Am. J. Med.* 68:683, 1980.

72. Nixon, D. W., Lawson, D., Kutner, M., et al. Hyperalimentation of the cancer patient with protein-calorie undernutrition. *Cancer Res.* 41:2038, 1981.

73. Nixon, D. W., Moffitt, S., Lawson, D. H., et al. Total parenteral nutrition as an adjunct to chemotherapy of metastatic colorectal cancer. *Cancer Treat. Rep.* 65(Suppl. 5):137, 1981.

74. Norton, J. A., Maher, M., Wesley, R., White, D., and Brennan, M. F. Glucose intolerance in sarcoma patients. *Cancer* 54:3022, 1984.

75. Oberlander, J., Crosby, L. O., Giandomenico, A., Stein, T., Mikuta, J., and Mullen, J. Total body water and whole body impedance. (Abstract) *Clin. Res.* 28:621A, 1980.

76. Pinsky, C. M., Diomieri, E. L., and Caronas, A. Delayed hypersensitivity reactions in patients with cancer. *Rec. Res. Cancer Res.* 47:37, 1974.

77. Popp, M. B., Brennan, M. F., and Morrison, S. D. Resting and activity energy expenditure during total parenteral nutrition in rats with methylcholanthrene-induced sarcoma. *Cancer* 49:1212, 1982.

78. Popp, M. B., Fisher, R. I., Wesley, R., Aamodt, R., and Brennan, M. F. A prospective randomized study of adjuvant parenteral nutrition in the treatment of advanced diffuse lymphoma: Influence on survival. *Surgery* 90:195, 1981.

79. Popp, M. B., and Wagner, S. C. Nearly identical oral and intravenous nutritional support in the rat: Effects on growth and body composition. *Am. J. Clin. Nutr.* 40:107, 1984.

80. Popp, M. B., Wagner, S. C., and Brito, O. J. Host and tumor responses to increasing levels of intravenous nutritional support. *Surgery* 94:300, 1983.

81. Popp, M. B., Wagner, S. C., Enrione, E. B., and Brito, O. J. Host and tumor responses to varying rates of nitrogen infusion in the tumor-bearing rat. *Ann. Surg.* 207:80, 1988.

82. Rombeau, J. L., Goldman, S. L., Apelgren, K. N., Sanford, I., and Frey, C. F. Protein-calorie malnutrition in patients with colorectal cancer. *Dis. Colon Rectum* 21:587, 1978.

83. Roth, J. A., Golub, S. H., Grimm, E. A., Eilber, F. R., and Morton, D. L. Effects of operation on immune response in cancer patients: Sequential evaluation of in vitro lymphocyte function. *Surgery* 79:46, 1976.

84. Russell, D. M., Shike, M., Marliss, E. B., et al. Effects of total parenteral nutrition and chemotherapy on the metabolic derangements in small cell lung cancer. *Cancer Res.* 44:1706, 1984.

85. Samuels, M. L., Selig, D. E., Ogden, S., Grant, C., and Brown, B. IV hyperalimentation and chemotherapy for stage III testicular cancer: A randomized study. *Cancer Treat. Rep.* 65:615, 1981.

86. Sauerwein, H. P., Pesola, G., Groeger, J. S., Jeevanandam, M., and Brennan, M. F. Relationship between glucose oxidation and FFA concentration in septic cancer-bearing patients. *Metabolism* 37:1045, 1988.

87. Segal, K. R., Gutin, B., Presta, E., Wang, J., and Van Itallie, T. B. Estimation of human body composition by electrical impedance methods: A comparative study. *J. Appl. Physiol.* 58:1565, 1985.

88. Serrou, B., Cupissol, D., Plagne, R., Boutin, P., Carcassone, Y., and Michel, F. B. Parenteral intravenous nutrition (PIVN) as an adjunct to chemotherapy in small cell anaplastic lung carcinoma. *Cancer Treat. Rep.* 65(Suppl. 5):151, 1981.

89. Shamberger, R. C., Brennan, M. F., Goodgame, J. T., et al. A prospective, randomized study of adjuvant parenteral nutrition in the treatment of sarcomas: Results of metabolic and survival studies. *Surgery* 96:1, 1984.

90. Shamberger, R. C., Pizzo, P. A., Goodgame, J. T., et al. The effect of total parenteral nutrition on chemotherapy-induced myelosuppression: A randomized study. *Am. J. Med.* 74:40, 1983.

91. Shaw, J. H. F., and Wolfe, R. R. Glucose and urea kinetics in patients with early and advanced gastrointestinal cancer: The response to glucose infusion, parenteral feeding and surgical resection. *Surgery* 101:181, 1987.

92. Shaw, J. H. F., and Wolfe, R. R. Fatty acid and glycerol kinetics in septic patients and in patients with gastrointestinal cancer: The response to glucose infusion and parenteral feeding. *Ann. Surg.* 205:368, 1987.

93. Shaw, J. H. F., and Wolfe, R. R. Whole body

protein kinetics in patients with early and advanced gastrointestinal cancer: The response to glucose infusion and total parenteral nutrition. *Surgery* 103:148, 1988.

94. Shike, M., and Brennan, M. F. Nutritional support. In V. T. DeVita, S. Hellman, and S. Rosenberg (eds.), *Principles and Practice of Oncology*, (3rd ed.). Philadelphia: J. B. Lippincott, 1989.

95. Shike, M., Russell, D. M., Detsky, A. S., et al. Changes in body composition in patients with small cell lung cancer: The effect of total parenteral nutrition as an adjunct to chemotherapy. *Ann. Intern. Med.* 101:303, 1984.

96. Shike, M., Schroy, P., Morse, R., and Ritchie, M. Percutaneous endoscopic jejunostomy in cancer patients with previous gastric resection. *Gastrointest. Endosc.* 33:372, 1987.

97. Shils, M. E., and Coiso, D. Report to the Medical Board on Nutritional Assessment of Hospitalized Adult Patients in Memorial Hospital. Memorial Sloan-Kettering Cancer Center, New York, 1979.

98. Shizgal, H. M. Total body potassium and nutritional status. *Surg. Clin. North Am.* 56:1185, 1976.

99. Simms, J. M., Oliver, E., and Smith, J. A. R. A study of total parenteral nutrition (TPN) in major gastric and esophageal resection for neoplasia. *J. Parenter. Enter. Nutr.* 4:422, 1980.

100. Sloan, G. M., Maher, M., and Brennan, M. F. Nutritional effects of surgery, radiation therapy, and adjuvant chemotherapy for soft tissue sarcomas. *Am. J. Clin. Nutr.* 34:1094, 1981.

101. Solassol, C., Joyeux, H., and DuBois, J. B. Total parenteral nutrition (TPN) with complete nutritive mixtures: An artificial gut in cancer patients. *Nutr. Cancer* 1(3):13, 1979.

102. Tayek, J. A., Bistrian, B. R., Hehir, D. J., Martin, R., Moldawer, L. L., and Blackburn, G. L. Improved protein kinetics and albumin synthesis by branched chain amino acid-enriched total parenteral nutrition in cancer cachexia: A prospective randomized crossover trial. *Cancer* 58:147, 1986.

103. Tellado-Rodriguez, J. M., Garcia-Sabrido, J. L., Shizgal, H. M., and Christou, N. V. NA$_e$/K$_e$ ratio is a better index of nutritional status than standard anthropometric and biochemical indices. *Surg. Forum* 38:56, 1987.

104. Thompson, B. R., Julian, T. B., and Stremple, J. F. Preoperative total parenteral nutrition in patients with gastrointestinal cancer. *J. Surg. Res.* 30:497, 1981.

105. Torosian, M. H., and Daly, J. M. Nutritional support in the cancer-bearing host: Effects on host and tumor. *Cancer* 58:1915, 1986.

106. Torosian, M. H., Mullen, J. L., Miller, E. E., Wagner, K. M., Stein, T. P., and Buzby, G. P. Adjuvant, pulse total parenteral nutrition and tumor response to cycle-specific and cycle-nonspecific chemotherapy. *Surgery* 94:291, 1983.

107. Torosian, M. H., Mullen, J. L., Stein, T. P., Miller, E. E., Zinsser, K. R., and Buzby, G. P. Enhanced tumor response to cycle-specific chemotherapy by pulse total parenteral nutrition. *J. Surg. Res.* 39:103, 1985.

108. Torosian, M. H., Tsou, K. C., Daly, J. M., et al. Alteration of tumor cell kinetics by pulse total parenteral nutrition: Potential therapeutic implications. *Cancer* 53:1409, 1984.

109. Valdivieso, M., Bodey, G. P., Benjamin, R. S., et al. Role of intravenous hyperalimentation as an adjunct to intensive therapy for small cell bronchogenic carcinoma: Preliminary observations. *Cancer Treat. Rep.* 65 (Suppl. 5):145, 1981.

110. Valerio, D., Overett, L., Malcolm, A., and Blackburn, G. L. Nutritional support for cancer patients receiving abdominal and pelvic radiotherapy: A randomized prospective clinical experiment of intravenous versus oral feeding. *Surg. Forum* 29:145, 1978.

111. Van Eys, J., Copeland, E. M., Cangir, A., et al. A clinical trial of hyperalimentation in children with metastatic malignancies. *Med. Pediatr. Oncol.* 8:63, 1980.

112. Veltri, R. W., Rodman, S. M., Maxim, P. E., Baseler, M. W., and Sprinkle, P. M. Immune complexes, serum proteins, cell mediated immunity and immune regulation in patients with squamous cell carcinoma of the head and neck. *Cancer* 57:2295, 1986.

113. Wagman, L. D., and Brennan, M. F. The effects of streptozocin-induced diabetes and weight-matched pair feeding on tumor growth and survival in Fischer rats. *J. Surg. Res.* 36:354, 1984.

114. Warnold, I., Lundholm, K., and Schersten, T. Energy balance and body composition in cancer patients. *Cancer Res.* 38:1801, 1978.

115. Warren, R. S., Starnes, H. F., Gabrilove, J. L., Oettgen, H. F., and Brennan, M. F. The acute metabolic effects of tumor necrosis factor administration in humans. *Arch. Surg.* 122:1396, 1987.

116. Waterhouse, C., and Kemperman, J. H. Carbohydrate metabolism in subjects with cancer. *Cancer Res.* 31:1273, 1971.

117. Watson, W. S., and Sammon, A. M. Body composition and cachexia resulting from malignant and non-malignant diseases. *Cancer* 46:2041, 1980.

Sepsis

Randall S. Moore
Frank B. Cerra

Sepsis is a common clinical problem that is often associated with the hypermetabolism and multiple-organ failure syndrome. Sepsis and hypermetabolism are unusual causes of death in and of themselves, as most patients survive the initial shock and resuscitation. Rather, the patients who die usually do so from hypermetabolism/multiple-organ failure. Hypermetabolism/multiple-organ failure is a clinical syndrome that can occur with, or follow, a number of different host tissue injuries, including trauma, burns, pancreatitis, and infection. While the initial event may vary, the events that follow are reasonably predictable and appear to be relatively independent of the inciting event. Although our understanding of the pathophysiology of the sepsis syndrome (hypermetabolism/multiple-organ failure in the absence of a demonstrable infectious etiology) has increased significantly over the past few decades, sepsis remains a major source of morbidity and mortality in the modern intensive care unit setting. The presence of patho-

genic organisms and their toxins in the host bloodstream and tissues (hypermetabolism/multiple-organ failure from invasive infection) evokes a variety of metabolic, hormonal, cardiovascular, and immunologic changes in the host. As physicians continue to more clearly define the pathophysiology of these changes, the ability to deliver improved patient care also improves. One such improvement has been the introduction of nutrition/metabolic support. This chapter reviews the pathophysiology and current treatment of hypermetabolism/multiple-organ failure as well as future directions for further research as they relate to nutrition/metabolic support in the sepsis syndrome.

THE CLINICAL SETTING

In 1942, Cuthbertson [22] described the metabolic response to sepsis as a series of ebb and flow states. Sepsis or another metabolic insult is associated with a short ebb period that is characterized by the activation of several systems, including the pituitary-adrenal axis, the autonomic nervous system, and monokine production, with resultant altered metabolism of protein, lipid, and carbohydrate. If adequate resuscitation is delivered, the patient enters a hypermetabolic period that peaks on day 3 and persists for 14 to 21 days. If the patient experiences recurrent inadequate perfusion, persistent areas of devitalized tissue, or uncontrolled infection, there can be a series of ebb and flow states associated with a sequential failure of lung, liver, and kidney over a 21- to 28-day period; this is known as the multiple-organ failure syndrome. The type of hypermetabolism/multiple-organ failure seen in sepsis is usually heralded by the adult respiratory distress syndrome (ARDS), with hepatic, renal, and gut failure occurring at the same time.

In patients, hypermetabolism/multiple-organ failure is heralded by the onset of fever, tachycardia, tachypnea, and an ARDS picture as demonstrated on chest radiograph. Insulin resistance and glucose intolerance occur. Protein catabolism, compared to anabolism, is markedly enhanced, resulting in negative nitrogen balance that can approach 20 to 30 g/day. Altered lipid metabolism is present, but less predictable due to the effect of variable tissue perfusion. A hyperdynamic response occurs with significantly increased cardiac output and low systemic vascular resistance in the 300 to 600 dyne/cm/sec range, associated with a high oxygen consumption and carbon dioxide production with a minute ventilation of 16 to 18 liters/min [13, 14, 74]. The clinical picture of starvation malnutrition occurs very rapidly and can rapidly become a comorbidity and comortality.

It is interesting to note that the traditional signs of perfusion, skin color, urine output, and mentation are proving to be unreliable predictors of the adequacy of perfusion. Rather, subclinical flow-dependent oxygen consumption and lactate release are probably better indicators of dysperfusion. Thus, through invasive cardiopulmonary monitoring, optimal perfusion and oxygen delivery can be realized until oxygen extraction peaks

Table 22-1. Metabolic Characteristics of Sepsis

	Starvation-Adapted	Sepsis
Resting energy expenditure	−	+ +
Gluconeogenesis	+	+ + +
Lipolysis	+ +	+ +
Ketonemia	+ + + +	+
Catabolism	+	+ + +
Anabolism	−	+ +
Lean body mass	−	− − −
Hepatic protein synthesis	+	+ + +
Oxidative fuel sources		
Glucose	+	+ +
Fat	+ + +	+ +
Amino acid	+	+ +

− = reduced; + = increased.

and excess lactate production has ceased. The end result is a decrease in morbidity, mortality, and hypermetabolism/multiple-organ failure [31, 45, 73]. Fink et al. [32] recently demonstrated one aspect of this phenomenon in a porcine study where endotoxin infusion resulted in gut ischemia despite normal cardiac output and mesenteric oxygen consumption. Decreased superior mesenteric artery perfusion and intestinal intraluminal acidosis were noted, suggesting that mesenteric $\dot{V}O_2$ was flow-limited and less than the metabolic requirement of the tissue [88].

In summary, the metabolic response to sepsis produces a hypermetabolic state that can ultimately result in multiple-organ failure and death. Metabolism is markedly different from that seen in classic starvation (Table 22-1). Control of starvation-induced malnutrition and individual nutrient deficiency with current nutritional support can reduce starvation-induced malnutrition as a comorbidity and comortality. The natural history of the sepsis syndrome requires close attention to early resuscitation and optimal metabolic support. Future research will attempt to further elucidate the underlying metabolic pathways, with modulation through specific nutrient effects (nutrient pharmacology), a capability currently in its infancy.

GENERAL NEUROENDOCRINE FEATURES

While much of the early research focused on the metabolic effects of the humoral mediator system, it is becoming increasingly clear that the cellular level should be the focus. The interactions of injury agents and injured tissue with cell recognition systems initiates the cell-mediated communication system. For instance, when the macrophage encounters the stimulus of pathogenic microbial components and toxins, it initiates the release of cytokines and other signals. This release initiates a cell-cell interaction that acts to initiate the paracrine system, which in turn activates systemic humoral mediators. Kelly et al. [47] found that rat hepatic macrophage activation by zymosan led to significant changes in liver weight, microsomal protein, cytochrome P_{450} content, and aniline hydroxylase activity.

Combined with the direct action of microbial toxins and components, the systemic response known as the sepsis syndrome develops. Cell-cell mediators such as the interleukin and leukotriene families, tumor necrosis factor (TNF), and other neuroendocrine factors interact in a complex fashion that remains less than fully elucidated. The circulating level of a given mediator may have little or no correlation with its actual effect at the cellular level.

These interactions can also induce further injury. Interleukin-1 at a site of local injury can be released into the systemic circulation and injure distant endothelium such as the lung endothelium. The close physical proximity of the hepatocyte and Kupffer cell when recreated in cell culture systems continues to demonstrate Kupffer cell modulation of hepatocyte function. Mazuski et al. [57] demonstrated that hepatocytes release factors that can enhance macrophage function and proliferation. Paracrine amplification may be a mechanism of hepatocellular injury.

Interleukins

Activation of the Kupffer cells and other macrophages results in the release of interleukins, TNF, and other cytokines. Interleukin-1 release from the activated macrophage results in a multitude of effects, including fever via resetting the hypothalamic temperature-regulating center; direct activation of other endocrine tissues resulting in increased catecholamines, glucagon, and corticosteroids; increased proteolysis; reprioritization of liver protein synthesis toward acute-phase reactants; and changes in lipid and carbohydrate metabolism. Interleukin-6 appears to be a key factor in initiating the hypermetabolism/multiple-organ failure response, particularly at the level of the CNS. Observed responses include fever, leukocytes, increased gluconeogenesis and proteolysis, and direct stimulation of the adrenal cortex. The mechanism is probably indirect, as recombinant interleukin-1 in cell culture does not elicit all expected responses.

Tumor Necrosis Factor

TNF is a cytokine released by the activated macrophage. It has been shown to be present in two forms: a free circulating entity and a larger membrane-bound form. An intact adrenal cortex is necessary to demonstrate the metabolic effects of endotoxin-stimulated TNF [59, 77]. General effects of TNF include fever, altered perfusion, intravascular coagulation, decreased activity of anticoagulant components in the serum, increased vascular permeability, and lactic acidosis. Starnes et al. [79] showed that the administration of TNF and interferon gamma to patients with disseminated cancer resulted in the initiation of the acute-phase response. Indomethacin blunted the febrile and rigor response, as well as enabled increased levels of TNF and interferon to be infused before higher levels of triglyceride were seen. This study suggested that the lipid substrate mobilization and utilization are augmented by the addition of interferon to TNF, resulting in higher levels than when either agent is administered alone. Significant levels of cortisol and C-reactive protein were found in the presence or absence of indomethacin. Tracey et al. [82] were able to show that by passively immunizing baboons prior to inducing *Escherichia coli* sepsis, many of the metabolic derangements of sepsis could be abrogated. Specifically, immunized animals showed inhibition of hypoglycemia, hypertriglyceridemia, and hyperaminoacidemia, as well as decreased levels of epinephrine, norepinephrine, and glucagon.

Endotoxin (Lipopolysaccharide)

Repeated injections of endotoxin can produce the hypermetabolic response [27]. Endotoxin may result in hepatotoxicity via lipid peroxidation [79]. Endotoxin administration also results in intestinal translocation of bacteria and toxins [25]. Macrophage-mediated microthrombosis can be mediated through an endotoxin-induced decrease in the activity of protein C-S complex [30]. Endotoxin can have many other effects of intermediary metabolism, with many mechanisms remaining to be defined. [*Editor's Note:* Recent work documented the ubiquitous presence of lipopolysaccharide. This suggests that most experimental animals and patients are in a state of chronic low-level activation. Experiments must be repeated using lipopolysaccharide-free reagents to gauge the true effect of lipopolysaccharide.]

Summary

The above discussion has only touched the surface of the altered hormonal milieu that is seen in sepsis. The role of counterregulatory hormones, thyroid hormones, complement, kinins, and so on, in their complex interaction remains to be defined. Summation of all of the changes adds up to the clinical changes that have been noted. Our understanding of the basic metabolic changes that occur as a result of the altered hormonal milieu is far from complete. A summary of the current understanding is presented in the following sections.

BASIC METABOLIC CHANGES

Carbohydrate Metabolism

Alterations in carbohydrate metabolism leading to hyperglycemia are characteristic of sepsis. Kinetic studies have demonstrated that the normal hepatic production of glucose is between 2 to 2.5 mg/kg of body weight/min, rising to values between 4.4 and 5.1 mg/kg/min, as reviewed by Nelson and Long [63]. The increase in production is commonly thought to be a result of an increase in available precursors such as alanine, glycerol, pyruvate, and lactate and the effect of the insulin counterregulatory hormones. The percentage of glucose oxidized appears to remain constant, resulting in an absolute increase in glucose oxidation [56, 71]. Another important aspect that was recently elucidated from studies using glucose labeled with radioactive carbon (^{14}C or ^{13}C) shows that glucose oxidation is decreased rather than increased, as suggested by indirect calorimetry [78]. Combining the results of these studies strengthens the clinical message to limit the carbohydrate calories to no more than 5 mg/kg/min.

This increased gluconeogenesis and glycogenolysis is refractory to exogenous glucose and insulin. Glucagon, insulin, and the glucagon-insulin ratio are all increased. Aerobic glycolysis results with a progressive reduction in the oxidation of glucose as a fraction of the total energy expenditure. Lactate and pyruvate releases from peripheral tissue are increased, as are those for alanine and glutamine. Carbohydrate metabolism is an important aspect of nutritional support of the septic patient because of serving as an obligate source of energy for certain tissue compartments, including the CNS, cells involved in host defense, and wound and granulation tissue. Obligate needs take on added significance because of the limited carbohydrate stores. The increased rate of glucose appearance seems to result primarily from gluconeogenesis at the expense of protein stores.

The role of the so-called "catabolic" or counterregulatory hormones, catecholamines, glucagon, and glucocorticoids, remains controversial. While some investigators used infusions of these hormones to study the altered metabolism of the septic state, others found evidence against their role. Blockade of the effects of these hormones does not appear to alter glucose kinetics in the septic model. Furthermore, using the mild hypermetabolic rat model, Spitzer et al. [75] were able to demonstrate enhanced glucose metabolism despite no significant elevation of glucagon or corticosteroids, and no change with adrenergic blockade.

TNF infusion mimics many of the effects of endotoxin-mediated shock and death, and glucose metabolism has been shown to be altered [81, 83]. Thus, cytokines like TNF may contribute to altered carbohydrate metabolism in the septic patient. However, cytokine changes alone do not account for all the changes of carbohydrate metabolism.

Protein Metabolism

Sepsis results in predictable changes in protein metabolism. Protein metabolism is characterized by a combination of significantly increased catabolism with a smaller increase in total body protein anabolism, with negative nitrogen balance frequently exceeding 20 gm/day, previously described as autocannibalism [17]. Inherent in the concept of autocannibalism is the auto-oxidation of branched-chain amino acids (BCAAs) by skeletal muscle. The loss of the skeletal muscle mass and redistribution of that nitrogen to the visceral compartment and areas of active inflammation and repair are relatively refractory to both regular and BCAA-enriched total parenteral nutrition (TPN). In part, this observation may be secondary to suppressed uptake of skeletal muscle amino acids as well as other potential contributing factors, such as having little effect on the mediators/hormones inducing catabolism, having a primary effect on synthetic rates, and being used as oxidative fuel sources [36–38].

In the absence of exogenous nitrogen support, lean body mass can become significantly depleted in 7 to 10 days. The control of protein metabolism in sepsis remains to be elucidated. The rate of catabolism can only be relatively reduced by an increase in synthetic rate induced by exogenous amino acids. Even in this regard, the dominant synthetic effects appear to be in the viscera, to be primarily hepatic tissue, and to come especially from the modified amino acid solutions. While early studies suggested that interleukin-1 and TNF may be responsible for the proteolysis of the hypermetabolism/multiple-organ failure response, separate studies by Moldawer et al. [60] and Goldberg et al. [34] presented evidence that individual factors and their antibodies have no effect in the in vitro setting. Thus, the precise factor controlling proteolysis remains unidentified. Proteolysis-inducing factor, a breakdown product of interleukin-1, may have a significant contribution toward muscle proteolysis. [Editor's Note: Hasselgren et al. [35] and others have had great difficulty in repeating the studies, described by Clowes et al. [20], in proposing a role for proteolysis-inducing factor.]

Hepatic uptake of amino acids is increased with preferential synthesis of acute-phase reactants instead of albumin and transferrin. Amino acids also appear to be increased in sites of active inflammation, wounds, and mononuclear cells. The increased flux of amino acids contributes to increased ureagenesis, which in turn contributes to prerenal azotemia as glomerular filtration decreases from other causes. The modified amino acids appear to induce less ureagenesis, presumably the result of a stimulation of protein synthesis.

In summary, altered protein metabolism results in lean body mass being redistributed to sites of active protein synthesis for oxidation and for conversion to other substrates such as glucose. More recent studies have added to the understanding of the kinetics related to nitrogen balance in septic patients. Shaw et al. [72] found that the increase in the difference in net protein catabolism was the result of sepsis leading to a 41% increase in whole-body protein catabolism, with a 36%

increase in whole-body protein synthesis, as compared to controls. Although catabolism was refractory to exogenous glucose or TPN, whole-body protein synthesis increased with progressive nutritional support. Prior studies by Long et al. [55] showed similar results. That muscle breakdown is refractory to exogenous protein indicates that proteolysis is a result of signals unresponsive to current nutritional formulas, and/or that the hormonal cytokine milieu is not approachable as yet by solely nutritional means. The clinical message is to increase infusion of exogenous amino acids until the rate of synthesis equals the rate of breakdown, as demonstrated by nitrogen balance being attained. Failure to provide adequate support, or progression of hypermetabolism/multiple-organ failure, results in hepatic protein synthesis failure. The former can be reversed with proper nutritional support, thereby eliminating malnutrition as an independent morbidity and mortality cofactor. In the latter setting, bilirubin rises, other hepatic enzymes remain relatively stable, the redox potential decreases, amino acid extraction decreases, and finally gluconeogenesis fails, with hypoglycemia as a preterminal event [13, 74].

Lipid Metabolism

Spitzer et al. [75] recently provided a concise review of lipid metabolism during sepsis. Lipid metabolism is increased and accounts for the majority of oxidative substrate utilization during the hypermetabolic phase of sepsis. There is a pronounced increase in the mobilization of fatty acids from adipose tissue, with elevated very-low-density-lipoprotein (VLDL) production by the liver and subsequent elevated serum triglyceride levels. VLDL triglycerides are then available for oxidative metabolism by other tissues. Adrenergic stimulation appears at least partially responsible for the increased fatty acid mobilization [91].

Although current research has led to an increased understanding of lipid metabolism, several areas remain uncertain. Lipoprotein lipase activity appears to favor the utilization of triglycerides and fatty acids as a primary fuel substrate by cardiac and skeletal muscle. Ketone bodies, although another potential source of oxidizable fuel, appear quantitatively insignificant. Furthermore, the formation of ketone bodies may be blunted in sepsis [28], trauma [8], and burns [1]. However, an alternative explanation may be rapid clearance of ketone bodies via oxidation. If rapid oxidation does take place, ketone bodies may provide an alternative fuel source, as discussed below.

It has been noted that as sepsis becomes more severe, at least three factors adversely affect the availability of lipid as a fuel source. First, impaired circulation to adipose tissue results in decreased mobilization of free fatty acids from adipose stores. The impairment increases as the degree of circulatory compromise increases, perhaps limited by availability of the carrier, albumin. Second, as the availability of substrate changes, individual tissues may preferentially utilize other fuels such as lactate. Finally, release of cytokines such as TNF and interleukin-1 by macrophages may result in decreased tissue lipoprotein lipase activity and subsequent decreased tissue utilization of free fatty acids and triglycerides [4]. Reduced lipoprotein lipase activity in skeletal muscle and adipose tissue has been documented in hypermetabolism/multiple-organ failure and correlates with the occurrence of spontaneous hypertriglyceridemia characteristic of the latter phases of the syndrome.

Whether there is increased or decreased clearance of triglycerides in the septic host remains controversial. However, most investigators stress the importance of monitoring triglyceride levels because elevated levels probably necessitate clearance by the macrophages. Lipid-laden macrophages appear to have decreased bacterial phagocytic capacity, thereby predisposing the host to further immune dysfunction. Excessive doses of the current omega-6-based lipid formulas have been associated with excess production of immunosuppressive prostaglandins and suppression on in vitro tests of immune functions. Excess administration has also been correlated with hypoxemia. Thus, our current understanding of lipid metabolism in septic patients does not indicate that nutritional support with lipids should be avoided. It does indicate that careful monitoring of triglyceride levels is necessary, with appropriate adjustment of therapy based on serum levels. [*Editor's Note:* I agree. One should add that under normal circumstances, fat is the preferred fuel of viscera. Thus, in sepsis, until we know otherwise, adequate fuel for the viscera in the form of fat should remain a priority.]

While increased lypolysis is the result of beta$_1$-adrenergic–stimulation in trauma, decreased lipolysis has been noted in the septic model. Meterissian et al. [58] concluded that this may account for the increased protein wasting that characterizes the early septic state.

Initial therapy at our institution is to supply 0.5 to 1 g of lipid/kg/day, provided by continuous infusion over 24 hours. The infusion is decreased if the serum level rises 10% over baseline values. Additional studies are needed to further define the proper use of different lipid moieties during nutritional support. Thus, metabolic changes during sepsis appear to enable the body to rely on lipid as a primary fuel source, while continuing to provide glucose for obligate glycolytic tissues.

In summary, many changes take place in lipid metabolism during sepsis. The ultimate balance and the type of fuel remain to be defined. As hypermetabolism/multiple-organ failure progresses, hepatic lipogenesis increases and peripheral triglyceride clearance decreases [13, 74]. Subsequent sections explore why alternative lipid sources not only may add to the possible fuel sources, but also may modulate the underlying metabolic changes.

EFFECT OF MALNUTRITION

Malnutrition, whether preexisting or acquired, adversely affects virtually all organ systems. The loss of mass, function, and reserve can result in a failure to initiate or maintain the necessary response to hypermetabolism/multiple-organ failure. Progressive malnutrition becomes an independent factor in morbidity and mortality. Effective nutritional and metabolic support becomes an important therapy to maximize the chance for resolution of the hypermetabolism/multiple-organ failure and the underlying disease process. Furthermore, nutritional support must be viewed in light of the pharmacologic potential of individual nutrients to alter the inflammatory and immunologic host response in hypermetabolism/multiple-organ failure, as discussed in subsequent sections.

It must be emphasized that the guidelines for nutritional/metabolic support are different from those for classic starvation (Table 22-2). Although measured energy expenditure may be 175 to 200% of the predicted basal energy expenditure, a nonprotein calorie load beyond 30 kcal/kg/day appears to be detrimental. In practical terms, this translates to about 5 g/kg/day for glucose, with a maximum lipid infusion of 0.5 to 1.0 g/kg/day, preferably infused over 24 hours. Whereas in classic starvation 1.0 to 1.5 g of protein/kg/day usually suffices for anabolism, 1.5 to 2.0 g/kg/day is the recommended starting dose of amino acid, with subsequent titration to maintain nitrogen balance. Survival appears to be correlated with achieving nitrogen balance, whereas achieving caloric equilibrium does not improve mortality figures [11, 16, 18, 26]. The differences in metabolic support are needed because of the redistribution of substrate metabolism with increased reliance on protein and glucose, rather than transitioning to a ketotic metabolism as is seen in simple starvation. Despite advances in understanding, at the present time there are insufficient clinical data to clearly identify optimal balance of substrate for the critically ill, septic patient [54].

Actual recommended daily allowances for vitamins and minerals are not well known, but there is no doubt that there are alterations in dosages in the setting of sepsis. Our guidelines include the provision of standard multivitamins and trace minerals as well as

Table 22-2. Characteristics of Metabolic Support

Characteristic	Nutrition Support	Metabolic Support
Focus	1. Support/build lean body mass	1. Minimize starvation effects
	2. Prevent specific nutrient deficiency	2. Do no harm
	3. Support/build organ function	3. Modulate disease
	4. Reduce starvation-related morbidity/mortality	4. Reduce distress-related morbidity/mortality
		5. Prevent substrate-limited metabolism
		6. Promote reparative processes
Basic nutrient requirements		
Glucose	As tolerated	< 5 mg/kg/day
Long-chain fat	As tolerated	< 1.0 g/kg/day
Amino acids	1.0–1.5 g/kg/day standard	1.5–2.0 g/kg/day
Achieve caloric balance	+	Not necessary for positive outcome
Achieve nitrogen balance	+	+

+ = Desired goal

additional vitamin C (500–1000 mg/day), thiamine (200 mg/day), and pyridoxine (20 mg/day). Potassium, magnesium, zinc, and phosphate are maintained at high normal levels. Iron is withheld because of its potential detrimental effect [61].

MONITORING

Monitoring is essential both to ensure efficacy and to avoid complications related to metabolic support. The ability to monitor efficacy, however, remains less than ideal. Traditional means of following serum protein levels, such as albumin and transferrin, can predict recovery but do not discriminate between resolution of the underlying disease process or therapeutic effect of metabolic support. For example, the well-nourished patient may have low visceral protein levels because of the shift in hepatic protein synthesis to acute-phase reactants. Alternatively, a malnourished patient may show an increase in visceral protein levels as the underlying disease process resolves, yet nutritional support may be suboptimal. Nevertheless, measurements of transferrin remain useful, in

that an increasing level is associated with improved survival.

It is important to follow nitrogen balance, since obtaining nitrogen equilibrium appears to be an important factor in optimizing nutritional support. Incremental addition of exogenous protein increases the rate of protein synthesis to equal the rate of catabolism (Fig. 22-1). Measurement of nitrogen balance in the stressed patient should probably be done by total urine nitrogen rather than urine urea nitrogen, because non-urea nitrogen is commonly substantial and a correction factor is not readily available. Thus, relying on the urine urea nitrogen would tend to result in a false-positive nitrogen balance [48].

When following and attempting to maintain nitrogen balance, one must keep in mind that the physiologic significance of attaining nitrogen balance is not known. As Russel and Jeejeebhoy [68] pointed out in regard to radionucleotide potassium studies, potassium retention does not equal nitrogen retention, which does not necessarily equal increased lean body mass. Whether positive nitrogen balance directly contributes to the host survival, or is simply an indication of the severity of the underlying process resolv-

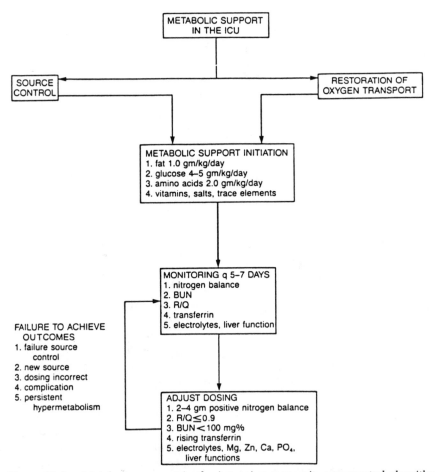

Figure 22-1. Metabolic support in the intensive care unit, a suggested algorithm.

ing, is not known. It may also be possible that anyone can be put into positive nitrogen balance without a net increase in lean body mass. Evidence for this includes studies that demonstrated that young healthy control subjects can be put into positive nitrogen balance by consuming 3 g of nitrogen/kg/day. Despite no change in lean body mass, their nitrogen balance remained positive over a period of 2 months [64]. Thus, high nitrogen infusion in the critically ill may represent the same phenomenon.

Another aspect of monitoring involves the use of indirect calorimetry. The most useful data in the critically ill involve defining the level of stress as well as making sure that the respiratory quotient remains below 0.9. Although the data obtained may indicate that the patient's caloric needs are greater than 30 kcal/kg, it must be remembered that additional calories may be more detrimental than beneficial. When interpreting data from an indirect calorimeter, one must keep in mind the limitations of the methodology in regard to calibration, the effect of mechanical ventilation, analgesia or neuromuscular blockage, or change in perfusion status.

One must always remember to continue to assess the underlying cardiopulmonary status. If the patient becomes hemodynamically unstable, inadequate tissue perfusion can limit the ability to metabolize substrate. To help prevent adverse effects on a compromised cardiac output, we recommend the infusion rate of TPN be cut by 50% until the patient is adequately resuscitated.

INSULIN

The alteration in carbohydrate metabolism in sepsis with hyperglycemia and insulin resistance raises the issue of the role of exogenous insulin. Studies utilizing the euglycemic pump in highly stressed patients have shown that amino acid flux from skeletal muscle can be significantly attenuated and nitrogen losses decreased by one-third to one-half [40, 41, 92]. A recent study in the rat cecal ligation and puncture model supports the hypothesis that insulin administration may inhibit myofibrillar breakdown in vitro in septic muscle as measured by 3-methylhistidine release [7]. Whether this phenomenon will be found to be true in vivo remains to be determined. Thus, exogenous insulin may inhibit muscle breakdown.

Current thought, however, does not support the aggressive use of exogenous insulin. Reasons against its use include the increased incidence of hepatic steatosis, the possibility that blocking amino acid mobilization may adversely affect outcome, and an inability to increase glucose oxidation despite lowering serum glucose concentrations. Exogenous insulin, then, should only be used to control serum glucose levels to some reasonable level (approximately 200 mg/dl) after decreasing the dextrose infusion to 2 mg/kg/mm has failed.

CONTROVERSIES WITH REFEEDING

There are many benefits of nutritional support of the septic patient, both realized and potential. However, many controversies exist. Teleologically, starvation may prove a beneficial adaptive response to infection or other stress. A reduction in lean body mass helps to minimize tissue substrate and oxygen demand. Starvation and nutrient deficiency may protect the host from infection by blunting the virulence of potential pathogens, especially intracellular organisms such as viruses [62]. Furthermore, many of the benefits of nutritional support may be counteracted by complications, including increased incidence of infection. We discuss some of these controversies before looking at future directions for metabolic support.

One area of controversy is whether there is a protective effect with hypocaloric or hyponitrogenous diets. Although most studies show survival with high nitrogen supplementation, some evidence in animal models questions this theory, as Peck et al. [65] showed in their recent experiment with protein modulation in guinea pigs with peritonitis. Control animals were fed diets of whey protein varying in 5% increments up to 20% of calories as protein, beginning 3 days after *E. coli* and *Staphylococcus aureus* infusions were started into their peritoneal cavities. In this setting of acute bacterial peritonitis, the 20% protein group was the only one to achieve nitrogen balance, although laboratory and pathologic studies indicated protein malnutrition in this group. It is interesting that the group receiving only 5% protein had the highest survival rate ($p < 0.05$). The only explanation offered by the authors was a possible increased bacterial virulence with increased protein load during the phase of active bacterial replication in this acute peritonitis model [65]. Again, the question raised is whether nutrients always favor the host, or does the pathogen sometimes benefit more? Furthermore, the timing of the support relative to the active peritonitis may be an additional critical factor.

Weinberg [87] found that withholding iron from nutritional support protected the host in bacterial sepsis. The addition of iron in nutritional support formulations results in increased iron being available to the invading organism, thereby augmenting the virulence [12]. Other studies support the rationale for iron restriction. For instance, interleukin-1 has been shown to cause increased leukocyte lactoferrin release [67].

The literature contains studies in animals and in humans showing that in certain situations, refeeding may add to the morbidity and mortality. Wing and Young [90] showed that acute starvation protects mice against *Listeria* monocytogenes. The message here is that our incomplete knowledge of the nutritional needs of humans as well as pathogens continues to limit therapy. As we continue to learn, we will continue in our ability to favor the host.

MODIFIED (BRANCHED-CHAIN) AMINO ACIDS

The use of branched-chain amino acid (BCAA)–enriched formulas remains an area of active investigation. There are several theoretic benefits for their use, as reviewed by Schlichtig and Ayres [70]. First, skeletal muscle consumes its own BCAAs, thereby potentially becoming depleted in its own preferred fuel. Second, BCAAs may be converted intracellularly to other fuels, such as ketones or glutamine. Third, BCAAs may stimulate muscle protein synthesis and decrease proteolysis. Fourth, a BCAA-enriched solution might increase the biologic value of the BCAA-poor protein that is being released from skeletal muscle. Finally, BCAA solutions might bypass metabolic blockades by directly entering oxidation pathways without the requirements for NAD.

The literature concerning efficacy of BCAA solutions was recently reviewed by Teasley and Buss [80]. They concluded that parenteral nutrition solutions with higher concentrations of BCAAs offer four benefits to patients with documented level 2 or greater stress (as defined by Cerra et al. [19]): (1) improved nitrogen retention, (2) increase in visceral protein status, (3) improvement in parameters of immune function, and (4) improvement in normalization of plasma amino acid profile [80]. Studies that did not show these changes omitted documentation of ob-

jective criteria of physiologic stress in their patients. Teasley and Buss [80] also pointed out the need for study of morbidity and mortality, as the studies done to date did not specifically study morbidity and mortality as outcome criteria.

Studies of BCAAs have not demonstrated a decreased catabolic rate, a distribution of nitrogen suggesting skeletal muscle sparing, a decrease in hypermetabolism, or a change in major morbidity or mortality. Examination of the efflux of amino acids out of skeletal muscle has not demonstrated any oxidation of exogenous BCAAs by skeletal muscle, even though they are taken up [10, 24]. In light of the increased cost of BCAA-enriched TPN, most institutions recommend their use only after conventional formulas have failed to achieve nitrogen balance. However, with nitrogen balance as the end point, the improved nutritional efficiency of these BCAA solutions may be cheaper on a per-gram basis, as nitrogen equilibrium is attained with less substrate [15].

In summary, the final answer on the use of BCAA solutions remains to be defined, and future studies need to specifically address morbidity and mortality using more statistical power. Although the theoretic benefits of BCAA solutions have not been fully realized, one must keep in mind the possibility of statistical type II error as an explanation for the lack of significant change in clinical outcome. The available data strongly support the position that these modified amino acid solutions are a more efficient "protein" source.

THE FUTURE

Enteral versus Parenteral Nutrition

Although the purpose of this text is to discuss the role of TPN in sepsis, it would be incomplete without mention of enteral nutrition. The gastrointestinal tract is still the preferred route of delivery of nutritional support, and it is more functional than initially thought. Most of the ileus is found in the stomach and colon. Intubation beyond the ligament of Treitz facilitates the use of enteral nutrition in a large percentage of patients, without excess morbidity.

The gastrointestinal tract contains enough organisms to kill the host many times over. Thus, maintaining gastrointestinal competence is essential. Enteral feeding of 0.6 kg/day of nitrogen via the gut appears to maintain gut integrity and immune function. Early refeeding via the gastrointestinal tract may decrease hypermetabolism/multiple-organ failure and endogenous flora bacteremia, while preserving gastrointestinal immuno-competence. Furthermore, glutamine or short-chain fatty acid supplementation of TPN may provide an ongoing preferred fuel source for the gastrointestinal tract, thereby preventing the mucosal breakdown that occurs several days after the cessation of oral feeding.

Early refeeding of the burned patient has been proposed to be safe and efficacious, blunting the hypermetabolic response, preserving gut integrity, and decreasing morbidity and mortality. Although some experimental data support this position, clinical applications are still in the data-gathering stage. The potential benefit appears to depend mainly on obtaining nitrogen balance rather than on obtaining energy balance. Indeed, feeding patients 40 to 60 kcal/kg results in excess morbidity and mortality.

The septic patient has been compared with the burned patient in terms of metabolic support and complications. This concept has been supported by a recent randomized study comparing the difference between early refeeding (< 12 hours after the burn) to controls (72 hours after the burn) in 17 burned patients. The early refeeding group showed statistically significant improvement in nitrogen balance, transferrin, and ceruloplasmin, as well as a respiratory quotient of 0.9 compared to 0.79 in the control group [44]. These data are in agreement with prior studies suggesting that early feeding and increased protein support decrease morbidity and mortality, particularly via the enteric route [2, 3]. Thus, until definitive data are available, in the TPN-supported patient, partial support by the enteral route should probably be attempted at the earliest possible time. Once hypermetabolism is established, there does not seem to be any benefit of the enteral route per se.

Gut and Translocation

The translocation of endotoxins and the translocation of bacteria from the bowel to the systemic circulation and extraintestinal tissues are recognized as a contributing factor in experimental sepsis and are hypothesized to be an important effector in human sepsis. The mechanism is not fully understood [25]. Two mechanisms have been proposed. First, there may be a direct role of the macrophage, which transports organisms across the mucosal barrier, without preceding gut injury being a necessary condition for the process to occur. Thus, organisms that are capable of surviving the intracellular milieu of the macrophage may invade tissues outside the bowel wall via this mechanism. Second, endotoxin, in conjunction with other insults such as ischemia, has been shown to be a contributing factor in direct damage to the bowel wall, resulting in a permeable pathway for organisms to directly migrate to surrounding tissues. Stimulants of gut mucosal growth, such as bombesin infusion, may preserve the gut mucosal barrier, thereby preventing bacterial translocation [21]. Glutamine or short-chain fatty acids, as discussed below, may provide protection from this second mechanism.

Future experimentation will continue to study the role of the gastrointestinal system as a factor in the control of the hypermetabolic state and the transition to organ failure. [*Editor's Note:* it is important to remember that the damaging material may be bacterial **products,** such as endotoxin in the portal blood, while most studies on translocation have concentrated on the presence of bacteria in mesenteric lymph nodes. The two may not be related. Translocation appears to be a natural process that occurs normally.]

Glutamine Hypothesis

Glutamine is an important fuel for entero-cytes, and its utilization is increased in the setting of various stress states. Standard TPN formulas lack glutamine. Two-percent glutamine-enriched formulas have been shown to maintain or increase intestinal growth [86]. The lack of glutamine may be partially responsible for the breakdown in the gut mucosal barrier. Fox et al. [33] recently provided additional support for the role of glutamine in nutritional support formulas, showing improved intestinal morphometry and mortality in the severe enterocolonic model. The glutamine hypothesis may even account for part of the theoretical benefit of BCAA solutions by their making more glutamine available for the enterocyte. However, it may also be that glutamine is acting as a "ketone" and that short-chain fatty acids may have the same effect. This latter phenomenon would obviate the dosing and utilization problems with glutamine.

Short-Chain Fatty Acids

Short-chain fatty acids are a preferred fuel source for the colonic mucosal cells. The combination of bowel rest and TPN results in colonic mucosal atrophy in experimental animals, probably as a result of decreased preferential fuel for the colonocyte. Kripke et al. [51] were able to show that provision of beta-hydroxybutyrate in TPN reduced the TPN-associated mucosal atrophy throughout the colon. Their data as well as that of others support the role for specific intravenous nutrient therapy in patients at bowel rest. This intervention may help to protect the vulnerable host from a possible source of sepsis [50].

Lipids and Alternative Fat Sources

The use of lipids in the setting of sepsis will undoubtedly change in the future. The administration of lipid emulsions can alter the membranes of cells within the body toward a composition similar to the administered lipid emulsion. Thus, by changing the composition of the infused lipid, one can change membrane phospholipids and, ultimately, the metabolic products of those lipids. The lipid emulsions currently in use are predominantly omega-6 fatty acids, the precursor of the even series of arachidonate metabolites. Several complications have been associated with their use. The use of alternative lipids, including omega-3 fatty acids, medium-chain triglycerides, and short-chain fatty acids, may provide both a decreased spectrum of toxicity and more desirable fuel substrates.

Complications of current lipid emulsions are well known. The liver may demonstrate steatosis, bile duct proliferation, periportal inflammation, and clinical cholestatic jaundice. Infusion of 3 g of lipid emulsion/kg/day has been associated with decreased pulmonary diffusion capacity. Detrimental changes in the immune system are inconsistent, but include reticuloendothelial system (RES) blockade with decreased particulate and bacterial clearance, decreased cell-mediated immunity, decreased C_2 synthesis, decreased phagocytosis, decreased bactericidal function, and decreased lymphoproliferation. Decreased clearance is associated with decreased lipoprotein lipase. The significance of the increase in lipoprotein X is not known.

Omega-3 fatty acids offer many potential benefits. They give rise to the 3 series of prostaglandins and the 5 series of leukotrienes, both possibly more favorable to the host by decreasing the inflammatory reponse and improving the immune responsiveness. Ultimately, the host's response is toward reduced thrombogenesis and blunted inflammation. Endres et al. [29] recently reported on the effect of omega-3 fatty acid supplementation in a group of nine normal subjects. They showed that oral supplementation resulted in changes in the composition of the macrophage membranes that persisted for up to 10 weeks after the 6-week period of supplementation. This was associated with a decreased production of interleukin-1 alpha, interleukin-1 beta, and TNF in response to lipopolysaccharide. Prostaglandin E, thought to be immunosuppressive, was similarly decreased from 612 to 302 pg ($p = 0.008$). It was hypothesized that changes may in part be mediated by the change in substrate availability for the lipoxygenase and cyclooxygenase pathways with decreased 5-lipoxygenate pathway products such as leukotriene B4, with increased production of the less active leukotriene B5 [29]. Other investigators found omega-3 fatty acid supplementation favorable in a variety of inflammatory conditions [9, 46, 49]. Since it is accepted that interleukin-1 and TNF probably have detrimental effects at high sustained tissue levels, providing part of the lipid calories as omega-3 fatty acids may have beneficial effects on altering the host's response in the sepsis and hypermetabolism syndrome.

Medium-chain triglycerides, fatty acids with eight to ten carbon atoms, may also play an important role in the future. Potential benefits include rapid clearance, with less interference in the RES pathways, carnitine independent uptake by the mitochondria, and protein-sparing effects at least equal to those of long-chain triglycerides. However, the therapeutic window may be narrow [39].

Short-chain triglycerides also offer potential benefits, but much investigation remains to be done. Short-chain fatty acids are produced and rapidly cleared in the septic patient. Providing lipid calories partially as short-chain moieties may provide an alternative, preferential fuel. Initial studies suggest efficacy and safety [5, 6], but further research is needed to clarify optimal delivery as well as possible toxicity. Additional potential benefits include the ability to provide fermentation products that may stimulate growth of the colon through polypeptides and act as a significant source of fuel for the colonocyte [42, 43, 69].

The lipid research demonstrated at present underscores the need for continuing research to define the optimal balance of lipid to be used in the septic patient. Structured lipid with well-defined components needs to be studied in more detail.

Growth Factors

Human growth hormone has been shown to result in a striking improvement in nitrogen balance in highly catabolic burned patients [89]. Glucose infusion appears to enhance hormone levels in septic and injured patients, which may provide a partial rationale for the ability of glucose to improve nitrogen balance [23]. Growth hormone also appears to enhance the ability of the stressed individual to utilize endogenous fat stores as a fuel source, thereby potentially improving nitrogen balance. In addition, human growth hormone may enhance both glucose uptake and oxidation. With ongoing research, the clinical use of growth hormone and other anabolic factors should be more clearly defined.

Immune System

Advances in parenteral nutrition have led to significant improvement in the care of the septic patient. However, sepsis continues to be a complication in patients managed with parenteral nutrition as compared with controls. Moreover, a systemic effect is suggested, as the excess in infection rates is more than simply an increase in access site infections. Studies on the role of nucleotides have added one area of insight into this phenomenon.

Dietary Nucleotides

The work of Van Buren and his group [85] focused on the role of dietary nucleotides in fully supporting the immune system rather than on the traditional focus of nitrogen balance. They found that the use of dietary nucleotides, specifically uracil, restores skin test response, enhances in vitro T-cell proliferation to interleukin-2 stimulation, corrects T-cell helper maturation arrest, and enhances induction of adenosine deaminase and purine nucleoside phosphorylase activities, both important in T-cell maturation and both decreased in animals fed nucleotide-free diets [52, 84]. In addition, they found that mice fed nucleotide-free diets are much more susceptible to lethal infections with *Candida albicans* and *S. aureus* than mice fed chow or nucleotide-supplemented diets. They also found that macrophage bactericidal activity was decreased in nucleotide-free animals [53].

Dietary nucleotides take on even more importance when one considers that virtually all parenteral and enteral nutritional support is free of nucleotides. Further, the individual patient may appear well nourished by traditional monitoring criteria, including positive nitrogen balance, yet have an immune deficiency secondary to the RNA-free diet.

Arginine

Another area of interest is the effect of arginine on the host immune system. While some investigated its role in modulation of the immune system, other investigators demonstrated that arginine has multiple effects, including acting as a secretagogue for growth hormone, improving wound healing, and demonstrating a thymotrophic effect with improved T-cell function. Some data support a role of supplemental arginine in the animal tumor model, but there is insufficient evidence to support the use of routine supplemental arginine in sepsis. A recent study by Peck et al. [66] showed that supplemental arginine at low levels had no effect on recovery from peritonitis in a guinea pig model, and that a high level of arginine (6%) adversely affected outcome. Thus, until further studies are available to demonstrate a beneficial effect of arginine, and at what level, arginine supplementation is not recommended in the setting of sepsis.

SUMMARY

The critically ill, septic patient presents a difficult management problem for the clinician. The early suggestion that starvation may have a short-term protective effect on the host in some types of infection has been demonstrated. However, it is also clear that the hypermetabolic state results in a rapid depletion of body nutrients and that, if left untreated, starvation-associated malnutrition becomes a separate cofactor of morbidity and mortality.

Immediate aggressive resuscitation of cardiopulmonary status should be followed as quickly as possible with nutritional support, with a goal of achieving early nitrogen balance. Total parenteral nutrition should probably be supplemented with and replaced by enteral supplements at the earliest possible time. Nonprotein calories should be limited to 25 to 30 cal/kg of body weight, with close monitoring for intolerance. Requirements for specific nutrients also change, as summarized in Table 22-2 and Figure 22-1.

The future requires a further expansion of our knowledge of the actions of specific nutrients, such as arginine, glutamine, and the omega-3 series of lipids. The interaction of nutrients with growth factors, hormonal manipulation, and solutions with better defined and tissue-specific fuels also needs elucidation. As we define the effects of nutrition on the host immune system, inflammatory response, and interaction with pathogens, we will be able to use substrate as pharmacologic agents as well as for the prevention of malnutrition.

Finally, the future should allow us to witness the results of current efforts to decrease the mortality resulting from the sepsis syndrome.

REFERENCES

1. Abbott, W. C., Schiller, W., Long, C. L., Birkhahn, R. H., and Blakemore, W. S. The effect of major thermal injury of plasma ketone body levels. *J. Parenter. Enter. Nutr.* 9:153, 1985.
2. Alexander, J. W., and MacMillan, B. G. Hospital infections in burns. In J. V. Bennett and P. Brachman (eds.), *Nosocomial Infections.* Boston: Little, Brown, 1979, P. 335.
3. Alexander, J. W., MacMillan, B. G., Stinnett, J. D., et al. Beneficial effects of aggressive protein feeding in severely burned children. *Ann. Surg.* 192:505, 1980.
4. Bagby, G. J., and Spitzer, J. A. Lipoprotein lipase activity in rat heart and adipose tissue during endotoxic shock. *Am. J. Physiol.* 238: H325, 1980.

5. Bailey, J. W., Rodriguez, N. R., Marsh, H., Haymond, M. W., and Miles, J. Metabolic effects of an intravenous short-chain triglyceride infusion in dogs. *J. Parenter. Enter. Nutr.* 11(1):6S, 1987.

6. Bailey, J. W., Rodriguez, N. R., Miles, J. M., and Haymond, M. W. Effect of an intravenous short-chain triglyceride infusion on leucine metabolism in dogs. (Abstract) *F.A.S.E.B. J.* 2:A431, 1988.

7. Benson, D. W., Hasselgren, P. O., James, J. H., Nelson, J. L., and Fischer, J. E. Inhibition by insulin of myofibrillar protein breakdown in septic skeletal muscle. *Surg. Forum* 39:36, 1988.

8. Birkhahn, R. H., Long, C. L., Fitkin, D. L., Busnardo, A. C., Geiger, J. W., and Blakemore, W. S. A comparison of the effects of skeletal trauma and surgery on the ketosis of starvation in man. *J. Trauma* 21:513, 1981.

9. Bittiner, S. B., Tucker, W. F. G., Cartwright, I., and Bleehen, S. S. A double-blind, randomised, placebo-controlled trial of fish oil in psoriasis. *Lancet* 1:378, 1988.

10. Bonau, R. A., Jeevanandam, M., Moldawer, L., Blackburn, G. L., and Daly, J. M. Muscle amino acid flux in patients receiving branched chain amino acid solutions after surgery. *Surgery* 10:400, 1987.

11. Bower, R. H., Muggia-Sullam, M., Vallgren, S., et al. Branched chain amino acid–enriched solutions in the septic patient: A randomized, prospective trial. *Ann. Surg.* 203:13, 1986.

12. Bullen, J. J. The significance of iron in infection. *Rev. Infect. Dis.* 3:1127, 1981.

13. Cerra, F. B. Hypermetabolism, organ failure, and metabolic support. *Surgery* 101:1, 1987.

14. Cerra, F. B. The syndrome of multiple organ failure. In F. B. Cerra and D. B. Binhari (eds.), *New Horizon Series: Cell Injury and Organ Failure.* Fullerton, CA: Society Critical Care Medicine, 1988.

15. Cerra, F. B., Blackburn, G., Hirsch, J., Mullen, K., and Luther, W. The effect of stress level, amino acid formula, and nitrogen dose on nitrogen retention in traumatic and septic stress. *Ann. Surg.* 205:282, 1987.

16. Cerra, F. B., Cheung, N. K., Fischer, J. E., et al. Disease-specific amino acid infusion (F080) in hepatic encephalopathy: A prospective, randomized, double-blind, controlled trial. *J. Parenter. Enter. Nutr.* 9:288, 1985.

17. Cerra, F. B., Siegel, J. H., Coleman, B., Border, J. R., and McMenamy, R. R. Septic autocannibalism: A failure of exogenous nutritional support. *Ann. Surg.* 192:570, 1980.

18. Cerra, F. B., Upson, D., Angelico, R., Wiles, C., Lyons, J., and Paysinger, J. Branched chains support postoperative synthesis. *Surgery* 92:192, 1982.

19. Cerra, F. B., Wiles, F. B., Siegel, J. H., Coleman, B., Border, J. R., and McMenamy, R. The best discriminators of sepsis are metabolic. *Crit. Care Med.* 8:230, 1980.

20. Clowes, G. H. A., Jr., George, B. C., Villee, C. A., Jr., and Saravis, C. A. Muscle proteolysis induced by a circulating peptide in patients with sepsis or trauma. *N. Engl. J. Med.* 308:545, 1983.

21. Coffey, J. A., Milhoan, R. A., Abdullah, A., Herndon, D. N., Townsend, C. M., and Thompson, J. C. Bombesin inhibits bacterial translocation from the gut in burned rats. *Surg. Forum* 39:109, 1988.

22. Cuthbertson, D. P. Post-shock metabolic response. *Lancet* 1:443, 1942.

23. Dahn, M. S., Jacobs, L. A., Lange, M. P., Smith, S., and Mitchell, R. A. Endocrine mediators of metabolism associated with injury and sepsis. *J. Parenter. Enter. Nutr.* 10:253, 1986.

24. Daly, J. M., Mihranian, M. H., Kehoe, J. E., and Brennan, M. F. Effects of post-operative infusion of branched chain amino acids on nitrogen balance and forearm muscle substrate flux. *Surgery* 94:151, 1983.

25. Deitch, E. A., Berg, R., and Specian, R. Endotoxin promotes the translocation of bacteria from the gut. *Arch. Surg.* 122:185, 1987.

26. Deitch, E. A., Winterton, J., Li, M., and Berg, R. The gut as a portal of entry for bacteremia: Role of protein malnutrition. *Ann. Surg.* 205:681, 1987.

27. Demling, R. H., Lalonde, C. C., Jin, L., Albes, J., and Fiori, N. The pulmonary and systemic response to recurrent endotoxin in the adult sheep. *Surgery* 100:876, 1986.

28. De Vasconcelos, P. R. L., Kettlewell, M. G. W., and Williamson, D. H. Time course of changes in hepatic metabolism in response to sepsis in the rat: Impairment of gluconeogenesis and ketogenesis in vitro. *Clin. Sci.* 72:683, 1987.

29. Endres, S., Ghorbani, R., Kelley, V. E., et al. The effect of dietary supplementation with n-3 polyunsaturated fatty acids on the synthesis of interleukin-1 and tumor necrosis factor by mononuclear cells. *N. Engl. J. Med.* 320:265, 1989.

30. Esmon, C. T. The regulation of natural anticoagulant pathways. *Science* 235:1348, 1987.

31. Eyer, S. D., and Cerra, F. B. Cost-effective use of the surgical intensive care unit. *World J. Surg.* 11:241, 1987.

32. Fink, M. P., Cohn, S. M., Lee, P. C., et al. Effect of lipopolysaccharide on intestinal intramucosal pH in pigs: Evidence of gut ischemia despite normal cardiac output and mesenteric oxygen consumption. *Surg. Forum* 39:80, 1988.

33. Fox, A. D., De Paula, J. A., Kripke, S. A., Glutamine-supplemented elemental diets re-

duce endotoxemia in a lethal model of enterocolitis. *Surg. Forum* 39:46, 1988.

34. Goldberg, A. L., Kettlehut, I. C., Furuno, K., Fagan, J. M., and Baracos, V. Activation of protein breakdown and prostaglandin E_2 production in rat skeleton muscle in fever is signaled by a macrophage product distinct from interleukin-1 or other known monokines. *J. Clin. Invest.* 81:1378, 1988.

35. Hasselgren, P. O., James, J. H., Benson, D. W., Li, S., and Fischer, J. E. Is there a circulating proteolysis-inducing factor during sepsis? *Arch. Surg.* 125:510, 1990.

36. Hasselgren, P. O., James, J. H., and Fischer, J. E. Inhibited muscle amino acid uptake in sepsis. *Ann. Surg.* 203:360, 1986.

37. Hasselgren, P. O., James, J. H., Warner, B. W., Ogle, C., Takehara, H., and Fischer, J. E. Reduced muscle amino acid uptake in sepsis and the effect in vitro of septic plasma and interleukin-1. *Surgery* 100:222, 1986.

38. Hasselgren, P. O., Talamini, M. A., James, J. H., and Fischer, J. E. Protein metabolism in different types of skeletal muscle during early and late sepsis in rats. *Arch. Surg.* 121:918, 1986.

39. Haymond, M. W., Tessari, P., Beaufrere, B., Rodriguez, N., Bailey, J., and Miles, J. M. Effects of parenteral lipid on leucine metabolism: Dependence on fatty acid chain length. *J. Parenter. Enter. Nutr.* 12(6):94S, 1988.

40. Iapichino, G., Gattinoni, L., Solca, M., et al. Protein sparing and protein replacement in acutely injured patients during TPN with and without amino acid supply. *Intens. Care Med.* 8:25, 1982.

41. Iapichino, G., Solca, M., Radrizzani, D., Zucchetti, M., and Damia, G. Net protein utilization during total parenteral nutrition of injured critically ill patients: An original approach. *J. Parenter. Enter. Nutr.* 5:317, 1981.

42. Jacobs, L. R., and Lupton, J. R. Effect of dietary fibers on rat large bowel mucosal growth and cell proliferation. *Am. J. Physiol.* 246:G378, 1984.

43. Jacobs, L. R., and White, F. A. Modulation of mucosal cell proliferation in the intestine of rats fed a wheat bran diet. *Am. J. Clin. Nutr.* 37:945, 1983.

44. Jenkins, M., Gottschlich, M., Alexander, J. W., and Warden, G. D. Effect of immediate enteral feeding on the hypermetabolic response following severe burn injury. *J. Parenter. Enter. Nutr.* 13(1):12S, 1989.

45. Jensen, J. A., Riggs, K., Vasconez, L. O., Goodson, W. H., Rabkin, J., and Hunt, T. K. Clinical assessment of postoperative peripheral perfusion. *Surg. Forum* 38:66, 1987.

46. Kelley, V. E., Ferretti, A., Izui, S., and Strom, T. B. A fish oil diet rich in eicosapentaenoic acid reduces cyclooxygenase metabolites, and suppresses lupus in MRL-1pr mice. *J. Immunol.* 134:1914, 1985.

47. Kelly, K., Price, R. M., Baxter, J. G., Steinberg, S., Lalka, D., and Hassett, J. M. In vivo macrophage activation alters hepatocyte metabolism. *Surg. Forum* 39:4, 1988.

48. Konstantinides, F. N., Konstantinides, N. N., Li, J. C., and Cerra, F. B. Can urinary urea nitrogen be substituted for total urinary nitrogen when calculating nitrogen balance in clinical nutrition? *J. Parenter. Enter. Nutr.* 12(1):18S, 1988.

49. Kremer, J. M., Jubiz, W., Michalek, A., et al. Fish-oil fatty acid supplementation in active rheumatoid arthritis: A double-blinded, controlled, crossover study. *Ann. Intern. Med.* 106:497, 1987.

50. Kripke, S. A., Fox, A. D., Berman, J. M., et al. Inhibition of TPN-associated intestinal mucosal atrophy with monoacetoacetin. *J. Surg. Res.* 44:436, 1988.

51. Kripke, S. A., Fox, A. D., Berman, J. M., De Paula, J. A., Rombeau, J. L., and Settle, G. Inhibition of TPN-associated colonic atrophy with beta-hydroxybutyrate. *Surg. Forum* 39:48, 1988.

52. Kulkarni, S. S., Bhateley, D. C., Zander, A. R., et al. Functional impairment of T-lymphocytes in mouse radiation chimeras by a nucleotide-free diet. *Exp. Hematol.* 12:694, 1984.

53. Kulkarni, A. D., Fanslow, W. C., Drath, D. B., Rudolph, F. B., and Van Buren, C. T. Influence of dietary nucleotide restriction on bacterial sepsis and phagocytic cell function in mice. *Arch. Surg.* 121:169, 1986.

54. Long, C. L. Fuel preferences in the septic patient: Glucose or lipid? *J. Parenter. Enter. Nutr.* 11(4):333, 1987.

55. Long, C. L., Jeevanandam, M., and Kinney, J. M. Whole body protein synthesis and catabolism in septic man. *Am. J. Clin. Nutr.* 30:1340, 1977.

56. Long, C. L., Spencer, J. L., Kinney, J. M., and Geiger, J. W. Carbohydrate metabolism in man: Effect of elective operations and major injury. *J. Appl. Physiol.* 31:110, 1971.

57. Mazuski, J. E., Bankey, P. E., Carlson, A., and Cerra, F. B. Hepatocytes release factors that can modulate macrophage IL-1 secretion and proliferation. *Surg. Forum* 39:13, 1988.

58. Meterissian, S., Saint Vil, D., and Forse, R. A. Decreased beta-adrenergic stimulated lipolysis with endotoxemia. *Surg. Forum* 39:38, 1988.

59. Michie, H. R., Spriggs, D. R., Rounds, J., and Wilmore, D. W. Does cachectin cause cachexia? *Surg. Forum* 38:38, 1987.

60. Moldawer, L. L., Svaninger, G., Gelin, J., and Lundholm, K. G. Interleukin-1 and tumor ne-

crosis factor do not regulate protein balance in skeletal muscle. *Am.J. Physiol.* 253:C766, 1987.

61. Murray, M. J., and Murray, A. B. Starvation suppression and refeeding activation and infection: An ecological necessity? *Lancet* 1:123, 1977.

62. Murray, M. J., and Murry, A. B. Anorexia of infection as a mechanism of host defense. *Am. J. Clin. Nutr.* 32:593, 1979.

63. Nelson, K. M., and Long, C. L. Physiologic basis for nutrition in sepsis. *Nutr. Clin. Pract.* 4:6, 1989.

64. Oddoye, E. A., and Margen, S. Nitrogen balance studies in humans: Long-term effect of high nitrogen intake on nitrogen accretion. *J. Nutr.* 109:363, 1979.

65. Peck, M. D., Alexander, J. W., Gonce, S. J., and Miskell, P. W. Low-protein diets improve survival from peritonitis in guinea pigs. *Surg. Forum* 39:31, 1988.

66. Peck, M. D., Gonce, S. J., Miskell, P. W., and Alexander, J. W. The effect of supplemental arginine on recovery from peritonitis in guinea pigs. *J. Parenter. Enter. Nutr.* 13(1):7S, 1989.

67. Powanda, M. C., and Beisel, W. R. Hypothesis: Leukocyte endogenous mediator/endogenous pyrogen/lymphocyte activating factor modulates the development of non-specific and specific immunity and affects nutritional status. *Am. J. Clin. Nutr.* 35:762, 1982.

68. Russel, D. M., and Jeejeebhoy, K. N. Radionucleotide assessment of nutritional depletion. In R. A. Wright and S. B. Heymsfield (eds.), *Nutritional Assessment.* London: Blackwell Scientific, 1984.

69. Sakata, T., and Yajima, T. Influence of short-chain fatty acids on the epithelial cell division of digestive tract. *Q. J. Exp. Physiol.* 69:639, 1984.

70. Schlichtig, R., and Ayres, S. M. *Nutritional Support of the Critically Ill.* Chicago: Year Book Medical, 1988, P. 116.

71. Shaw, J. H. F., Klein, S., and Wolfe, R. R. Assessment of alanine, urea, and glucose interrelationships in normal subjects and in patients with sepsis with stable isotopic tracers. *Surgery* 97:557, 1985.

72. Shaw, J. H. F., Wildbore, M., and Wolfe, R. R. Whole body protein kinetics in severely septic patients: The response to glucose infusion and total parenteral nutrition. *Ann. Surg.* 205:288, 1987.

73. Shoemaker, W. Hemodynamic and oxygen transport patterns in septic shock: Physiologic mechanisms and therapeutic implications. In W. Sibbald and C. Sprung (eds.), *Prospectives in Sepsis and Septic Shock.* Fullerton, CA: Society of Critical Care Medicine, 1985. P. 203.

74. Siegel, J. H., Cerra, F. B., Coleman, B., et al.

Pathophysiological and metabolic correlations in human sepsis. *Surgery* 86:163, 1979.

75. Spitzer, J. J., Bagby, G. J., Mészáros, K., and Lang, C. H. Alterations in lipid and carbohydrate metabolism in sepsis. *J. Parenter. Enter. Nutr.* 12(6):53S, 1988.

76. Starnes, H. F., Larchian, W. A., McHugh, N. E., Gabrilove, J. L., and Brennan, M. F. Metabolic effects of tumor necrosis factor and gamma-interferon are not abrogated by indomethacin. *Surg. Forum* 39:1, 1988.

77. Starnes, H. F., Warren, R. S., Conti, P. S., Calvano, S. E., and Brennan, M. F. Redistribution of amino acids in rat liver and muscle induced by tumor necrosis factor requires the adrenal response. *Surg. Forum* 38:41, 1987.

78. Stoner, H. B., Little, R. A., Frayn, K. N., Elebute, A. E., Tresadern, J., and Gross, E. The effect of sepsis on the oxidation of carbohydrate and fat. *Br. J. Surg.* 70:32, 1983.

79. Sugino, K., Dohi, K., Yamada, K., and Kawasaki, T. The role of lipid peroxidation in endotoxin-induced hepatic damage and the protective effect of antioxidants. *Surgery* 101:746, 1987.

80. Teasley, K. M., and Buss, R. L. Do parenteral nutrition solutions enriched with high concentrations of branched chain amino acids offer significant benefits to stressed patients? *Ann. Pharmacol.* 23:411, 1989.

81. Tracey, K. J., Beutler, B., Lowry, S. F., et al. Shock and tissue injury induced by recombinant human cachectin. *Science* 234:470, 1985.

82. Tracey, K. J., Fong, Y., Hesse, D. G., et al. Cachectin (tumor necrosis factor-alpha) participates in the metabolic derangements induced by gram-negative bacteremia. *Surg. Forum* 39:8, 1988.

83. Tracey, K. J., Lowry, S. F., Fahey, T. J., et al. Cachectin/tumor necrosis factor induces lethal shock and stress hormone response in the dog. *Surg. Gynecol. Obstet.* 164:415, 1987.

84. Van Buren, C. T., Kulkarni, A. D., Fanslow, W. C., and Rudolph, F. B. Dietary nucleotides, a requirement for helper/inducer T lymphocytes. *Transplantation* 40:694, 1985.

85. Van Buren, C. T., Kulkarni, A. D., Schandle, V. B., and Rudolph, F. B. The influence of dietary nucleotides on cell mediated immunity. *Transplantation* 36:350, 1983.

86. Wang, X., Jacobs, D. O., O'Dwyer, S. T., Smith, R. J., and Wilmore, D. W. Glutamine-enriched parenteral nutrition prevents mucosal atrophy following massive small bowel resection. *Surg. Forum* 39:44, 1988.

87. Weinberg, E. D. Iron withholding: A defense against infection and neoplasia. *Physiol. Rev.* 64:65, 1984.

88. Wiles, J. B., Cerra, F. B., Siegel, J. H., and

Border, J. R. The systemic septic response: Does the organism matter? *Crit. Care Med.* 8:55, 1980.

89. Wilmore, D. W., Moylan, J. A., Bristow, B. F., Mason, A. D., Jr., and Pruitt, B. A., Jr. Anabolic effects of human growth hormone and high caloric feedings following thermal injury. *Surg. Gynecol. Obstet.* 138:875, 1974.

90. Wing, E. J., and Young, J. R. Acute starvation protects mice against Listeria monocytogenes. *Infect. Immun.* 28:771, 1980.

91. Wolfe, R. R., and Shaw, J. H. F. Glucose and FFA kinetics in sepsis: Role of glucagon and sympathetic nervous system activity. *Am. J. Physiol.* 248:E236, 1985.

92. Woolfson, A. M. J., Heatley, R. V., and Allison, S. P. Insulin to inhibit protein catabolism after injury. *N. Engl. J. Med.* 300:14, 1979.

III

Supplemental Techniques

Home Parenteral Nutrition

Robert H. Bower

Parenteral nutrition is utilized extensively in the treatment of malnutrition in hospitalized patients. Most of these patients recover and are able to return to oral or enteral nutrient intake. A small subsegment of these patients may have inadequate gastrointestinal reserve to resume enteral intake, but have otherwise had a satisfactory convalescence. For those patients who would remain hospitalized solely for the provision of parenteral nutrition, techniques have been developed to provide parenteral nutrition at home. Although less expensive than hospitalization, this therapy accounted for an estimated $480 million expended in 1987 [33]. Due to its economic cost and requirement for intensive training and monitoring, it is not to be undertaken lightly or without full knowledge of procedures, techniques, and complications. Such therapy draws extensively on the skills of the nutrition support team. Likewise, close cooperation must exist among referring physicians, the nutrition support team, hospital staff, and professionals from the home care

vendor. As such, this therapy is best undertaken in medical centers with experience in this form of therapy.

INDICATIONS

The most recent data concerning patients receiving home parenteral and enteral nutrition are derived from the most current annual report of the OASIS Home Nutrition Support Patient Registry for the year 1987 [33]. This report is a cooperative project of the Oley Foundation and the American Society for Parenteral and Enteral Nutrition that is designed to collect and analyze data on these patients and to maintain a data bank for specialized nutrition support research.

During 1987, the most recent year for which data are available, 2466 patients were reported to be receiving home nutrition support: 1627 were receiving home parenteral nutrition and 839 were receiving home enteral nutrition by tube [33]. These figures, compared with 1986 data, represent a 10% increase in the number of patients reported to be receiving home parenteral nutrition [32]. Based on figures derived from national reimbursement sources, this voluntary registry represents approximately 10% of the estimated population receiving home parenteral nutrition in the United States, and is thus an insignificant portion of home nutritional support practices. Nevertheless, it gives the best estimate of available usage of home parenteral nutrition and allows a comparison between actual use and ideal indications for use [3, 4].

DISEASE STATES FOR WHICH HOME PARENTERAL NUTRITION IS ROUTINELY INDICATED

Severe Short-Bowel Syndrome

Most patients with short-bowel syndrome who have an ileocecal valve and colon in-continuity with the small bowel can be managed by enteral nutrition. However, massive small-bowel loss (> 70%) likely results in the inability to absorb adequate nutrients to meet normal requirements. Patients who have had resections of more than 200 cm of small bowel or those who have lost less small bowel but have also undergone colectomy will likely need parenteral nutrition along with a graduated program of change in nutrient source as adaptation occurs. Patients who have less than 60 cm of small bowel remaining will need home parenteral nutrition indefinitely [25]. [Editor's Note: This is close to the limit, but should not be taken as gospel. I have had experience with patients with shorter small bowel who stopped needing total parenteral nutrition (TPN).] Oral intake of some kind is encouraged to provide a stimulus to the gastrointestinal tract to adapt. Patients initially require home parenteral nutrition to meet virtually all fluid, electrolyte, and nutritional needs. As adaptation occurs, patients may progress to a defined formula enteral diet as home enteral nutrition or may maintain nutritional requirements by an oral diet of solids while still receiving home par-

enteral fluids and electrolytes. Eventually, with adaptation periods of months to years, patients may be able to maintain body weight and fluid and electrolyte status, and control diarrhea by eating a near-normal diet separating solids and liquids [25].

Cholestyramine may be helpful to control the diarrhea that results from ileal resection. Parenterally administered vitamin B_{12} may be necessary if abnormal absorption is demonstrated. In addition to routine replacement of trace elements, zinc losses in diarrhea may require additional supplementation. Wolman and associates [51] suggested the need for 12 to 15 mg/day of zinc in the presence of intestinal loss and diarrhea.

Disease states that frequently result in massive small-bowel loss include mesenteric vascular thrombosis or embolization. Patients with these conditions accounted for 12.1% of patients receiving home parenteral nutrition in 1987 (Fig. 23-1) [32]. Mid-gut volvulus, internal herniation with infarction of bowel, and abdominal trauma involving extensive small-bowel injury likewise result in short-bowel syndrome. In such instances, the remaining small bowel is generally healthy. In other disease states such as Crohn's disease, radiation enteritis and intraabdominal malignancies may require resections of small bowel of variable size, although the portion that remains is still diseased and incapable of adequate absorption. These conditions may require home parenteral nutrition and are discussed separately.

DISEASE STATES FOR WHICH HOME PARENTERAL NUTRITION IS USUALLY INDICATED

Crohn's Disease

A small number of patients with Crohn's disease may be unable to maintain adequate nutrition by oral intake or defined formula enteral diets. Patients may suffer from short-bowel syndrome due to multiple resections, just mentioned. However, generally small-bowel loss is accompanied by persistent inflammation in the remaining bowel, which

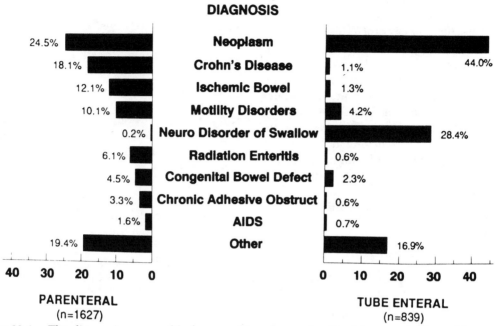

Figure 23-1. The diagnosis responsible for use of home parenteral and home enteral nutrition, reported as a percentage of total patients registered in 1987. (From *OASIS Home Nutrition Support Patient Registry, Annual Report 1987.* Albany, NY: Oley Foundation; and Silver Spring, MD: American Society for Parenteral and Enteral Nutrition, 1989. Reprinted with permission.)

prevents adequate absorption. Occasionally, patients may be able to absorb macronutrients but need parenteral fluids, electrolytes, and trace elements [17]. In such conditions, reduction by 50% of numbers of patients hospitalized has been reported [14]. Despite achievement of improved nutritional status and decreased number of hospitalizations, the progression of the disease is not arrested. Patients may later develop fistulous disease and require further operative therapy while receiving home parenteral nutrition [14, 38].

The OASIS registry reported Crohn's disease as its most frequently reported diagnosis in 1985. However, for 1987 it is the second most reported diagnosis, representing 18.1% of patients receiving home parenteral nutrition [33]. Of those reported, 88% were already reported in the registry, testifying to the long-term nature of home parenteral nutrition in these patients. At year's end, two-thirds of 399 patients remained on therapy,

with fewer than one-fourth having resumed oral intake. Very few patients died while receiving therapy.

Patients with chronic inflammatory bowel disease often adapt to home parenteral nutrition more readily than do patients who are previously healthy but undergo massive resection due to an intraabdominal catastrophe. One possible explanation suggests that chronically debilitated patients accept the increased responsibilities since the therapy helps them to feel better. On the other hand, previously healthy patients view the new therapy as a burden that is now imposed on them.

Chronic Radiation Enteritis

Radiation therapy to the abdomen or pelvis for treatment of malignancy may cause significant damage to the gastrointestinal tract, including malabsorption, chronic obstruction, bleeding, fistulas, and steatorrhea. Mild diarrhea during therapy usually subsides rapidly. However, radiation scarring develops months later and may be followed still later by vascular changes including telangiectasias and obliterative endarteritis [44, 48]. Although cured of the malignancy, such patients may be unable to maintain adequate nutrition. In such instances, home parenteral nutrition may be helpful. The OASIS registry identifies 6.1% of patients who receive home parenteral nutrition as having radiation enteritis [33]. Less than 1% of patients receiving home enteral nutrition are in this diagnostic category, attesting to the limited use of defined formula diets in this condition.

Motility Disturbances

Patients with collagen vascular diseases, especially scleroderma, and other hereditary or acquired diseases of intestinal motility may experience intestinal pseudo-obstruction, which results in distension, nausea, vomiting, and resultant fluid and electrolyte disorders. Those patients who are refractory to dietary management, have no evidence of mechanical obstruction, and are unable to maintain nutritional or fluid status may require home parenteral nutrition. Such patients comprise 10.1% of those receiving home parenteral nutrition [33]. Most of such patients require it indefinitely.

Congenital Bowel Defects

Many patients with congenital bowel defects such as atresias and malformations may have malabsorption due to short-bowel syndrome. In treating such patients, home parenteral nutrition may be necessary for variable periods of time. Most of such patients are children. This diagnosis is present in 4.5% of patients receiving home parenteral nutrition. Congenital bowel defects account for 2.3% of those patients receiving home enteral nutrition, accounting for patients with less severe short-bowel syndrome [33].

Chronic Intestinal Obstruction

Patients who have developed extensive or repeated postoperative intestinal obstructions may need to have operative correction delayed due to extensive peritoneal inflammation and nutritional depletion. Such patients who have no vomiting when NPO or who have stable modest gastrostomy drainage and are otherwise doing well may benefit from receiving home parenteral nutrition during the period of waiting, as an alternative to hospitalization. In such cases, the period of therapy is at least 60 to 90 days, following which operative correction may be undertaken. We have had at least one patient who spontaneously resolved his obstruction during home parenteral nutrition therapy and remained cured for more than 2 years. Patients with this diagnosis constituted 3.3% of those receiving home parenteral nutrition [33].

Enterocutaneous and Enteroenteric Fistulas

Home parenteral nutrition may be beneficial to allow spontaneous closure of enterocutaneous fistulas that are the result of operative complications or trauma. Causes of fistula nonclosure must be excluded and fistula output must be stable and of a level that is manageable in terms of fluid and electrolyte replacement [1]. In conditions such as malignancy or inflammatory bowel disease in which spontaneous closure may be unlikely, home parenteral nutrition may be helpful to allow metabolic and nutritional stabilization and repletion prior to operative correction. No percentage of patients in this disease category is listed in the OASIS registry. Such patients constitute less than 1.6% of cases (the lowest disease percentage reported) and are grouped in the classification "Other."

Carefully Selected Patients with Malignancy

Malignancy represents the most frequent diagnosis among patients receiving either home parenteral (24.5%) or enteral (44.0%) nutrition [33]. This diagnostic category has shown a steady rise since 1985 and surpassed Crohn's disease in 1986 [32]. Large- and small-bowel malignancies, genitourinary malignancies, and abdominal malignancies were responsible for the need for home parenteral nutrition in 62% of patients. In contrast to other diagnostic categories, 80% of patients receiving home parenteral nutrition for complications of malignancy have had therapy for less than 12 months. At the end of 1987, approximately 30% of patients receiving home parenteral or enteral nutrition for malignancy remained on therapy, less than 15% resumed oral intake, and the remainder had died [33]. This group was rehospitalized less often than other groups for complications of their home parenteral nutrition, but more often than any other diagnostic groups for complications of their disease. In addition to the relatively short duration of therapy as well as the rapidly rising number of patients receiving home parenteral nutrition for malignancy, there is concern over the stimulation of tumor growth by parenteral nutrition. Several investigators demonstrated stimulation of growth of tumor cells [9, 10, 45], increase in tumor mass [9, 36], or increase in the ratio of tumor mass to host mass in animal models of tumors [9, 36]. Although caution must be observed in extrapolating from animal experiments to humans, there are anecdotal observations of increased tumor growth in humans receiving large amounts of parenteral nutrition.

With this in mind, it has been my practice to be extremely conservative in the use of home parenteral nutrition in patients with malignancy. To avoid the harm of stimulating tumor growth, home parenteral nutrition in patients with malignancy should be part of a program of antitumor therapy. It should be used to help support the patient during a prolonged period of intensive chemotherapy or radiation therapy that results in significant gastrointestinal toxicity. Brief periods of outpatient chemotherapy should be managed by oral supplements or enteral nutrition. In ad-

dition, complications of surgical therapy that require weeks of parenteral nutrition may occasionally be treated in the ambulatory setting. Utilizing these criteria, we have treated very few patients with malignancy with home parenteral nutrition. Most patients with malignancy have done well with alterations in diet, oral supplements, and enteral nutrition at home.

AIDS

Patients with AIDS constituted 1.6% of those receiving home parenteral nutrition and 0.7% of those requiring home enteral nutrition in 1987 [33]. These percentages were little changed from the previous year. However, a greater percentage of patients with AIDS are now receiving enteral rather than parenteral therapy.

Malnutrition frequently accompanies AIDS, although the effect of nutritional restoration on disease outcome is as yet unknown. Oral supplementation and enteral formulas are often effective for supplementation. Patients who have severe diarrhea or intestinal disease, or who receive therapy that renders them unable to take nutrients via the gastrointestinal tract may be candidates for home parenteral nutrition [27, 49]. Patients or their care-givers must be willing to learn procedures and maintain aseptic technique to avoid further complicating the disease by increasing the risk of catheter-related infection. Due to the nature of the disease, the OASIS registry reported no patients receiving therapy for longer than 18 months. Most patients received the therapy for significantly less than 1 year [33].

Other Disorders of Malabsorption or Diarrhea

Occasional patients with disorders other than those just discussed are candidates for home parenteral nutrition. These include patients with sprue, carcinoid tumor, chronic pancreatitis, cystic fibrosis, and graft-versus-host disease secondary to bone marrow transplantation.

DISEASE STATES FOR WHICH HOME PARENTERAL NUTRITION IS USUALLY NOT INDICATED

Home parenteral nutrition generally is not indicated in certain circumstances. There are individual exceptions to such guidelines. However, one must carefully weigh the benefits versus the risks and costs in these situations.

Patients who require extremely complex care and require frequent changes in fluids, electrolytes, and nutrient formulas should be treated in a hospital. Patients whose gastrointestinal tract is functional or will only be unavailable for a few days should receive enteral nutrition support. No benefit of parenteral nutrition over enteral nutrition, when both are satisfactory alternatives, has been observed.

Patients whose disease is untreatable, such as a widely metastatic malignancy, in general are not candidates for home parenteral nutrition. If patients and their families are incapable of managing home parenteral nutrition or are unwilling to do so, therapy should not be started. Finally, whenever the risks of home parenteral nutrition are thought to outweigh its benefits, it should be withheld [4].

PATIENT SELECTION

Selection of patients should be performed in consultation with members of the nutritional support team. The absence of such a multidisciplinary team should be a consideration for referral to a major center having such a team, due to the specialized approach to patients that is necessary for successful home parenteral nutrition programs.

Once the patient has been determined to have a condition or disease for which home parenteral nutrition is appropriate therapy, the individual patient must be evaluated for psychosocial suitability. Patients must have

adequate intelligence to understand and be willing to participate in the program and basic procedures. Literacy is not mandatory if the patient can follow instructions on audiotape. However, the mastery of procedures is facilitated by literacy of the patient or caregiver. Likewise, patients or care-givers need adequate eyesight and manual dexterity to manage infusion pumps, to add selected additives to infusions, to administer set tubing connections, and to care for the catheter. These procedures need to be performed by the patient as much as possible. If the patient is unable to do so, another member of the patient's household may be a suitable substitute. However, the program is usually not as successful if individuals from outside the home are required to perform the procedures.

Financial status should be evaluated thoroughly. Patients and their families should understand the coverage and limitations of their insurance programs. Need for declaration of disability or application for public assistance should be covered in detail if applicable.

As mentioned above, patients who have experienced chronic disease often have better acceptance of the program than those patients who were previously well and have had a catastrophic event. The former patients are willing to accept the changes in life-style in order to feel better. The latter, who have not experienced sequelae of chronic illness, may view the therapy as a burden and intrusion into their daily lives. Education by nutritional support team members and enlistment of the aid of psychologists or psychiatrists can facilitate acceptance [37].

Patients with chronic illness who have abused narcotics or patients who have a history of drug abuse are expected to have problems with compliance. The magnitude of the drug abuse problem should be a major consideration in the decision to use home parenteral nutrition.

Patients with small children may have difficulty adapting to home parenteral nutrition. Such patients may have poor compliance, as the needs of their children may assume primary importance. Compliance may also be low if marital or family problems were present prior to the decision to use parenteral nutrition at home [46].

Home parenteral nutrition requires storage of significant quantities of supplies. Even with careful inventory of supplies and weekly deliveries, storage may be a problem in small apartments or crowded living situations. The nutrition support team or vendor can help patients arrange for minimal disruption. The home environment should also allow easy ambulation of the patient from bedroom to bathroom and living areas during periods of infusion. Stairs and varying floor surfaces may make the maneuvering of the infusion container, pump, and pole difficult.

Every effort is made to make the home parenteral nutrition as small an intrusion into the life-style of the patient as possible. Rehabilitation to the patient's previous vocation and family life is the goal.

VENOUS ACCESS SYSTEMS

Following the decision to initiate home parenteral nutrition, appropriate long-term venous access must be established. The access system should satisfy a number of requirements. Since parenteral nutrition formulas have a high osmolality, the access should allow infusion into a vein where there is a high rate of flow and rapid dilution to avoid phlebitis, pain, and thrombosis of the vein. Such flow rates are achieved only when the tip of the infusion catheter is located in the vena cava, right atrium, or a surgically created arteriovenous shunt similar to that utilized for hemodialysis. In addition, the system should be comfortable and must not limit joint mobility or interfere with normal activity or the ability to exercise. The site of access should allow infusion and maintenance procedures to be performed safely and comfortably under direct vision by the patient. Finally, the access system should minimize the development of infection.

Devices

In their original description of an "artificial gut" system, Scribner et al. [41] suggested the use of an arteriovenous shunt for access to the circulation for infusion of parenteral nutrition. It was believed that infusion of the nutrient solution into the shunt rather than a vein, coupled with the high rate of blood flow through the shunt, would prevent phlebitis and thrombosis [40]. Despite these theoretic advantages, the shunts were difficult to construct in malnourished patients and patients had the complications of thrombosis as well as infection [40]. For these reasons, this technique was abandoned for routine access in parenteral nutrition patients, although shunts or arteriovenous graft fistulas may be of benefit even today in certain patients who have no adequate central venous access or who may require parenteral nutrition for a relatively short time [21].

Tunneled External Catheters

Most catheters currently in use are similar to that described by Broviac et al., later modified by Hickman [8]. Their original right atrial catheter incorporated the subcutaneous tunnel and the Dacron (polyester fiber) tunnel cuff of the Tenckhoff peritoneal dialysis catheter. The subcutaneous tunnel allowed for separation of the site of vein entry from the site of skin exit. In addition to the tunnel, the Dacron cuff allowed ingrowth of fibrous tissue to serve both as a means of anchoring the catheter and as a barrier to infection ascending the tunnel from the skin site. Initial catheters were associated with thrombosis of the vena cava due to the stiffness of the catheter itself. Silicone rubber proved to be pliable enough to prevent such complications. The Hickman 9.6-French catheter, an enlarged version of the Broviac 6.6-French catheter, was subsequently developed to allow easier infusion of blood products and withdrawal of blood for laboratory sampling [23]. Experience has shown these catheters to be safe and effective means of long-term venous access for administering parenteral nutrition [18, 19, 39].

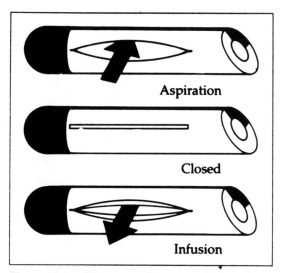

Figure 23-2. Diagrammatic representation of the Groshong three-position valve, which requires active aspiration or infusion to open the valve. (Reprinted with permission from Davol, Inc., Cranston, RI.)

Most long-term central venous catheters used for parenteral nutrition share the common features of tip placement in the superior vena cava or proximal part of the right atrium, a Dacron cuff for anchoring and a barrier against infection, and a subcutaneous tunnel that separates the skin wound from the point of catheter entry into the vein. A recent modification involves the construction of a rounded, blunt catheter tip that incorporates a three-way valve. The Groshong catheter (C. R. Bard, Inc.) utilizes a three-position pressure-sensitive valve (Fig. 23-2) that remains closed at normal vena caval pressure, thereby restricting either entrainment of air into the venous system or backflow of blood from the catheter. Application of vacuum with a syringe allows the valve to open inward for blood aspiration. Positive pressure into the catheter by the infusion forces the valve to open outward. Theoretic advantages of this type of catheter include:

1. Decreased risk of bleeding or air embolization.

2. Resultant elimination of catheter clamping.
3. Use of heparin in the catheter irrigant is unnecessary.
4. Reduced requirement for irrigation between uses.

However, position of the catheter tip is critical for proper function of the valve. The tip must be situated in the midsuperior part of the vena cava [30]. Position of the tip in the right atrium may result in thrombus formation around the catheter tip, which may cause malfunction and loss of competence of the valve. Such malfunction may result in the backflow of blood or air entrainment. Occasionally, use of a thrombolytic agent may restore valve function. If not, the patient needs to initiate clamping and irrigation with heparin similar to that which is required to maintain nonvalved catheters.

Subcutaneous Infusion Ports

Early in the 1980s, subcutaneous infusion ports were introduced to provide venous access, primarily for intermittent infusions in patients with cancer. Such a system generally utilizes a silicone rubber catheter whose tip is positioned in the superior vena cava or proximal part of the right atrium and whose opposite end terminates in a reservoir or port with a self-sealing silicon rubber diaphragm. The port may be constructed of stainless steel, titanium, or plastic, and comes in a variety of configurations including single- and double-lumen devices. The catheter may be preattached to the port or attachment may be performed by the surgeon at the time of implantation. Access to the central venous system is obtained by percutaneous cannulation of the port through its diaphragm.

The major advantage of the system is that it is totally implanted. Whereas tunneled catheters require the maintenance of a sterile, occlusive dressing at the exit site, subcutaneous infusion ports require no dressing. Intermittent violation of the skin theoretically carries a lower risk of infection. In addition, they require less frequent irrigation than do tunneled catheters. Initial experience in cancer patients involved access to the ports by professional staff in an outpatient clinical setting at intervals of a week or longer [6, 7, 31]. Transfer of this technology to patients receiving parenteral nutrition at home has been slow, probably due to concern over the ability of patients to perform the daily needle entry without introduction of infection or injury to the skin or port diaphragm. Recent experience indicates that the subcutaneous infusion port is an acceptable alternative to tunneled external catheters and may even be superior in certain patients [5, 24, 35, 52].

Choice of Access System

Howard et al. [24] reviewed 5 years' experience with both implanted reservoirs and external catheters in 58 patients who were involved in selection of their access systems. Those patients who had subcutaneous ports had significantly fewer complications than did those patients who had external catheters. However, this may have been due to patient factors such as motivation and procedure competence. Further analysis of patients who had experienced both systems indicated that patients who experienced complications with one system tended likewise to experience complications with the other. Similarly, patients who did well had few complications with either system. In their experience, 80% of patients who had used both systems preferred the port.

In general, the subcutaneous port system should be offered to patients about to begin home parenteral nutrition. Such a system may allow a more active life-style and greater rehabilitation. For patients who have experienced problems with devices already or who are reluctant to attempt nightly percutaneous access, the external catheter is preferred.

Techniques of Insertion

Tunneled External Catheters
Early descriptions of the method of catheter placement recommended use of cephalic or jugular vein cutdown with selection of a catheter exit site over the sternum or on the ipsilateral side of the chest [22]. In patients treated at University of Cincinnati Medical Center, we have avoided the use of cephalic vein cutdown in the deltopectoral groove because: (1) Patients are likely to receive parenteral nutrition for prolonged periods and will likely require more than one catheter. (2) Once utilized, the cephalic vein cannot be reused through the same wound. We utilized two alternative approaches, both of which allow subsequent catheters to be replaced via the original wound. The first uses small branches of the axillary vein through an axillary approach. The second involves introduction of a percutaneous catheter using a peelaway introducer. The former is suitable for external catheters only, while the latter is suitable for implantation of both ports and external catheters.

The chest as a site for catheter exit has been abandoned. We prefer the ipsilateral upper quadrant of the abdomen (Fig. 23-3) for several reasons:

1. It is more easily accessible under direct vision for self-care.
2. It facilitates maintenance of an occlusive dressing, especially in women with large breasts.
3. It interferes less with sexual intimacy.

Such considerations are less important when considering access for chronically or terminally ill patients than they are for home parenteral nutrition patients who are rehabilitated to resume normal daily activities.

Use of Branches of the Axillary Vein
The patient is positioned supine with the arm abducted and a cloth roll elevating the axilla 10 to 15 degrees. The procedure may be performed under general or local anesthesia. An incision is made in the anterior axillary fold, parallel to and slightly behind the lateral border of the pectoralis major muscle (Fig. 23-4). The axillary vein and its branches are identified. The distal end of the vein branch is li-

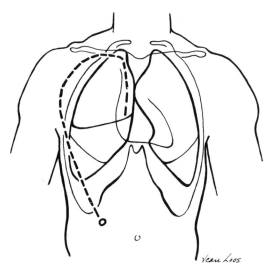

Figure 23-3. Position of the tunneled right atrial catheter inserted via the right subclavian vein. Placement of the catheter exit site in the right upper quadrant of the abdomen facilitates self-care. (From Freund, H. R., Benson, D. W., Bower, R. H., and Fischer, J. E. Enteral and parenteral nutrition. In F. G. Moody, L. C. Carey, R. S. Jones, K. A. Kelly, D. L. Nahrwold, and D. B. Skinner (eds.), *Surgical Treatment of Digestive Disease* (2nd ed.). Chicago: Year Book Medical, 1990. P. 864. Reprinted with permission.)

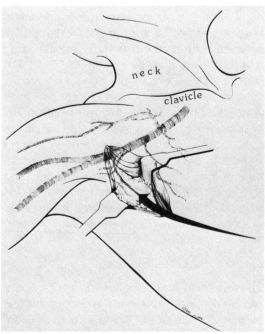

Figure 23-4. Incision and operative exposure of branches of the right axillary vein. (From Freund, H. R., Benson, D. W., Bower, R. H., and Fischer, J. E. Enteral and parenteral nutrition. In F. G. Moody, L. C. Carey, R. S. Jones, K. A. Kelly, D. L. Nahrwold, and D. B. Skinner (eds.), *Surgical Treatment of Digestive Disease* (2nd ed.). Chicago: Year Book Medical, 1990. P. 864. Reprinted with permission.)

gated and the proximal end is encircled. Next, the exit site previously selected and marked on the upper quadrant of the abdomen is incised transversely to allow passage of a long alligator forceps subcutaneously from the exit site into the axillary wound. A No. 2 silk suture is drawn with the forceps from the axillary wound out the exit site and tied to the catheter tip, which is then pulled into the axillary wound a sufficient length to seat the Dacron cuff in the subcutaneous tunnel 1 to 2 cm from the exit site. The distance from the site of venotomy to the superior vena cava is estimated and the catheter tip trimmed at an oblique angle accordingly. A transverse venotomy is made in the vein branch, following which the previously flushed catheter is threaded into the superior vena cava and its position confirmed by fluoroscopy (Fig. 23-5A, B). The proximal suture is then tied, taking care not to compromise

the catheter lumen (Fig. 23-5C). The wound is closed in layers. A running subcuticular absorbable suture and Steri-strips complete the skin closure. A 5-0 stainless-steel suture at the exit site anchors the catheter for at least 2 weeks until fibrous ingrowth at the subcutaneous cuff has occurred. The exit site is dressed with a standard occlusive central venous catheter dressing supplied in a kit designed by the nutrition support team to comply with patient procedures.

Some modification of this procedure is necessary if the Groshong valved catheter is used rather than the Hickman-type catheter. The Groshong catheter's valve prevents trimming the tip to achieve proper length. Thus, the catheter is first threaded into the superior vena cava and confirmed fluoroscopically. The catheter is then tunneled to the exit site

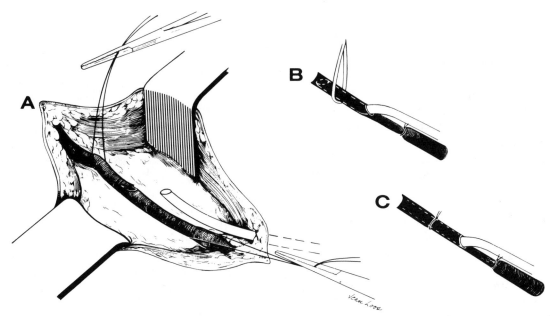

Figure 23-5. *A*, Pectoral branch of the right axillary vein is controlled proximally and distally, following which a transverse venotomy is made. *B*, The catheter tip is introduced into the venotomy. *C*, Following fluoroscopic confirmation of proper position of the tip, the catheter is tied in place.

with the tunneling device provided, following which the external end of the catheter is trimmed to length and the hub attached [30]. However, the extra-long length of the Groshong catheter is frequently too short to reach the upper quadrant of the abdomen.

Percutaneous Catheter Insertion

Prior to this procedure, patients should be adequately hydrated and have normal coagulability. The patient is in Trendelenberg position with a cloth roll placed beneath the thoracic spine to allow the shoulders to drop back. The procedure is usually performed under local anesthesia with intravenous sedation. The subclavian vein or internal jugular vein is cannulated with an 18-gauge needle provided in the introducer kit. Observing air embolism precautions, the angiography guidewire is threaded into the vena cava and confirmed by fluoroscopy. The needle is withdrawn and a 1.0- to 1.5-cm skin incision is made from the site of wire entry laterally. The 9.6-French Hickman catheter is then tunneled as described previously so that the tip

exits lateral to the guidewire. The catheter is then trimmed to the appropriate length and irrigated. The vein dilator and peel-away introducer sheath are then threaded over the guidewire as a unit and confirmed fluoroscopically to lie within the superior vena cava. While air embolism precautions are observed, the wire and dilator are withdrawn from the introducer sheath and the catheter tip is threaded into the introducer. The catheter should be threaded fully into the introducer. The two halves of the introducer are then distracted and peeled away while the catheter is held in place. Occasionally, resistance is encountered if the introducer bends passing beneath the clavicle. In such case it will be difficult to thread the soft catheter. The catheter should be advanced until it can be advanced no further. The introducer should then be peeled away slowly in 5-mm increments until the catheter threads easily. The wound is closed, and the catheter is secured and dressed as previously described. The procedure is modified for the use of the Groshong catheter, as described above.

Following insertion by either technique, the catheter should be irrigated with sodium heparin (10 U/ml) and gradually clamped while actively irrigating. A volume equal to approximately 0.5 ml greater than the capacity of the catheter should be used. The cap may then be applied to the catheter and the clamp opened. Neither heparinized solution nor clamping is required when irrigating and capping valved catheters. The catheters may be used for infusion immediately if needed.

Implantation of Subcutaneous Ports

Subcutaneous ports have several advantages for patients receiving home parenteral nutrition. They require neither dressings nor maintenance between infusions; they are totally implanted, allowing bathing and swimming; and they may be less likely to become infected since they do not traverse the skin. The disadvantage centers around the difficulty and discomfort of needle cannulation prior to each infusion.

Choice of port involves consideration of surgeon preference, other intravenous infusions, and probable need for future radiographic studies. Valved and nonvalved port catheters are available, depending on the preference of the implanting surgeon and the nutrition support service. Dual-lumen ports are available for patients who require frequent prolonged infusions of medication in addition to parenteral nutrition. Such infusions, if given through a single-lumen port before or after parenteral nutrition, may extend the period of daily infusion to unacceptable lengths. In such cases a dual-lumen port is an option, although the devices are considerably larger than single-lumen ports. Finally, titanium ports cause less artifact on radiographic and MRI studies than do stainless-steel ports. This artifact can be reduced to almost negligible levels if plastic ports are used rather than titanium. No differences in infection rate or useful life have been reported based on material used for construction.

The same precautions of hydration, posi-

tioning, anesthesia, and sedation are observed for subcutaneous port placement as those described for percutaneous catheter insertion. The usual approach is percutaneous cannulation of the subclavian vein or, less often, cutdown of the cephalic vein since venous access and port implantation can be accomplished through a single skin incision. Percutaneous cannulation of the internal jugular vein may also be used, although it requires a small additional incision over the vein and tunneling of the catheter to the port implantation site, which is generally on the upper part of the chest beneath the clavicle near the deltopectoral groove. Pectoral branches of the axillary vein may be used, although this approach is generally less satisfactory since it requires two working incisions, one for the cutdown and one for the port.

The subclavian vein is cannulated with an 18-gauge needle following adequate infiltration of the skin and subcutaneous tissue with local anesthetic. While air embolism precautions are observed, the angiography guidewire is threaded into the vena cava and confirmed by fluoroscopy. If cannulation is unsuccessful, the internal jugular vein or contralateral veins may be cannulated. Confirmation of appropriate guidewire position prior to the creation of a subcutaneous pocket for the port prevents the unnecessary creation of a pocket at a site where venous cannulation was impossible.

The subcutaneous port pocket is then created. In general, the incision is placed so that the port pocket is inferior to the incision and the site of port cannulation is separated from the incision by a few centimeters. The procedure is facilitated by including the guidewire entrance wound as the medial end of the incision. Doing so allows proximity of the venipuncture site and the port pocket without a long subcutaneous tunnel. The pocket is created by sharp and blunt dissection within the subcutaneous tissue, taking care to make the overlying tissue sufficiently thin to allow easy palpation of the port. The pocket should be sufficiently large to accommodate the port and allow closure of the skin wound without tension. However, the pocket should not be excessively large since rotation of the device or migration can result. Hemostasis must be complete.

Following creation of the subcutaneous pocket, the dilator and percutaneous introducer are inserted as a unit over the guidewire until fully inserted. Their position within the vena cava should be confirmed by fluoroscopy and the guidewire should slide back and forth easily within the lumen of the dilator. The port and catheter should be flushed with saline solution and cleared of all air. The preattached port and catheter should be trimmed to the appropriate length to allow the tip to be in the superior vena cava. Catheters that are not attached to the port should be clamped at the end opposite the tip after flushing. While air embolism precautions are observed, the dilator and guidewire are removed as a unit, following which the port catheter tip is inserted into the introducer and threaded into position in the vena cava. Position is confirmed fluoroscopically and the introducer is peeled away as it is withdrawn.

If the port and catheter were preattached, the port is then inserted into the pocket. If a nonattached system is used, the catheter must be trimmed to a length that allows easy attachment to the port while the catheter remains clamped on the venous side until attachment is complete. The procedure for attachment differs among manufacturers.

To anchor the port in the pocket, manual pressure is used to hold the port deep in its pocket while the diaphragm is entered percutaneously with the Huber needle. This maneuver both holds the port in its pocket during suturing and allows confirmation of proper functioning by both aspirating and infusing. Sutures should anchor the port to the underlying tissue in at least two separate places. The subcutaneous tissue is approximated, following which the skin is closed with a running subcuticular absorbable closure followed by Steri-strips.

The port is then irrigated with approximately 5 ml of heparin, 100 U/ml. To avoid

subsequent thrombosis of the port, the Huber needle is withdrawn rapidly while the last half milliliter of heparin is infused. A sterile occlusive dressing is maintained for 24 hours.

The subcutaneous port access system may be used immediately if necessary. However, there may be less discomfort if the first use is delayed for 48 to 96 hours postoperatively. Brothers et al. [7] noted a higher incidence of complications if the first use of the port occurred 5 or more days postoperatively than if ports were used within the first 4 days.

Placement of the port at a site on the upper part of the chest may necessitate the use of a mirror for the patient to access the port. When this is necessary, the patient may identify the outline of the port more readily by applying gentle traction to the skin adjacent to the subcutaneous port. Such traction causes the metallic portion of the port to blanche the skin overlying it while the skin over the port entry retains its natural color. The effect is one of a "bull's-eye," which allows for easier access.

Subsequent entries into the port should be performed at different skin sites around the port diaphragm. Such rotation helps to avoid excessive trauma to one area of skin. In theory, the septum should withstand approximately 5 years of nightly access with the 22-gauge huber needle [24]. If leakage occurs, a new port may be attached to an existing catheter.

Rarely, patients will need venous access by routes other than the jugular or subclavian veins. Long-term catheterization may lead to thromboses of the aforementioned veins and the superior vena cava. Patients who have patent veins in the lower extremity may have the catheter placed in the inferior vena cava just below the right atrium by means of a saphenous vein cutdown in the groin. The catheter exit site we have used is the lower abdomen, although exit sites in the thigh have been reported [46, 50]. In one such patient treated at University of Cincinnati Hospital, thrombosis of a renal vein developed. Although the thrombosis was not proved to be caused by inferior vena caval catheter placement, it was temporally related.

Patients in whom upper and lower extremity venous access is exhausted may have catheters placed directly into the right atrium by means of a limited thoracotomy [34]. One of our patients required removal of such a catheter, which was accomplished by traction with thoracotomy. No complications resulted. He subsequently underwent placement of a second right atrial catheter by limited thoracotomy.

Contrast venography is particularly helpful in planning the operative approach in patients with limited access. It should be performed before any such procedure to help develop the operative plan and alternative plans. Since thrombosed veins recannulize over time, obtaining a contrast study prior to a major operation for access may demonstrate an easily accessible vessel that had previously been thrombosed.

FORMULA SELECTION AND PREPARATION

The patient's daily infusion is formulated to provide amino acids in balanced mixture to meet daily protein needs; adequate substrate as dextrose and lipid emulsion to meet daily energy needs; maintenance plus replacement fluid; and electrolytes, vitamins, and trace elements.

Formulations differ little from those used for hospitalized patients. Modified amino acid formulas are rarely necessary, but may be needed in patients with altered protein or fluid requirements due to cardiac or renal insufficiency. Substrate is mixed using both dextrose and lipid emulsion as total nutrient admixture (TNA) when feasible [2, 12, 13]. Advantages to such a system are many. It is easier for home use and allows all components of the mixture to be infused simultaneously with one infusion pump. A stability of 4 to 7 days allows larger volumes to be premixed and stored. Disadvantages include difficulty visualizing particulate matter and inability to filter the final infusion. Of greatest concern is the limitation on addition of certain minerals or amino acid mixtures to avoid damage to the emulsion. Patients with large electrolyte, mineral, or fluid requirements may need to receive the lipid infusion sequentially, extending the infusion period but allowing the use of one pump; or simultaneous infusion of separate units of lipid by means of a Y-connector using two pumps or by means of simultaneous infusion using both lumina of a two-lumen catheter and two pumps.

The formula is prepared by the home care vendor and delivered to the patient in weekly quantities. Despite early enthusiasm for teaching patients to compound their own formulation [46], few patients continue to do so. The original impetus for such a system was cost savings. However, current practices of home care vendors compounding for many patients in a geographic area have allowed for cost reductions. Disadvantages of such a system include the need for extensive storage space within the home, a dedicated clean area where compounding takes place, a large commitment of time, and meticulous technique to avoid errors or microbial contamination. Premixture of formulations requires less storage space, greater freedom of the patient and time for rehabilitation, and better quality control of the final product. Patients need only be taught to add selected nutrients or insulin that may be unstable in formulations stored for 1 week.

ADMINISTRATION

Although early systems of home parenteral nutrition were continuous, most patients now utilize a system of nocturnal infusion usually over a 12-hour period. This allows the majority of the infusion period to occur during sleep. The patient is disconnected from the infusion apparatus during the other 12 hours, allowing mobility for rehabilitation, return to vocation, and a life-style that is more nearly normal.

The infusion is administered by battery-powered infusion pump. Infusion devices for home patients need to have additional safety features, alarms, and programming, which might be considered unnecessary in hospital settings but is appropriate for infusion during sleep without the attendance of professional medical personnel. To allow accommodation to the large dextrose load, infusion is initiated at 60 ml/hr for 1 hour (see Appendix). At the beginning of the second hour, the infusion rate is increased to 200 ml/hr for 9 hours, in the case of a typical 1980-ml infusion. The final 2 hours include 1 hour at 80 ml/hr and a final hour of 40 ml/hr. Tapering the infusion prevents hypoglycemia or a rapid fall in blood glucose that may produce unpleasant symptoms for the patient. Certain pumps now commercially available allow programming of a gradual initial increase in rate followed by a final tapering of the rate without a manual change, simplifying the infusion procedure and minimizing patient sleep disruption.

All procedures involving catheter connections to administration tubing and care of the catheter site are performed using aseptic technique, masks, sterile gloves, and a sterile field. Even after healing of the catheter exit site has occurred, sterile techniques continues to be required (see Appendix).

Patient Training

Procedures specific to each patient's individual infusion equipment, rates of infusion, supplies, and handedness are prepared (see Appendix). Patient training is accomplished as a collaborative effort among the nurses of the nutrition support team, the nurse of the home care vendor company, and the nurses caring for the patient in the hospital if such is the case. At each session of infusion administration, the procedures are read as written and aloud, explaining as an analogy of the airline pilot's use of a checklist. The first phase of training is observation. During this phase, the patient observes the nurse per-forming the procedures while they are read aloud. When the patient indicates comprehension, the second phase, supervision, is begun. During this phase the patient performs the procedures under the supervision of nursing personnel. Breaks in technique thus can be caught and corrected. Once mastery has been demonstrated, the patient progresses to the phase of independence, during which procedures are performed with the patient reading all procedures and performing them without supervision. If additional family members are to assist with care, all are required to participate in all phases of training.

Emergency procedures taught include the management of damaged or ruptured catheters. Patients are instructed in techniques of clamping and occlusion. Proper application of these techniques appears not to lead to increased incidence of sepsis [29]. Repair is carried out by trained personnel usually in the Emergency Department.

If the patient is hospitalized prior to the transition to home parenteral nutrition, teaching is carried out in the hospital as soon as the patient is sufficiently alert and able to receive instruction. Occasionally, the decision to initiate home parenteral nutrition is made while the patient is being cared for in the outpatient setting. Teaching can be accomplished in the home with minimal hospitalization if patients are properly motivated and there is cooperation with the home care vendor. Sterile technique and gloving may be taught prior to implantation of the venous access device. Likewise, catheter care may be taught prior to catheter or port implantation, but mock catheter teaching aids may be necessary. Implantation may then be undertaken on an outpatient basis, following which catheter care procedures may be resumed. The length of time required for adequate training varies with the patient. It rarely takes less than a week to train patients adequately. Most patients will achieve competence within 7 to 14 days.

The initial infusions of the nutrient solutions are generally best accomplished in a hospital. Blood glucose levels during and following infusion can be monitored, as can electrolyte levels and tolerance to fluid. To monitor fluid changes at home, patients are trained to record weight, intake and output, temperature, urine glucose determinations, and other pertinent events in a clinical diary on a daily basis. The diary is helpful in dealing with difficulties in the home, either by telephone or in the physician's office.

MONITORING

Monitoring consists of clinical observations and laboratory measurements. Home clinical self-monitoring is accomplished by means of the diary. In addition to the recording of values, patients are trained to call the physician's office for abnormalities. Urine outputs below 600 ml for 2 days prompt the patient to notify the physician. Similarly, excessive urine output or weight gain is cause for notification, and may require reduction in infused volume or reformulation. Slow chronic weight gain may indicate adaptation and require a consequent reduction in calories. Urine glucose levels are monitored. If patients spill 1+ or 2+ transiently during their infusion, it is usually known from in-hospital monitoring prior to dismissal. Blood sugar levels are checked to determine the renal threshold. Subsequent glycosuria above the patient's usual level is reported to the physician. In addition, fever, chills, and sweats are reported as possible indicators of catheter-associated sepsis or infection related to the underlying disease. Nausea, vomiting, muscle weakness, tingling, symptoms of neuropathy, or other untoward events are reported.

Laboratory monitoring may be accomplished in the home by certain home care vendors, at a clinic near the patient's home, or at the physician's office. Visits with laboratory monitoring typically occur weekly for the first month, then every 2 weeks for the next month. Determinations may then be performed monthly or bimonthly if the pa-

tient's status is stable. Patients who have been stable for many months need determinations only approximately every 3 months. Parameters measured include complete blood count, prothrombin time, liver enzyme function, and levels of electrolytes, glucose, BUN, creatinine, cholesterol, triglycerides, uric acid, calcium, phosphorus, magnesium, albumin, transferrin, prealbumin, and retinol-binding protein. Trace element levels and vitamin levels may be checked yearly, but clinical monitoring for deficiency syndromes occurs at each visit.

COMPLICATIONS

Catheter Complications

Catheter-associated sepsis is the most common catheter complication and the most common home parenteral nutrition complication necessitating rehospitalization [33], representing 54% of such hospitalizations. Percentages of patients developing sepsis were highest in those with congenital bowel disease (36%), presumably due to the greater incidence of sepsis in children, patients with motility disorders (26%), and those with ischemic bowel disease (25%). Figures for 1986 had indicated an increase in the number of infections in patients whose indication was neoplasm; however, 1987 figures returned to the 1985 levels (9%). Current statistics indicate a rise in rates of catheter-related sepsis overall in nearly all age groups and disease categories. Our own results indicate a catheter life of approximately 7 years and increasing. Catheters are being changed more often for material fatigue than for sepsis.

The best treatment of catheter-related sepsis is prevention. Proper teaching, reinforcement of aseptic technique, and prompt recognition of problems are essential. When sepsis occurs, it is generally caused by gram-positive organisms, especially *Staphylococcus epidermidis* or *Staphylococcus aureus*, or by *Candida* species. In the presence of florid sepsis or hemodynamic instability, immediate removal of the catheter is mandatory. Symptoms and signs of sepsis often resolve with institution of appropriate antibiotics. Antibiotics alone, however, rarely obliterate but merely mask the catheter-related infection. Such failure of antibiotics alone may be due to failure to clear an infected thrombus or fibrin sheet surrounding the catheter [47]. Use of thrombolytic agents to treat catheter-related infection has met with variable results [11, 16, 20]. We have now successfully treated five patients using a combination of antibiotics and systemic thrombolytic therapy [28]. Such therapy should be reserved for patients with limited access and infections that respond promptly to antibiotic therapy.

Catheter thrombosis occurs with variable frequency. Occlusion secondary to a clot or failure to be able to withdraw blood due to a fibrin or clot "ball-valve" may be treated with low-dose thrombolytic therapy. The catheter volume is measured or estimated. Urokinase solution, 5000 U/ml, is injected in volume equal to the catheter volume, following which the catheter is clamped. If such instillation does not open the catheter after 30 minutes, it may be repeated [15]. Very small syringes and excessive pressure should be avoided since high pressure may rupture the catheter above the occlusion. Occlusions caused by precipitation of minerals or incompatible drugs will not be cleared by urokinase and may require catheter replacement.

Catheter occlusion has been rare in our series of home patients. One possible explanation is that our patients are instructed to clamp catheters slowly while actively infusing the heparinized saline flush. By so doing, rather than clamping after the flush is completed, the clamping causes less aspiration of blood at the catheter tip and may result in a lower incidence of thrombosis. Similarly, infusion of irrigant actively while withdrawing the port needle may reduce the incidence of port thrombosis.

Catheter injury or breakage may be repaired, as described above, both temporarily and permanently. Catheters so repaired function well for indefinite periods.

Metabolic Complications

Patients receiving home parenteral nutrition may experience any or all of the metabolic complications of deficiency states or disorders of glucose metabolism that can occur with hospitalized patients receiving parenteral nutrition.

Problems unique to receiving nutrient needs entirely by vein include vitamin and trace element deficiencies. These can be evaluated by serum levels and by clinical observation for signs and symptoms of deficiency. They are best treated by prevention through providing adequate replacement from the beginning of therapy.

A metabolic bone disease has been reported in patients receiving long-term parenteral nutrition [26, 42]. Features of this disorder included increased serum calcium levels, excessive losses of calcium and phosphorus in the urine, low normal plasma levels of parathyroid hormone (PTH), and low plasma levels of 1,25-dihydroxyvitamin D. These and further studies [43] demonstrated fundamental abnormalities of bone remodeling with varied manifestations. Severe osteopenia has been observed in patients although fractures were uncommon and bone pain was mild to moderate. The significance of the condition, its exact cause, and treatment are unclear, although it is likely multifactorial.

COST

The cost of home parenteral nutrition must be considered in the light of cost of therapy, cost of home therapy versus hospital inpatient therapy, and reversal of disability with return to meaningful life. Many of the figures necessary to determine the above costs are difficult to derive.

Figures from Blue Cross/Blue Shield of South Carolina Medicare Part B indicate allowed parenteral charges for 1987 to be $100,110,476. It is estimated that this carrier processed 70% of Medicare Part B claims. Thus, the total estimated allowable charges for Medicare equal $143 million. Assuming that Medicare represented 30% of total national payments, the total national home parenteral nutrition expenditure is an estimated $480 million. Using the same assumptions, it is estimated that 17,300 persons receive home parenteral nutrition. Simple division, assuming equal therapy in all patients, yields an average $27,500/patient [33].

For 1987, 38% of patients were not readmitted to a hospital. Of the 2026 total rehospitalizations, 44% were due to complications of home parenteral nutrition, 43.4% were due to the primary disease process, and 12.7% were for other reasons [33].

The same report indicates that the degree of rehabilitation of patients is related primarily to the primary diagnosis. Most patients with benign disorders experienced complete or partial rehabilitation, while most patients with malignancy or AIDS achieved only partial remission [33]. Disability and employment figures remain difficult to assess since disability from healthy conditions is relatively common in the United States. Likewise, patients able and willing to work may be denied employment due to the potential negative impact their therapy may have on the company's health insurance costs. Others may remain unemployed because they must remain "totally disabled" to retain Medicare coverage. Many home care vendors now employ teams of reimbursement specialists who are able to help obtain or retain benefits while allowing patients to lead a productive life.

APPENDIX

University Surgical Associates of Cincinnati Nutritional Support Home Division

Start procedure—Hickman catheter

1. Clean table with alcohol, put on mask, and wash hands.
2. Open start kit, creating sterile field.
3. Remove tape anchoring catheter to dressing.
4. Open sterile towel and place on lap.
5. Remove tape covering catheter junction and drop junction onto sterile towel without touching junction.
6. Put on gloves and open iodine swabs and two gauze pads.
7. Pick up catheter on ridge and cleanse junction with iodine swab for 15 seconds; let junction dry for 2 minutes in fold of gauze pad.
8. Clamp catheter.
9. Untwist catheter cap and discard. Do not set catheter down.
10. Remove cover from filter tubing.
11. Check for air in end of tubing.
12. Unclamp catheter.
13. Insert tubing into catheter, twisting securely for a tight fit.
14. Cleanse junction with iodine swab for 15 seconds; let junction dry for 2 minutes in fold of gauze pad.
15. Turn on pump, set rate and volume to be infused, and push start button.
16. Check screen to be sure pump is actually infusing.
17. Remove gloves.
18. Prepare two strips of tape and tab ends. Tape catheter junction crosswise; then place catheter along length of tape and pinch closed. Do not touch adhesive back of tape.
19. Reanchor catheter to skin.

Dressing change procedure

1. Clean table with alcohol, put on mask, and wash hands.
2. Open dressing kit, creating a sterile field.
3. Remove tape anchoring catheter to dressing, and at bottom of dressing.
4. Remove dressing, starting at bottom and pulling up gently.
5. Put on gloves, then open alcohol and iodine swabs.
6. Cleanse skin with each alcohol swab; start in center at catheter and move in a circle out beyond area dressing will cover. Let dry.
7. Now cleanse with each iodine swab; start in center at catheter and move in a circle out beyond area dressing will cover. Let air-dry for 2 minutes.

8. Put ointment on center of 2 × 2 inches gauze and place over catheter site.
9. Take window off Tegaderm transparent dressing and remove backing; center over catheter site; and apply, starting at center and moving out, first to one side, then to the other. Now remove paper border.
10. Remove gloves.
11. Take strip of tape and slit to the center; place it under catheter, at lower edge of dressing. Do not touch back of tape.
12. Take another strip of tape and place over the slit and catheter.
13. Using long strip of tape, make a "loop."
14. Anchor catheter to dressing. Remember "tape on tape" only.

Stop procedure—Hickman catheter

1. Clean table with alcohol, put on mask, and wash hands.
2. Open package; remove and open kit, creating a sterile field.
3. Prepare heparin syringe by removing clear cap, insert plunger rod, and twist. Remove blue cap and push plunger gently until heparin comes out tip of syringe. Expel all air. (5 ml of 100-U/ml heparin)
4. Place syringe tip inward on sterile field.
5. Remove tape anchoring catheter to dressing.
6. Open sterile towel and place on lap.
7. Remove tape covering catheter junction and drop junction onto sterile towel without touching junction.
8. Put on gloves and open iodine swabs and gauze pads. Stand Luer-lock cap up on gauze pad for stability and remove cap cover. Do not touch inside of cap.
9. Prepare two short strips of tape and tab ends. Place adhesive side up on sterile field.
10. Pick up catheter on ridge and cleanse junction with iodine swab for 15 seconds; let junction dry for 2 minutes in fold of gauze pad.
11. Clamp catheter and immediately turn off pump.
12. Check to make certain clamp is secure.

Grasp catheter on the ridge (do not set catheter down), remove tubing by untwisting, and discard.
13. Pick up syringe and fill cap with heparin. Re-check to make sure all air has been removed from syringe and attach syringe to catheter, twisting securely for a tight fit.
14. Gently begin injecting heparin and immediately unclamp catheter. After 3 ml is injected, and before syringe is empty, clamp catheter while still pushing forward on plunger.
15. Untwist syringe and discard.
16. Pick up heparin-filled cap; do not touch inside of cap.
17. Place catheter into cap and screw cap on for a tight fit.
18. Unclamp catheter.
19. Cleanse junction with iodine swab for 15 seconds; let junction dry for 2 minutes in fold of gauze pad.
20. Tape catheter junction crosswise; then place catheter junction into center of tape, fold tape over end, and pinch closed to completely cover tubing. Do not touch adhesive back of tape.
21. Reanchor catheter to skin.
22. Record volume infused in daily diary. Zero the pump: (1) Turn on pump; (2) set rate and volume to be infused to zero; (3) push volume infused button. Turn off pump.

REFERENCES

1. Aguirre, A., and Fischer, J. E. Intestinal fistulas. In J. E. Fischer (ed.), *Total Parenteral Nutrition* (1st ed.). Boston: Little, Brown, 1976, P. 203.
2. Albrecht, J., Camson, S., and Elias, J. Total parenteral nutrient admixtures (3-in-1 or all-in-one solutions). In J. Rombeau, M. Caldwell, L. Forlaw, and P. Guenter (eds.), *Atlas of Nutritional Support Techniques*. Boston: Little, Brown, 1989, P. 306.
3. American Society for Parenteral and Enteral Nutrition. Standards for home nutrition support. *Nutr. Clin. Pract.* 3:202, 1988.
4. American Society for Parenteral and Enteral Nutrition Board of Directors. Guidelines for use of home total parenteral nutrition. *J. Parenter. Enter. Nutr.* 11:342, 1987.

5. Beck, S. L., Rose, N. R., and Zagoren, A. J. Home total parenteral nutrition utilizing implantable infusion ports: A retrospective review. *Nutr. Clin. Pract.* 2:26, 1987.

6. Bothe, A., Piccione, W., Ambrosino, J. J., Benotti, P. N., and Lokich, J. J. Implantable central venous access system. *Am. J. Surg.* 147:565, 1984.

7. Brothers, T. E., Von Moll, L. K., Niederhuber, J. E., Roberts, J. A., Walker-Andrews, S., and Ensminger, W. D. Experience with subcutaneous infusion ports in three hundred patients. *Surg. Gynecol. Obstet.* 166:295, 1988.

8. Broviac, J. W., Cole, J. J., and Scribner, B. H. A silicone rubber right atrial catheter for prolonged parenteral alimentation. *Surg. Gynecol. Obstet.* 136:602, 1973.

9. Cameron, I. L. Effect of total parenteral nutrition on tumor-host responses in rats. *Cancer Treat. Rep.* 65(Suppl.):93, 1981.

10. Cameron, I. L., and Pavlat, W. A. Stimulation of growth of a transplantable hepatoma in rats by parenteral nutrition. *J. Natl. Cancer Inst.* 56:597, 1976.

11. Curnow, A., Idowu, J., Behrens, E., Toomey, F., and Georgeson, K. Urokinase therapy for Silastic catheter-induced intravascular thrombi in infants and children. *Arch. Surg.* 120:1237, 1985.

12. Deitel, M. Total nutrient admixtures: An NSS symposium in three parts. *Nutr. Supp. Serv.* 7(10):14, 7(12):11, 1987; 8(1):22, 1988.

13. Flaatelen, H. Long-term parenteral nutrition using a mixture of fat, amino acids and carbohydrates in a single three-litre bag. *Acta Anaesthesiol. Scand.* 29:81, 1985.

14. Fleming, C. R., Beart, R. W., Jr., Berkner, S., McGill, D. B., and Gaffron, R. Home parenteral nutrition for management of the severely malnourished adult patient. *Gastroenterology* 79:11, 1980.

15. Forlaw, L. Clearing obstructed Broviac/Hickman catheters in adult patients. In J. Rombeau, M. Caldwell, L. Forlaw, and P. Guenter (eds.), *Atlas of Nutritional Support Techniques.* Boston: Little, Brown, 1989.

16. Glynn, M. F. X., Langer, B., and Jeejeebhoy, K. N. Therapy for thrombotic occlusion of long-term intravenous alimentation catheters. *J. Parenter. Enter. Nutr.* 4:387, 1980.

17. Greenberg, G. Inflammatory bowel disease. In J. Kinney, K. Jeejeebhoy, G. Hill, and O. Owen (eds.), *Nutrition and Metabolism in Patient Care.* Philadelphia: W. B. Saunders, 1988, P. 266.

18. Grunfest, S., and Steiger, E. Experience with the Broviac catheter for prolonged parenteral alimentation. *J. Parenter. Enter. Nutr.* 3:45, 1979.

19. Grundfest, S., and Steiger, E. Home parenteral nutrition. *J.A.M.A.* 244:1701, 1980.

20. Haffar, A. A. M., Rench, M. A., Ferry, G. D., Seavy, D. E., and Edwards, M. S. Failure of urokinase to resolve Broviac catheter-related bacteremia in children. *J. Pediatr.* 104:256, 1984.

21. Havill, J. H., and Blair, R. D. Home parenteral nutrition using shunts. *J. Parenter. Enter. Nutr.* 8:321, 1984.

22. Heimbach, D. M., and Ivey, T. D. Technique for placement of a permanent home hyperalimentation catheter. *Surg. Gynecol. Obstet.* 143:635, 1976.

23. Hickman, R. D., Buckner, C. D., Clift, R. A., Sanders, J. E., Stewart, P., and Thomas, E. D. A modified right atrial catheter for access to the venous system in bone marrow recipients. *Surg. Gynecol. Obstet.* 148:871, 1979.

24. Howard, L., Claunch, C., McDowell, R., and Timchalk, M. Five years of experience in patients receiving home nutrition support with the implanted reservoir: A comparison with the external catheter. *J. Parenter. Enter. Nutr.* 13:478, 1989.

25. Jeejeebhoy, K. Short bowel syndrome. In J. Kinney, K. Jeejeebhoy, G. Hill, and O. Owen (eds.), *Nutrition and Metabolism in Patient Care.* Philadelphia: W. B. Saunders, 1988, P. 259.

26. Klein, G. L., Targoff, C. M., Ament, M. E. et al. Bone disease associated with total parenteral nutrition. *Lancet* 2:1041, 1980.

27. Kotler, D. P. Malnutrition in HIV infection and AIDS. *AIDS* 3(Suppl.):5175, 1989.

28. Lewis, J., LaFrance, R., and Bower, R. H. Treatment of an infected silicone right atrial catheter with combined fibrinolytic and antibiotic therapy: Case report and review of the literature. *J. Parenter. Enter. Nutr.* 13:92, 1989.

29. Montague, N., Srp, F., and Steiger, E. Emergency catheter repairs in the home parenteral nutrition patient. (Abstract) *J. Parenter. Enter. Nutr.* 4:597, 1980.

30. Nicholson, L., and Groshong, C. V. *Catheter Nursing Procedure Manual.* Salt Lake City: Catheter Technology, 1989. P. 3.

31. Niederhuber, J. E., Ensminger, W., Gyves, J. W., Liepman, M., Doan, K., and Cozzi, E. Totally implanted venous and arterial access system to replace external catheters in cancer treatment. *Surgery* 92:706, 1982.

32. *OASIS Home Nutrition Support Patient Registry, Annual Report 1986.* Albany, NY: Oley Foundation; and Silver Spring, MD: American Society for Parenteral and Enteral Nutrition, 1988.

33. *OASIS Home Nutrition Support Patient Registry, Annual Report 1987.* Albany, NY: Oley Foundation; and Silver Spring, MD: American Society for Parenteral and Enteral Nutrition, 1989.

34. Oram-Smith, J., Mullen, J., Harken, A., and Fitts, W. Direct right atrial catheterization for total parenteral nutrition. *Surgery* 83:274, 1978.

35. Pomp, A., Caldwell, M. D., and Albina, J. Subcutaneous infusion ports for administration of parenteral nutrition at home. *Surg. Gynecol. Obstet.* 169:329, 1989.

36. Popp, M. B., Wagner, S. C., and Brito, O. J. Host and tumor responses to increasing levels of intravenous nutritional support. *Surgery* 94:300, 1983.

37. Price, B., and Levine, E. Permanent total parenteral nutrition: Psychology and social responses of the early stages. *J. Parenter. Enter. Nutr.* 3:48, 1979.

38. Quayle, A., Griffith, C., Mangnall, D., et al. Long-term parenteral nutrition in the management of severe Crohn's disease. *Clin. Nutr.* 4:195, 1985.

39. Riella, M. C., and Scribner, B. H. Five years' experience with a right atrial catheter for prolonged parenteral nutrition at home. *Surg. Gynecol. Obstet.* 143:205, 1976.

40. Scribner, B. H., and Cole, J. J. Evolution of the technique of home parenteral nutrition. *J. Parenter. Enter. Nutr.* 3:58, 1979.

41. Scribner, B. H., Cole, J. J., and Christopher, T. C. Long-term total parenteral nutrition: The concept of an artificial gut. *J.A.M.A.* 212:457, 1979.

42. Shike, M., Harrison, J. E., Sturtridge, W. C., et al. Metabolic bone disease in patients receiving long-term total parenteral nutrition. *Ann. Intern. Med.* 92:343, 1980.

43. Shike, M., Shils, M. E., Heller, A., et al. Bone disease in prolonged parenteral nutrition: Osteopenia without mineralization defect. *Am. J. Clin. Nutr.* 44:89, 1986.

44. Smith, A. N., Douglas, M., McLean, N., Ruckley, C. V., and Bruce, J. Intestinal complications of pelvic irradiation for gynecologic cancer. *Surg. Gynecol. Obstet.* 127:721, 1968.

45. Steiger, E., Oram-Smith, J., Miller, E., Kuo, L., and Vars, H. M. Effects of nutrition on tumor growth and tolerance to chemotherapy. *J. Surg. Res.* 18:455, 1975.

46. Steiger, E., Srp, F., Helbby, M., et al. Home parenteral nutrition. In J. Rombeau and M. Caldwell (eds.), *Clinical Nutrition*. Vol. 2: Parenteral Nutrition. Philadelphia: W. B. Saunders, 1986. P. 654.

47. Stillman, R. M., Soliman, F., Garcia, L., and Sawyer, P. N. Etiology of catheter-associated sepsis: Correlation with thrombogenicity. *Arch. Surg.* 112:1497, 1977.

48. Tankle, H., Clark, D., and Lee, F. Radiation enteritis with malabsorption. *Gut* 6:560, 1965.

49. Task Force on Nutrition Support in AIDS. Guidelines for nutrition support in AIDS. *Nutrition* 5:39, 1989.

50. Wilson, S., and Owens, M. (eds.). *Vascular Access Surgery*. Chicago: Year Book Medical, 1980, P. 24.

51. Wolman, S. L., Anderson, G. H., Marliss, E. B., and Jeejeebhoy, K. N. Zinc in total parenteral nutrition: Requirements and metabolic effects. *Gastroenterology* 76:458, 1979.

52. Yakoun, M., Armynol du Chatelet, A., and Quillon, A. Reduction of catheter related sepsis in long-term catheters: A prospective study on 44 patients. (Abstract) *J. Parenter. Enter. Nutr.* 11:39, 1987.

Peripheral Amino Acids

Harry M. Shizgal
Jarol B. Knowles

The incidence of hospital morbidity and mortality is profoundly affected by the nutritional state. Preventing the development of malnutrition in the hospitalized patient and maintaining a normal nutritional state are associated with improved wound healing, fewer infectious complications, and decreased postoperative morbidity [27]. The combination of starvation and stress-induced catabolic state is associated with a loss of body protein, as evidenced by a negative nitrogen balance, which if sufficiently severe and prolonged may lead to life-threatening malnutrition. In a variety of clinical situations, the use of amino acid–dextrose solutions administered by a peripheral vein can decrease this loss of body protein. This chapter describes the rationale for the infusion of amino acids by a peripheral vein, commonly referred to as "protein-sparing therapy."

STARVATION

Most hospitalized patients with a restricted oral intake receive some form of intravenous fluid during their hospitalization. Traditionally, a dilute solution of dextrose with electrolytes is infused to meet the requirements for water and electrolytes. This usually provides approximately 400 kcal/day. Gamble [19] demonstrated that 100 g of glucose has a protein-sparing effect in the starving human. This effect has been confirmed by others in both normal subjects [8, 28] and in the obese [15].

With either total or partial starvation, endogenous sources must supply the required energy. The body stores of carbohydrate, in the form of muscle and hepatic glycogen, are minimal. In the reference 70-kg man, there are 150 g and 75 g of glucogen in skeletal muscle and liver, respectively [7]. Glycogen stores are depleted within the first 24 to 48 hours of starvation. Subsequently, the body relies on triglycerides from adipose tissue and amino acids from body protein [29]. One of the primary functions of adipose tissue is the provision of endogenous calories during either partial or total starvation. As a labile pool of body protein is unavailable, all of the

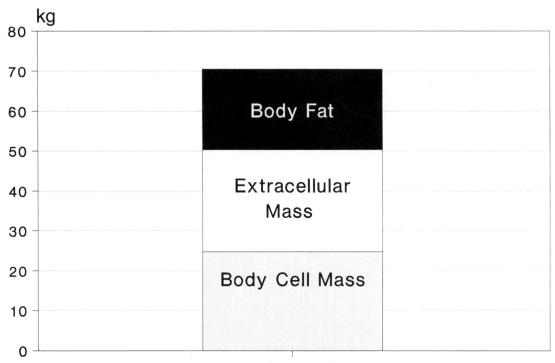

Figure 24-1. Mean body composition (with standard error of mean) of 25 normal volunteers. Body weight or total body mass in kilograms is divided into three major compartments: body fat, body cell mass, and extracellular mass. The lean body mass is the sum of the extracellular mass and body cell mass.

protein broken down during periods of starvation serve either a structural or a functional role. The skeletal muscles are the major source of this protein, but some protein is also derived from the breakdown of the viscera. This breakdown of body protein, as reflected by a net loss of body nitrogen, is responsible for a significant loss of body cell mass. The body cell mass is the total mass of living cells in the body. It is the metabolically active component of the body that performs all the work, both the physical and chemical work. It is that component which is responsible for all the oxygen consumed and carbon dioxide produced. In contrast, the extracellular mass is not metabolically active, does not consume any oxygen or produce any carbon dioxide, and performs no work. The lean body mass is the sum of the body cell mass and the extracellular mass, and is therefore the fat-free mass of the body (Fig. 24-1).

During the initial few days of total starvation, the nonstressed, normally nourished, resting 70-kg man breaks down approximately 75 g of protein/day, primarily from skeletal muscle, and 160 g/day of adipose tissue, which provides 1800 cal [7]. This breakdown of body protein provides amino acids, which are converted to the glucose required by those tissues, principally the CNS, for which glucose is their primary fuel. A negative nitrogen balance of approximately 12 g/day results. In the absence of a catabolic stress, an adaptive process occurs, mediated primarily by the plasma concentrations of insulin and glucagon. With fasting, the plasma levels of insulin fall, while the concentration of glucagon progressively rises. This results in increased release of free fatty acids (FFAs) and the formation of ketone bodies by the liver. FFAs and ketone bodies replace glucose as the major fuel for muscle.

The Cori and the glucose-alanine cycles are important components of this adaptation to starvation, as both cycles are involved in the shuttling of energy, as carbohydrate, be-

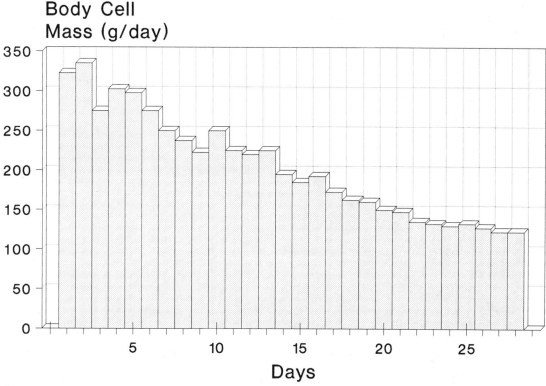

Figure 24-2. Daily loss of body cell mass with total starvation in a normally nourished, unstressed, 70-kg man. (Data adapted from Owen, O. E., Felig, P., Morgan, A. P., Wahren, J., and Cahill, G. F. Liver and kidney metabolism during prolonged starvation. *J. Clin. Invest.* 48:574, 1969.)

tween the liver and skeletal muscle. The Cori cycle involves the production of lactate by muscle from glycolytic sources, which is released and converted by the liver to pyruvate and glucose. The glucose so formed is cycled back to the muscle where it can again be broken down to lactate. The "glucose-alanine" cycle is also responsible for the provision of energy as carbohydrate to the carcass. Alanine and glutamine each account for 30 to 40% of the total amino acid nitrogen released from the muscle of fasting subjects [11]. Half the glutamine is converted to alanine by the intestine, which along with the alanine released from the periphery is the substrate for gluconeogenesis by the liver. The glucose so formed also becomes available to muscle. The energy requirements of the brain may account for up to 25% of the resting energy expenditure of the adult. These must be met by substrates that can cross the blood-brain barrier, namely, glucose in the normally fed

subject and ketone bodies in the starvation-adapted individual. As starvation is prolonged for several weeks, proteolysis of muscle with the release of alanine diminishes, as less glucose is made in the liver and ketone bodies take over as the major fuel for the brain.

With time, the rate of gluconeogenesis from protein therefore decreases, and the daily urinary nitrogen loss decreases from 12 g/day, early in starvation, to 3 to 5 g/day by the fourth week of starvation. The rate at which the body cell mass is lost decreases significantly as this adaptive process develops. During the initial days of total starvation, the body cell mass is lost at a rate of 300 g/day, which by the fourth week is reduced to 125 g/day (Fig. 24-2). The cumulative loss of body cell mass during this 4-week period of total starvation is 5.7 kg (Fig. 24-3), which in the normally nourished, 70-kg man represents 38% of the skeletal muscle mass, or 23%

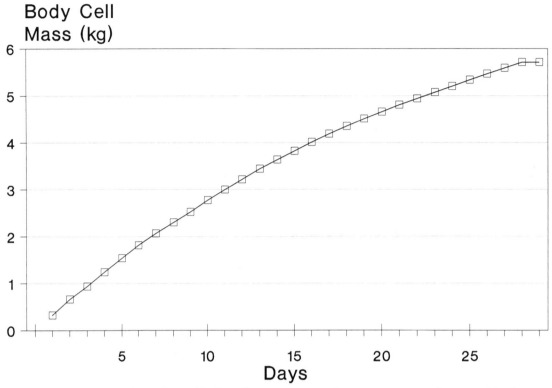

Figure 24-3. The cumulative loss of body cell mass, expressed as a percentage of a normal body cell mass for a 70 kg man (25 kg), with stress and starvation resulting in a nitrogen loss of either 10, 20, or 30 g/day.

of the body cell mass. It has been estimated that a loss of 50 to 60% of body cell mass is incompatible with survival. Infusing glucose at a rate of 150 g/day reduces nitrogen loss by about one-half, but does not totally abolish the breakdown of protein [36]. For most healthy, well-nourished patients the imposed state of starvation is short term, and this loss of body protein is well tolerated.

STRESS AND STARVATION

The rapid catabolism of body protein is one of the most dramatic features of the metabolic response to trauma. In the patient who is not receiving nitrogen from any source, the breakdown of body protein is directly reflected by the loss of nitrogen in the urine. The majority of this nitrogen originates from a breakdown of skeletal muscle. Cuthbertson [10] was one of the first to report a direct

relationship between the magnitude of trauma and the severity of muscle wasting and urinary loss of nitrogen, phosphorus, and sulfur, and correctly concluded that skeletal muscle was the major source of these intracellular elements.

Marked tissue wasting and weight loss occur following trauma and/or sepsis because of the combined presence of both starvation and the catabolic processes that result from the initiating event. Regional amino acid flux studies indicate that there is accelerated breakdown of skeletal muscle protein, with a release of amino acids that are taken up centrally, especially by the splanchnic bed [3]. Protein turnover studies have demonstrated increased protein catabolism. In the unfed patient, protein synthesis remains normal, while with either parenteral or enteral feeding, protein synthesis increases to approach or match the catabolic rate [24]. In the traumatized patient there is a parallel increase in the resting metabolic rate and negative nitrogen balance, which is directly proportional to the severity of trauma. The daily nitrogen loss ranges from 10 to 15 g/day, following an uncomplicated operation of moderate severity [25]. When injury is complicated with sepsis, the daily nitrogen loss increases to 15 to 25 g/day. With severe injury and sepsis (i.e., major thermal burns), it may rise to 35 g/day. The traumatized patient, in contrast to the unstressed starved individual, does not adapt, with an increased reliance on endogenous lipids and a subsequent decrease in the rate of gluconeogenesis from protein. The large nitrogen losses that develop result in an extensive erosion of the body cell mass. The cumulative loss of body cell mass with various degrees of catabolic stress are depicted in Figure 24-3. A nitrogen loss of 10 g/day for 1 month results in a 7-kg loss of body cell mass, which is equivalent to 47% of the skeletal muscle mass or 28% of the body cell mass. With a negative nitrogen balance of 30 g/day, there is a 5.3-kg loss of body cell mass by the end of 1 week. At this rate, by 2.5 weeks, over 50% of the body cell mass is lost. Thus starvation and injury, especially when complicated with sepsis, result in a rapid erosion of the cellular mass. The body cell mass impacts significantly on morbidity and mortality. As skeletal muscle is lost, the ability to cough and clear pulmonary secretions becomes impaired, leading eventually to pulmonary infection. In addition, malnutrition is associated with impaired wound healing, decreased resistance to infection, and impaired synthesis of many other important acute-phase proteins. As a result, numerous attempts have been made to prevent or at least to decrease the massive protein wasting that accompanies significant stress.

PROTEIN-SPARING EFFECT OF INTRAVENOUS AMINO ACIDS

Blackburn et al. [4, 5] were the first to report a significant reduction in nitrogen loss in the stressed and starved patient when amino acids rather than the usual glucose solutions were infused. They postulated that the infusion of glucose increases plasma insulin concentration which, because of its antilipolytic action, would decrease fat mobilization and ketosis. In the absence of an adequate caloric intake, the patient must therefore rely on endogenous energy sources, leading to increased breakdown of the body cell mass to furnish a supply of amino acids for gluconeogenesis by the liver. The patient receiving a hypocaloric glucose infusion must therefore rely on the catabolic breakdown of body protein for energy.

To test their hypothesis, Blackburn and his group randomized, in a crossover routine, 10 surgical patients to receive each of the following three intravenous solutions for 4 days: (1) 5% glucose at 100 g of glucose/24 hr, (2) 3% crystalline amino acids at 90 g/24 hr, and (3) 5% glucose and 3% amino acid to deliver in each 24-hour period 70 g of amino acids and 100 g of glucose. An additional group of obese volunteers received either only water, minerals, and vitamins, or in addition 1 g of protein/kg of body weight. There was an inverse correlation between the daily nitrogen balance and the serum FFA concentration. The nitrogen balance was most negative with the lowest serum FFA concentration, which typically occurred in the group receiving the 5% dextrose solution. When the same patients received the amino acid solution without glucose, the FFA levels increased and the net nitrogen losses decreased. The changes in ketone body concentration paralleled the FFA levels. There was a direct correlation between the plasma glucose and insulin levels. The highest glucose and insulin levels were seen in the patients receiving 100 g of glucose/day, and was associated with the greatest net nitrogen losses. Adequate levels of insulin during amino acid infusion in the surgical patients and protein ingestion by the obese were associated with the maintenance of nitrogen balance. The addition of amino acids to the glucose infusate improved nitrogen retention with a mean net cumulative nitrogen balance over 4 days of 15 ± 6 g as compared to 28.9 ± 4.0 g in the patients who

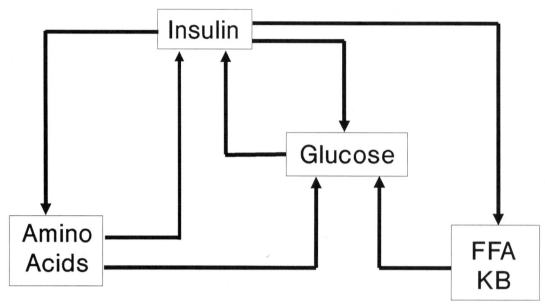

Figure 24-4. The model proposed by Flatt and Blackburn [14] describing the interplay between the plasma concentration of metabolic fuels and insulin. Upward pointing arrows indicate an increase in concentration, while a downward pointing arrow indicates a decrease in concentration. FFA = free fatty acids; KB = ketone bodies.

received only dextrose. When only amino acids were infused, the net cumulative nitrogen balance approached zero. [*Editor's Note:* It should be pointed out that there were differences in amino acid infusion at 20 g/24 h between Groups 2 and 3, which probably account for the differences in nitrogen balance. This fact seems to have been overlooked by most authors quoting Blackburn et al.'s article.] A similar response to amino acid infusion was reported by this group in 17 patients immediately following major urologic operations [34].

Flatt and Blackburn [14] proposed a model describing the interplay between the metabolism of carbohydrates, fat, and amino acids, which they claim is consistent with their observations. According to their model, the infusion of either glucose alone or in combination with amino acids elicits insulin release, and because of its antilipolytic action, fat mobilization is reduced to such an extent that the infused glucose and amino acids are all oxidized to support energy production (Fig. 24-4). The infusion of amino acids without glucose permits the development of fasting

ketosis, permitting energy requirements to be met entirely from endogenous FFAs and ketones. The infused amino acids may then replenish the amino acid pools and are in addition available for protein synthesis.

Hoover et al. [22] reported similar findings to that of Blackburn's group. Patients undergoing either head-and-neck or abdominal surgery were randomly allocated to receive immediately following operation either a 3% solution of crystalline L-amino acid (n = 9) or 5% dextrose solution (n = 11). The infusions were started immediately after operation and continued for a minimum of 6 days. The amino acid infusion significantly reduced nitrogen losses. The mean cumulative negative nitrogen balance was significantly reduced from 74 ± 7 g in the control glucose group, to 42 ± 5 g in the patients receiving amino acid. In the patients receiving the amino acid infusion the serum insulin and glucose levels were significantly reduced, while the ketone bodies rose.

Numerous other studies confirmed that nitrogen balance is maintained by the intravenous infusion of amino acid solutions, but the data have often not supported the hormonal-substrate interrelations proposed by Flatt and Blackburn. The protein-sparing effect of amino acid solutions, with or without additional glucose, was evaluated by Wolfe et al. [37] in totally fasting, healthy, adult male volunteers. During an 8-hour period, they infused 3 liters/day of a 3.4% crystalline amino acid solution with (four subjects) or without (four subjects) an additional 150 g of glucose/day. The addition of glucose significantly improved nitrogen balance. The mean nitrogen balance with additional glucose was -0.9 ± 1.0 g $\cdot$ sq m^{-1} $\cdot$ day^{-1} compared to -3.0 ± 0.2 g $\cdot$ sq m^{-1} $\cdot$ day^{-1} with amino acids alone. Plasma glucose and immunoreactive insulin levels were not increased by the addition of glucose. The glucose infusion did prevent the ketosis that developed with the amino acid infusion.

Similar findings were reported by Elwyn et al. [12], who compared the protein-sparing effect of an amino acid infusion with or without additional glucose following abdominal surgery. Starting on the second day following operation, 12 patients received, in a random crossover design, a 3.5% crystalline L-amino acid solution with or without an additional 100 g of glucose/day, each for 4 days. The order was reversed in half of the patients. The addition of glucose increased net nitrogen retention by 3.4 g/day. Surprisingly, the addition of glucose also decreased energy expenditure. Although carbohydrate oxidation increased, the energy derived from fat and protein decreased. These changes in energy metabolism were attributed to the anabolic effects of insulin, which increased in the patients receiving additional glucose.

Freeman et al. [17] also failed to demonstrate a relationship between insulin and the protein-sparing effect of peripherally administered amino acids. Eight morbidly obese patients following abdominal surgery received amino acid infusions, with and without additional glucose, for sequential 4-day study periods in a crossover design. The infusion of 3 liters/day of a 5% amino acid solution, when compared to a dextrose control period, increased the serum FFA and ketone body levels, while the serum insulin levels fell. Nitrogen balance improved from -12.3 ± 4.7 g/day to -1.3 ± 1.8 g/day. The addition of 150 g of glucose/day to the amino acid infusate returned the insulin, FFA, and ketone body levels to those observed during the dextrose control period. In spite of these changes, nitrogen balance was essentially unchanged at -0.8 ± 1.2 g/day. They concluded that the protein sparing occurred because of the availability of a supply of exogenous amino acids and the ability to mobilize endogenous lipid, and that it was not mediated by changes in insulin secretion. Foster et al. [16] evaluated the protein-sparing effects of amino acid with glucose, with and without exogenous insulin, in postoperative patients. They concluded that the protein-sparing effects of amino acids were due to increased protein synthesis rather than decreased protein breakdown.

Greenberg et al. [21] demonstrated that the protein-sparing effect of amino acids is related to the infused amino acids alone and is not related to the degree of endogenous fat mobilization. Thirty patients undergoing elective abdominal surgery were randomized to receive daily, during the initial 4 postoperative days, either (1) 150 g of carbohydrate as 5% glucose, (2) 5% amino acids to provide 1 g/kg/day, (3) 1 g/kg/day of amino acids plus 500 ml of a 10% soybean oil emulsion, or (4) 1 g/kg/day of amino acids plus 150 g of glucose. In the patients receiving either glucose alone or amino acids plus glucose, the plasma glucose and insulin levels were higher, while the plasma FFA and ketone body concentrations were lower. Nitrogen balance was significantly more negative in the control patients receiving only glucose compared to those who received amino acids. Despite the variability of the plasma levels of insulin and substrate, nitrogen balance was not significantly different among the groups receiving amino acids (Fig. 24-5).

A relationship between plasma insulin and the protein-sparing effect of intravenous amino acids was also not observed by Rowlands and Clark [30], who compared the use of amino acid solution with conventional in-

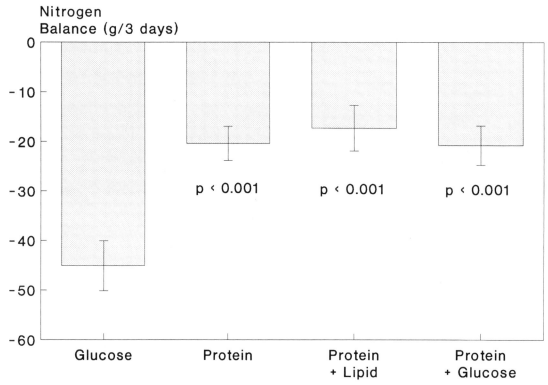

Figure 24-5. Mean (± standard error of mean) 3-day cumulative nitrogen balance following elective abdominal surgery with the intravenous infusion of either glucose, amino acids, or amino acids plus either lipid or glucose.

travenous therapy following an elective operation of moderate severity in 16 male patients. During the initial 4 postoperative days, each patient received either an amino acid infusion (0.23 g of nitrogen/kg/day) or a dextrose solution (1.43 g/kg/day) for 16 hours each day followed by an 8-hour infusion of saline solution. The plasma hormone and substrate concentrations during the infusion of either amino acids or glucose were compared with the levels during the infusion of saline solution. The infusion of amino acids reduced the negative nitrogen balance in the postoperative period when compared with a 5% dextrose infusion. Their data also demonstrated that the protein-sparing effect was related to the infused amino acids alone and was not related to a change in substrate patterns and endogenous fat mobilization.

Freund et al. [18] demonstrated that the protein-sparing effect of intravenous amino acids was independent of the amino acid composition. Thirty-five patients undergoing elective surgery of moderate severity were randomized to receive, for the first 5 postoperative days, one of the following solutions: (1) 5% dextrose, (2) 3% crystalline amino acids containing 22% branched-chain amino acids (BCAAs) with 5% dextrose, (3) 3% crystalline amino acids with 35% BCAAs with 5% dextrose, or (4) 3% crystalline amino acids consisting entirely of BCAAs with 5% dextrose. The mean nitrogen balance in the control group receiving only 5% dextrose was −6.6 ± 0.6 g/day, while all three groups receiving amino acid solutions were either in nitrogen equilibrium or in slightly positive nitrogen balance. [*Editor's Note:* It is by no means clear that the results in Group 3 would have been the same with any three amino acids. As coauthor of that article, I had always interpreted the results as supporting the anticatabolic properties of the BCAAs.]

A relationship between the nitrogen sparing of intravenous amino acids and the magnitude of the catabolic stress was demonstrated by Ching et al. [9], who evaluated the protein-sparing effects of the peripheral infusion of crystalline amino acids in surgical patients subjected to various degrees of stress. They infused a solution containing 4.2% crystalline amino acids with 5% glucose. All the patients remained in negative nitrogen balance. However, there was a relationship between the loss of nitrogen and the magnitude of the stress. The greatest loss of nitrogen occurred in the patients subjected to the most stress. Serum albumin level, which fell in all the patients, was only preserved when additional calories were provided.

Young and Hill [38] compared the protein-sparing effects of hypocaloric amino acid infusion with total parenteral nutrition (TPN). Thirty patients undergoing resection of the rectum received for 13 days in the immediate postoperative period either (1) no nutrition, (2) 4.25% amino acid solution providing a mean of 0.23 ± 0.02 g of nitrogen/kg of body weight, or (3) amino acids with 25% glucose providing 0.23 ± 0.02 g of nitrogen/kg of body weight. In the control group, which received no nutritional therapy, body weight, total body nitrogen, body fat, and plasma albumin and transferrin levels were all decreased by 15 days after surgery. Amino acids alone caused some sparing of body tissues, but the decrease in body weight and in plasma albumin and transferrin was not prevented. In contrast, the infusion of the hypertonic dextrose solution prevented the decrease in all of the above variables, while weight and prealbumin increased.

In addition to measuring nitrogen balance to evaluate the protein-sparing effect of amino acid infusion, Skillman et al. [33] also measured the albumin synthesis rate in 10 patients following major abdominal surgery. Patients were randomized to receive postoperatively either a 3.5% amino acid or a 5% glucose solution. Although the patients receiving glucose received more calories, they were in negative nitrogen balance, while the patients who received amino acids were in nitrogen equilibrium. The albumin synthesis

rate was significantly greater in the patients receiving the amino acid infusion (237 ± 24 mg/kg/day). The infused amino acids appeared to be more effective than glucose in promoting albumin synthesis.

The protein-sparing effect of hypocaloric amino acid infusions was assessed by determining body composition, via multiple isotope dilution, before and on the fifth postoperative day in patients undergoing elective surgery of moderate severity [32]. The patients were randomized to receive either the usual glucose-containing intravenous solutions, or a 5% casein hydrolysate, and caloric intake was similar in the two groups. In both groups there was a statistically significant loss of body weight postoperatively. The mean weight loss was 2.6 ± 0.6 kg in the glucose patients and 2.0 ± 0.5 kg in the protein group (Fig. 24-6). In the glucose group, this weight loss resulted from a loss of both body fat (1.8 ± 0.9 kg) and body cell mass (3.2 ± 0.6 kg), while the extracellular mass increased by 2.4 ± 0.5 kg; a body composition typical of mild malnutrition. The mean Na_e/K_e, which is a sensitive index of the nutritional state, increased significantly ($p < 0.05$) from 1.04 ± 0.08, which is within the normal range, to 1.29 ± 0.11, which denotes mild malnutrition. In contrast, in the patients who received amino acids, the only change postoperatively was a loss of body fat (4.1 ± 0.8 kg), while the body cell mass and extracellular mass remained unchanged (see Fig. 24.6). The Na_e/K_e remained normal (1.00 ± 0.03). The intravenous infusion of amino acids at a daily rate of 1.8 ± 0.2 g/kg of body weight effectively prevented the malnutrition that developed when only a glucose solution was administered.

The data in the literature clearly demonstrate that in the starving patient, with or without additional mild to moderate stress, significant protein sparing may be achieved with the infusion of intravenous amino acids. It is also clear that this protein-sparing effect is not related to changes in the plasma insulin concentration, but rather appears to be related simply to the availability of exogenous amino acids. The protein sparing that is

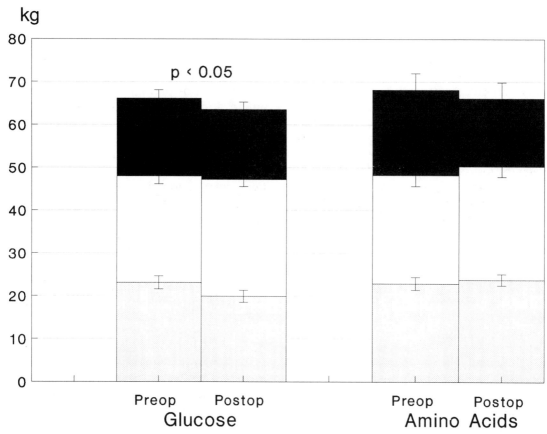

Figure 24-6. Mean (± standard error of mean) body composition before and on the fifth postoperative day following major elective surgery in patients who received all of their postoperative intravenous fluids with either glucose- or amino acid–containing solutions. Body weight is divided into the three major compartments: body fat (solid), extracellular mass (clear), and body cell mass (bottom).

achieved appears to be related to the magnitude and duration of the stress and the additional nonprotein calories infused with the amino acids. The infusion of amino acids either decreases the loss of nitrogen or, at best, nitrogen equilibrium is achieved. Positive nitrogen balance indicative of net protein synthesis is only achieved when significant additional nonprotein calories are infused with the amino acids.

PROTEIN AND ENERGY INTERRELATIONSHIP

The interaction between energy intake and protein intake has been studied extensively in both animals and humans and may be summarized as follows: (1) With energy intake constant, the efficiency of protein retention improves as protein intake is increased. (2) Conversely, with protein intake constant, increasing energy intake improves the efficiency of protein retention. (3) Efficiency of protein retention is greater in the malnourished. (4) There is less protein retention, at any given protein and energy intake, in the hypermetabolic patient.

The relationship between energy and nitrogen retention was evaluated by Elwyn et al. [13] in 10 depleted hospitalized patients, who were maintained on intravenous amino acids and glucose. The nitrogen intake was maintained constant at 0.173 g/kg/day with three different energy intakes (15.4, 37.6, and 58.5 kcal/kg/day) administered sequentially for 4 days each. The resting energy expenditure did not increase as the energy intake was increased as long as the energy balance was negative. However, as the energy intake increased and energy balance became positive, the resting energy expenditure increased at a rate of 1 kcal for each additional intake of 5 kcal. The following linear relationship existed between nitrogen balance and energy intake:

Nitrogen balance (mg of nitrogen/kg
of body weight)
$$= -24.3 + 1.4 \text{ kcal/kg}$$

This regression demonstrates the linear relationship between caloric intake and nitrogen retention.

Similar data were obtained in a group of patients receiving TPN who were randomized to receive either (1) 25% dextrose with 2.5% crystalline L-amino acids; (2) 25% dextrose with 5% amino acids; or (3) 2.5% amino acids, 12.5% dextrose, and a 5% lipid emulsion [31]. The response to TPN was evaluated by determining body composition, via multiple isotope dilution, at 2-week intervals. Data analysis was restricted only to patients with malnutrition as defined by their body composition. This is essential, as an increase in the body cell mass, which is equivalent to positive nitrogen balance, occurs only in the malnourished. In the normally nourished, the body cell mass increases only with normal growth or in response to an exercise program designed specifically to increase muscle mass. As expected, with the three solutions, the body cell mass was maintained in the normally nourished and increased in the malnourished. The mean daily change in the body cell mass (in g/day) was correlated with the carbohydrate, lipid, and protein calories infused, and with the nutritional state as assessed by the Na_e/K_e ratio, a sensitive index of the nutritional state. The following statistically significant multiple linear regression was obtained:

This multiple linear correlation [...] cally significant ($p < 0.01$), as we [...] gression coefficients associated with [...] K_e ratio and with the carbohydrate an[...] calories infused. However, the coefficien[...] sociated with the protein infused was not si[...] nificant. The regression equation demonstrates that the rate at which a malnourished body cell mass was restored was (1) proportional to the caloric intake and the degree of malnutrition, (2) occurred more rapidly with carbohydrate rather than lipid calories, and (3) was unaffected by increasing the amino acid concentration from 2.5 to 5%. These data are essentially similar to the Elwyn data described above. The response to the lipid infusion is consistent with the view proposed by Moore [26], who emphasized the importance of differentiating the energy for work from that required for protein synthesis. Although the energy derived from the oxidation of endogenous fat can supply all of the energy required by the body cell mass to perform its various functions, it cannot support the requirements for protein synthesis. Thus, during periods of starvation there is a gradual wasting away of the body cell mass, despite adequate stores of endogenous lipid in the form of body fat. In contrast, carbohydrates, even in relatively small amounts, provide the energy required for protein synthesis, with a significant reduction in the net loss of body protein. The nitrogen-sparing effect of intravenous lipid emulsions in the normal starving subject can be accounted for by the glycerol content of the emulsion [6].

The experience with children recovering from malnutrition is similar [35]. Traditionally, a high protein diet was the recommended treatment for the child recovering from malnutrition. This arose because of the emphasis on protein deficiency as the main cause of malnutrition in underdeveloped countries, and on the observation that kwashiorkor could be effectively treated with milk. A number of recent reports demon-

Body cell mass/day = $-348.5 + 4.9 \text{ CHO}^* + 3.2 \text{ lipid}^* + 4.7 \text{ protein}^* + 98.7 \text{ Na}_e/\text{K}_e$
*Cal/kg of body weight/day.   ($p < 0.005$)   ($p < 0.05$)   (not significant)   ($p < 0.001$)

is neither nec-
]. The protein
growing in-
of the total
tes the pro-
covery from
providing
...us amount.

...worth and coworkers [2] randomized a group of malnourished infants to receive one of two similar liquid diets with different caloric and protein contents. A multiple linear correlation was performed between weight gain (as the dependent variable) and caloric and protein intakes (as independent variables). In the resultant regression, the relationship between weight gain and calories was significant, while that between protein intake and weight gain was not significant:

$$\text{Weight gain (g/kg/day)} = 0.072 \text{ calories (cal/kg/day)} + 0.283 \text{ protein (g/kg/day)} - 3.57 \ (p < 0.01) \text{ (not significant)}$$

This relationship is similar to the others described above and demonstrates the relatively greater importance of calories as opposed to protein. This can be illustrated by the following example. With an intake of 100 cal/kg/day and 3 g/kg/day of protein, the weight gain according to the regression would be 4.5 g/kg/day. Increasing the caloric intake by 50% to 150 cal/kg/day, the weight gain would increase to 8.1 g/kg/day, an 80% increase. However, if instead the protein intake was increased by 50%, the weight gain would only increase to 4.9 g/kg/day, a 9% increase. The use of high caloric and low protein feeding has resulted in growth rates in malnourished children which are 15 times normal. These high growth rates have resulted in much shorter stays in hospital, in contrast to the long hospitalizations which were the norm with the traditional high protein diets [35].

CLINICAL IMPLICATIONS

The metabolic adaptation to starvation is intended to minimize the loss of body protein. In contrast, the metabolic and hormonal responses to stress and starvation initiate a catabolic response that is characterized by a release of amino acids from the body cell mass, primarily from the skeletal muscles, which is proportional to the magnitude of the trauma. Malnutrition may therefore develop rapidly. In the healthy, nonstressed, 70-kg individual, starvation initially results in a daily nitrogen loss of 12 to 15 g, which is equivalent to a body cell mass loss of 300 g/day. With stress and starvation, losses of 500 to 1000 g/day of body cell mass are not uncommon. An elective operation of moderate severity results in a mean body cell mass loss of 3.2 kg during the initial 5 postoperative days. In contrast, the recovery from malnutrition, as demonstrated above, both in the hospitalized patient and in the malnourished child, is a slow process and requires a relatively high caloric intake. The prevention of malnutrition should therefore be the primary therapeutic objective. This is probably the major role for the infusion of hypocaloric amino acid solutions.

Thrombophlebitis is a common complication of a dextrose–amino acid infusion, and is thought to be related to the irritating effect of the mildly acidic amino acid solution on the peripheral veins. Protein-sparing peripheral parenteral nutrition is limited on two accounts: (1) the development of thrombophlebitis, and (2) the low calorie density of the infusion. Clearly, peripheral hypocaloric amino acid infusions are for those patients in whom short-term nutritional support is required, and whose nutritional status may be maintained by low caloric intake. The simultaneous infusion of a lipid emulsion presents a number of advantages. The neutral pH of the lipid solution tends to neutralize the acidic pH of the amino acid solution and may therefore improve the tolerance of the peripheral veins. In addition, because of the high caloric density of lipid emulsions, additional calories may be infused.

The published reports clearly demonstrate that intravenous amino acids effectively spare protein. The majority of these studies were carried out in normally nourished individuals who were exposed to trauma of moderate severity. The results of these studies cannot therefore be extrapolated to the malnourished, the severely traumatized, or patients subjected to a prolonged catabolic stress. Further studies are required to evaluate the role of protein sparing with intravenous amino acids in these patients.

Our present practice is to administer hypocaloric amino acid infusions, for the purpose of protein sparing, to patients who require nutritional support, but who are not as yet candidates for TPN. This includes the severely malnourished patient who had just undergone corrective surgery and is expected to resume a normal oral intake in a few days. Because of preexisting malnutrition and therefore a decreased reserve, this individual cannot tolerate an additional loss of nutritional reserve, especially if a postoperative complication develops and the resumption of oral intake is further delayed. Protein sparing is similarly indicated for the extensively traumatized patient in whom there is uncertainty regarding the return of normal gastrointestinal function. In such a patient, amino acids are administered until oral intake is resumed or until it is obvious that dietary intake will be unduly delayed. When it becomes obvious that there is a prolonged delay in the resumption of gastrointestinal function, TPN is initiated. Generally, therefore, protein sparing with intravenous amino acids is used when indications for TPN do not exist, but it is anticipated that TPN might be required. To achieve protein sparing, amino acids are administered at a rate of 1.5 to 2.9 g/kg of body weight using a solution containing 5% amino acids with either 5 or 10% dextrose. However, the infusion of a protein-sparing solution cannot replace TPN, especially in the malnourished. To correct a malnourished state, net protein synthesis must be initiated, and this can only be achieved by the simultaneous intake of amino acid with adequate nonprotein calories.

REFERENCES

1. Ashworth, A. Growth rates of children recovering from protein-calorie malnutrition. *Br. J. Nutr.* 23:835, 1969.
2. Ashworth, A., Bell, R., James, W. P. T., and Waterlow, J. C. Calorie requirements of children recovering from protein-calorie malnutrition. *Lancet* 2:600, 1968.
3. Aulik, L. H., and Wilmore, D. W. Increased peripheral amino acid release following burn injury. *Surgery* 85:560, 1979.
4. Blackburn, G. L., Flatt, J. P., Clowes, G. H. A., Jr., O'Donnell, T. F., and Hensle, T. E. Protein sparing therapy during periods of starvation with sepsis or trauma. *Ann. Surg.* 177:588, 1973.
5. Blackburn, G. L., Flatt, J. P., Clowes, G. H. A., Jr., and O'Donnell, T. Peripheral amino acid feeding with isotonic amino acid solutions. *Am. J. Surg.* 125:447, 1973.
6. Brennan, M. F., Fitzpatrick, G. F., Cohen, K., and Moore, F. D. Glycerol. *Ann. Surg.* 182:386, 1975.
7. Cahill, G. F., Jr. Starvation in man. *N. Engl. J. Med.* 282:668, 1970.
8. Calloway, D. M., and Spector, H. Nitrogen balance as related to calorie and protein intake in active young men. *Am. J. Clin. Nutr.* 2:405, 1954.
9. Ching, N., Millis, C. J., Grossi, C., et al. The absence of protein-sparing effects utilizing crystalline amino acids in stressed patients. *Ann. Surg.* 190:565, 1979.
10. Cuthbertson, D. P. The metabolic response to injury and its nutritional implications: Retrospect and prospect. *J. Parenter. Enter. Nutr.* 3:107, 1979.
11. DiFronzo, R. A., and Felig, P. Amino acid metabolism in uremia: Insights gained from normal and diabetic man. Symposium on Nutrition in Renal Disease, Proceedings of the Second International Congress on Nutrition in Renal Disease. *Am. J. Clin. Nutr.* 33:1378, 1980.
12. Elwyn, D. H., Gump, F. E., Iles, M., Long, C. L., and Kinney, J. M. Protein and energy sparing of glucose added in hypocaloric amounts to peripheral infusions of amino acids. *Metabolism* 27:325, 1978.
13. Elwyn, D. H., Gump, F. E., Munro, H. N., Iles, M., and Kinney, J. M. Changes in nitrogen balance of depleted patients with increasing infusions of glucose. *Am. J. Clin. Nutr.* 32:1597, 1979.
14. Flatt, J. P., and Blackburn, G. L. The metabolic fuel regulatory system: Implications for protein sparing therapies during caloric deprivation and disease. *Am. J. Clin. Nutr.* 27:175, 1974.
15. Forbes, G. B., and Drenick, E. J. Loss of body

nitrogen on fasting. *Am. J. Clin. Nutr.* 32:1570, 1979.

16. Foster, K. J., Alberti, K. G. M. M., Binder, C., et al. Metabolic effects of the use of protein-sparing infusions in postoperative patients. *Clin. Sci.* 58:507, 1980.

17. Freeman, J. B., Stegink, L. D., Wittine, M., Danny, M., and Thompson, R. Lack of correlation between nitrogen balance and serum insulin levels during protein sparing with and without dextrose. *Gastroenterology* 73:31, 1977.

18. Freund, H. R., Hoover, H. C., Atamian, S., and Fischer, J. E. Infusion of the branched chain amino acids in postoperative patients: Anticatabolic properties. *Ann. Surg.* 190:18, 1979.

19. Gamble, J. L. *Chemical Anatomy, Physiology and Pathology of Extracellular Fluids: A Lecture Syllabus* (5th ed.). Cambridge, MA: Harvard University Press, 1947.

20. Graham, G. G., Cordano, A., and Baeril, J. M. Studies in infantile malnutrition. II. Effect of protein and calorie intake on weight gain. *J. Nutr.* 81:249, 1963.

21. Greenberg, G. R., Marliss, E. R., Anderson, H., et al. Protein-sparing therapy in postoperative patients: Effects of added hypocaloric glucose and lipid. *N. Engl. J. Med.* 294:1411, 1976.

22. Hoover, H. C., Grant, J. P., Gorschboth, C., and Ketcham, A. S. Nitrogen-sparing intravenous fluids in postoperative patients. *N. Engl. J. Med.* 293:172, 1975.

23. Kerr, D., Ashworth, A., Picou, D., et al. Accelerated recovery from infant malnutrition with high calorie feeding. In L. I. Gardner and P. Amacher (eds.), *Endocrine Aspects of Malnutrition*. Santa Ynez, CA: The Kroc Foundation, 1973. P. 467.

24. Kien, C. L., Young, V. R., Rohrbaugh, D. K., and Burke, J. F. Increased rates of whole body protein synthesis and breakdown in children recovering from burns. *Ann. Surg.* 187:383, 1978.

25. Kinney, J. M. Energy requirements of the surgical patient. In American College of Surgeons Committee on Pre- and Postoperative Care (eds.), *Manual of Surgical Nutrition*. Philadelphia: Saunders, 1975. P. 223.

26. Moore, F. D. Energy and the maintenance of the body cell mass. *J. Parenter. Enter. Nutr.* 4:223, 1980.

27. Mueller, J. M., Brenner, U., Dienst, C., and Pichlmaier, H. Preoperative parenteral feeding in patients with gastrointestinal carcinoma. *Lancet* 1:68, 1982.

28. Munroe, H. N. Carbohydrate and fat as factors in protein utilization. *Physiol. Rev.* 31:449, 1951.

29. Owen, O. E., Felig, P., Morgan, A. P., Wahren, J., and Cahill, G. F. Liver and kidney metabolism during prolonged starvation. *J. Clin. Invest.* 48:574, 1969.

30. Rowlands, B. J., and Clark, R. G. Postoperative amino acid infusions: An appraisal. *Br. J. Surg.* 65:384, 1978.

31. Shizgal, H. M., and Forse, R. A. Protein and calorie requirements with total parenteral nutrition. *Ann. Surg.* 192:562, 1980.

32. Shizgal, H. M., Milne, C. A., and Spanier, A. H. The effect of nitrogen-sparing intravenously administered fluids on postoperative body composition. *Surgery* 85:496, 1979.

33. Skillman, J. J., Rosenoer, V. M., Smith, P. C., and Fang, M. S. Improved albumin synthesis in postoperative patients by amino acid infusion. *N. Engl. J. Med.* 295:1037, 1976.

34. Solomon, M. J., Smith, M. F., Dowd, J. B., Bistrian, B. R., and Blackburn, G. L. Optimal nutritional support in surgery for bladder cancer: Preservation of visceral protein by amino acid infusions. *J. Urol.* 119:350, 1978.

35. Waterlow, J. C. The rate of recovery of malnourished infants in relation to the protein and calorie levels of the diet. *J. Trop. Pediatr.* 7:16, 1961.

36. Wolfe, B. M., Culebras, J. M., Sim, A. J. W., Ball, M. R., and Moore, F. D. Substrate interaction in intravenous feeding. *Ann. Surg.* 186:518, 1977.

37. Wolfe, B. M., Culebras, J. M., Tweedle, D., and Moore, F. D. Effect of glucose on the nitrogen-sparing effect of amino acids given intravenously. *Surg. Forum* 27:39, 1976.

38. Young, G. A., and Hill, G. L. A controlled study of protein sparing therapy after excision of the rectum. *Ann. Surg.* 192:183, 1980.

Lipid Emulsions

Khursheed N. Jeejeebhoy

ENERGY SUPPLY IN TOTAL PARENTERAL NUTRITION

Nutrients are ingested or infused to provide the basic needs for growth, maintenance, and repair of normal body constituents. In addition, ingested nutrients are used as fuels, which are oxidized to provide energy for the aforementioned processes and for such vital functions as heat production, respiration, locomotion, and blood circulation. The living organism is constantly consuming fuel and generating energy to remain alive. In the absence of nutrients, the organism draws primarily on disposable stores—glycogen and fat in the human—but it also consumes essential tissues by utilizing structural proteins for energy. This last source is undesirable because, if excessive or prolonged, it consumes lean tissue and ultimately results in death. Hence, the provision of energy sources is essential to prevent protein "autophagy" and to preserve essential tissues. These sources also provide tissues with sufficient energy to function. However, it is equally axiomatic that protein equilibrium and synthesis require that exogenous protein be provided.

SOURCES OF ENERGY

The human body can utilize many sources of energy, each through its own set of metabolic pathways. However, in the administration of total parenteral nutrition (TPN), certain constraints make only a few sources suitable for the provision of energy on a large scale.

Constraints

Caloric Density
The ability to provide a high calorie–fluid volume ratio is critical so that the patient can receive sufficient calories without having to be infused with excessive volumes of fluid.

Complete Utilization and Negligible Excretion
As a corollary to the first constraint, it is clear that even if a calorie-dense solution can be

infused, the loss of a substantial part of such an infusion into the urine or by accumulation in the body fluids effectively prevents the patient from utilizing the infused nutrient.

Freedom from Toxicity in the Dose Required to Meet Energy Needs

The nutrient or its metabolic products should not adversely affect the function of any organ.

Osmolality

The osmolar concentration of the solution influences its effect on veins. Hypertonic solutions are injurious to veins and certainly cannot be given into peripheral veins. Thus any regimen involving the use of peripheral veins cannot tolerate markedly hypertonic solutions. This has been offset by the use of central venous infusions. However, even with this route there is a significant incidence of caval injury and thrombosis, which may be reduced by the use of infusions having a lower tonicity and containing lipid [18, 51, 61]. [Editor's Note: There is little evidence that it is the infused solution, which I calculate as being diluted 2700 times by blood flow, which is injurious. Most evidence suggests that it is the material of the catheter that plays a major role in caval thrombosis.]

When all these criteria are met, it is clear that at present only two sources of energy are suitable. They are glucose and triglyceride-containing lipid emulsions. These two, and others, are discussed in this chapter.

Glucose

Ordinarily, this physiologic carbohydrate fuel is readily and completely utilized, and has no known direct toxic effects. When endogenous insulin secretion is insufficient, insulin can be infused in order to control hyperglycemia and glycosuria. On the other hand, the high osmotic pressure of glucose solutions that are sufficiently calorie dense to meet energy requirements is a disadvantage because hypertonic solutions can injure the endothelium of veins. It is also poorly utilized in states of insulin resistance and does

not supply essential fatty acids. Furthermore, recent studies indicated that total energy needs are not met by oxidation of infused glucose only, and a significant amount of the infused glucose may be synthesized into fatty acids instead of being oxidized for energy. This process increases carbon dioxide output. Since fatty acid synthesis is an energy-requiring process, there is a decrease in the net energy available for other purposes. These aspects are discussed later in the text. Recent evidence has shown that in injured septic patients, glucose infusion increases oxygen consumption and catecholamine excretion.

Fat

Fat emulsions are made up of three groups of constituents: triglyceride, an emulsifying agent, and an agent added to give an acceptable osmolar concentration. Wretlind and his colleagues [26] developed and perfected a lipid emulsion, Intralipid (Vitrum, Stockholm, Sweden), which is made up of soya bean triglyceride, purified egg phospholipid as emulsifier, and glycerol to make the final emulsion isotonic. This emulsion could be infused in dogs over a 4-week period to provide total caloric replacement without any untoward reaction [24]. The particle size of this emulsion and its clearance from the plasma after intravenous infusion are comparable to those of chylomicrons [27]. In addition, its elimination characteristics are comparable to those of chylomicrons [25], and it has a neglible (deleterious) effect on the function of the reticuloendothelial system [47]. Furthermore, it is hydrolyzed by lipoprotein lipase in the same way as chylomicrons [11]. More recently, Ota et al. [49] showed that this lipid actually enhances the reactivity of lymphocytes to antigens and does not depress immunity. Two other emulsions with very similar characteristics have become available in North America: Liposyn (Abbott, Chicago, IL) and Soyacel (Baxter Travenol, Des Moines, IL). They have the same clearance and utilization characteristics as Intralipid and appear to be similarly free of toxicity. Recently it was shown that fat emulsions made up of a mixture of triglycerides of long- (16–18 carbon) and medium- (8–10 carbon) chain fatty acids can be infused in humans without significant toxicity. Preliminary results suggested that these emulsions are cleared more rapidly than those of existing long-chain triglycerides [15, 16, 70].

Amino Acids

After amino acids are transaminated or deaminated, the resulting carbon skeletons are oxidized either directly via subsequent conversion to pyruvate or entry into the tricarboxylic acid cycle, or indirectly by prior conversion to glucose (gluconeogenesis). However, this is a costly way of providing energy. Furthermore, the infusion of amino acids in quantities sufficient to provide a substantial part of the total energy requirements of an individual would result in massive urea production, osmotic diuresis, and azotemia.

Alcohols, Polyols, and Other Mono- and Disaccharides

Ethanol can be used as a source of calories, but its utilization is limited by CNS effects, altered redox state, and risk of hepatic damage. Sorbitol has been advocated as a source of calories, but studies have shown that between 20 and 40% of the infused sorbitol is excreted through the kidneys [34]. Furthermore, in a controlled study, 10% sorbitol was not less thrombogenic than 10% glucose when infused into a peripheral vein [34]. Xylitol is another polyol used as a source of energy, but it causes oxaluria and oxalosis of the kidney. [Editor's Note: In early studies in other countries, it may have been responsible for a number of deaths from hepatotoxicity.] Maltose, the disaccharide of glucose, has half the osmolality of glucose, but its metabolic availability when it is given intravenously is controversial. Fructose has been advocated because its intracellular transport is not insulin dependent. However, in large doses it depletes hepatic adenosine triphosphate (ATP), raises lactate (and hence uric acid) levels, and

has been claimed to result in relatively higher plasma triglyceride levels than glucose. Although the last may not be the case, it does not have sufficient merit to be used in preference to glucose.

METABOLIC FATE AND INTERRELATIONSHIPS

A scheme of these relationships is given in Figure 25-1. The three major nutrients—carbohydrate, fat, and protein—are interrelated metabolically in three ways. First, all these nutrients can provide substrates for oxidation in the Krebs cycle (see Fig. 25-1, 1). Second, biosynthesis of one of these nutrients can occur from others in specified ways. In this regard, alpha-keto-acids can be synthesized into nonessential amino acids (see Fig. 25-1, 2) by transamination, with glutamic acid as the nitrogen donor. In muscle, alanine is synthesized from pyruvate (see Fig. 25-1, 3), with the amino acid group being derived by transamination from other amino acids originating from muscle protein catabolism, especially the branched-chain amino acids—valine, leucine, and isoleucine. Recently [62, 63] it was shown that by providing the keto or hydroxy analogue of certain essential amino acids exogenously, one can cause biosynthesis of essential amino acids to occur, thus showing that it is the carbon skeleton of these amino acids that is essential. Fatty acid synthesis occurs in the liver from acetyl-CoA (see Fig. 25-1, 4A) derived from pyruvate, a product of carbohydrate metabolism. This pathway is a major source of fatty acids in patients infused with large amounts of carbohydrate. Likewise, the glycerol for triglyceride synthesis (see Fig. 25-1, 4B) can be derived from dihydroxyacetone phosphate, a metabolite of glucose. Glucose, on the other hand, can be synthesized via the gluconeogenic pathway (see Fig. 25-1, 5) from substrates derived from amino acid metabolism. Although it is currently popular to consider "the" gluconeogenic amino acid to be alanine, Figure 25-1 shows that what is gluconeogenic is the carbon skeleton derived

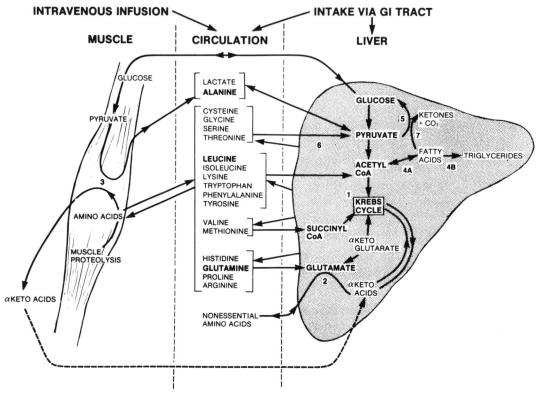

Figure 25-1. Interrelationships of energy sources and their metabolites.

from pyruvate, which in turn is derived primarily from glucose. Hence the "alanine-glucose cycle" does not lead to net glucose synthesis from amino acid precursors unless the pyruvate is derived from other amino acids (see Fig. 25-1, 6). In this respect, alanine and lactate are analogous as gluconeogenic precursors, since no net new glucose is produced from lactate derived from glucose and recycled (via the Cori cycle) back to glucose in the liver. Experimental studies have shown that in fasted animals, pyruvate derived from amino acids in muscle is quantitatively of minor importance as a source of pyruvate for gluconeogenesis. Thus, alanine can equally be regarded as no more than an amino group carrier to rid muscle of otherwise potentially toxic ammonia, which the liver synthesizes into urea for subsequent excretion. Lastly, while the naturally occurring fatty acids themselves cannot be converted to glucose, it should be recognized that the energy-requiring gluconeogenic pathway is

"fueled" by fatty acid oxidation (see Fig. 25-1, 7). Hence, energy from oxidation of one substrate supports the biosynthesis of others.

In the case of fatty acid oxidation by the liver, the "by-products" are the ketone bodies, acetoacetate, and 3-hydroxybutyrate. Thus, in states in which fat-derived fuels are the primary energy source, elevation in ketone body levels is expected. This occurs whether fatty acids are derived from endogenous lipid stores or from infusion of triglyceride emulsions. When gluconeogenesis is accelerated as a primary event (as in certain forms of trauma), again this link between gluconeogenesis and fatty acid oxidation results in accelerated ketogenesis. A fundamental principle of control of all the foregoing processes is that the pathways do not usually operate in both directions simultaneously. Thus, in states of isocaloric provision of glucose exogenously, that glucose is oxidized and used as substrate for fatty acid synthesis, and gluconeogenesis and fatty acid oxidation are shut off. In the opposite direction, with fat as the principal energy source, gluconeogenesis to provide the necessary fuel for obligate glycolytic tissue (erythrocytes, CNS, skin, etc.) is active. But when both glucose and lipid are available, the net adjustment of these pathways is determined by the proportion of each provided. However, these relationships may be disturbed by sepsis and injury where there may be insulin resistance and high levels of cortisol, catecholamines, and glucagon [3, 7, 52, 66].

These interrelationships are important in recognizing that there is nothing exclusive about any one substrate, and that infusion of any one energy source influences the utilization of other sources. A discussion of the hormonal mediation of these responses follows.

UTILIZATION OF ENERGY SOURCES IN PATHOLOGIC STATES

Malnutrition

In malnutrition and fasting, there is mobilization of fatty acid from adipose tissue stores to provide energy for peripheral tissues, including muscle. In addition, there is an obligatory release of amino acids from muscle protein, and this leads to wasting. The carbon skeletons of the released amino acids are used for gluconeogenesis to provide fuel for the CNS and other glucose-utilizing tissues. In prolonged fasting, ketogenesis becomes well established, and ketones are used as fuels by the CNS, displacing glucose in part. Additionally, associated with increased ketonemia and a rise in plasma free fatty acid levels, the mobilization of amino acids from muscle is reduced. Hence, in malnutrition and starvation, endogenous lipids are selectively utilized as fuel, and protein loss is curtailed but does persist [10]. If carbohydrates are administered in this state, the insulin levels will rise and protein catabolism and consequent release of amino acids will be suppressed. In addition, the utilization of

glucose for energy increases in proportion to the amount given in relation to total needs. The administered glucose also decreases gluconeogenesis from protein and, hence, protein catabolism. This protein-sparing effect of carbohydrate has been known for a century, but popularized in the past several decades [19]. [*Editor's Note:* The classic "life raft" studies of Gamble are simple yet exquisite, despite the fact that they are not entirely correct at higher glucose levels.] In otherwise normal individuals, exogenous fat given with amino acids as energy also spares protein, although without elevating insulin levels.

Trauma

In trauma, the metabolic rate is increased and energy expenditure rises. Kinney et al. [37] estimated that the increase may be 25% above normal for multiple fractures and as much as 40 to 100% with burns. However, in both animal models and in humans, a significant part of the increased metabolic rate in burns is due to the thermogenic effect of feeding [1, 69]. The enhanced thermogenic effect of feeding may be related to the effects of increased catabolic hormones including cortisol, catecholamines, and glucagon [7]. However, Wolfe et al. [69] found no relationship between the thermogenic effect of glucose and any alteration in the hormonal milieu.

Associated with a rise in metabolic rate in the injured patient, there is increased gluconeogenesis, increased nitrogen loss, and insulin resistance. Despite this increased flow of glucose, it is clearly not used as the primary metabolic fuel [68] since the respiratory quotient in these patients is only 0.70 to 0.75, indicating that fat oxidation still provides the primary energy substrate [37, 66]. Furthermore, in burned patients, during glucose infusion with or without insulin, the proportion of glucose oxidized fell as uptake increased, showing that the availability of this substrate as the primary source of energy is limited and is not enhanced by insulin [68]. In these patients, it is of interest that the high rate of gluconeogenesis cannot be curtailed by glucose infusions alone [23]. In trauma, the muscle appears to completely oxidize only 50% of the glucose extracted from the circulation, the remainder being released, after only partial oxidation, as lactate [12, 66]. The increase in muscle lactate output and the consequent increase in blood lactate are associated with increased gluconeogenesis. Clowes et al. [12] indicated that in the traumatized subject, muscle also does not use fatty acids effectively and thus increases the need to oxidize amino acids as a source of fuel. The nitrogen released by oxidation of endogenous amino acids from muscle flows out as alanine, resulting in a further increase in the availability of substrate for gluconeogenesis. The enhanced rate of gluconeogenesis derives its energy needs from fatty acid oxidation. Hence, fatty acid utilization is enhanced, and the respiratory quotient falls to 0.70 to 0.75. Viewed in another way, it can be shown that in such patients, despite the increased nitrogen wasting, 80% of the total metabolic energy is derived from fat [37, 66].

In contrast to the findings of Clowes et al. [12], and a concordant conclusion drawn from selected literature by Ryan [54] that fatty acid mobilization and ketogenesis are impaired in trauma, are the findings of Batstone et al. [6] and Carlson [11] in patients with burns. In these studies, fatty acid mobilization and ketogenesis did occur during the early phase of injury, but the levels fell after the first few days. Barton [5] showed in experiments that ketone body production early after injury was normal, but peripheral utilization was increased.

Infection

Infection is associated with only a modest increase in metabolic rate [3, 52]. Recently the metabolic effects of infection have been simulated by the effects of a cytokine, cachectin [59]. Studies of this cytokine demonstrated increased protein turnover, increased lipolysis with an increased triglyceride level, and increased fatty acid oxidation [58]. [*Editor's Note:* The authors do not intend by this statement to attribute all of the metabolic effects

of infection to tumor necrosis factor (TNF)/cachectin. Recent studies [24a] from a variety of laboratories, including our own, suggest that cofactors, including steroids, are required for at least some of the effects attributed to TNF/cachectin.] In contrast, the presence of septic shock is associated with a fall in metabolic rate owing to poor perfusion and, possibly, the effect of endotoxin on the oxidative mechanism of the cell [12].

The uptake of glucose by muscle is increased by infection, but lactate output rises to a degree that suggests that only 25% of the glucose is being fully oxidized. This finding, together with the observation that free fatty acid utilization is only one-seventh that of the fasting patient despite only a 50% reduction in free fatty acid levels, suggests that the muscle must obtain a significant part of its energy from amino acid oxidation. This assumption is supported by the higher nitrogen loss seen in these patients and the greater release of alanine and glutamine from muscle, which may amount to two to three times the output in controls [12, 58]. Gluconeogenesis is increased, as expected from the hormonal milieu (inappropriately low insulin and high glucagon, corticosteroids, catecholamines, and growth hormone), and the increase in lactate and alanine output by muscle makes substrates available for gluconeogenesis by the liver. However, with septic shock and endotoxemia, gluconeogenesis falls, lactate and alanine levels rise, and blood glucose levels approach normal [12, 66]. In extreme septic shock, hypoglycemia may occur.

Recently we showed that patients with sepsis and pancreatitis who failed to utilize glucose and fats, and who also had a low metabolic rate, rarely survived [60]. Therefore, it appears that with serious infection no exogenous substrate is utilized and muscle continues to rely on endogenous protein as a source of energy, despite the availability of glucose and fatty acids. Hence, in such patients the traditional sources of nonprotein energy may not be of any value, and in fact it is not clear whether any nutrient can be metabolized without side effects such as hy-

perglycemia, hypertriglyceridemia, and azotemia. [*Editor's Note:* This may be the one
group of patients in whom use of a high
branched-chain amino acid (BCAA) solution
may be justified, as the BCAAs may be utilized by muscle without the necessity of going through glucose. Azotemia is also reduced [9].]

Lipoprotein Abnormalities

In type I and type V hyperlipoproteinemias,
the utilization of circulating triglycerides is
impaired because of reduced or absent lipoprotein lipase activity, preventing the hydrolysis of the circulating triglyceride into fatty
acids. In type IV hyperlipoproteinemia, increased carbohydrate intake is associated
with a rise in circulating triglyceride levels,
presumably from increased hepatic very-
low-density-lipoprotein (VLDL) –triglyceride
synthesis from the glucose provided.

Liver and Renal Diseases

In liver disease, especially cirrhosis and
chronic liver failure, there is insulin resistance with carbohydrate intolerance. In consequence, hyperglycemia and hyperinsulinemia occur with carbohydrate infusions. In
contrast, there is no evidence for impaired
utilization of lipids. [*Editor's Note:* Caution
must be exercised in hepatic failure, as nonesterified fatty acids may displace tryptophan
from decreased serum albumin, making more
free tryptophan available for transport across
the blood-brain barrier.]

In chronic renal disease, there are impaired
tolerances of carbohydrate and fat, both of
which are corrected by dialysis. Furthermore,
it has been shown that infused lipid emulsions do not adversely affect the dialysis
membrane in its ability the clear the blood of
such waste products as urea and electrolytes.

Diabetes Mellitus

Since insulin is a primary regulator of the responses to altered nutritional states and has
been described as a factor in several of the
aforementioned abnormal states, predicted
responses of diabetics to parenteral nutrition
and to these pathologic states are correspondingly exaggerated. Absolute insulin deficiency, in insulin-dependent (juvenile-onset
type) diabetics, has been described as a "su-
perfasted state" in which all early fasting
metabolic adjustments are amplified (fat mobilization, gluconeogenesis, and protein
mobilization) and are exacerbated by the
inability to generate a "fed-state" response
to exogenous nutrients. Thus, utilization of
both exogenous and endogenously overpro-
duced nutrients is impaired. The administration of either glucose or lipid, or mixes
of both, to such diabetics would thus produce catastrophic effects unless appropriate
amounts of insulin (determined by the nutrient composition and its rate of delivery) are
concurrently provided. This is easily done by
merely adding insulin to infusates, titrating
the amount against glycemia, glucosuria, and
ketone levels. When this is done, there is no
contraindication to the use of any nutrient
mix considered appropriate to the state being
treated.

In the non–insulin-dependent (maturity-
onset type) diabetic, the metabolic state is the
integrated result of the magnitude of insulin
deficiency and insulin resistance present. The
majority of such patients are obese, and their
insulin levels may range from low compared
with normal weight or obese nondiabetics,
all the way to high compared with normal
weight or even obese nondiabetics. The requirement for parenteral nutrition in such individuals is most often associated with stress
states, in which insulin secretory capacity is
further suppressed. These states often convert such diabetics into "apparent" insulin-
dependent diabetics, now termed "insulin-
requiring." Without insulin treatment, marked
hyperglycemia and its consequences—or
even ketoacidosis—may appear. Therefore,
in any case of isocaloric or hypercaloric parenteral nutrition in such individuals, insulin
therapy should be introduced at the outset
and continued throughout treatment, again
with careful monitoring. Without it, the risk
of hyperosmolar, hyperglycemic states is significant.

Often in the course of acute illness in previously undiagnosed diabetics, hyperglycemia develops, precipitated by suppression of insulin secretion and elevation of anti-insulin hormone levels. If unrecognized, marked hyperglycemia may rapidly evolve, with all its untoward consequences. Therefore, all candidates for TPN must be tested for diabetes at the outset and at intervals during treatment. Especially vulnerable are individuals with renal failure and those receiving high-dose corticosteroids, or any drug known to be capable of impairing insulin secretion (e.g., diazoxide, phenytoin) or previously described as being associated with hyperglycemia (e.g., some diuretics, l-asparaginase, azathioprine, lithium, pentamidine).

On the other hand, our observations have shown that providing 50% of the total caloric input as lipid emulsion frequently abolishes or greatly reduces the degree of hyperglycemia [3, 52] and thus obviates the need to add exogenous insulin. The introduction of fat does not adversely alter nitrogen balance when compared with an all-glucose infusion [3, 33, 52]. Hence, mixed lipid-glucose infusions are recommended for these patients.

PROTEIN-SPARING ACTION OF ENERGY SUBSTRATES

Concept of Protein Sparing and Factors Modifying the Protein-Sparing Effect of Energy Sources

In 1946 Gamble [18], in his now classic "life raft" studies, showed that the infusion of glucose reduced by 50% the nitrogen loss (as urea) due to protein catabolism. This effect was referred to as the protein-sparing effect of glucose. Subsequently, Cahill [10] showed that in prolonged fasting, a rise in circulating nonprotein fuels, such as fatty acids and ketones, was associated with a fall in urinary nitrogen, one interpretation of which is that fuels derived from fat can inhibit the breakdown of muscle protein.

These effects demonstrate that availability of nonprotein energy, both as glucose and as fat, can inhibit the breakdown of endogenous protein in the absence of exogenous protein. Since the early 1900s, it has been known that with a fixed protein intake, nitrogen balance improved with the addition of energy as either carbohydrate or fat [42]. More recently, Blackburn et al. [8] and others, including ourselves [42], showed that infusing amino acids alone results in a reduced net negative balance of nitrogen, indicating that exogenous amino acids are also protein-sparing. The key finding in all these studies has been the inability to attain positive nitrogen balance when one energy substrate was used alone or when amino acids were combined with hypocaloric (i.e., < metabolic needs) amounts of carbohydrate or fat.

By contrast, modest amounts of amino acids combined with carbohydrate, in quantities exceeding the energy requirements of the patient, have resulted in positive nitrogen balance. Similarly, the use of fat has also been associated with positive nitrogen balance [33]. Hence, protein anabolism can only be attained by combining amino acids with an energy source in amounts sufficient to meet or exceed the energy requirements of the patient.

In addition to positive nitrogen balance, it can be shown that such a combination indeed results in an increase in total body nitrogen measured by the gamma emission of neutron bombardment, and in total body potassium measured by whole-body counting of potassium 40 (Fig. 25-2) [41]. It is the universal experience that such patients gain body weight and tissue as assessed by a variety of measures.

Role of Carbohydrate versus Fat in Nitrogen Sparing: The Modifying Effects of Malnutrition, Infection, and Trauma

It appears that in both malnutrition and trauma, the major part of the oxidized fuel is fat [12, 37, 66]. Furthermore, Holroyde et al. [29] showed that even when glucose is infused as the sole exogenous energy substrate, 30 to 50% of the carbon dioxide ex-

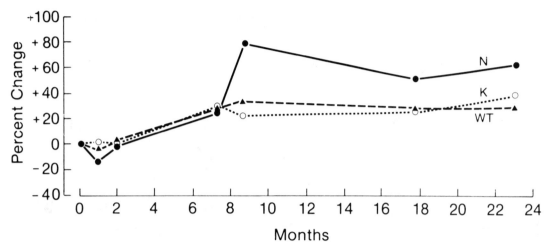

Figure 25-2. Course with time of one patient's changes in body weight (WT), total body potassium (naturally occurring potassium 40 determined in whole-body counter) (K), and total body nitrogen (N) (as determined by neutron capture gamma analysis).

creted comes from sources other than glucose, indicating that glucose fails to provide all the carbon required for oxidation in the situations examined. Fat might be expected to be the natural substrate for the provision of the nonprotein energy in these situations. In contrast to this simple theory, however, the results of experimental studies comparing the relative efficacy of carbohydrate and fat in promoting positive nitrogen balance are controversial. The weight of evidence now supports the equivalence of fat and carbohydrate in many clinical situations. On the other hand, studies by Long et al. [40] and McDougal et al. [43] on critically ill burned patients suggested that despite excellent utilization of exogenously infused lipid, this substrate did not reduce nitrogen loss. In contrast, the infusion of glucose did significantly reduce nitrogen excretion. The maximum reduction in nitrogen excretion was found to occur when the infusion rate of glucose was equal to the metabolic requirements for energy. These studies were widely interpreted as suggesting that lipid had no role in promoting nitrogen retention during parenteral nutrition.

Nevertheless, another controlled crossover trial of glucose and lipid sources [33] of nonprotein energy in patients with malnutrition and a variety of gastrointestinal disorders, including those with infection and inflammation such as Crohn's disease, pancreatitis, and peritonitis, showed that lipids and carbohydrates were comparable in promoting nitrogen retention. In this study, a mixture of 5% amino acid and 5% dextrose solution, delivering 1 g/kg of ideal body weight, was infused throughout the study. On an average, these patients therefore received a constant intake of 60 g of amino acids and 60 g of dextrose. In addition, the patients were randomized to receive either glucose or lipid at 40 kcal/kg of ideal body weight. After a week of this regimen, the additional nonprotein energy source was switched, making each patient his or her control for comparing the two substrates. By randomizing the order, the effect of any change due to improvement in the clinical state was minimized. It is seen in Figures 25-3 to 25-5 that the glucose infusion resulted in higher levels of pyruvate and lactate, both glucose-derived substrates, and that the circulating concentrations of free fatty acids and ketones were suppressed. Plasma glucose levels were not different, but they had higher insulin and lower glucagon levels. In contrast, during lipid infusion there were lower pyruvate and lactate levels with higher concentrations of fat-derived substances, namely free fatty acids and ketones, with lower insulin and higher glucagon lev-

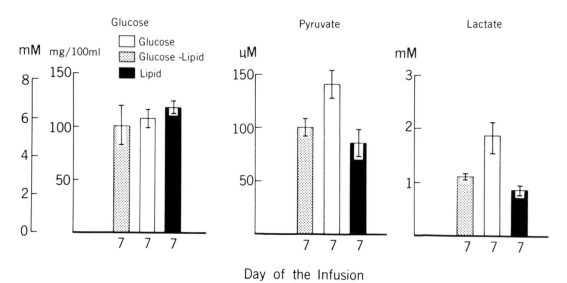

Figure 25-3. Serum concentrations of glucose, pyruvate, and lactate during 24-hour infusions of total parenteral nutrition containing 1 g of amino acids/kg of ideal body weight. The nonprotein calories, prescribed to maintain normal body weight, were randomly given in turn for 1 week at a time as 100% glucose; 50% glucose, 50% lipid (Intralipid); or 17% glucose, 83% lipid (Intralipid).

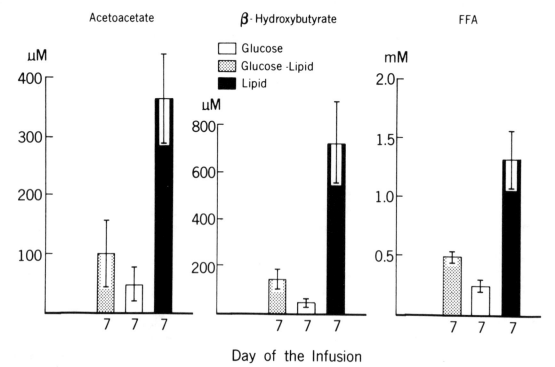

Figure 25-4. Serum concentrations of acetoacetate, beta-hydroxybutyrate, and plasma free fatty acids (FFA) under the conditions noted in Figure 25-3.

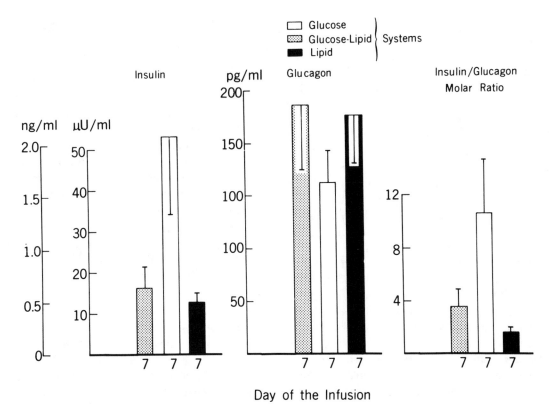

Figure 25-5. Plasma immunoreactive insulin and glucagon and their molar ratio, under the conditions noted in Figure 25-3.

els. Despite these very different substrate-hormone profiles, the nitrogen balances were comparable after the initial 3 days of study on each substrate. During the initial 3 days of infusion, there was slightly higher nitrogen retention with glucose. However, after the initial 3 days, nitrogen retention was comparable. In addition, it was noted that during lipid infusion, a higher free fatty acid level was associated with a lower nitrogen excretion, showing the nitrogen-sparing effect of exogenous fatty acids and indicating that during exogenous fat infusions, addition of agents such as heparin improves nitrogen retention. Subsequently, in critically ill septic patients, Roulet et al. [52], Baker et al. [3], and Shaw and Holdaway [56] showed that net protein balance was comparable when nonprotein calories were given as glucose alone or as a glucose-fat mixture. However, the latter mixture resulted in the need for less infusion of insulin to maintain euglycemia and a lower carbon dioxide output [3, 52].

Other investigators also noted that fat and carbohydrate are comparable in promoting nitrogen balance in patients in a variety of conditions similar to those studied by us [6, 20, 71]. Wannemacher et al. [64] showed that in monkeys infected with *Pneumococci*, exogenous glucose and lipid had equal protein-sparing actions and both were clearly superior to amino acids alone. Data on whole-body composition by MacFie et al. [41] indicate that total body nitrogen may increase only when lipid is added to the TPN regimen.

TECHNIQUES OF INFUSING LIPID AS AN ENERGY SOURCE

Metabolic Considerations

Over the years numerous studies have shown that nutrients are most effectively utilized when given simultaneously. Hence, it is appropriate that intravenous fat be infused concurrently with the other nutrients. Also, by infusing nutrients gradually, the circulating substrate profile remains at near steady-state levels, and rapid and marked increases in triglyceride or fatty acid levels are thereby avoided.

Despite dogmatic pronouncements about the danger of mixing fat with glucose and amino acids, because of the risk of breaking the emulsion, experimental and practical experience has shown otherwise. When lipid has been infused concurrently with a glucose-amino acid solution through a Y-connector in the manner to be described later in this chapter, no untoward effects have been reported from the experience of infusing 36,000 U over 10 years at the Toronto General Hospital. Furthermore, published metabolic studies indicated excellent utilization of fat when it is given this way. More recently, 3-in-1 mixtures of amino acids, glucose, and lipid emulsion have been shown to be stable for several days and have been used in clinical practice without any untoward effects [48]. The only restriction concerning such mixtures is the amount of divalent ions that can be added. There is therefore no evidence to support the alleged requirements for separately infusing fat and dextrose–amino acid mixtures.

The next metabolic consideration is the most appropriate ratio of fat to carbohydrate. It is clear from what has been noted earlier that nitrogen balance is comparable in many studies, irrespective of the nature of the non-protein energy source, the only exception being patients with severe burns, who do not constitute the majority given parenteral nutrition. This being the case, a decision regarding the type of infusion is based mainly on other criteria. These are the (1) route of administration, (2) substrate-hormone profile, (3) need for specific factors only available in lipid, (4) effect of infusion on fluid and electrolyte balance, (5) effect on ventilatory load, and (6) maintenance of normal biochemical parameters. These criteria are discussed when we present the advantages and disadvantages of fat as a caloric source compared with glucose.

Peripheral Infusion Technique

Solutions Used

Amino acids, dextrose, electrolytes, vitamins, and trace elements in a mix are infused. A 5% amino acid solution with 12.5% dextrose is made by mixing equal volumes of commercially available 10% amino acids with 25% dextrose. In most adults, about 1500 ml/24 hr is sufficient to meet amino acid requirements. Electrolytes are added to this infusion to provide about 115 to 120 mEq of sodium, 80 to 100 mEq of potassium, 20 mEq of calcium, 25 to 30 mEq of magnesium, and 500 to 600 mg of phosphorus per 24 hours. Vitamins are added as indicated previously [32]. Trace elements are likewise introduced as required [31].

Lipid Emulsion

Concurrently with the amino acid–dextrose mix just described, 1500 ml of 10% lipid emulsion is infused. With 20% lipid more calories can be given in the same volume at a lower osmolality by infusing 1000 ml of this lipid and diluting the amino acid–dextrose mixture with 500 ml of distilled water.

Method of Infusion

The success of the peripheral venous infusion depends on strict adherence to the method to be described. The amino acid–dextrose mixture must be infused concurrently and at the same rate as the lipid through a Y-connector to avoid thrombophlebitis [18, 51, 61]. [*Editor's Note:* This experience of avoiding thrombophlebitis is not universal.] The entire success of the method depends on the lipid mixing and diluting the amino acid–dextrose mixture to a near-isotonic state. It is desirable to use a two-channel pump so as to ensure uniform infusion of the viscous lipid and the dextrose–amino acid mixture.

Nutrient Prescription

The infusion described above provides 75 g of amino acids, 659 kcal of dextrose, and 1650 kcal of lipid, giving a total caloric input of

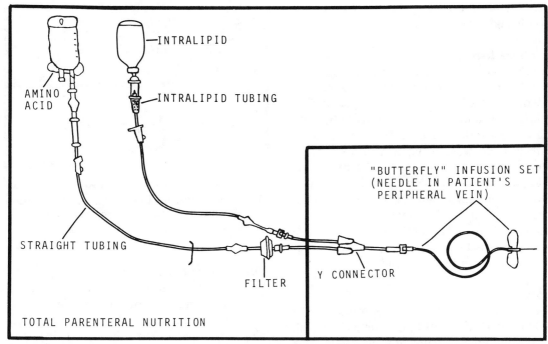

Figure 25-6. Peripheral venous infusion for total parenteral nutrition.

about 2300 kcal in 3000 ml of fluid. From these figures, it is apparent that sufficient calories and protein can be given by this system to induce anabolism. Thus, such a peripheral system can provide sufficient calories to restore tissue proteins. If more fluids should be given, as in patients with fistulas, the caloric input can be increased further. Also, with 20% lipid the lipid input can be increased.

Equipment Required (Fig. 25-6)
1. A 19-gauge butterfly needle or 18-gauge Angiocath Teflon intravenous catheter placement unit (Deseret Company, Sandy, UT).
2. 500 ml of normal saline solution (initially).
3. Straight intravenous tubing.
4. Intralipid tubing (if Intralipid is to be given).
5. Alcohol swabs.
6. Povidone-iodine 10% solution. (PI).
7. Tourniquet.
8. Y-connector (to allow mixing of lipid with the other solutions as close to point of entry as possible).
9. Filter.

Procedure
Note: The intravenous nurse or doctor should insert the butterfly needle or catheter.

1. Explain to the patient what is to be done and why.
2. Bring all the necessary equipment to the bedside and connect and flush the intravenous tubing with saline solution.
3. Place the tourniquet on the arm; clean the skin with alcohol and apply povidone. Insert the butterfly needle or catheter. Release the tourniquet and connect the tubing.
4. Open the control clamp on the intravenous tubing to run quickly at first, then regulate.
5. Tape the butterfly needle or catheter securely.
6. When the saline flush is running properly, the nutrient mixture can be started (see Fig. 25-6).

Central Venous Infusion Technique

The central venous catheter is inserted and cared for in the usual way [53]. To infuse lipids, the central route is used with minor modifications as follows.

Solutions Used

Amino acids, dextrose, electrolytes, vitamins, and trace elements in a mix are infused. The solutions used consist of 5% amino acids and 25% dextrose made by mixing commercially available 10% amino acids with 50% dextrose in equal volumes. In an average adult, 1.5 to 2.0 liters/24 hr of this solution are infused with lipid. Electrolytes, vitamins, and trace elements are added to the solution as indicated under the peripheral infusion system. Details of these additives have been published elsewhere [31] and can be reviewed by the interested reader.

Lipid Emulsion

The aforementioned mixture is infused with 1000 or 1500 ml of 10% lipid or 500 to 1000 ml of 20% lipid concurrently by means of a Y-connector, as described previously.

Method of Infusion

The two solutions are infused concurrently by means of a standard drip system. No pumps are necessary. The dextrose concentration in the final infusate using this technique is diluted by the lipid emulsion to about 16%, reducing the danger of hypoglycemia in the event that the drip is discontinued abruptly.

Nutrient Prescription

This system provides 100 g of amino acids, 1250 to 1700 kcal of glucose, and 1100 to 1650 kcal of lipid, giving a total of 2350 to 3350 kcal/24 hr.

Technique

The hub of the central venous line is attached to a connecting length of intravenous tubing (e.g., Extension Set 30", Abbott Hospital Supplies, Abbott Laboratories, North Chicago, IL), which is then connected to the Y-connector (Fig. 25-7). The remaining connections are as given under peripheral infusion (see Fig. 25-6).

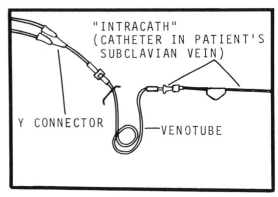

Figure 25-7. Proximal modifications of Figure 25-6 for central venous infusion for total parenteral nutrition.

Three-In-One Infusion

As an alternative to the above method, there is an increasing tendency to consider the use of a three-in-one complete amino acid, dextrose, and lipid mixture in which the pharmacy mixes a complete mixture of a composition described previously [48]. The main consideration is to avoid excess of divalent ions: calcium (up to 2.3 mmol), magnesium (up to 10 mmol), and zinc (up to 20 mg) [48].

ADVANTAGES AND DISADVANTAGES OF FAT AS A CALORIE SOURCE COMPARED WITH GLUCOSE

Substrate-Hormone Profile

It is seen from Figures 25-3 to 25-5 that the substrate-hormone profile depends on the nature of the nonprotein calories infused. It is quite clear that the substrate-hormone profile is closest to the postprandial state when half the calories are given as glucose and half as lipid (glucose-lipid). The insulin levels are largely within the postprandial range. Hence, this ratio of calories provides the system closest to that observed in the postabsorptive state. The modest insulin response required to utilize the substrate infused makes it attractive for non–insulin-dependent diabetics and when there is insulin resistance. Using this ratio of calories, or when more fat is infused, as in a peripheral system, we have rarely had to give insulin to our patients, thus improving the simplicity of the method and reducing the need for frequent monitoring. Correspondingly, the reduced glucose concentration required when lipid is given as a caloric source has simplified the technique for ambulatory patients who receive parenteral nutrition at home. The lower circulating levels of insulin, with a glucose-lipid infusion, reduce the need to use pumps or to carefully taper the infusion in order to avoid hypoglycemia on its termination. Toleration of abrupt stoppage or change of infusion is useful in case of mishap or sudden alteration in circumstances, and allows ambulatory patients to take the infusion in units that can be easily discontinued, thus giving the system a flexibility that can suit the social needs of the patient.

Fluid and Sodium Balance

It was shown by Spark et al. [57] and by others that high insulin levels and carbohydrate feeding result in marked sodium retention, an undesirable development for patients prone to pulmonary complications and for those with heart failure. This theoretic possibility has been confirmed by Hill et al. [28] and Yeung et al. [72] who showed through careful body composition studies that during glucose-based hyperalimentation, a major part of the increase in body weight was due to water. In our own unpublished studies using a glucose-lipid based system, such water retention has not occurred.

Respiratory Quotient and Carbon Dioxide Load

When carbohydrate alone is infused, the respiratory quotient (RQ) (carbon dioxide excreted/oxygen consumed) rises to 1.0, or higher if fat synthesis occurs. With a mixed intake of lipid and carbohydrate, the RQ is between 0.80 and 0.85. Hence, there is at least a 15 to 20% lower carbon dioxide load to

be excreted when lipid is infused. Recently, using an all-glucose system, Askanazi et al. [2] showed that glucose infusion increases the carbon dioxide load and especially increases oxygen consumption and the ventilatory effort in hypermetabolic patients. The same group also noted difficulty in weaning patients from respirators because of this high carbon dioxide load and could only do so by reducing the caloric intake. Respiratory failure with high glucose loads has also been described [13]. We demonstrated that in critically sick patients the carbon dioxide output was lower with a mixed lipid-glucose system than with glucose alone, provided that at least 50% of calories was in the form of lipid [3, 52].

Potential Complications of Lipid Infusion: Fact and Fiction

In older literature, the use of earlier lipid preparations (such as Lipomul), which proved to be toxic by reason of the particular lipid or emulsifier used, led to the accumulation of references that are often quoted to indicate the hazards of lipid infusions. It is important to emphasize that modern lipid sources, available in North America, do not show these effects.

Utilization of Fat in Trauma

It is often claimed that fat is not utilized in the traumatized patient. This appears not to be the case. Wilmore et al. [67] showed increased clearance of infused fat in catabolic patients, as did Hallberg [25].

Utilization of Fat in Sepsis

Fat clearance has been shown to be reduced in septic animals, and hence it was concluded that fat is not utilized in septic patients. However, a controlled study by Wannemacher et al. [64] showed that while triglyceride levels were higher in infected animals infused with lipid, there was no difference in nitrogen retention or recovery from the infection when compared with glucose-infused animals. Recent studies with an experimental cachectin infusion which mimics the effects of sepsis showed that both triglyceride levels and fat oxidation were increased. This finding indicates that high triglycerides in sepsis are not due to nonutilization but to increased mobilization and oxidation. Thus, the increased triglyceride levels seen in septic patients must not be construed necessarily as indicating nonutilization. In a recent study of septic patients with pancreatitis, we showed that patients who died exhibited high plasma glucose, triglyceride, and urea levels, and a low metabolic rate, and that these events thus appear to form an end-stage phenomenon [60].

Effect of Fat Emulsions on the Reticuloendothelial System

It is commonly believed that fat emulsions are taken up by the reticuloendothelial system, reducing the ability to combat infection. Previous studies did not uniformly support this concept [21, 55], and recent studies also failed to show any adverse effects on macrophage activity and polymorphonuclear leukocyte function [17, 47, 50]. Furthermore, Huth et al. [30] showed that while Lipomul-like emulsions using cottonseed oil reduced tolerance to endotoxin, the same phenomenon was not observed with soya oil emulsions such as Intralipid.

Effect of Fat Emulsions on the Coagulation System

Disseminated intravascular coagulation has been reported after the use of cottonseed oil emulsions, but no such effect and, indeed, no abnormality of coagulation in vivo has been reported during infusion of soya bean oil emulsions.

Effect of Fat Emulsions on Liver and Renal Disease

Liver disease is commonly believed to be a contraindication to the use of lipid emul-

sions. However, on theoretic and practical grounds, this cannot be justified. The lipid emulsions are hydrolyzed by lipoprotein lipase, mainly situated outside the liver, and the fatty acids thus released are taken up largely by muscle and adipocytes. In contrast, excess carbohydrate has to be converted to fatty acids in the liver [R. R. Wolfe, personal communication, 1977] and then excreted as lipoproteins. Hence, carbohydrates place a greater load on the liver than do fats. This is attested to by the observation that a high carbohydrate infusion reproducibly induces a fatty liver [35, 36, 44], whereas high fat infusions rarely do so. Furthermore, Jeejeebhoy et al. [35, 36] showed that isocaloric replacement of carbohydrate with lipid to the extent of 30 to 50% of total calories reproducibly clears the liver of the fat observed when an all-glucose system has been infused.

In practice, Zohrab et al. [73] found that when lipid was given in a TPN mixture in an amount of up to 2 mg/kg of ideal body weight/day in patients with jaundice and abnormal results of liver function tests, no adverse effect was seen, and in fact the liver function abnormalities improved during infusion. Similar results were reported by Lee [38], Michel et al. [45], and Zumtobel and Zehle [74]. More recently, a controlled trial by Glynn et al. [22] showed that a large infusion of lipid may even have beneficial effects on encephalopathy. [*Editor's Note:* The issue is not whether fat is utilized in liver disease, but rather the effect on fat displacing tryptophan from albumin, increasing its penetration across the blood-brain barrier. See Naylor et al. [46].]

In renal disease, both glucose and lipid utilization are reduced [14, 65], but this abnormality is corrected by dialysis. Furthermore, lipids do not influence the clearance of electrolytes and dialyzable nitrogenous products during hemodialysis [39].

Partial Parenteral Nutrition

In a number of gastrointestinal conditions, the patient may be able to tolerate only a limited amount of normal or elemental diet. Under these circumstances, balances of the nutritional requirements (after taking into account any energy reserves as fat) can be easily made up through peripheral parenteral nutrition, using the technique described earlier. This is especially useful in selected patients with esophageal and gastric obstruction, intractable diarrhea, anorectal disease, and partial bowel obstruction, as a temporary measure pending definitive treatment. By means of this method, optimal nutrition can be provided by all available routes and by simple techniques.

CONCLUSION

In conclusion, lipid is an important energy source for parenteral nutrition, and may be the preferred substrate in some situations.

REFERENCES

1. Allard, J. P., Jeejeebhoy, K. N., Whitwell, J., et al. Factors influencing energy expenditure in patients with burns. *J. Trauma* 28:199, 1988.
2. Askanazi, J., Carpentier, Y. A., Elwyn, D., et al. Influence of total parenteral nutrition on fuel utilization in injury and sepsis. *Ann. Surg.* 191:40, 1980.
3. Baker, J. P., Detsky, A. S., Stewart, S., Whitwell, J., Marliss, E. B., and Jeejeebhoy, K. N. Randomized trial of total parenteral nutrition in critically ill patients: Metabolic effects of varying glucose:lipid ratios as the energy source. *Gastroenterology* 87:53, 1984.
4. Bark, S., Holm, I., Hakansson, I., and Wretlind, A. Nitrogen-sparing effects of fat emulsion compared with glucose in the postoperative period. *Acta Chir. Scand.* 142:423, 1976.
5. Barton, R. N. Ketone body metabolism after trauma. In R. Porter and J. Knight (eds.), *Energy Metabolism in Trauma* (Ciba Foundation Symposium). London: Churchill-Livingstone, 1970. P. 173.
6. Batstone, G. F., Alberti, K. G. M. M., Hinks, L., et al. Metabolic studies in subjects following thermal injury: Intermediary metabolites, hormones, and tissue oxygenation. *Burns* 2:207, 1976.
7. Bessey, P. Q., Watters, J. M., Aoki, T. T., and Wilmore, D. W. Combined hormonal infusion simulates the metabolic response to injury. *Ann. Surg.* 200:264, 1984.
8. Blackburn, G. L., Flatt, J-P., Clowes, G. H. A., and O'Donnell, T. F. Peripheral intravenous feeding with isotonic amino acid solutions. *Am. J. Surg.* 125:447, 1973.
9. Bower, R. H., Muggia-Sullam, M., Vallgren, S., et al. Branched chain amino acid–enriched solutions in the septic patient: A randomized, prospective trial. *Ann. Surg.* 203:13, 1986.
10. Cahill, G. F., Jr. Starvation in man. *N. Engl. J. Med.* 282:668, 1970.
11. Carlson, L. A. Mobilization and utilization of lipids after trauma: Relation to caloric homeostasis. In R. Porter and J. Knight (eds.), *Energy Metabolism in Trauma* (Ciba Foundation Symposium). London: Churchill-Livingstone, 1970. P. 155.
12. Clowes, G. H. A., Jr., O'Donnell, T. F., Blackburn, G. L., and Maki, T. N. Energy metabolism and proteolysis in traumatized and septic man. *Surg. Clin. North Am.* 56:1169, 1976.
13. Covelli, H. D., Black, W. J., Olsen, M. S., and Beckman, J. F. Respiratory failure precipitated by high carbohydrate loads. *Ann. Intern. Med.* 95:579, 1981.
14. Cramp, D. G., Moorhead, J. F., and Wills, M. R. Disorders of blood lipids in renal disease. *Lancet* 1:672, 1975.
15. Crowe, P. J., Dennison, A. R., and Royle, G. T. A new intravenous emulsion containing medium-chain triglyceride: Studies of its metabolic effects in the perioperative period compared with a conventional long-chain triglyceride emulsion. *J. Parenter. Enter. Nutr.* 9:720, 1985.
16. Dawes, R. F. H., Royle, G. T., Dennison, A. R., Crowe, P. J., and Ball, M. Metabolic studies of a lipid emulsion containing medium-chain triglyceride in perioperative and total parenteral nutrition infusions. *World J. Surg.* 10:38, 1986.
17. Escudier, E. F., Escudier, B. J., Henry-Amar, M. C., et al. Effects of infused Intralipids on neutrophil chemotaxis during total parenteral nutrition. *J. Parenter. Enter. Nutr.* 10:596, 1986.
18. Fujiwara, T., Kawarasaki, H., and Fonkalsrud, E. W. Reduction of postinfection venous endothelial injury with Intralipid. *Surg. Gynecol. Obstet.* 158:57, 1984.
19. Gamble, J. L. Physiological information gained from studies on the life raft ration. Harvey Lectures (Harvey Society of New York) Lancaster, PA: Science Press Printing Co., 1946/47, Series 42, P. 247.
20. Gazzaniga, A. B., Bartlett, R. H., and Shobe, J. B. Nitrogen balance in patients receiving either fat or carbohydrate for total intravenous nutrition. *Ann. Surg.* 182:163, 1975.
21. Gigon, J. P., Enderlein, F., and Scheidegger, S. Über das Schicksal infundierter Fettemulsionen in der menschlichen Lunge. *Schweiz. Med. Wochenschr.* 96:71, 1966.
22. Glynn, M. J., Powell-Tuck, J., Reaveley,

D. A., and Murray-Lyon, I. M. High lipid parenteral nutrition improves portasystemic encephalopathy. *J. Parenter. Enter. Nutr.* 12:457,
1988.

23. Gump, F. E., Long, C. L., Killian, P., and Kinney, J. M. Studies of glucose intolerance in
septic, injured patients. *J. Trauma* 14:378, 1974.

24. Håkansson, I. Experience in long-term studies
on nine intravenous fat emulsions in dogs.
Nutr. Diet 10:54, 1968.

24a. Hall-Angerås, M., Angerås, V., Zamir, O.,
Hasselgren, P., and Fischer, J. E. Interaction
between corticosterone and tumor necrosis
factor stimulated protein breakdown in rat
skeletal muscle, similar to sepsis. *Surgery*
100:460–466, 1990.

25. Hallberg, D. Elimination of exogenous lipids
from the blood stream: An experimental meth-
odological and clinical study in dog and man.
Acta Physiol. Scand. Suppl. 259:1, 1965.

26. Hallberg, D., Schuberth, O., and Wretlind, A.
Experimental and clinical studies with fat
emulsion for intravenous nutrition. *Nutr. Diet.*
8:245, 1966.

27. Hallberg, D., and Wersall, J. Electron-micro-
scopic investigation of chylomicrons and fat
emulsions for intravenous use. *Acta Chir.
Scand. Suppl.* 325:23, 1964.

28. Hill, G. L., McCarthy, I. D., Collins, J. P., and
Smith, A. H. A new method for the rapid measurement of body composition in critically ill
surgical patients. *Br. J. Surg.* 65:732, 1978.

29. Holroyde, C. P., Myers, R. N., Smink, R. D.,
Putnam, R. C., Paul, P., and Reichard, G. A.
Metabolic responses to total parenteral nutrition in cancer patients. *Cancer Res.* 37:3109,
1977.

30. Huth, K. W., Schoenborn, W., and Börner,
J. Zur Pathogenese der Unverträglichkeitser-
scheinungen bei parenteraler Fettzufuhr. *Med.
Ernähr.* 8:146, 1967.

31. Jeejeebhoy, K. N. Enteral and parenteral nu-
trition. In J. M. Civetta, R. W. Taylor, and
R. R. Kirby (eds.), *Critical Care.* Philadelphia:
Lippincott, 1988.

32. Jeejeebhoy, K. N. Total parenteral nutrition
(TPN)—A review. *Ann. R. Coll. Phys. Surg.
Canada* 9:287, 1976.

33. Jeejeebhoy, K. N., Anderson, G. H., Na-
khooda, A. F., Greenberg, G. R., Sanderson,
I., and Marliss, E. B. Metabolic studies in total
parenteral nutrition with lipid in man: Comparison with glucose. *J. Clin. Invest.* 57:125,
1976.

34. Jeejeebhoy, K. N., Anderson, G. H., Sanderson, I., and Bryan, M. H. Total parenteral
nutrition. In J. G. G. Ledinghan (ed.), *Tenth
Symposium on Advanced Medicine.* London: Pitman Medical, 1974. P. 132.

35. Jeejeebhoy, K. N., Langer, B., Tsallas, G.,

Chu, R. C., Kuksis, A., and Anderson, G. H.
Total parenteral nutrition at home: Studies in
patients surviving 4 months to 5 years. *Gastroenterology* 71:943, 1976.

36. Jeejeebhoy, K. N., Zohrab, W. J., Langer, B.,
Phillips, M. J., Kuksis, A., and Anderson,
G. H. Total parenteral nutrition at home for 23
months without complication and with good
rehabilitation. A study of technical and metabolic features. *Gastroenterology* 65:811, 1973.

37. Kinney, J. M., Long, C. L., and Duke, J. H.
Carbohydrate and nitrogen metabolism after
injury. In R. Porter and J. Knight (eds.), *Energy Metabolism in Trauma* (Ciba Foundation
Symposium). London: Churchill-Livingstone,
1970. P. 103.

38. Lee, H. A. The rationale for using a fat emulsion (Intralipid) as part energy substrate during intravenous nutrition. In J. M. Greeps,
P. B. Soeters, R. I. C. Wesdorp, C. W. R. Phaf,
and J. E. Fischer (eds.), *Current Concepts in Parenteral Nutrition.* The Hague: Martinus Nijhof,
1977. P. 261.

39. Lee, H. A., Sharpstone, P., and Ames, A. C.
Parenteral nutrition in renal failure. *Postgrad.
Med. J.* 43:81, 1967.

40. Long, J. M., Wilmore, D. W., Mason, A. D.,
Jr., and Pruitt, B. A., Jr. Fat-carbohydrate interaction: Effects on nitrogen-sparing in total
intravenous feeding. *Surg. Forum* 25:61, 1974.

41. MacFie, J., Smith, R. C., and Hill, G. L. Glucose or fat as a non-protein energy source? A
controlled clinical trial. *Gastroenterology* 80:103,
1981.

42. Marliss, E. B. An overview of amino acid metabolism: the determinants of protein homeostasis in parenteral nutrition. In H. L. Greene,
M. A. Holliday and H. N. Munro (eds.), *Clinical Nutrition Update: Amino Acids.* Chicago:
American Medical Association, 1977. P. 34.

43. McDougal, W. S., Wilmore, D. W., and Pruitt,
B. A., Jr. Effect of intravenous near isosmotic
nutrient infusions on nitrogen balance in critically ill injured patients. *Surg. Gynecol. Obstet.*
145:408, 1977.

44. Messing, B., Bitoun, A., Galian, A., Mary,
J. Y., Goll, A., and Bernier, J. J. La stéatose
hépatique au cours del la nutrition parentérale
dépendelle de l'apport calorique glucidique?
Gastroenterol. Clin. Biol. 1:1015, 1977.

45. Michel, H., Raynaud, A., Crastes de Paulet,
Mme., et al. Tolerance du cirrhotique aux lip-
ides intra-veineux. Presented at the Congress
International de Nutrition Parenterale, Mont-
pellier, France, September 12–14, 1974.

46. Naylor, C. D., O'Rourke, K., Detsky, A. S.,
and Baker, J. P. Parenteral nutrition with
branched-chain amino acids in hepatic encephalopathy: a meta-analysis. *Gastroenterology* 97:1033, 1989.

47. Nishiwaki, H., Iriyama, K., Asami, H., et al. Influences of an infusion of lipid emulsion on phagocytic activity of cultured Kupffer cells in septic rats. *J. Parenter. Enter. Nutr.* 10:614, 1986.

48. O'Keefe, S. J. D., Bean, E., Symmonds, K., Smit, R., Delport, I., and Dicker, J. Clinical evaluation of a "3-in-1" intravenous nutrient solution. *S. Afr. Med. J.* 68:82, 1985.

49. Ota, D. M., Copeland, E. M., III, Corriere, N. J., Jr., Richie, E. R., Jacobson, K., and Dudrick, S. J. The effects of a 10% soya-bean oil emulsion on lymphocyte transformation. *J. Parenter. Enter. Nutr.* 2:112, 1978.

50. Palmblad, J., Brostrom, O., Lahnborg, G., Uden, M.-A., and Venizelos, N. Neutrophil functions during total parenteral nutrition and Intralipid infusion. *Am. J. Clin. Nutr.* 35:1430, 1982.

51. Pithie, A., Soutar, J. S., and Pennington, C. R. Catheter tip position in central venous thrombosis. *J. Parenter. Enter. Nutr.* 12:13, 1988.

52. Roulet, M., Detsky, A. S., Marliss, E. B., et al. A controlled trial of the effect of parenteral nutritional support on patients with respiratory failure and sepsis. *Clin. Nutr.* 2:97, 1983.

53. Ryan, J. A., Jr. Complications of total parenteral nutrition. In J. E. Fischer (ed.), *Total Parenteral Nutrition* (1st ed.). Boston: Little, Brown, 1976. P. 55.

54. Ryan, N. T. Metabolic adaptations for energy production during trauma and sepsis. *Surg. Clin. North Am.* 56:1073, 1976.

55. Scholler, K. L. Transport and Speicherung von Fettemulsion-Teilichen. *Z. prakt. Anästh. Wiederbel.* 3:193, 1968.

56. Shaw, J. H. F., and Holdaway, C. M. Protein-sparing effect of substrate infusion in surgical patients is governed by the clinical state and not by the individual substrate infused. *J. Parenter. Enter. Nutr.* 12:433, 1988.

57. Spark, R. F., Arky, R. A., Boulter, P. R., and Saudek, C. D., and O'Brian, J. T. Renin, aldosterone and glucagon in the natriuresis of fasting. *N. Engl. J. Med.* 292:1335, 1975.

58. Starnes, H. F., Warren, R. S., Jeevanandam, M., et al. Tumor necrosis factor and the acute metabolic response to tissue injury in man. *J. Clin. Invest.* 82:1321, 1988.

59. Tracey, K. J., Beutler, B., Lowry, S. F., et al. Shock and tissue injury induced by recombinant human cachectin. *Science* 234:470, 1986.

60. Van Gossum, A., Lemoyne, M., Greig, P. D., and Jeejeebhoy, K. N. Lipid-associated total parenteral nutrition in patients with severe acute pancreatitis. *J. Parenter. Enter. Nutr.* 12:250, 1988.

61. Wakefield, A., Cohen, Z., Craig, M., Connolley, P., Jeejeebhoy, K. N., Silverman, R., and Levy, G. A. Thrombogenicity of total parenteral nutrition. I. Effect on induction of monocyte/macrophage procoagulant activity. *Gastroenterology* 97:1210, 1989.

62. Walser, M. Therapeutic aspects of branched-chain amino and keto acids. *Clin. Sci.* 66:1, 1984.

63. Walser, M. Rationale and indications for the use of α-keto analogues. *J. Parenter. Enter. Nutr.* 8:37, 1984.

64. Wannemacher, R. W., Kaminski, M. V., Jr., Neufeld, H. A., Dinterman, R. E., Bostian, K. A., and Hadick, C. L. Protein-sparing therapy during pneumococcal infection in rhesus monkeys. *J. Parenter. Enter. Nutr.* 2:507, 1978.

65. Westerveit, F. B., and Schreiner, G. E. The carbohydrate intolerance of uremic patients. *Ann. Intern. Med.* 57:266, 1962.

66. Wilmore, D. W. Alterations in intermediary metabolism. In T. King and K. Reemtsma (series eds.), *The Metabolic Management of the Critically Ill: Reviewing Surgical Topics.* New York: Plenum Press, 1977. P. 129.

67. Wilmore, D. W., Moylan, J. A., Helmkamp, G. M., and Pruitt, B. A., Jr. Clinical evaluation of a 10% intravenous fat emulsion for parenteral nutrition in thermally injured patients. *Ann. Surg.* 78:503, 1973.

68. Wolfe, R. R., Durkot, M. J., Allsop, J. R., and Burke, J. F. Glucose metabolism in severely burned patients. *Metabolism* 28:1031, 1979.

69. Wolfe, R. R., Miller, H. I., Elahi, D., and Spitzer, J. J. Effect of burn injury on glucose turnover in guinea pigs. *Surg. Gynecol. Obstet.* 144:359, 1977.

70. Wolfram, G. Medium-chain triglycerides (MCT) for total parenteral nutrition. *World J. Surg.* 10:33, 1986.

71. Woolfson, A. M. J., Heatley, R. V., and Allison, S. P. Insulin to inhibit protein catabolism after injury. *N. Engl. J. Med.* 300:14, 1979.

72. Yeung, C. K., Smith, R. C., and Hill, G. L. Effect of an elemental diet on body composition: Comparison with intravenous nutrition. *Gastroenterology* 77:652, 1979.

73. Zohrab, W. J., McHattie, J. D., and Jeejeebhoy, K. N. Total parenteral nutrition with lipid. *Gastroenterology* 64:583, 1973.

74. Zumtobel, V., and Zehle, A. Postoperative parenterale Ernährung mit Fettemulsionen bei Patienten mit Leberschaden. *Langenbecks Arch. Chir. Suppl. Chir. Forum*, 1972. P. 179.

Enteral Nutrition

John L. Rombeau
Scott A. Kripke

Enteral nutrition is the provision of liquid formula diets by tube or mouth into the gastrointestinal tract. Recent advances in access, delivery systems, nutrient formulations, and patient monitoring, combined with experimental evidence that enteral nutrition is essential for maintenance of gastrointestinal mucosal growth and function, have led to increased usage of enteral nutrition. Enteral nutrition is significantly less expensive than total parenteral nutrition (TPN) [145] and this economic advantage is an additional factor leading to greater usage of enteral nutrition.

This chapter describes the rationale, assessment and patient selection, access and delivery, nutrient formulations, patient monitoring, and gastrointestinal complications for the use of enteral nutrition. Recent rationale and experiments for providing organ-specific fuels for the gut are also included. Finally, the use of enteral nutrition in the critically ill and the prevention of bacterial translocation and transmigration of endotoxin by direct feeding into the gut are described.

RATIONALE

The rationale for using enteral nutrition rather than TPN is primarily based on two findings: (1) the significant benefit of enteral nutrition to gut growth and function, and (2) the marked reduction in cost of enteral nutrients.

The gastrointestinal tract is commonly regarded as an organ system that is involved solely with the digestion and absorption of nutrients. However, recent investigations demonstrated that this system also regulates and processes substrates circulating through the splanchnic vasculature and is a major component of host defenses [146]. In addition, it is a potent source of peptides, endocrine and paracrine hormones, and peptide neurotransmitters.

The most important stimulus for mucosal cell proliferation is the presence of nutrients in the intestinal lumen [73]. The transit of a meal through the gastrointestinal tract increases epithelial desquamation and enhances mucosal cell renewal. Bowel rest due to starvation or the administration of TPN leads to villus atrophy [85], decreased cellularity, and a reduction in intestinal disaccharidase activities [46]. Further effects of nutrients on the gastrointestinal tract are mediated by enterohormones such as gastrin, enteroglucagon, peptide YY, and urogastrone [128, 143], and by nonenteric hormones such as growth hormone and epidermal growth factor [4].

The cost of enteral diets is significantly less than parenteral solutions because of the manufacturing expense required to meet the stringent requirements for intravenous formulations. Based on previously published data [111], extrapolated daily costs for enteral nutrition in 1990 were about $40 [123]. This compares quite favorably to the projected daily costs of standard hospital diets and TPN at $25 and $325, respectively. In two prospective, controlled trials, the costs for enteral nutrition were significantly less than equivalent amounts of parenteral feeding [19, 22].

In one of these trials reported in 1985 [22], feedings of modified amino acid diets in septic patients resulted in daily costs (including pump and tubing) for enteral and parenteral feedings of $54 and $160, respectively.

Finally, enteral nutrition is not only as clinically efficacious as and less expensive than TPN, it also does not require the extensive sterile techniques needed for parenteral feedings, and there is less need for a trained pharmacist.

ASSESSMENT AND PATIENT SELECTION

Enteral nutrition is the preferred method of feeding patients with both an inability to ingest adequate nutrients by mouth and a gastrointestinal tract that can be used safely and effectively. Before initiating nutritional therapy, the physician must first perform a baseline nutritional assessment by means of a thorough medical history, dietary review, complete physical examination, and labora-

tory tests including serum electrolytes, albumin, iron and total iron-binding capacity (or true transferrin, if available), liver function tests, coagulation parameters, cholesterol, and triglycerides.

To establish the need for supplementary enteral feedings, the nutritional assessment should demonstrate that the patient's volitional intake is sufficient to meet his or her nutrient needs. The major objective of nutritional support must be clearly identified as either nutritional maintenance or repletion. In critically ill or stressed patients, the goal should be to maintain the nutritional status. Repletion of nutritional deficits is indicated in malnourished nonstressed patients and in critically ill individuals when the stress resolves and the patient is able to assimilate greater nutrient intakes. Most patients are given 1500 to 2000 kcal via the enteral route.

Once it has been shown that oral volitional intake is inadequate and the patient's need for nutritional maintenance or repletion has been evaluated, the route for nutrient delivery must be determined (see Access and Delivery, below). The gastrointestinal tract is evaluated through an appropriate history to determine whether it is functioning normally and can be used safely. Safe use of the gastrointestinal tract is clinically defined as the absence of diarrhea, intestinal hemorrhage, or obstruction. Even if the gastrointestinal tract is not wholly intact, a sufficient length may be available for absorption of a defined formula diet. The need for at least 100 cm of functioning jejunum or 150 cm of ileum, preferably with some colon and intact ileocecal valve, has been suggested [49]. [*Editor's Note:* If the ileocecal valve is intact, many patients can support themselves with food with 65 to 75 cm of either ileum or jejunum. They may need supplementation from TPN on a long-term basis, but usually will manifest gut hypertrophy to the point where patients can survive on oral intake alone.]

The specific indications and contraindications for enteral feeding, developed by the American Society for Parenteral and Enteral Nutrition (ASPEN) [6] are listed in Table 26-1. The conditions listed in the table serve as

Table 26-1.   Guidelines for the Use of Enteral Nutrition in the Adult Patient*

Routine indications
   Protein-calorie malnutrition with inadequate oral intake of nutrients for the previous 5 days
   Normal nutritional status with < 50% of required nutrient intake orally for the previous 7 days
   Severe dysphagia
   Major burn injury
   Massive small-bowel resection in combination with TPN
   Low-output (< 500 cc/day) enterocutaneous fistulas
Relative indications
   Major trauma
   Radiation therapy with anorexia
   Mild chemotherapy with anorexia
   Liver failure, renal insufficiency
Relative contraindications
   Immediate postoperative or poststress period (< 12 hr)
   Acute severe enteritis
   < 10% remaining small intestine
Contraindications
   Complete mechanical intestinal obstruction
   Ileus
   Severe diarrhea
   High-output external fistulas (> 500 cc/day)
   Severe acute pancreatitis

*From American Society for Parenteral and Enteral Nutrition Board of Directors. Guidelines for the use of enteral nutrition in the adult patient. *J. Parenter. Enter. Nutr.* 11:435, 1987. Reprinted with permission.

a general guideline; however, good clinical judgment must be applied as well.

ACCESS AND DELIVERY

Enteral nutrition is delivered by mouth, nasoenteric tube, or tube enterostomy. Detailed descriptions of these access and delivery techniques have been published [120]. Adequate oral supplementation of calories, protein, and micronutrients is possible in many hospitalized patients and should be the preferred route of nutrient delivery. Evidence suggests that the oral route provides the most complete dietary utilization when compared to intragastric or intravenous feeding [99]. Nutritional support by the oral route must meet the metabolic needs of disease or trauma, correct prior deficiencies, and satisfy requirements of palatability. Palatability, the hedonic response of the individual to the flavor (smell, taste, texture, and temperature) of the food to be ingested, is an important

determinant of oral consumption [132]. Most elemental diets are unpalatable; however, flavor modifications with various additives (fruit flavors, gelatin) can improve patient ratings [33, 59, 131]. In addition to problems with palatability, diet repetition (monotony), negative environmental stimuli (noxious odors), and other factors (e.g., radiation to the oropharynx) limit a patient's ability to ingest adequate nutrients. In these instances, and when oral nutrition is impossible (head-and-neck surgery, disorders of swallowing, patient refusal to eat), feeding by nasoenteric tube or tube enterostomy should be instituted.

Feeding by Nasoenteric Tube

Access by nasoenteric tube is the preferred method of delivery for those patients in need of enteral nutrition for less than 4 weeks (Fig. 26-1). The soft, pliable, small-bore tubes composed of nonreactive materials such as polyurethane or silicone elastomer (Silastic) have

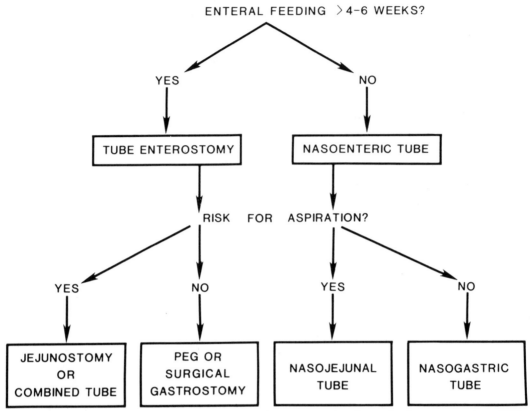

Figure 26-1. Decision approach for feeding access by nasoenteric tube and tube enterostomy. PEG = percutaneous endoscopic gastrostomy.

improved patient tolerance to nasoenteric tubes. These tubes, weighted with a bolus of tungsten, usually pass into the duodenum or jejunum in noncritically ill patients. The new nasoenteric feeding tubes with smaller diameters may decrease the risk for aspiration because there is less compromise of the lower esophageal sphincter than with the larger tubes, and the feeding is delivered beyond the pylorus. Additionally, these tubes enable the patient to continue to swallow around the tube so that some oral intake can be maintained if desired [91]. Techniques for insertion of nasoenteric tubes are well described [52].

When a nasoenteric tube is placed for enteral feeding, verification of tube location is mandatory. Simple insufflation of air into the tube is not sufficient to verify the distal position of the tube. Auscultation over the epigastrium while air is being injected into the tube can pick up sound transmitted through a tube that has been inadvertently passed into the tracheobronchial tree. Many of these tubes are small enough to pass through the glottis and trachea without markedly interfering with phonation or respiration. Enteral solutions delivered through a misplaced tube into the bronchial tree can cause severe pneumonitis and death. The safest means of confirming proper tube placement within the gut is by the aspiration of gastrointestinal contents through the tube with a syringe. If intestinal contents cannot be aspirated through the tube, radiographic confirmation of tube location is necessary before enteral feedings are started. Because feeding tubes are often radiopaque, a simple plain film of the abdomen is usually adequate to identify the tube location. If the exact location of the tube is still in doubt, a small amount of contrast material is injected through the tube.

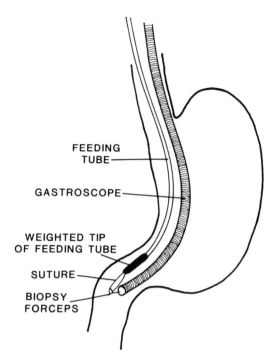

FEEDING TUBE

GASTROSCOPE

WEIGHTED TIP OF FEEDING TUBE

SUTURE

BIOPSY FORCEPS

GASTROSCOPE AIDED PASSAGE OF FEEDING TUBE

Figure 26-2. Endoscopic placement of nasoenteric tube beyond the pylorus.

In patients with an increased risk for aspiration, feeding should be administered beyond the pylorus, preferably beyond the ligament of Treitz (see Fig. 26-1). It is my clinical impression that the incidence of aspiration is reduced when feeding beyond the stomach; however, this observation awaits confirmation with controlled clinical trials. Critically ill patients often require either endoscopic (Fig. 26-2) or radiologic techniques for tube placement beyond the pylorus.

Feeding by Tube Enterostomy

Tube enterostomy refers to the operative, endoscopic, or radiologic placement of a tube or catheter into any segment of the gastrointestinal tract, from the pharynx to the colon. Access by tube enterostomy is the preferred method of delivery for those patients in need of enteral nutrition for greater than 4 weeks (see Fig. 26-1). Detailed descriptions of tech-

niques of tube enterostomy have been published [120]. Enterostomy tubes are most commonly placed into the pharynx, cervical esophagus, stomach, and jejunum [144]. Tube enterostomy is also commonly performed concomitantly with gastrointestinal surgery when the need for long-term nutritional support is anticipated. Examples of these conditions are major esophageal or gastric resections [121].

Gastrostomy

Gastrostomy is performed surgically or endoscopically. Comprehensive descriptions of surgical gastrostomies have been published [121]. The indications for surgical gastrostomies are for patients in need of either a concomitant abdominal operation or in whom a percutaneous gastrostomy cannot be performed. Gauderer and Ponsky [51, 107] described the percutaneous endoscopic gastrostomy (PEG), later modified by Russell et al. [125]. The Russell, or single endoscopy technique, which is gaining wide acceptance, eliminates the insertion of the feeding tube through the bacteria-laden oral pharynx. The procedure requires only mild sedation and local anesthesia and is usually performed in the endoscopy suite. Substantial cost savings, with less morbidity and mortality, have been demonstrated with the PEG over traditional surgically placed gastrostomies. Detailed descriptions of the single and double endoscopic techniques have been published [31].

Jejunostomy

Jejunostomy feedings are administered in patients with carcinoma of the esophagus or stomach, peptic ulcer disease, gastric outlet obstruction, or gastric trauma, and after gastric resection [115]. Jejunostomy feeding decreases gastroesophageal reflux and, hence, potentially reduces the risk of aspiration when compared to intragastric tube feeding [53, 87]. If feedings are to be started soon after surgery, the jejunal route is preferred because return of normal small intestine motility may occur within 12 to 14 hours, and paralytic ileus is usually limited to the stomach and colon [152, 157].

There are two basic types of feeding jejunostomy: Witzel and needle catheter. These techniques have been described in detail [120]. We favor the Witzel technique because it enables the placement of a larger tube for delivery of more viscous formulas and there are fewer episodes of tube blockage.

Intermittent versus Continuous Feeding

The feeding pattern is in part determined by the route of administration. Intermittent feedings are tolerated when delivered into the stomach but not the small intestine [34, 35, 102, 103, 119]. [Editor's Note: The reason for this is that the stomach can dilute a hypertonic load by secretion while the pylorus retains the hypertonic bolus. When the feed becomes isosmotic, transfer across the pylorus begins. No such capacity exists in the small bowel.] Therefore, nasoenteric or jejunostomy delivered feedings should be given continuously. The question of whether to feed intermittently or continuously arises only when intragastric feedings are at issue. Intermittent, bolus, or meal-type feeding is convenient and inexpensive and may be more physiologic than continuous feeding. There is no need for infusion pumps or controllers, and, if the nasogastric tube is of a large bore, viscous formulas or blenderized foods flow through readily. In addition, intermittent feedings more closely simulate the normal feeding pattern and the distension caused by bolus feeding may stimulate digestion. In patients with normal gastric emptying or those who are receiving home enteral nutrition regimens, intermittent feedings may be more desirable than continuous feedings [102, 105]. Intermittent feedings should not be infused at rates greater than 30 ml/min, and small volumes should be given initially [61].

There are several advantages to continuous feeding, including the decreased risk of abdominal distension and aspiration [102]. Furthermore, small gastric residuals and improved tolerance are seen in patients who are fed continuously [60]. Unfortunately, continuous feeding requires an infusion apparatus to which the patient is "tied" for many hours. This can be inconvenient even if the patient is only fed continuously for 12 hours. Another liability of continuous feeding is the cost of the pump.

Physiologic superiority has not been assigned to either of the two techniques. Comparative effects on nutrient utilization in humans are unclear. In one study, infants with different intestinal diseases had significantly greater protein synthesis and mineral absorption, associated with a greater weight gain, when fed intragastrically and continuously compared to infants fed the same formula intermittently and orally [104]. Adult burn patients who received continuous feedings had significantly decreased stool frequency and required significantly less time to achieve their nutritional goals than those fed intermittently [60]. Nacht et al. [98] administered a milkshake to six healthy volunteers either as a single bolus or continuously over 3 hours using a nasogastric tube. Resting energy expenditure, respiratory quotient, plasma glucose, and insulin concentrations increased sooner and steeper, and plasma free fatty acid levels decreased earlier with the meal ingested as a single bolus than with continuous administration. Nutrient-induced thermogenesis was significantly greater with the single dose; however, overall nutrient balance was not affected by the mode of enteral nutrient administration.

In summary, intermittent and continuous intragastric feeding methods are roughly equivalent, and the choice of one technique should be determined by patient tolerance, tube location, convenience, and cost. In our experience, critically ill patients tolerate continuous feedings better than intermittent delivery.

ENTERAL DIET FORMULATIONS

Most standard commercial enteral formulas contain 55% carbohydrate, 30% fat, and 15% protein, with a total calorie-nitogen ratio of

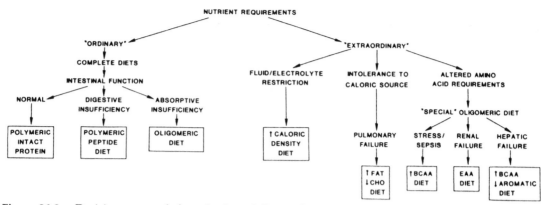

Figure 26-3. Decision approach for selection of dietary formulas. CHO = carbohydrates; BCAA = branched-chain amino acids; EAA = essential amino acids; aromatic = aromatic amino acids.

150:1. Detailed descriptions of the contents of enteral diets have been published [88].

Once the decision to provide enteral nutrition is made, the proper formula must be selected. Several clinical criteria must be considered when selecting an enteral formula: (1) caloric requirements (maintenance versus repletion), (2) digestive and absorptive function, and (3) extraordinary disease-specific nutrient requirements. A decision tree for the selection of an initial dietary formula is depicted in Figure 26-3.

The current rapid proliferation of commercial enteral formulas mandates the classification of these products to assist the clinician in selecting the proper diet. In addition to clinical criteria, several dietary characteristics must be considered when selecting an enteral formula: (1) caloric density, (2) nutrient source and content, (3) osmolality, (4) complexity, (5) route of administration, (6) residue content, and (7) cost. Many classifications of enteral diet formulations have been proposed [109, 134, 141]. The classification scheme used at our institution is based on nutrient composition: polymeric, oligomeric, or modular [77] (Table 26-2). Approximately 95% of our patients who receive enteral nutrition are given polymeric diets. These diets are relatively inexpensive and reasonably well tolerated by most patients. Recent attention has focused on providing liquid formula diets that are formulated to meet the metabolic needs of patients with hepatic, renal,

and pulmonary dysfunction, and burns or trauma.

Hepatic Failure

Patients with chronic liver disease are frequently malnourished. Poor dietary intake, increased rate of protein breakdown, pancreatic exocrine insufficiency, and malabsorption of vitamins contribute to malnutrition in these patients [135].

Enteral formulas enriched with branched-chain amino acids (BCAAs)—valine, leucine, and isoleucine—have been developed to improve the nutritional and mental status of patients with hepatic encephalopathy. Three controlled trials have addressed the question of whether BCAA supplementation has a beneficial effect on hepatic encephalopathy. Two small trials [43, 92] reported no appreciable improvement in mental status. [*Editor's Note:* Erickson et al.'s trial is noteworthy because it is not negative in that 30 g of additional protein equivalent were ingested (as BCAAs) without encephalopathy. In the McGhee et al. "trial" four patients were used—a type II statistical error.] Analysis of a larger prospective, double-blind, randomized study suggested that a BCAA-enriched formula was as effective at inducing positive nitrogen balance as an equivalent amount of whole protein. Encephalopathy was induced far less often with the BCAA-enriched formula than with the whole-protein enteral diet

Table 26-2. Classification of Enteral Formulas

Polymeric	Oligomeric	Modular
1 kcal/ml	Elemental	Carbohydrate
Ensure/HN	Vivonex TEN	Polycose
Osmolite/HN	Low residue	Medical
Isocal	Precision LR	Sumacal
Sustacal	Precision HN	Hycal
1.5 kcal/ml	Flexical	Calplus
Ensure Plus/HN	Vital	Fat
Sustacal HC	Special	Microlipid
2 kcal/ml	Hepatic encephalopathy	Lipomul
Isocal HCN	Hepatic-Aid	MCT
Magnacal	Travasorb Hepatic	Protein
	Renal failure	Casec
	Aminaid	Promix
	Travasorb Renal	Propac
	Stress/trauma	EMF
	Trauma-aid	Aminess
	Stresstein	Minerals
	Criticare	Complete
		Modular
		Nutrisource

[66]. Based on this study, patients with hepatic encephalopathy must benefit from specialized formulas with high quantities of BCAAs and low quantities of aromatic amino acids (phenylalanine, tyrosine, tryptophan, methionine) to induce positive nitrogen balance without worsening the encephalopathy.

Renal Failure

The goal of enteral nutrition in acute renal failure is to provide caloric requirements without accumulating nitrogenous by-products, fluid, or electrolytes. Based on these needs, specialized renal failure formulas that contain crystalline essential amino acids, minimal sodium and potassium, and high caloric densities are available. These products are expensive, hyperosmolar, and unpalatable.

The value of providing essential amino acids as the sole nitrogen source is controversial (see Chap. 13). Early studies demonstrated favorable utilization of essential amino acids by tissues with control of BUN to the extent that dialysis could be deferred [1, 151]. It was postulated that these formulas

promoted the reutilization of urea nitrogen through liver transamination for the synthesis of nonessential amino acids [1]. More recent studies found no difference in the metabolic and therapeutic effects of essential amino acids versus a low-strength general amino acid formula [12, 94]. Further studies are needed to determine the importance of essential amino acid–based enteral diets in renal failure.

The use of specialized renal formulas during acute renal failure is recommended when attempting to avoid or delay the onset of dialysis. Standard or high calorie formulas are provided for patients undergoing dialysis.

Pulmonary Failure

The critically ill patient with respiratory insufficiency requires meticulous attention to nutritional status, because these patients are often malnourished from poor nutrient intake. Several investigators reported an enhanced ability to wean patients from mechanical ventilation with nutritional supplementation [29, 84]. Moreover, additional reports suggested an advantage of fat-based formulas versus carbohydrate-based formulas for patients suffering from respiratory failure. When fat calories replaced carbohydrate calories in enteral feedings, significant reductions of carbon dioxide production, minute ventilation, arterial carbon dioxide tension ($PaCO_2$, and oxygen consumption were achieved [50, 63]. These findings suggest that patients may be more rapidly weaned from mechanical ventilation with fat-based formulas.

Our approach to the patient with pulmonary insufficiency is based on the degree of respiratory compromise as measured by pulmonary function tests. Those patients with mild to moderate deficits in pulmonary reserve and those patients dependent on chronic respirator support are prescribed standard polymeric formulas with about 50% of their total calories as carbohydrate and 30% as fat. Those patients with severely compromised pulmonary function, or those experiencing difficulty weaning from mechanical ventilation, are provided the more expensive fat-based formulas (55% fat with 28% carbohydrate or 40% fat with 38% carbohydrate). However, many of these critically ill patients have difficulty absorbing this high fat intake and diarrhea is potentiated. [*Editor's Note:* As stated elsewhere, the significance of the article by Askanazi and Kinney is to make people aware of the possible problem of increased CO_2 production. In my experience, this rarely happens. (See Chapter 4)]

Stress and Trauma

The metabolic response to trauma, sepsis, and burn injuries is characterized by increased energy expenditure, early mobilization of skeletal muscle protein and adipose tissue for energy substrates, negative nitrogen balance, insulin resistance, and later decreased immunocompetence and hepatic protein synthesis [16, 75, 148]. An important aspect of the metabolic response to stress is an increased hydrolysis of BCAAs in skeletal muscle [149].

The enteral diets formulated for stressed patients are high in BCAAs (approximately

50% of total amino acids compared to 30% in standard formulas) and have a low calorie-nitrogen ratio (80–100:1 compared to 150:1 in standard formulas). Several investigators reported a more rapid return to positive nitrogen balance and improved nitrogen retention in both parenterally and enterally administered high-BCAA diets compared to standard formulas [13, 21, 39]. In a randomized, prospective trial in 37 stressed surgical patients receiving TPN, Bower et al. [18] compared the nutritional efficacy of a standard amino acid solution and two BCAA-enriched formulas, one enriched primarily with valine and the other with leucine. Nitrogen retention was significantly better on days 5, 7, and 10 in both groups of patients receiving the BCAA-enriched solutions, but differences in cumulative nitrogen balance were not statistically significant. Improved clinical outcome was not seen in the groups receiving the BCAA-enriched solutions. Recent controlled clinical studies showed no significant benefit in protein metabolism and nitrogen balance when BCAA-enriched formulas were used [15, 30]. Most important, there has been no convincing proof of improved clinical outcome due to providing enriched BCAA formulas in stressed patients. Presently, we recommend these controversial stress formulas only for patients with markedly negative nitrogen balance or intolerance to standard polymeric formulas.

MONITORING

Patients who receive enteral feedings require the same careful monitoring as those who receive parenteral nutrition. This is especially true in the critically ill patient. Routine monitoring is best accomplished by following a protocol that ensures complete and detailed surveillance of the patient, reducing the possibility of error in formula choice, nutrient administration, and assessment of progress toward nutritional goals (Table 26-3). Appropriate monitoring is best achieved when enteral nutrition is administered under the

Table 26-3. Monitoring Protocol for Hospitalized Patients Receiving Enteral Nutrition

Feeding tube location: _____

Check items to be done:

_____ 1. Confirm placement of tube by aspiration of gastric contents prior to the administration of feeding. If no gastric aspirate, obtain abdominal x-ray to confirm tube location.

_____ 2. Elevate head of bed to 30 degrees when feeding into stomach.

_____ 3. Name of formula _____
to be given over _____ hr. Rate of feeding _____ ml/hr.

_____ 4. Do not hang formula for more than 8 hr.

_____ 5. Check for gastric residual every _____ hr. Withhold feedings for _____ hr. if residual is 50% greater than ordered volume.

_____ 6. Weigh patient Monday, Wednesday, Friday. Chart on graph.

_____ 7. Record intake and output daily, and chart on graph.

_____ 8. Change administration tubing and feeding bag daily.

_____ 9. Irrigate feeding tube with 20–30 ml of water or saline every 4 hr, or if feeding is stopped for any reason.

_____ 10. Calorie counts daily for first 5 days, then weekly.

_____ 11. Complete blood count, SMA-12, total iron-binding capacity, serum iron, magnesium, every Monday.

_____ 12. SMA-6 twice weekly.

_____ 13. 24-hr urine collection for urea (for nitrogen balance calculation) once per week on stable dietary regimen.

SMA-6 = Na, K, Cl CO_2, Glu, BUN
SMA-12 = SMA-6 + Cr, Ca, Bilirubin, SGPT, SGOT, ALKPTASE

direction of a multidisciplinary nutritional support team [108].

COMPLICATIONS

Clinically significant complications of enteral alimentation, although few, should be promptly recognized and aggressively treated. An organized monitoring protocol, as already described, aids in the early detection of possible problems. Complications of enteral feeding are grouped into four major categories: gastrointestinal, metabolic, infectious, and mechanical. Gastrointestinal complications occur most frequently; the discussion is limited to these problems. A comprehensive review of the remaining types of enteral nutrition complications has been published [136].

Gastrointestinal complications of enteral feeding include nausea, vomiting, diarrhea, and constipation. Diarrhea is the most frequent and difficult-to-treat gastrointestinal complication of enteral nutrition.

Diarrhea is defined as an increase in stool weight of more than 150 g/24 h or an increase in stool water of more than 1500 ml/24 hr. Diarrhea occurs in at least 10 to 20% of patients on tube feeding regimens [62] and is more prevalent in the critically ill [76]. Diarrhea results from decreased intestinal absorptive capacity (celiac sprue, lactase deficiency, short-bowel syndrome) and/or increased intestinal secretion (cholera, laxatives, bile acids, fatty acids). Dietary factors include formula hyperosmolality, lactose-containing formulas in the presence of relative lactase deficiency, high fat content when there is some degree of fat malabsorption (pancreatic exocrine insufficiency, biliary obstruction, ileectomy, ileitis), and bacterial contamination of the enteral products and delivery systems [67, 129, 130, 150]. Finally, diarrhea is commonly caused by enterally administered medications including antibiotics, hyperosmolar drug solutions, and magnesium-containing antacids [118].

Treatment of diarrhea is directed at the underlying etiology. However, the cause of diarrhea is frequently difficult to identify. When there is no clearly identifiable cause of the diarrhea, several options are available. Decreasing the delivery rate may alleviate diarrhea by allowing time for intestinal mucosal adaptation to occur in patients in whom the gastrointestinal tract has not been used for an extended period of time (starvation, TPN-induced intestinal atrophy) [46, 74, 86]. The flow rate is then slowly increased over several days. Parenteral supplementation of nutrients may be necessary during this interval. Decreasing the osmolality of the formula can be helpful as well. Nonspecific treatment with antidiarrheal agents (Lomotil, Imodium) and paregoric can also be tried cautiously. The addition of a bulking agent to the formula may help solidify the stool and slow transit time [20].

CLINICAL STUDIES COMPARING ENTERAL AND PARENTERAL NUTRITION

Clinical studies have demonstrated that diets given via the enteral route resulted in improved nitrogen retention when compared to the identical diets given intravenously [3, 65]. In postsurgical neonates, enteral nutrition increased amino nitrogen flux, protein synthesis, and breakdown by 40% compared to parenteral nutrition [36]. In infants with intractable diarrhea and malabsorption, continuous enteral nutrition with an elemental formula was compared to TPN. Enteral nutrition and TPN produced similar correction of malnutrition, but enteral nutrition was associated with faster resolution of malabsorption and diarrhea, fewer complications, and less expensive hospitalization than TPN [101]. Enteral and parenteral nutrition have also been compared in the postoperative patient. Muggia-Sullam et al. [97] found that the two nutrient modalities promoted positive nitro-

gen balance, preserved body weight, maintained serum protein levels, and were equally safe, but the enteral feeding was much less expensive. Bower et al. [19] also concluded that postoperative enteral feeding was as efficacious as TPN and significantly less expensive. In another study in patients after abdominal aortic surgery, enteral and parenteral nutrition both equivalently reduced the postoperative negative nitrogen balance compared to standard intravenous fluids [45]. Enteral nutrition was also found to be safe and efficacious after laparotomy for multiple trauma, and reduced septic complications in critically injured patients when compared to TPN [2, 96].

GUT-SPECIFIC FUELS

Bowel Rest

Bowel rest is the provision of substrates, fluid, minerals, and vitamins either intravenously as parenteral nutrition or into the gut as an elemental diet. Despite the widespread clinical practice of bowel rest, there is little physiologic evidence to support its use. In fact, most studies show that bowel rest is associated with adverse gastrointestinal sequelae [85]. For example, bowel rest produces significant gut atrophy in just 3 days in the rat [69] and these changes are followed by functional deficits such as decreases in brush-border enzyme production. Attention has therefore been directed to using enteral nutrition to preserve gut structure and function [122]. Furthermore, specific fuels such as glutamine and short-chain fatty acids have been identified as the preferential respiratory fuels of the enterocyte [154] and colonocyte [113], respectively. These fuels are now being added to intravenous and liquid formula diets.

Glutamine

General Characteristics and Functions
Glutamine is the most abundant amino acid in plasma and skeletal muscle, and constitutes

more than 60% of the total free amino acid pool in muscle tissue [10]. Glutamine is synthesized by many tissues; hence, it is considered by classic definition to be a "nonessential" amino acid. Glutamine is unique in that it has two amine moieties: a standard alpha-amino group and an additional amide group. Due to the polarity of the terminal amide group, glutamine is easily hydrolyzed to produce glutamate and ammonia. This initial step in glutamine degradation is central to whole-body nitrogen exchange and is regulated by the activity of glutaminase enzymes. Glutamine is synthesized from its precursors—glutamate and ammonia—in the presence of glutamine synthetase. Skeletal muscle is the main producer of glutamine and has high levels of glutamine synthetase, whereas the intestine, being a major glutamine consumer, has high glutaminase activity.

Glutamine provides nitrogen for a number of biosynthetic pathways, serving as a precursor to the purine and pyrimidine rings of nucleic acids and nucleotides, and is also an important constituent of proteins and a precursor of amino acids [80]. Furthermore, it is the most important substrate for renal ammoniagenesis (Fig. 26-4), as well as a potential substrate for hepatic gluconeogenesis, a regulator of hepatic glycogen synthesis, and possibly a regulator of muscle protein degradation [137].

Although it has been known for many years that glutamine is essential for growth of many types of rapidly dividing cells in culture [37], it has only recently become apparent that enterocytes preferentially metabolize this amino acid [54, 153]. In the enterocyte, greater than 50% of the glutamine carbon taken up by the small intestine is completely oxidized to carbon dioxide (see Fig. 26-4) [154].

Experimental and Clinical Investigations

Glutamine is absent from all of the currently available parenteral nutrient solutions. It has been omitted from all but a few enteral diets, and when it is present, it is in suboptimal concentrations. Therefore, when normal en-

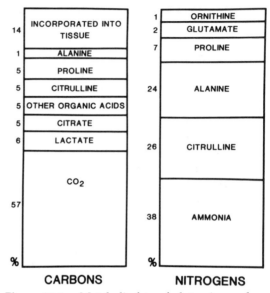

Figure 26-4. Metabolic fate of glutamine and carbon, and nitrogen breakdown in the small-bowel mucosa [154].

teral intake is inadequate and/or parenteral feeding is required, current therapy fails to provide this essential nutrient.

Several animal studies examined the effects of glutamine-supplemented liquid formula diets on gut structure and function. In the rat, following 60% resection of the small bowel, a glutamine-supplemented defined formula diet provided significantly greater weight gain, as well as hyperplasia of the jejunum and ileum [70]. The trophic effect of glutamine was limited to the villi, without significant change in crypt depth or alteration in thickness of the other layers of the intestinal wall. In a model of 5-fluorouracil-induced intestinal injury, glutamine-supplemented liquid formula diets improved mucosal cellularity and nitrogen balance [71]. In a similar experiment performed in our laboratory with methyltrexate-induced enterocolitis, glutamine-supplemented elemental diets significantly reduced the incidence of enteric bacteremia and endotoxemia, prolonged survival, and decreased mortality [47, 48].

Several reports noted benefit in postoperative patients receiving glutamine-supplemented intravenous diets. Postoperative patients receiving TPN supplemented with glutamine-alanyl dipeptide had significant increases in nitrogen balance when compared to individuals receiving TPN without glutamine [142]. In another recent study, glutamine-supplemented intravenous diets preserved intracellular glutamine concentration and protein synthesis in skeletal muscle and improved nitrogen balance in postoperative patients [55]. [*Editor's Note*: It is important to note that these differences were probably too small to affect outcome.]

Short-Chain Fatty Acids

General Characteristics and Functioning

The short-chain fatty acids (SCFAs), also called the volatile fatty acids, are the C1-6 organic fatty acids. These are formed in ruminants and in the cecum and ascending colon in humans by microbial fermentation of fiber polysaccharides (Fig. 26-5) [138]. The bacterial flora use less than 10% of the energy available from fiber fermentation for their metabolic activity [93]. Acetate, propionate, and butyrate account for 83% of the SCFAs so formed [31] and are usually produced in nearly constant molar ratios of 60:25:15 [25]. Among their various properties, SCFAs are readily absorbed by intestinal mucosa [26], are relatively high in caloric content [159], are readily metabolized by intestinal epithelium in liver [23], stimulate sodium and water absorption in the colon [11, 114], and are trophic to the intestinal mucosa [82, 127].

As mentioned previously, SCFAs are produced in the mammalian intestinal tract as a by-product of anaerobic bacterial metabolism of carbohydrate. The straight-chain fatty acids—acetate, propionate, and butyrate—are the major end-products of bacterial carbohydrate metabolism in the colon. Hydrogen gas, carbon dioxide, methane, and water are also produced [155].

Carbohydrates reach the large bowel in at least three forms: (1) nonstarch polysaccharides (dietary fiber—plant-cell wall polysac-

FIBER FERMENTATION

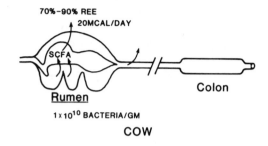

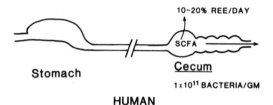

Figure 26-5. Similarity between rumen and cecum as to microbial fermentation of fiber with the production of short-chain fatty acids (SCFA). REE = resting energy expenditure.

charides that are resistant to the digestive enzymes of the upper gastrointestinal tract), including cellulose, pectins, and hemicellulose; (2) other polysaccharides that resist digestion, such as resistant starch [42]; and (3) simple carbohydrates that escape absorption in the small bowel [110].

The pathways by which acetate, propionate, and butyrate are formed from carbohydrate have been reviewed in detail [156]. In general, these SCFAs are generated by the metabolism of pyruvate, which is produced by oxidation of glucose via the glycolytic Embden-Meyerhof pathway [156].

Inasmuch as SCFAs are produced by endogenous bacterial fermentation, concentrations are highest where the bacterial population is most abundant. Interestingly, in the large intestine of man, SCFA concentrations are roughly equivalent to those found in the rumen (approximately 75 mM acetate, 30 mM propionate, and 20 mM butyrate), reflecting the similarity in bacterial flora between these two organs [23].

Colonic absorption rates for the three principal SCFAs in several nonruminent species are similar [24]. The small intestine, as well as the colon, has the capacity to absorb SCFAs. Although normal SCFA concentrations within the small bowel are low, small-intestinal mucosa can absorb these acids as efficiently as the colonic and ruminal epithelia [140].

The exact mechanism for the absorptive process is unknown, but recent investigations elucidated several important characteristics. First, absorption occurs in both the ionized and the nonionized forms [23]. Second, transport from the lumen is invariably associated with the luminal accumulation of bicarbonate ion [147]. Third, SCFA absorption stimulates sodium absorption [8, 11]. Fourth, a luminal source of hydrogen ion appears to be important for absorption of the proteinated (nonionized) form [41].

The three major SCFAs, once absorbed, are metabolized by the cecal and colonic mucosa. In human colonocyte suspensions prepared from either proximal or distal colonic mucosa, added butyrate suppressed glucose oxidation by about 50% [112]. Approximately 75% of the oxygen consumed by the colonocytes was attributable to butyrate oxidation when butyrate was the only substrate available. Butyrate is preferentially oxidized by colonocytes in vitro when compared to several common fuels. The preferential descending order of utilization of respiratory fuels by colonocytes is: butyrate, acetoacetate, L-glutamine, d-glucose [6, 113].

SCFAs not metabolized by the mucosal epithelium are transported to the liver in the portal blood. Portal blood concentrations are four to ten times higher than systemic levels, indicating a substantial clearance function for the liver [68].

Experimental and Clinical Investigations

One result of production, absorption, and metabolism of the SCFAs is the provision of energy to the host [133]. It has been estimated that the absorption of SCFAs from fiber fermentation may provide from 5 to 30% of the daily energy requirement [158]. Co-lonic luminal profusion studies estimated that the human colon has the ability to absorb up to 540 kcal/day in the form of SCFAs [124]. Other studies indicated that in humans, colonic absorption of SCFAs may normally supply 5 to 10% of daily energy requirements, depending on the quantity of fiber and resistant starch in the diet [24, 68]. In addition to the simple provision of a caloric source to the host, SCFA production in the cecum and colon of nonruminants may strongly influence normal gastrointestinal function by increasing colonic blood flow [83], stimulating pancreatic enzyme secretion [57], promoting sodium and water absorption [11, 124], and by potentiating intestinal mucosal growth [78, 82].

Potential clinical indications for the use of SCFAs include those patients with intestinal dysfunction who require nutritional support [133]. The stimulatory effects of SCFAs on the intestinal mucosa suggest that they may be used in the treatment of various forms of intestinal dysfunction such as short-bowel syndrome, TPN-induced small-bowel atrophy, and colitis. Rolandelli et al. found that the intracolonic infusion of SCFAs in rats receiving a fiber-free enteral diet enhanced the healing of colonic anastomoses as measured by a significant increase in the bursting strength of the anastomosis [116]. In rats deprived of both endogenous and exogenous SCFA production, intracolonic infusion of either combined SCFAs or butyrate significantly increased colonic mucosal DNA concentration [82]. Koruda et al. also showed that following massive small-bowel resection in the rat, TPN supplemented with SCFAs significantly reduced the mucosal atrophy associated with TPN, and thus facilitated adaptation to small-bowel resection [79]. A recent study in patients with diversion colitis showed a signficant reduction in inflammation of the defunctionalized colon when SCFAs were routinely instilled into the diverted colon [58]. Thus, either the enteral or the parenteral provision of SCFAs may provide useful adjuvant therapy in patients with intestinal disease, injury, or loss.

SCIENTIFIC BASIS FOR THE USE OF ENTERAL NUTRITION IN CRITICAL ILLNESS

The gastrointestinal mucosa normally is an efficient barrier that prevents migration of microorganisms and their by-products into the systemic circulation. The epithelial cells of the intestinal mucosa are in constant renewal and thus are markedly affected by nutrient availability, hormonal environment, and intestinal blood flow.

Nutrients taken up by enterocytes for cellular metabolism may enter the intestine through either the luminal side or the basolateral membrane via the mesenteric arteries. Enterocytes extract glutamine, which is oxidized in preference to glucose, fatty acids, or ketone bodies in the small intestine [154]. Glutamine becomes available to the small intestine from mucosal absorption or systemically as a result of muscle proteolysis.

As discussed previously, colonocytes use *n*-butyrate, an SCFA, in preference to glutamine, glucose, and ketone bodies [113]. In contrast to glutamine, which is synthesized by the body, butyrate is not produced by mammalian tissues and is only available to the colonic mucosa as a result of bacterial fermentation in the colonic lumen. SCFAs, primarily butyrate but also acetate and propionate, are used for energy-consuming cellular processes in the colon such as sodium absorption and cell proliferation and growth [114].

In the absence of the physical stimulus of a meal and the lack of intestinal fuels (e.g., glutamine and *n*-butyrate), the small [40] and large bowel [126] atrophy. This atrophy affects not only absorptive cells but also mucus-secreting cells, the gut-associated lymphoid tissue, and brush-border enzymes. While brush-border enzymes and absorptive cells are essential for nutrient assimilation, mucus cells and the gut-associated lymphoid tissue are key components of the intestinal barrier. Bacteria, endotoxins, and other antigenic macromolecules are contained in the intestinal lumen by this barrier (see section on enteral nutrition and critical illness).

Parenteral delivery of nutrients avoids the gastrointestinal tract, reduces the stimulus for pancreatic-biliary and hormonal secretions, and therefore produces intestinal atrophy. TPN-associated atrophy of intestinal structure and function and its reversal by enteral nutrition are well-known phenomena, proved in many animal studies [38, 44, 46, 85, 86]. In addition, experiments in animals suggested that enteral nutrition, when compared to TPN, may enhance survival after peritonitis [106], blunt the postburn hypermetabolic response [95], and better maintain gastrointestinal immunity conferred by secretory IgA [5].

The number and type of bacteria also influence the efficacy of the intestinal barrier. The upper gastrointestinal tract is essentially devoid of bacteria as the result of the bactericidal action of hydrochloric acid and the intestinal motility that transports any surviving bacteria toward the colon. In the human colon, bacteria exist in counts as high as 10^{11}, and the homeostasis of these bacteria is closely controlled by the availability of energy substrate, physicochemical conditions of the colonic lumen, and interactions among microorganisms and with the nonmicrobial environment [64].

The disruption of the intestinal barrier and alteration of the bacterial microflora allow increased translocation of bacteria and absorption of endotoxins from the gut lumen [9]. Bacterial translocation is the process of bacterial migration or invasion across the intestinal mucosa into mesenteric lymph nodes and the portal bloodstream. Bacterial translocation has been studied most extensively in animal models. For example, the translocation of indigenous enteric bacteria into mesenteric lymph nodes occurred in rats following scald burns of 40% of total body surface area [89].

Bacterial translocation has also been observed in patients. Life-threatening infections from gut-associated bacteria have been documented in patients with multiple-organ failure syndrome [90], in those with cancer who have had chemotherapy [14], and in those with major burns [72]. [*Editor's Note:* Translocation is probably a normal process that may not be damaging. The deleterious process may be the absorption of bacterial toxins into the portal blood, about which there are much fewer data, and which in our hands has been extraordinarily difficult to prove.]

Bacterial endotoxins may also migrate across the gut mucosa. Endotoxins are lipo-polysaccharide components of the bacterial cell wall that are normally absorbed in small quantities into the portal bloodstream and are usually detoxified by hepatic Kupffer cells [100]. In rabbits receiving either a single dose of endotoxin, temporary occlusion of the superior mesenteric artery, or 30% scald burn, a fatal endotoxic shock ensued within 12 hours [54]. If the animals were pretreated, and gram-negative bacteria either were absent or present in reduced amounts in the intestinal tract, these injuries were not lethal. Endotoxins given intraperitoneally to mice produced bacterial translocation from the gut to the mesenteric lymph nodes in a dose-dependent manner [27]. The combination of malnutrition with endotoxemia was associated with a significantly higher number of translocated bacteria to systemic organs than was seen in normally nourished animals receiving endotoxin [28].

CRITICAL ILLNESS, ENTERAL NUTRITION, AND THE GUT BARRIER

Many factors affect both the intestinal barrier and the bacterial microflora in critically ill patients (Fig. 26-6). When the cause of critical illness is extensive or prolonged, the gastrointestinal tract may be affected in a sequential manner as depicted in Figure 26-7. In the immediate postinjury phase, the intestinal mucosa atrophies due to many factors including the lack of intraluminal nutrients and a redistribution in the interorgan exchange of metabolic substrates. The inability to tolerate enterally delivered nutrients was a major determinant of adverse clinical outcome in a recent study of critically ill patients [17].

The intestinal consumption of glutamine

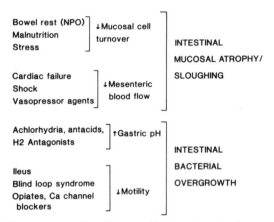

Figure 26-6. Conditions affecting intestinal mucosal integrity and bacterial overgrowth. (From Rolandelli, R. H., and Rombeau, J. L. Scientific basis and clinical utility of enteral nutrition in critically ill patients. *Perspect. Crit. Care* 2:1, 1989. Reprinted with permission.)

increases with stress [139], and the demand for glutamine in the intestine may exceed its production from muscle proteolysis. Glutamine-supplemented elemental diets significantly reduced enteric bacteremia and endotoxemia and prolonged survival in a rat model of enteritis [47, 48]. [*Editor's Note:* Recent clinical trials [55, 142] suggested that glutamine supplied as a peptide in TPN formulations may better maintain muscle glutamine stores and result in improved nitrogen balance in postoperative patients. Other studies [71] suggested that gut chemotherapy toxicity may be prevented by intravenously administered glutamine-containing TPN.]

The large bowel also suffers a deficit of fuels as fasting is prolonged and systemic antibiotics decrease bacterial fermentation of polysaccharides in the colon. In a later phase, the small intestine becomes colonized with bacteria and the equilibrium of the colonic microflora is disrupted. The most severe phase of this spectrum is when the intestinal barrier fails and becomes more permeable to bacteria and endotoxins.

The initial phase of gut atrophy and dysfunction is reversed or ameliorated by the administration of early enteral feedings, as shown by a series of experiments performed

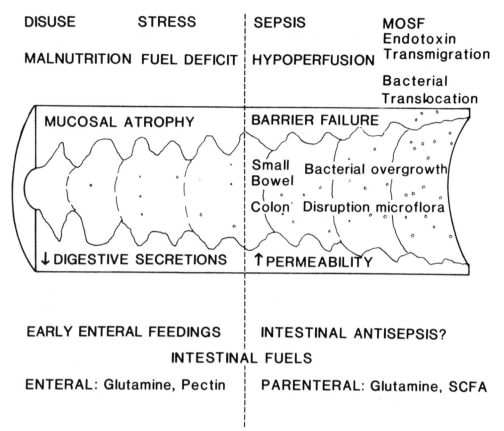

Figure 26-7. The effects of critical illnesses on the gastrointestinal tract. On the upper part of the figure, various noxious stimuli are listed in order of severity as the critical illness progresses. In the lower part of the figure, potential therapeutic interventions are indicated during the progression of critical illness. The dotted vertical line represents an arbitrary point of irreversibility of the intestinal compromise where the therapeutic approach changes from intraluminal nutrition to intestinal antisepsis and intravenous provision of intestinal fuels. MOSF = multiple-organ failure syndrome; SCFA = short chain fatty acids. (From Rolandelli, R. H., and Rombeau, J. L. Scientific basis and clinical utility of enteral nutrition in critically ill patients. *Perspect. Crit. Care* 2:1, 1989. Reprinted with permission.)

in animal models of stress [95]. Intestinal fuels added to the enteral diet may further increase intestinal trophism [82]. On the other end of the spectrum, it is unlikely that a hyperpermeable small bowel populated by bacteria may benefit from enteral nutrition. Moreover, it may be postulated that intraluminal nutrients increase bacterial overgrowth and worsen the situation. The nutritional management of these patients is still highly controversial and experimental work is underway to determine whether intestinal fuels (glutamine, SCFAs, and ketone bodies) could reverse the situation when given parenterally rather than enterally [70, 79, 81].

SUMMARY

There has been renewed interest in the use of enteral nutrition as a result of confirmed benefits to gastrointestinal mucosal structure and function; reduced costs; and improvements in formulas, equipment, and delivery methods. Specific conditions exist for which these feedings are preferred over other routes of nutrient administration. Enteral feedings are efficacious in selected patients who do not ingest sufficient nutrients and have gastrointestinal tracts that can be used safely. Strict adherence to a monitoring protocol prevents most potential complications and enables achievement of specified nutritional goals. The provision of enteral feedings supplemented with gut-specific fuels to maintain the gastrointestinal barrier is an exciting new area of investigation. Investigations are underway to identify the indications for enteral nutrition in critically ill patients.

REFERENCES

1. Abel, R. M., Shih, V. E., Abbott, W. M., Beck, C. H., and Fischer, J. E. Amino acid metabolism in acute renal failure: Influence of intravenous essential L-amino acid hyperalimentation therapy. *Ann. Surg.* 180:350, 1974.

2. Adams, S., Dellinger, E. P., Wetz, M. J., Oreskovich, M. R., Simonowitz, D., and Johansen, K. Enteral versus parenteral nutritional support following laparotomy for trauma: A randomized prospective trial. *J. Trauma* 26:882, 1986.

3. Allardyce, D. B., and Groves, A. D. A comparison of nutritional gains resulting from intravenous and enteral feedings. *Surg. Gynecol. Obstet.* 139:180, 1974.

4. Al-Nafussi, A. J., and Wright, N. A. The effect of epidermal growth factor (EGF) on cell proliferation of the gastrointestinal mucosa in rodents. *Virchows Arch. (Cell Pathol.)* 40:63, 1982.

5. Alverdy, J., Chi, H. S., and Sheldon, G. F. The effect of parenteral nutrition on gastrointestinal immunity: The importance of enteral stimulation. *Ann. Surg.* 202:681, 1986.

6. American Society for Parenteral and Enteral Nutrition Board of Directors. Guidelines for the use of enteral nutrition in the adult patient. *J. Parenter. Enter. Nutr.* 11:435, 1987.

7. Ardawi, M. S. M., and Newsholme, E. A. Fuel utilization in colonocytes of the rat. *Biochem. J.* 231:713, 1985.

8. Argenzio, R. A., and Whipp, S. C. Interrelationship of sodium, chloride, bicarbonate and acetate transport by the colon of the pig. *J. Physiol.* 295:365, 1979.

9. Berg, R. D. Promotion of the translocation of enteric bacilli from the gastrointestinal tracts of mice by oral treatment with penicillin, clindamycin, or metronidazole. *Infect. Immun.* 33:854, 1981.

10. Bergstrom, J., Furst, P., Noree, L., and Vinnars, E. Intracellular free amino acid concentration in human muscle tissue. *J. Appl. Physiol.* 36:693, 1974.

11. Binder, H. J., and Mehta, P. Short-chain fatty acids stimulate active sodium and chloride absorption in vitro in the rat distal colon. *Gastroenterology* 96:989, 1989.

12. Blackburn, G. L., Etter, G., and Mechenzie, T. Criteria for choosing amino acid therapy in acute renal failure. *Am. J. Clin. Nutr.* 31:1841, 1978.

13. Blackburn, G. L., Moldawer, L. L., Usui, S., Bothe, A., O'Keefe, S. J., and Bistrian, B. R. Branched chain amino acid administration and metabolism during starvation, injury and infection. *Surgery* 86:307, 1979.

14. Bodey, G. P. Antibiotic prophylaxis in cancer patients: Regimens of oral nonabsorbable antibiotics for prevention of infection during induction of remission. *Rev. Infect. Dis.* 3 (Suppl.)259:S268, 1981.

15. Bonau, R. A., Daly, J. M., Moldawer, L., and Blackburn, G. Muscle amino acid flux in patients receiving BCAA solutions. (Abstract) *J. Parenter. Enter. Nutr.* 9:116, 1985.

16. Border, J. F., Chenier, R., and McMenamy, R. H. Multiple systems organ failure: Muscle fuel deficit with visceral protein malnutrition. *Surg. Clin. North Am.* 56:1147, 1976.

17. Border, J. R., Hassett, J., LaDuca, J., et al. The gut origin septic states in blunt multiple trauma (ISS = 40) in the ICU. *Ann. Surg.* 206:427, 1987.

18. Bower, R. H., Muggia-Sullam, M., Vallgren, S., et al. Branched chain amino acid–enriched solutions in the septic patient: A randomized, prospective trial. *Ann. Surg.* 203:13, 1986.

19. Bower, R. H., Talamini, M. A., Sax, H. C., Hamilton. F., and Fischer, J. E. Postoperative enteral vs parenteral nutrition: A randomized controlled trial. *Arch. Surg.* 121:1040, 1986.

20. Brown, P. E. The role of fiber in liquid formula diets. In *The Clinical Role of Fiber.* Montreal: Ross Laboratories, 1985. Pp. 53–64.

21. Cerra, F. B., Shronts, E., Konstantinides, N., et al. Enteral modified amino acids (MAA) are efficacious in ICU stress. (Abstract) *J. Parenter. Enter. Nutr.* 9:108, 1985.

22. Cerra, F. B., Shronts, E., Konstantinides, N., et al. Enteral feeding in sepsis: A prospective, randomized, double-blind trial. *Surgery* 98:632, 1985.

23. Cummings, J. H. Short chain fatty acids in the human colon. *Gut* 22:763, 1981.

24. Cummings, J. H. Colonic absorption: The importance of short chain fatty acids in man. *Scand. J. Gastroenterol.* 20:88, 1984.

25. Cummings, J. H., and Branch, W. J. Fermentation and the production of short chain fatty acids in the human large intestine. In G. B. Vahouny and D. Kritchevsky (eds.), *Dietary Fiber: Basic and Clinical Aspects.* New York: Plenum Press, 1986. Pp. 131–152.

26. Cummings, J. H., Pomare, E. W., Branch, W. J., Naylor, C. P., and McFarlane, G. T. Short chain fatty acids in human large intes-

tine, portal, hepatic and venous blood. *Gut* 28:1221, 1987.

27. Deitch, E. A., Berg, R., and Specian, R. Endotoxin promotes the translocation of bacteria from the gut. *Arch. Surg.* 122:185, 1987.

28. Deitch, E. A., Winterton, J., Li, M., and Berg, R. The gut as a portal of entry for bacteremia: Role of protein malnutrition. *Ann. Surg.* 205: 681, 1987.

29. Deitel, M., Williams, V. P., and Rice, T. N. Nutrition and the patient requiring ventilatory support. *J. Am. Coll. Nutr.* 2:25, 1983.

30. DeJung, K. P., Von Meyenfeldt, R., and Rouflart, M. The effect of branched chain amino acids (BCAA) on organ functioning in septic and stressed patients. *Clin. Nutr.* 4(Suppl.):71, 1985.

31. Demigne, C., and Remesy, C. Stimulation of absorption of volatile fatty acids and minerals in the cecum of rats adapted to a very high fiber diet. *J. Nutr.* 115:53, 1985.

32. Deveney, K. Endoscopic gastrostomy and jejunostomy. In J. L. Rombeau and M. D. Caldwell (eds.), *Clinical Nutrition*, Vol. I: Enteral Nutrition (2nd ed.). Philadelphia: W. B. Saunders, 1990.

33. Dewys, W. D., and Herbst, S. H. Oral feeding in the nutritional management of the cancer patient. *Cancer Res.* 37:2429, 1977.

34. Dobbie, R. P., and Butterick, O. D., Jr. Continuous pump-tube enteric hyperalimentation: Use in esophageal disease. *J. Parenter. Enter. Nutr.* 1:100, 1977.

35. Dobbie, R. P., and Hoffmeister, J. A. Continuous pump-tube enteric hyperalimentation. *Surg. Gynecol. Obstet.* 143:273, 1976.

36. Duffy, B., and Pencharz, P. The effect of feeding route (IV or oral) on the protein metabolism of the neonate. *Am. J. Clin. Nutr.* 43:108, 1986.

37. Eagle, H., Oyama, V. I., Levy, M., Horton, C. L., and Fleischman, R. The growth response of mammalian cells in tissue culture to L-glutamine and L-glutamine acid. *J. Biol. Chem.* 218:607, 1956.

38. Eastwood, G. L. Small bowel morphology and epithelial proliferation in intravenously alimented rabbits. *Surgery* 82:613, 1977.

39. Echenique, M. M., Bistrian, B. R., Moldawer, L. L., Palombo, J. D., Miller, M. M., and Blackburn, G. L. Improvement in amino acid use in the critically ill patient with parenteral formulas enriched with branched chain amino acids. *Surg. Gynecol. Obstet.* 159:233, 1984.

40. Ecknauer, R., Sircar, B., and Johnson, L. R. Effect of dietary bulk on small intestinal morphology and cell renewal in the rat. *Gastroenterology* 81:781, 1981.

41. Englehardt, W., and Rechkemmer, G. Ab-

sorption of inorganic ions and short chain fatty acids in the colon of mammals. In M. Gilles-Baillein and R. Gilles (eds.), *Intestinal Transport: Fundamental and Comparative Aspects.* Berlin: Springer, 1983. Pp. 26–45.

42. Englyst, H. N., Trowell, H., Southgate, D. A., and Cummings, J. H. Dietary fiber and resistant starch. *Am. J. Clin. Nutr.* 46: 873, 1987.

43. Erickson, L. S., Person, A., and Wahren, J. Branched chain amino acids in the treatment of chronic hepatic encephalopathy. *Gut* 23: 801, 1983.

44. Feldman, E. J., Dowling, R. H., McNaughton, J., and Peters, T. J. Effects of oral versus intravenous nutrition on intestinal adaptation after small bowel resection in the dog. *Gastroenterology* 70:712, 1976.

45. Fletcher, J. P., and Little, J. M. A comparison of parenteral nutrition and early postoperative enteral feeding on the nitrogen balance after major surgery. *Surgery* 100:21, 1986.

46. Ford, W. D. A., Boelhouwer, R. U., King, W. W. K., de Vries, J. E., Ross, J. S., and Malt, R. A. Total parenteral nutrition inhibits intestinal adaptive hyperplasia in young rats: Reversal by feeding. *Surgery* 96:527, 1984.

47. Fox, A. D., De Paula, J. A., Kripke, S. A., et al. Glutamine-supplemented elemental diets reduce endotoxemia in a lethal model of enterocolitis. *Surg. Forum* 39:46, 1988.

48. Fox, A. D., Kripke, S. A., De Paula, J. A., Berman, J. M., Settle, R. G., and Rombeau, J. L. Effect of a glutamine-supplemented enteral diet on methotrexate-induced enterocolitis. *J. Parenter. Enter. Nutr.* 12:325, 1988.

49. Freeman, H. J., Kim, Y. S., and Sleisenger, M. H. Protein digestion and absorption in man. Normal mechanisms and protein-energy malnutrition. *Am. J. Med.* 67:1030, 1979.

50. Garfinkel, F., Robinson, S., and Price, C. Replacing carbohydrate calories with fat calories in enteral feeding for patients with impaired respiratory function. *J. Parenter. Enter. Nutr.* 9:106, 1985.

51. Gauderer, M. W., and Ponsky, J. L. A simplified technique for constructing a tube feeding gastrostomy. *Surg. Gynecol. Obstet.* 152:83, 1981.

52. Guenter, P. A., Jones, S., and Rombeau, J. L. Administration and delivery of enteral nutrition. In J. L. Rombeau and M. D. Caldwell (eds.), *Clinical Nutrition*, Vol. I: Enteral Nutrition (2nd ed.). Philadelphia: W. B. Saunders, 1990.

53. Gutske, R. F., Varma, R. R., and Soergel, K. H. Gastric reflux during perfusion of the proximal small bowel. *Gastroenterology* 59: 890, 1970.

54. Hamer-Hodges, D., Woodruff, P., Cuevas, P., Kaufman, A., and Fine, J. Role of the intraintestinal gram-negative bacterial flora in response to major injury. *Surg. Gynecol. Obstet.* 138:599, 1974.

55. Hammarqvist, F., Wernerman, J., Ali, R., von der Decken, A., and Vinnars, E. Addition of glutamine to total parenteral nutrition after elective abdominal surgery spares free glutamine in muscle, counteracts the fall in muscle protein synthesis, and improves nitrogen balance. *Ann. Surg.* 209:455, 1989.

56. Hanson, H. P. J., and Parsons, D. S. Metabolism and transport of glutamine and glucose in vascularly perfused small intestine of the rat. *Biochem. J.* 166:509, 1977.

57. Harada, E., and Kato, S. Effect of short-chain fatty acids on the secretory response of the ovine exocrine pancreas. *Am. J. Physiol.* 244:G284, 1983.

58. Harig, J. M., Soergel, K. H., Komorowski, R. A., and Wood, C. M. Treatment of diversion colitis with short chain fatty acid (SCFA) irrigation. *N. Engl. J. Med.* 320:23, 1989.

59. Harrah, J. D., Stephens, N. D., and Hawes, M. C. Prospective sensory evaluation of preparatory methods of elemental diets. *J. Parenter. Enter. Nutr.* 4:303, 1980.

60. Heibert, J. M., Brown, A., Anderson, R. G., Halfacre, S., Rodeheaver, G. T., and Edlich, R. F. Comparison of continuous vs intermittent tube feedings in adult burn patients. *J. Parenter. Enter. Nutr.* 5:73, 1981.

61. Heitkemper, M. E., Martin, D. L., Hansen, B. C., Hanson, R., and Vanderburg, V. Rate of volume of intermittent enteral feeding. *J. Parenter. Enter. Nutr.* 5:125, 1981.

62. Heymsfield, S. B., Bethel, R. A., Ansley, J. D., Nixon, D. W., and Rudman, D. Enteral hyperalimentation: An alternative to central venous hyperalimentation. *Ann. Intern. Med.* 90:63, 1979.

63. Heymsfield, S. B., Head, C. A., McManus, C. B., Seitz, S., Staton, G. W., and Grossman, G. D. Respiratory, cardiovascular, and metabolic effects of enteral hyperalimentation: Influence of formula dose and composition. *Am. J. Clin. Nutr.* 40:116, 1984.

64. Hill, M. J. Factors affecting bacterial metabolism. In M. J. Hill (ed.), *Microbial Metabolism in the Digestive Tract.* Boca Raton: CRC Press, 1986. Pp. 22–29.

65. Hindmarsh, J. T., and Clark, R. G. The effects of intravenous and intraduodenal feeding on nitrogen balance after surgery. *Br. J. Surg.* 60:589, 1973.

66. Horst, D., Grace, N. D., Conn, H. O., et al. Comparison of dietary protein with an oral, branched chain-enriched amino acid supplement in chronic portal-systemic encephalopathy: A randomized controlled trial. *Hepatology* 4:279, 1984.

67. Hostetler, C., Lipman, T. O., Geraghty, M., and Parker, R. H. Bacterial safety of reconstituted continuous drip tube feeding. *J. Parenter. Enter. Nutr.* 6:232, 1982.

68. Hoverstad, T. Studies of short chain fatty acid absorption in man. *Scand. J. Gastroenterol.* 21:257, 1986.

69. Hughes, C. A., and Dowling, R. H. Speed of onset of adaptive mucosal hypoplasia and hypofunction in the intestine of parenterally fed rats. *Clin. Sci.* 59:317, 1980.

70. Hwang, T. L., O'Dwyer, S. T., Smith, R. J., and Wilmore, D. W. Preservation of small bowel mucosa using glutamine-enriched parenteral nutrition. *Surg. Forum* 37:56, 1986.

71. Jacobs, D. O., Evans, D. A., O'Dwyer, S. T., Smith, R. J., and Wilmore, D. W. Disparate effects of 5-fluorouracil on the ileum and colon of enterally fed rats with protection by dietary glutamine. *Surg. Forum* 38:45, 1987.

72. Jarrett, F., Balish, E., Moylan, J. A., and Ellerbe, S. Clinical experience with prophylactic antibiotic bowel suppression in burn patients. *Surgery* 83:523, 1978.

73. Johnson, L. R. (ed.), *Regulation of Gastrointestinal Growth in Physiology of the Gastrointestinal Tract*, Vol. 1 (2nd ed.). New York: Raven Press, 1987. Pp. 301–333.

74. Johnson, L. R., Copeland, E. M., Dudrick, S. J., Lichtenberger, L. M., and Castro, G. A. Structural and hormonal alterations in the gastrointestinal tract of parenterally fed rats. *Gastroenterology* 68:1177, 1975.

75. Kahan, B. D. Nutrition and host defense mechanisms. *Surg. Clin. North Am.* 61:557, 1981.

76. Kelly, T. W., and Hillman, K. M. Study of diarrhea in critically ill. *Crit. Care Med.* 11:7, 1983.

77. Koruda, M. J., Guenter, P. A., and Rombeau, J. L. Enteral nutrition in the critically ill. *Crit. Care Clinics* 3:133, 1987.

78. Koruda, M. J., Rolandelli, R. H., Settle, R. G., Zimmaro, D. M., Hastings, J., and Rombeau, J. L. The effect of short chain fatty acids on the small bowel mucosa. (Abstract) *J. Parenter. Enter. Nutr.* (Suppl.):8s, 1987.

79. Koruda, M. J., Rolandelli, R. H., Settle, R. G., Zimmaro, D. M., and Rombeau, J. L. Effect of parenteral nutrition supplemented with short-chain fatty acids on adaptation to massive small bowel resection. *Gastroenterology* 95:715, 1988.

80. Krebs, H. A. Glutamine metabolism in the animal body. In J. Mora and R. Palacios (eds.), *Glutamine: Metabolism, Enzymology and Regulation.* New York: Academic Press, 1980. Pp. 319–329.

81. Kripke, S. A., Fox, A. D., Berman, J. M., De Paula, J. A., Rombeau, J. L., and Settle, R. G. Inhibition of TPN-associated colonic atrophy with β-hydroxybutyrate. *Surg. Forum* 39:48, 1988.

82. Kripke, S. A., Fox, A. D., Berman, J. M., Settle, R. G., and Rombeau, J. L. Stimulation of intestinal mucosal growth with intracolonic infusion of short-chain fatty acids. *J. Parenter. Enter. Nutr.* 13:109, 1989.

83. Kvietys, P. R., and Granger, N. D. Effect of volatile fatty acids on blood flow and oxygen uptake by the dog colon. *Gastroenterology* 80:962, 1981.

84. Larca, L., and Greenbaum, D. M. Effectiveness of intensive nutritional regimens in patients who fail to wean from mechanical ventilation. *Crit. Care Med.* 10:297, 1982.

85. Levine, G. M., Deren, J. J., Steiger, E., and Zinno, R. Role of oral intake in maintenance of gut mass and disaccharide activity. *Gastroenterology* 67:975, 1974.

86. Levine, G. M., Deren, J. J., and Yezdimir, E. Small bowel resection: Oral intake is the stimulus for hyperplasia. *Dig. Dis. Sci.* 21:542, 1976.

87. Liffman, K. E., and Randall, H. T. A modified technique for creating a jejunostomy. *Surg. Gynecol. Obstet.* 134:663, 1972.

88. MacBurney, M., See-Young, L., and Russell, C. Enteral nutrition formulas. In J. L. Rombeau and M. D. Caldwell (eds.), *Clinical Nutrition,* Vol. I: Enteral Nutrition (2nd ed.). Philadelphia: W. B. Saunders, 1990.

89. Maejima, K., Deitch, E. A., and Berg, R. D. Bacterial translocation from the gastrointestinal tracts of rats receiving thermal injury. *Infect. Immun.* 43:6, 1984.

90. Marshall, J. C., Christou, N. V., Horn, R., and Meakins, J. L. The microbiology of multiple organ failure: The proximal gastrointestinal tract as an occult reservoir of pathogens. *Arch. Surg.* 123:309, 1988.

91. Matarese, L. E. Enteral alimentation: Equipment, Part III. *Nutr. Supp. Serv.* 2:48, 1982.

92. McGhee, A., Henderson, J. M., Millikan, W. J., et al. Comparison of the effects of Hepatic-Aid and a casein modular diet on encephalopathy, plasma amino acids, and nitrogen balance in cirrhotic patients. *Ann. Surg.* 197:288, 1983.

93. Miller, T. L., and Wolin, M. J. Fermentations by sacharolytic intestinal bacteria. *Am. J. Clin. Nutr.* 32:164, 1976.

94. Mirtallo, J. M., Schneider, P. J., Mavko, K., Ruberg, R. L., and Fabri, P. J. A comparison of essential and general amino acid infusions in the nutritional support of patients with compromised renal function. *J. Parenter. Enter. Nutr.* 6:109, 1982.

95. Mochizuki, H., Trocki, O., Dominoni, L., Brackett, K. A., Joffe, S. N., and Alexander, J. W. Mechanism of prevention of postburn hypermetabolism and catabolism by early enteral feeding. *Ann. Surg.* 200:297, 1984.

96. Moore, E. E., and Jones, T. N. Benefits of immediate jejunostomy feeding after major abdominal trauma: A prospective randomized study. *J. Trauma* 26:874, 1986.

97. Muggia-Sullam, M., Bower, R. H., Murphy, R. F., Joffe, S. N., Kern, K. A., and Fischer, J. E. Postoperative enteral versus parenteral nutritional support in gastrointestinal surgery: A matched prospective study. *Am. J. Surg.* 149:106, 1985.

98. Nacht, C. A., Schutz, Y., Vernet, O., Christin, L., and Jequier, E. Continuous versus single bolus enteral nutrition: Comparison of energy metabolism in humans. *Am. J. Physiol.* 251:E524, 1986.

99. Nicolaidis, S. Intravenous self-feeding: Long-term regulation of energy balance in rats. *Science* 195:589, 1977.

100. Nolan, J. P. The contribution of gut-derived endotoxins to liver injury. *Yale J. Biol. Med.* 52:127, 1979.

101. Orenstein, W. R. Enteral versus parenteral therapy for intractable diarrhea of infancy: A prospective, randomized trial. *J. Pediatr.* 109:227, 1986.

102. Orr, G., Wade, J., Bothe, A., and Blackburn, G. L. Alternatives to total parenteral nutrition in the critically ill patient. *Crit. Care Med.* 8:29, 1980.

103. Page, C. P., Ryan, J. A., and Haff, R. C. Continued catheter administration of an elemental diet. *Surg. Gynecol. Obstet.* 142:184, 1976.

104. Parker, P., Stroop, S., and Green, H. A controlled comparison of continuous versus intermittent enteral feeding in the treatment of infants with intestinal disease. *J. Pediatr.* 99:360, 1981.

105. Parrish, R. A., and Cohen, J. Temporary tube gastrostomy. *Am. Surg.* 38:168, 1972.

106. Petersen, S. R., Kudsk, K., Carpenter, G., and Sheldon, G. F. Malnutrition and immunocompetence: Increased mortality following an infectious challenge during hyperalimentation. *J. Trauma* 21:528, 1984.

107. Ponsky, J. L., and Gauderer, M. W. Percutaneous endoscopic gastrostomy: A nonoperative technique for feeding gastrostomy. *Gastrointest. Endosc.* 27:9, 1981.

108. Powers, D. A., Brown, R. O., Cowan, G. S., Luther, R. W., Sutherland, D. A., and Drexler, P. G. Nutritional support team vs nonteam management of enteral nutritional support in a Veterans Administration Medical Center teaching hospital. *J. Parenter. Enter. Nutr.* 10:635, 1986.

109. Randall, H. T. Enteral nutrition: Tube feeding in acute and chronic illness. *J. Parenter. Enter. Nutr.* 8:113, 1984.

110. Ravich, W. J., Bayless, T. M., and Thomas, M. Fructose: Incomplete intestinal absorption in humans. *Gastroenterology* 84:26, 1983.

111. Roberts, D., Thelen, D., and Weinstein, S. Parenteral and enteral nutrition: A cost-benefit audit. *Minn. Med.* 65:707, 1982.

112. Roediger, W. E. W. Role of anaerobic bacteria in the metabolic welfare of the colonic mucosa in man. *Gut* 21:793, 1980.

113. Roediger, W. E. W. Utilization of nutrients by isolated epithelial cells of the rat colon. *Gastroenterology* 83:424, 1982.

114. Roediger, W. E. W., and Rae, D. A. Trophic effect of short chain fatty acids on mucosal handling of ions by the defunctionalized colon. *Br. J. Surg.* 69:23, 1982.

115. Rogers, J. C. T. Jenonostomy in the high-risk gastrectomy patient. *Surg. Gynecol. Obstet.* 126:333, 1967.

116. Rolandelli, R. H., Koruda, M. J., Settle, R. G., and Rombeau, J. L. Effects of intraluminal infusion of short-chain fatty acids on the healing of colonic anastomosis in the rat. *Surgery* 100:198, 1986.

117. Rolandelli, R. H., and Rombeau, J. L. Scientific basis and clinical utility of enteral nutrition in critically ill patients. *Perspect. Crit. Care* 2:1, 1989.

118. Rolandelli, R. H., and Rombeau, J. L. Enteral nutrition and diarrhea. In G. L. Blackburn and S. J. Bell (eds.), *Clinical Nutrition: A Case Management Approach.* Philadelphia: W. B. Saunders, 1989.

119. Rombeau, J. L., and Barot, L. R. Enteral nutrition therapy. *Surg. Clin. North Am.* 61:605, 1981.

120. Rombeau, J. L., Caldwell, M. D., Forlaw, L., and Guenter, P. (eds.), *Atlas of Nutritional Support Techniques.* Boston: Little, Brown, 1989.

121. Rombeau, J. L., and Palacio, J. C. Feeding by tube enterostomy. In J. L. Rombeau and M. D. Caldwell (eds.), *Clinical Nutrition,* Vol. I: Enteral Nutrition (2nd Ed.). Philadelphia: W. B. Saunders, 1990.

122. Rombeau, J. L., and Rolandelli, R. H. Enteral and parenteral nutrition in patients with enteric fistulas and short bowel syndrome. *Surg. Clin. North Am.* 67:551, 1987.

123. Rombeau, J. L., Rolandelli, R. H., and Wilmore, D. W. Nutritional support in pre- and postoperative care. In D. W. Wilmore (ed.), *Care of the Surgical Patient.* New York: Scientific American, 1989.

124. Ruppin, H., Bar-Meir, S., Soergel, K. H., Wood, C. M., and Schmitt, M. G. Absorption of short-chain fatty acids by the colon. *Gastroenterology* 78:1500, 1980.

125. Russell, T. R., Brotman, M., and Norris, F. Percutaneous gastrostomy: A new simplified and cost-effective technique. *Am. J. Surg.* 148:132, 1984.

126. Ryan, G. P., Dudrick, S. J., Copeland, E. M., and Johnson, L. R. Effects of various diets on colonic growth in rats. *Gastroenterology* 77:658, 1979.

127. Sakata, T. Stimulatory effect of short chain fatty acids on epithelial cell proliferation in the rat intestine: A possible explanation for the trophic effects of fermentable fiber, gut microbes, and luminal trophic effects. *Br. J. Nutr.* 58:95, 1987.

128. Savage, A. P., Adrian. T. E., Carolan, G., Chatterjee, V. K., and Bloom, S. R. Effects of peptide YY (PYY) on mouth to caecum intestinal transit time and on the rate of gastric emptying in healthy volunteers. *Gut* 28:166, 1987.

129. Schreiner, R. L., Eitzen, H., Gfell, M. A., et al. Environmental contamination of continuous drip feedings. *Pediatrics* 63:232, 1979.

130. Schroeder, P., Fisher, D., Volz, M., and Paloucek, J. Microbial contamination of enteral feeding solutions in a community hospital. *J. Parenter. Enter. Nutr.* 7:364, 1983.

131. Seltzer, M. H., and Quarantillo, E. P., Jr. The taste of commercially available supplemental elemental diets. *Milit. Med.* 140:471, 1975.

132. Settle, R. G. Defined formula diets: Palatability and oral intake. In J. L. Rombeau and M. D. Caldwell (eds.), *Clinical Nutrition,* Vol. I: Enteral and Tube Feedings. Philadelphia: W. B. Saunders, 1984. P. 212.

133. Settle, R. G. Short chain fatty acids and their potential role in nutritional support. *J. Parenter. Enter. Nutr.* 12:104s, 1988.

134. Shils, M. E., Block, A. S., and Chernoff, R. *Liquid Formulas for Oral and Tube Feeding* (2nd ed.). New York: Memorial Sloan-Kettering Cancer Center, 1972. Pp. 1–10.

135. Silk, D. B. Branched chain amino acids in liver disease: Fact or fantasy? *Gut* 27(Suppl. 1):103, 1986.

136. Silk, D. B. Complications of enteral nutrition. In J. L. Rombeau and M. D. Caldwell (eds.), *Clinical Nutrition,* Vol. I: Enteral Nutrition (2nd ed.). Philadelphia: W. B. Saunders, 1990.

137. Smith, R. J. Regulation of protein degradation in differentiated skeletal muscle cells in monolayer culture. In E. Khairallah, J. Bond, and J. C. Bird (eds.), *Intracellular Protein Catabolism.* New York: Liss, 1985. Pp. 633–635.

138. Soergel, K. H. Absorption of fermentation products from the colon. In H. Kaspar and

H. Goebell (eds.), *Colon and Nutrition*. Lancaster: MTP Press, 1982.

139. Souba, W. W., and Wilmore, D. W. Postoperative alteration of arteriovenous exchange of amino acids across the gastrointestinal tract. *Surgery* 94:342, 1983.

140. Smyth, D. H., and Taylor, C. B. Intestinal transfer of short chain fatty acids in vitro. *J. Physiol.* 141:73, 1958.

141. Steffee, W. P., and Krey, S. H. Enteral hyperalimentation for patients with head and neck cancer. *Otolaryngol. Clin. North Am.* 13:437, 1980.

142. Stehle, P., Zander, J., Mertes, N., et al. Effect of parenteral glutamine peptide supplements on muscle glutamine loss and nitrogen balance after major surgery. *Lancet* 1:231, 1989.

143. Thompson, J. S., Sharp, J. G., Saxena, S., and McCullagh, K. G. Stimulation of neomucosal growth by systemic urogastrone. *J. Surg. Res.* 42:402, 1987.

144. Torosian, M. H., and Rombeau, J. L. Feeding by tube enterostomy. *Surg. Gynecol. Obstet.* 150:918, 1980.

145. Twomey, R. L. Cost effectiveness of enteral nutrition support. In J. L. Rombeau and M. D. Caldwell (eds.), *Clinical Nutrition*, Vol. I: Enteral Nutrition, Philadelphia: W. B. Saunders, 1990.

146. Udall, J. N., and Walker, W. A. Mucosal defense mechanisms. In M. N. March (ed.), *Immunopathology of the Small Intestine*. New York: Wiley & Sons, 1987. Pp. 3–20.

147. Umesaki, Y., Yajima, T., Yokokura, T., and Mutai, M. Effect of organic acid absorption on bicarbonate transport in rat colon. *Pflugers Arch.* 379:43, 1979.

148. Waterlow, J. C., Golden, M., and Picou, D. The measurement of rates of protein turnover, synthesis and breakdown in man and the effects of nutritional status and surgical injury. *Am. J. Clin. Nutr.* 30:1333, 1972.

149. Wedge, J. H., De Campos, R., Kerr, A., et al. Branched-chain amino acids, nitrogen excretion and injury in man. *Clin. Sci. Mol. Med.* 50:393, 1976.

150. White, W. T., Acuff, T. E., Sykes, T. R., and Dobbie, R. P. Bacterial contamination of enteral nutrient solution: A preliminary report. *J. Parenter. Enter. Nutr.* 3:459, 1979.

151. Wilmore, D. W., and Dudrick, S. J. Treatment of acute renal failure with intravenous essential L-amino acids. *Arch. Surg.* 99:669, 1969.

152. Wilson, J. P. Postoperative motility of the large intestine in man. *Gut* 16:689, 1975.

153. Windmueller, H. G. Glutamine utilization by the small intestine. *Adv. Enzymol.* 53:201, 1982.

154. Windmueller, H. G., and Spaeth, A. E. Uptake and metabolism of plasma glutamine by the small intestine. *Biol. Chem.* 249:5070, 1974.

155. Wolin, M. J. Interactions between the bacterial species of the rumen. In I. W. McDonald and A. C. Warner (eds.), *Digestion and Metabolism in the Ruminant*. Armidale, Australia: University of New England Publications, 1974. Pp. 134–148.

156. Wolin, M. J., and Miller, T. L. Interactions of microbial populations in cellulose fermentations. *Fed. Proc.* 42:109, 1983.

157. Woods, J. H., Erickson, L. W., Concon, R. E., Schulte, W. J., and Sillin, L. F. Postoperative ileus: A colonic problem? *Surgery* 84:527, 1978.

158. Wrong, O. M. Carbohydrates. In O. M. Wrong, C. J. Edmonds, and V. S. Chadwick (eds.), *The Large Intestine: Its Role in Mammalian Nutrition and Homeostasis*. New York: Halsted Press, 1981. Pp. 107–112.

159. Yang, M. D., Manoharen, K., and Mickelsen, O. Nutritional contributions of volatile fatty acids from the cecum of rats. *J. Nutr.* 100:545, 1970.

Future Considerations for Nutrition

J. Wesley Alexander
Michael D. Peck

Nutritional support has become an increasingly important aspect of health care during the past several decades because it has been learned that outcome of both medical and surgical therapy can be altered by dietary manipulation. While prevention and/or correction of malnutrition has continued to be the major concern for nutritional support, new and exciting areas of nutritional therapy are emerging, perhaps the most important of which is nutritional pharmacology—achievement of a therapeutic effect well beyond correction of a deficiency.

Despite many advances, a staggering number of questions remain to be answered, and the influence of specific nutrients, nutrient-nutrient, and nutrient-drug interactions on outcome in specific disease states is only now beginning to be studied in a meaningful way. The purpose of this chapter is to provide an admittedly biased overview as to where improvements in nutritional therapy might occur in the next few years, based on observations of the recent past.

DELIVERY SYSTEMS

The entire field of total parenteral nutrition (TPN) and enteral tube feeding has depended on satisfactory delivery systems. Because of this, both industry and academia have developed innovative methods that are currently satisfactory. However, continued improvements will be made. Perhaps more importantly, it should be possible to provide new and innovative complexes of nutrients such as amino acids (e.g., glutamine complexed with arginine or another amino acid) or structured lipids that are stable and compatible with currently available products and delivery systems. Such innovations may be critically important for parenteral hyperalimentation products since current formulations do not provide adequate support for hypermetabolism or stressed states. Improved catheters will undoubtedly result in reduced morbidity with prolonged hyperalimentation. Prepackaged total delivery systems will make the delivery of enteral nutrition not only easier for the personnel involved, but also safer because of reduction in microbial contamination. Appreciation of the importance of delivery of nutrients via the gut has encouraged practitioners to master the skills necessary for safe and effective enteral alimentation in patients who previously either were not fed or were fed intravenously.

EFFECTS OF SPECIFIC NUTRIENTS

To better understand how diet modifications can influence specific disease outcome, it is desirable to briefly examine the effect of specific nutrients on biologic and immunologic functions. Perhaps the greatest amount of information is on the effect of specific nutrients on immunologic variables.

Amino Acids

Protein supplementation is the keystone on which nutritional support systems depend. Adequate protein repletion has had dramatic effects on wound healing, outcome from trauma and burns, and recovery from major illness. However, the protein or amino acid content of nutritional support systems has generally been prepared empirically. Accumulated evidence indicates that modification of individual amino acid concentrations can affect host defenses, metabolism, and ultimately outcome. In addition, there may be some advantage to using intact protein as opposed to free amino acid solutions for enteral feeding [153].

Branched-Chain Amino Acids
There is considerable experience with the branched-chain amino acids (BCAAs)—valine, leucine, and isoleucine—in the treatment of hepatic encephalopathy [26]. In addition, the metabolism of this triad of amino acids is increased in peripheral muscle during states of hypercatabolism, such as sepsis and trauma, and administration of BCAAs in this setting decreases protein breakdown [63]. Although trials of supplementation with BCAAs have generally shown improvement

in nitrogen balance, they have not demonstrated beneficial effects on outcome [109] (with exception of hepatic encephalopathy), in some instances perhaps because the numbers of patients studied were too small to detect an effect [23].

Arginine
Arginine has also attracted attention in the last decade. Once thought to be a nonessential amino acid, the requirement for arginine was first appreciated in immature rodents. It was then established that arginine is necessary for both weight gain and wound healing in injured rats [140], and that it improves nitrogen retention in these animals [143]. Subsequent work by Barbul and colleagues demonstrated that arginine has a powerful thymotropic effect, able to increase thymic weight, thymic lymphocyte count, and mitogen-induced lymphoproliferation [15–19].

More information is now available regarding the site of action of arginine on the immune response. Dietary supplementation with arginine significantly enhances cytotoxic T-lymphocyte development, helper cell subsets, natural killer cell activity, and the kinetics of interleukin-2 receptor expression on activated T cells [36, 130]. In addition, arginine is required for expression of the activated macrophage cytotoxic effector mechanism that causes inhibition of metabolic activity in tumor cells [67]. The effect of arginine supplementation may be multifactorial, through the increase in ornithine levels and through the modulation of insulin, glucagon, and growth hormone.

This information has suggested that improved cell-mediated immunity could alter outcome from disease. Indeed, Rettura et al. [129] subsequently showed that resistance to murine sarcoma virus tumor was increased by arginine supplementation. Similarly, Madden et al. [101] presented evidence that survival was increased by arginine supplementation given orally prior to sepsis, or started intravenously after cecal ligation and puncture in rats.

Arginine supplementation also has an important role in the care of patients with severe burns. First shown to improve cell-mediated immunity and survival in burned guinea pigs [137], arginine supplementation now plays a pivotal role in the improved results from using an arginine-enriched diet formulation for burned patients at the University of Cincinnati and the Cincinnati Shriners Burns Institute [2].

However, some cautions must be raised. Although arginine has marked effects in vitro on immune function, these may not apply in the more complex living organism. For example, Gonce et al. showed that in guinea pigs with prolonged peritonitis, arginine supplementation has no effect on survival at low levels (i.e., 2–4% of total calories), and in fact supplementation with higher levels (i.e., 6% of total calories) worsens both nitrogen balance and mortality [59]. Arginine may be degraded to form toxic products such as nitrates and nitrites, which are damaging to cells [5]. Although this may be detrimental in some patient populations, this toxic effect may be turned to advantage in the treatment of solid tumors.

Thus, although arginine has potent immunostimulatory effects, its role in the treatment of the patient with injury, infection, or cancer has not yet been clearly defined.

Glutamine
Preservation of the integrity of intestinal mucosa has become a topic of increasing importance as the implications of bacterial translocation have become evident. Enteral administration of nutrients can diminish the rate of bacterial translocation [22], as can a single bolus feeding after thermal trauma [71]. Although the mechanisms of these benefits are not yet fully understood, selective nutrition for gut mucosal cells has become an important consideration.

Intestinal epithelial cells preferentially utilize glutamine and short-chain fatty acids for energy metabolism [158]. Whether the glutamine is absorbed from the gut lumen or from the bloodstream appears to have no effect on its metabolism by mucosal cells [157], and indeed glutamine-enriched parenteral solutions have led to increased mucosal mass [70,

75]. Intravenous supplementation with glutamine was not shown to improve nutritional or metabolic status of burned guinea pigs during the first week after thermal injury, perhaps because of low glutaminase content of the gut mucosa in guinea pigs [72]. However, a glutamine-supplemented enteral diet significantly improved nutritional status, decreased intestinal injury, decreased bacterial translocation, and resulted in improved survival in a lethal model of enterocolitis in rats [55].

Equally intriguing is the hypothesis recently advanced by Newsholme et al. from Oxford [114]. They postulated that the purpose of increased protein catabolism during trauma, sepsis, surgery, and burns is to supply alanine to the liver and glutamine to the gut and leukocytes for energy and synthesis of nucleotide precursors. This theory attempts to develop a teleologic explanation for skeletal muscle consumption of BCAAs, the keto-acids of which provide the precursors for alanine and glutamine. In addition, it emphasizes the potential importance of glutamine to the cells of the immune system.

The possibility that nutrient-assisted protection of mucosal integrity may help limit the severity of illness in the compromised host has stimulated interest in the use of glutamine in parenteral solutions. However, a cautionary note should be raised. Popp et al. [125] demonstrated that growth of implantable methylcholanthrene (MCA) sarcoma in rats is dependent on availability of asparagine and glutamine. In the same model, Chance et al. [29] showed that tumor growth is limited by the glutamine antimetabolite acivicin. Thus, glutamine supplementation should be used thoughtfully in patients with neoplastic disease until more information about tumor utilization of substrates is available.

Lipids

The importance of essential fatty acid supplementation was first recognized in patients fed for long periods on intravenous nutrition. Addition of small amounts of soybean oil (Intralipid) was routinely employed to avert signs of essential fatty acid deficiency. However, the adverse effects of Intralipid on polymorphonuclear cell function and survival in animal models were soon recognized [21, 52, 76, 115]. These findings heightened awareness of the potential influence dietary fats might have on patient outcome.

Recently, concern has arisen that long-chain triglycerides (LCTs), such as those found in safflower and soybean oils, may not be utilized optimally in the septic patient because of a relative carnitine deficiency, which blocks their entry into the mitochondria for beta oxidation. Medium-chain triglycerides (MCTs) are absorbed directly into the portal system, do not require chylomicron formation, and are metabolized as rapidly as glucose in the septic patient [11]. Besides the metabolic advantages of MCTs, they may also have an ameliorative effect on immune function.

Studies from the New England Deaconess Hospital provide evidence for the superiority of MCTs. Burned rats fed TPN solutions with LCTs showed impaired reticuloendothelial clearance of bacteria compared to those fed MCT solutions [145]. In another experiment, rats with bilateral septic femoral fractures had decreased bacteremia when given MCT diets [61]. Some tendency toward improved nitrogen balance has been noted, but the animals also lost more weight due to increased thermogenesis [111].

In order to supply the necessary essential fatty acids (approximately 4% of total calories), MCTs have been combined with linoleic acid in structured lipids, which are rearranged triglycerides with both fatty acid types on the same glycerol molecule [22]. When structured lipids were used in the experimental designs described above, results similar to those obtained with MCT were noted [104]. Future clinical studies may confirm the importance of MCTs, possibly in the form of structured lipids which could have other advantages.

Similarly, there has been an explosion in the understanding of the role of eicosanoids (prostaglandins, thromboxanes, and leuko-

trienes) in the pathophysiology of illness and injury. Evidence came to light that dietary fatty acid composition clearly affects eicosanoid metabolism [50, 53, 68, 69, 84, 103, 152]. Specifically, diets rich in linoleic acid result in increased amounts of dienoic prostaglandin and thromboxane production (such as prostaglandin E_2 [PGE_2] and thromboxane A_2 [TXA_2]), and of tetraenoic leukotriene production (such as leukotriene B_4 [LTB_4]). On the other hand, diets enriched with fish oils are high in omega-3 fatty acids, the precursors to trienoic prostaglandins (e.g., PGE_3) and pentaenoic leukotrienes (e.g., LTB_5). This diversion of the metabolites of arachidonic acid has tremendous implications for modification of the immune response after injury, since PGE_2 has more potent immunosuppressive effects than its trienoic counterpart [112], and TBA_3 has much less biologic potency than TXA_2.

Based on this appreciation of the role of dietary fatty acids in prostaglandin production, we performed several animal experiments. Guinea pigs recovering from flame burns over 30% of their total body surface area were enterally fed isocaloric and isonitrogenous diets differing only in lipid type. When compared to those fed safflower oil (75% linoleic acid) or linoleic acid alone, the animals fed fish oil benefited from less weight loss, better skeletal muscle mass, lower resting metabolic expenditure, better cell-mediated immune responses, better opsonic indices, higher splenic weight, lower adrenal weight, higher serum transferrin, and lower serum C_3 levels [4].

These studies formed the basis for a clinical trial in burned patients. In a preliminary report, 50 patients over 3 years old with burns over more than 10% of their total body surface area were randomized to receive either Osmolite/Promix, Traumacal (high in linoleic acid), or a modular tube feeding which contained 23% calories as protein and 15% nonprotein calories as fat, 50% of which was fish oil. All three groups of children tolerated the formulas equally well, although there was more diarrhea in the Traumacal group. The children who received the modular tube feeding had a significantly lower incidence of wound infection and pneumonia, and had significantly reduced hospital stay. Mortality in the group receiving the modular tube feeding was lower than that in the Traumacal group, but not different from the Osmolite group [2]. Thus, diets enriched with omega-3 fatty acids may improve outcome after burn injury, largely due to their effects on prostaglandin synthesis.

Another area of research has yielded seemingly contradictory results. For 2 to 3 weeks, mice were fed diets with different amounts and types of fats, including fish oil and safflower oil (high in linoleic acid). They were then subjected to flame burn over 20% of their total body surface area and infected with *Pseudomonas aeruginosa*. Survival in the group fed a diet high in safflower oil (40% of total calories) was significantly higher than that in the group fed a diet high in fish oil [119]. Subsequent studies indeed confirmed that the fish oil diet did suppress splenic macrophage production of PGE, but not LTB_4 or TXA_2 [119]. The results of this study can perhaps be reconciled with those of the former studies if it is postulated that the immunosuppression of PGE_2 at the time of thermal injury acts to down-regulate the many stimulated arms of the host inflammatory system, especially the production of tumor necrosis factor and interleukin-1. It is also probable that linoleic acid–derived eicosanoids are crucial to cell activation. For example, LTB_4 is a major mediator of leukocyte inflammation, capable of producing cell aggregation, lysosomal enzyme release, and chemotaxis [117]. Unpublished results from our laboratory have in fact shown that although T-cell and B-cell functions are not affected in the burned animal prefed the high fat diets, serum from rats fed for 2 weeks on diets high in safflower oil provided much better opsonization for bacterial killing by normal neutrophils when compared to animals fed fish oil diets. Diets high in omega-3 fatty acids may be important to the burned patient later in the course of recovery by alleviating the continued immunosuppression by PGE_2.

Clearly, manipulation of dietary fatty acids can have a profound effect on outcome after injury. Its effects on survival in the animal with peritoneal sepsis are currently under investigation. It is obvious that this is a fertile area for future research, since these early findings imply the importance of dietary fats in thermal or traumatic injury, sepsis, recovery from surgery, response to neoplastic disease, and correction of malnutrition.

Carbohydrates

Little is known about the interaction of carbohydrates with host immunity, metabolism, or wound healing. It is clear that overfeeding animals results in worsened mortality in models of infection [1,159], although the energy needs of septic patients are unmistakably increased [142]. Whether the deleterious effects of overfeeding are due to increased amounts of carbohydrate calories or to the excess of some other nutrient is not known.

The type of carbohydrate may also influence outcome. In general, carbohydrates are supplied as simple sugars, especially in intravenous formulas, or as more complex carbohydrates, such as cornstarch or dextrins (which are partially hydrolyzed starches). It is known that hepatic lipogenesis in rats is increased when dietary starch is replaced by sucrose, and that this effect can be somewhat abrogated by the addition of linoleic acid to the diet [77]. It may also hold true that energy utilization and the protein-sparing effects of carbohydrates during sepsis and other states of hypermetabolism may be similarly affected.

Fibers

Although it is of central interest in the management and prevention of myriad disease states such as diabetes mellitus, hypercholesterolemia, diverticulosis, and colon cancer, dietary fiber has received little attention in the care of the critically ill patient, except as an adjunct for the treatment of diarrhea [57, 62]. However, dietary fiber may provide the gut mucosa with important nutrients (see discussion of glutamine above).

Dietary fibers, especially the fermentable polysaccharides such as pectins and gums, are metabolized by gut flora to short-chain fatty acids. Butyric acid is the preferred respiratory fuel source for colonic enterocytes [133], and instillation of short-chain fatty acids into the colon stimulates mucosal growth and decreases the growth of colonic tumors [91, 138]. Just as glutamine-enriched solutions may provide additional mucosal protection against bacterial translocation, so may diets enriched with fermentable fibers fortify colonic defenses against invasion.

Metals

Iron
Host withholding of iron from bacteria has long been thought to play a significant role in host defense [156]. Whereas iron-free diets improved survival in mice after parenteral challenge with *Salmonella typhimurium* [123], there was no effect in guinea pigs with prolonged peritonitis [30]. Although there is no evidence for removing iron from diets for patients in clinical practice, iron supplementation may be hazardous. Hyperferremia can increase bacterial virulence, alter polymorphonuclear cell function, and increase host susceptibility to infection [123, 156]. Therefore, addition of iron to the diets of critically ill patients should not be undertaken lightly.

Selenium
Selenium is an integral component of the enzyme glutathione peroxidase, and thus has antioxidant properties, as it participates in the dismutation of hydrogen peroxide and organic hydroperoxides [30, 116, 134]. Although an essential nutrient in some species, selenium deficiency is well tolerated in human populations in Finland and New Zealand, without adverse effects. However, a recent epidemiologic review of dietary selenium and cancer rates suggests a relationship. Both the studies of the geographic distribution of plant selenium levels and regional cancer rates, and the retrospective studies of selenium blood levels in cancer patients, support the hypothesis that decreased levels of selenium increase susceptibility to cancer in subjects exposed to carcinogens [31].

The needs for selenium in the critically ill patient are not known. Selenium supplementation to selenium-deficient, but otherwise healthy, Finnish adults had no effect on lymphoproliferation or antibody production, but did increase in vitro killing of bacteria by polymorphonuclear cells [9]. It is important to note that human cells have more catalase than glutathione peroxidase, and may thus be less dependent on selenium for protection from free radical damage [146].

Zinc
Zinc deficiency can clearly depress immune function, as shown in those patients suffering from alcoholism, renal disease, burns, gastrointestinal tract disorders, and acrodermatitis enteropathica. A suboptimal intake of zinc in mice results in thymic atrophy, peripheral lymphopenia, and reduction in antibody-mediated, cell-mediated, and delayed-type hypersensitivity responses [56]. Although zinc repletion in the zinc-deficient host is clearly important, the role of zinc supplementation in patients with normal zinc levels has not been established. "Megadose" zinc supplementation may impair T-cell and granulocyte function [105]. Thus, as with many other nutrients, the role of zinc supplementation in the augmentation of host defenses is yet undefined, and, as with iron, overzealous administration should be avoided.

Copper
Copper deficiency leads to a number of changes in immune function [88]. These include decreased antibody production, diminished natural killer cell function, inhibition of lymphoproliferation, and increased susceptibility to infection. However, it is not clear that supplementation with copper beyond the minimum daily requirement will improve immune function.

Vitamins

Vitamin A

Vitamin A refers to several biologically active compounds including the retinols (vitamins A_1 and A_2), retinal (the active form of vitamin A in vision), and the carotenoids with pro-vitamin A activity. Many physiologic functions, including stabilization of lysosomes, are affected by vitamin A. Experimental studies show that vitamin A supplementation is related to survival after various challenges. Rodents supplemented with vitamin A had increased survival after cecal ligation and puncture [41] or after parenteral challenge with organisms [34]. In addition, vitamin A supplementation has long been known to restrict the tumor process in experimental models [34].

Vitamin A does not have direct toxic effects on tumor cells or bacteria, but is thought to act as an adjuvant to the immune system. The effect of vitamin A on antibody production has been well studied and is known to increase stimulated antibody production in most models [33, 45, 80, 100, 148]. Other studies have documented the effect of vitamin A on T-cell proliferation and function. Acquired tolerance to allogeneic skin grafts or tumors can be overcome with vitamin A [102, 118], and lymphoproliferation is enhanced in vitro [35, 54, 58, 108, 113], possibly through increased production of interleukin-2 and interferon gamma [87].

A randomized, prospective, placebo-controlled, double-blind clinical trial of the effect of prophylactic vitamin A on tumor development in a cohort of 22,071 male physicians in the United States is currently underway [66]. In addition, more animal research on the potential applications of vitamin A in stimulating the immune response should soon increase interest in this micronutrient as an adjuvant in the treatment of disease.

Vitamin C

Ascorbic acid is a powerful reducing agent that can be synthesized by most species, but not by humans or guinea pigs. It is involved with several hydroxylation reactions, including those involving proline and lysine in the synthesis of collagen. As such, it has traditionally attracted attention as a necessary cofactor for satisfactory wound healing.

However, ascorbic acid also has antioxidant effects, which may protect host tissues from free radical damage. For example, free radical suppression of monocyte proliferation can be overcome by ascorbic acid [6]. Vitamin C has other effects on immune function in vitro, such as improved polymorphonuclear cell adherence, delivery and motility [7, 153], increased antibody production [49], and enhanced lymphoproliferative response [7, 39, 40, 85]. However, meaningful experimental trials of host metabolic or immune response in vivo are sparse. Future roles for vitamin C are undefined, and may in fact be related to its synergism with other nutrients, such as vitamin E.

Vitamin E

Unresolved questions remain regarding the mode of action of vitamin E. Although some believe that so vital a compound as vitamin E must be a component of an enzyme or transport system in an action unrelated to its antioxidant function, most agree that the primary role of vitamin E is as a biologic antioxidant that protects cellular membranes from oxidative destruction [48]. The requirements for vitamin E are in fact related to the amount of long-chain polyunsaturated fatty acids, since they are the major source of lipid peroxides [107]. Similarly, although the adverse effects of vitamin E deficiency are well known, the beneficial effects of supplementation in clinical settings are not well documented.

Some animal studies have shown that vitamin E supplementation prior to infection improves outcome [47, 64, 65, 98], although this same protective effect is lost when given after injury [101] and cannot be reproduced in other murine models of infection [122]. Results of in vitro tests are contradictory when lymphoproliferation is measured [99, 106, 127, 135, 149], but indicate clearly enhanced antibody production [25, 64, 98, 131, 150, 151].

Some of these effects may be due to the influence of vitamin E on prostaglandin synthesis. Not only is the synthesis of dienoic prostanoids (such as PGE_2) suppressed, but vitamin E also locks activation of neutrophils by LTB_4, suggesting that vitamin E can inhibit both cyclo-oxygenase- and lipo-oxygenase-dependent pathways [98, 106, 153].

A note of caution is necessary. As a potent antioxidant, vitamin E is capable of depressing hydrogen peroxide production in normal human neutrophils [12, 13]. Perhaps as a consequence, vitamin E has been noted to impair bacterial killing of neutrophils, as well as to diminish release of lysosomal enzymes and reduce adherence [12, 13, 60, 96, 127]. Whether this is an important effect in vivo is not known, but certainly high doses of vitamin E should not be employed without serious consideration of this problem.

EFFECT OF NUTRIENT MODIFICATION ON SPECIFIC CONDITIONS

Cardiovascular Disease

Epidemiologic studies from the mid-1970s demonstrated that age-adjusted mortality from myocardial infarction was significantly lower among the Greenland Eskimos than their North American neighbors [92]. The principal components of the Eskimo diet were marine mammals which fed on fish, leading to consumption of 5 to 10 g/day of long-chain polyunsaturated omega-3 fatty acids [14, 46]. Although a causal relationship was not established, these findings stimulated several studies on the antiatheromatous effects of omega-3 fatty acids, recently reviewed by Kinsella [86], and by Leaf and Weber [97].

Briefly, omega-3 fatty acids exert marked effects on risk factors related to vascular disease. Omega-3 fatty acids reduce hyperlipidemia and production of cholesterol and the low-density lipoproteins (low-density lipo-

proteins and very-low-density lipoproteins). Preferential production of the antiaggregatory trienoic prostacyclin (PGI_3) and suppression of the chemotactic platelet adhesion-promoting eicosanoid LTB_4 enhances antiaggregatory and antiadhesive activity. On the one hand, these effects are responsible for the easy bruisability and prolonged bleeding time observed in Eskimos, but on the other hand they undoubtedly contribute to the protection from atherosclerotic disease.

These epidemiologic and biophysiologic studies have exciting implications in the treatment of patients with cardiovascular disease. Clinical trials are currently underway to evaluate the benefit of fish oil supplementation on regression of atheromatous plaques (J. D. Davies, personal communication, 1990). The most recent study details the results of a randomized, nonblinded study comparing aspirin and dipyridamole alone with a similar regimen supplemented with eicosapentaenoic acid (EPA; 20:5 omega-3) in the prevention of restenosis in 82 male patients after coronary angioplasty [37]. The incidence of early restenosis was 36% in the control group and 16% in the treatment group, a statistically significant difference. These findings suggest that long-chain polyunsaturated omega-3 fatty acids, such as those found in fish oils, may prevent restenosis of endarterectomized sites, vascular grafts, and arteriovenous fistulas for hemodialysis.

Cancer

Some of the major problems confronting this field of research are that the immunologic responses of the host are often altered by products of the tumor, by tumor interaction with the host, and by interactions among dietary components. For example, it has been long appreciated that increased nutritional support results in increased tumor growth in some models. Popp et al. [125, 126] recently showed that growth of the MCA sarcoma is dependent on total nitrogen substrate, and in particular on the amino acids asparagine and glutamine. However, results of clinical studies are equivocal, with the majority demonstrating no increased survival rate or duration for patients with neoplastic disease assigned to parenteral nutrition while hospitalized for chemotherapy [89]. [*Editor's Note:* On the contrary, what most workers are concerned about is that TPN may actually benefit the tumor rather than the host [51, 126, 141].

Nonetheless, the possibility remains that dietary manipulation can affect progression of disease, response to therapy, and length of disease-free remission. Arginine increases nonspecific host defense mechanisms and has been shown in certain experimental situations to increase the resistance to the growth of malignant tumors [129]. Vitamin A supplementation has also long been known to restrict the tumor process in experimental models [100]. The epidemiologic association between dietary fiber and colon cancer may prove related to protective nourishment of gut mucosa by short-chain fatty acids, an effect which may be supplemented with glutamine. [*Editor's Note:* On the other hand, glutamine is a principal fuel of many tumors, and blocking glutamine metabolism may benefit the host by directing substrate from the tumor to the host [28].]

The relationship of dietary fat to neoplastic disease is complex, and a comprehensive review is beyond the scope of this chapter. However, an excellent, up-to-date review is available [73]. To summarize, several epidemiologic studies suggested that there exists a link between dietary fat and cancers of the breast and colon, among others. Animal models of carcinogenesis support this concept, as do studies of cellular interaction. The Diet and Cancer Branch of the National Cancer Institute is sponsoring two human clinical trials to determine whether a reduced fat diet will reduce the incidence and recurrence of breast cancer [24].

Although diets high in fat generally predispose to neoplastic transformation, diets high in omega-3 fatty acids may be protective. Rats with induced or transplanted mammary tumors and fed diets high in fish oils had reduction in tumor incidence, prolongation of the tumor latent period, and suppression of tumor growth [74, 81, 83]. These findings have not been tested in the clinical setting, but stand with the aforementioned studies to indicate that dietary manipulation of total energy intake, protein level and amino acid content, specific vitamin supplementation, and alteration of fatty acid profiles may benefit patients with neoplastic disease.

Trauma and Burn Response

Aggressive enteral hyperalimentation is routinely used at most burn centers. Part of the rationale for this approach is derived from a prospective study of children with burns averaging 60% of their total body surface area who were fed diets supplemented with protein [3]. These children had higher levels of total serum protein, transferrin, C_3, and IgG than the group fed a standard enteral formulation. Of importance is that there was no mortality in this group, compared to 44% in controls.

These data stimulated a series of animal experiments using gastrostomized guinea pigs with flame burns over 30% of their total body surface area [43]. The hypermetabolic response typical of thermal injury in guinea pigs was abrogated by initiation of enteral feedings within the first two hours [44]. When compared to animals given only lactated Ringer solution per gastrostomy during the first 24 hours, early enteral feedings enhanced jejunal mucosal weight, suggesting a protective effect on the gut mucosal barrier. In addition, there was a highly significant inverse correlation between the serum hormones, cortisol and glucagon, and gut mucosal weight. These findings suggested that early feeding prevented translocation of bacteria and endotoxin across the mucosal barrier, thus excluding some of the initiating factors for the hypermetabolic response. [*Editor's Note:* Translocation of bacteria is probably a naturally occurring process. It is still a hypothesis that translocation results in disease. On the other hand, endotoxin is deleterious, but it has proved very difficult to isolate even picogram quantities of endotoxin in the portal blood.]

Subsequent studies have indeed demonstrated that a single enteral feeding given soon after thermal injury can diminish the magnitude of translocation of *Candida albicans* [22], but that this protective effect is not achieved with intravenous feedings [136]. These findings have been confirmed in otherwise normal rats fed intravenous or enteral solutions for 2 weeks [22]. Moreover, endotoxin administered directly into the portal vein results in the development of a hypermetabolic state whereas similar doses given peripherally do not [8].

These findings are being translated into clinical benefits. An ongoing study in severely burned patients has revealed that patients fed immediately after burn injury compared to those with delayed feeding have reduced incidence of diarrhea and infection as well as improvements in total serum levels of proteins, albumin, ceruloplasmin, and IgG, when measured 7 days after the burn [78, 79].

The composition of the diet also profoundly influences outcome following burn injury. Free amino acids given enterally do not preserve weight and nitrogen balance as well as whey protein, nor do they prevent hypermetabolism when given soon after injury [154]. BCAAs have no beneficial effect [110], but arginine in the amount of 2% of total energy reduced mortality and improved delayed hypersensitivity responses and clearance of bacteria from intradermal injection sites [137]. Diets with more than 15% of nonprotein calories as lipids had an adverse effect on carcass weight, nitrogen content of the liver, and serum transferrin and C_3 levels [136]. At this level of fat, animals receiving fish oil had significantly greater body weight, greater carcass weight, greater spleen weight, improved opsonic index, and preservation of delayed-type hypersensitivity, compared with animals receiving linoleic acid [4].

These laboratory studies led to the development of a new dietary formulation for patients with severe thermal injury. This diet had 20% of total calories supplied by whey protein, 2% by arginine, and 0.5% each by histidine and cysteine. Fat content of the diet was limited to 15% of nonprotein calories, half provided by fish oil (MaxEPA) and half by a product rich (78%) in linoleic acid (Microlipid). A complex carbohydrate (Sumacal) provided 85% of nonprotein calories. Minerals and vitamins were added based on an estimated increased need of two to five times the recommended daily allowance (RDA) in burn patients.

This new burn diet has been tested in seriously burned patients in a prospective randomized trial. Fifty patients have thus far entered the trial, with two control groups. Group I received Osmolite enriched with Promix to bring the protein content of the diet up to 22% of calories. Group II received the modular burn diet described above, and Group III received diluted Traumacal. Measurement of outcome variables has shown that patients in Group II had fewer wound infections, shortened hospital stay, and less mortality [2].

These observations in both experimental animals and humans show that nutrition can make a difference in outcome for victims of thermal injuries. Timing and route of administration as well as dietary composition are all important factors in the seriously burned patient. A prospective, randomized, blinded trial is currently underway to test a new product (Impact) of similar composition for the nutritional support of intensive care patients.

Infection

The point cannot be made too frequently that the optimal route for the administration of nutrients is through the gut. The enteral route has the theoretic advantages of blunting the hypermetabolic response after thermal injury, improving mucosal growth, and decreasing the rate of translocation. In addition, clear benefits in animal studies of mortality have also been demonstrated. In a series of papers, Sheldon and associates showed that rats challenged with *Escherichia coli*/hemoglobin peritonitis had lower mortality rates when fed enterally [94, 95, 124].

However, a recent clinical study from the University of Minnesota indicated that the route of nutrient delivery did not affect the incidence of multiple-organ system failure or mortality after sepsis or surgery [27]. It is important to note that the patients in this study were randomized to the treatment groups after persistent hypermetabolism had been demonstrated for 4 to 6 days. Thus, although enteral feedings started ex post facto may not influence outcome, early institution of gut-delivered alimentation may prevent some of the metabolic and infectious complications of injury and surgery.

With this orientation in mind, a series of animal experiments were conducted to elucidate the best combination of nutrients for the septic state. Guinea pigs were provided with gastrostomies, and bacterial peritonitis was then induced with the implantation of an osmotic pump which allows for the effusion of viable *E. coli* and *Staphylococcus aureus* for 1 week. The tube feedings can be continued for a 2-week period of time, resulting in a unique model that allows for the investigation of dietary manipulation during sepsis [1].

Initial findings showed that diets lower in total energy than the diets fed burned, hypermetabolic guinea pigs (125 kcal/kg/day versus 175 kcal/kg/day) significantly improved survival [1]. Subsequent studies revealed the surprising finding that diets low in protein (5% of total calories, equivalent to approximately 0.5 g/kg/day in an adult human) resulted in markedly improved survival rates [120]. In addition, the effect of iron withholding and supplementation was examined. Guinea pigs were given diets stripped of iron, containing one times the RDA or ten times the RDA. After 2 weeks of enteral feeding, survival was similar in the iron-deficient and control groups. Although survival in the iron-supplemented group was higher, there was inadequate statistical power to establish whether or not this was a real difference [123].

Arginine supplementation has been shown to be thymotropic in vivo and in vitro, and has also been shown to improve outcome in models of animal injury and infection. How-

ever, when arginine supplementation at levels of 2%, 4%, and 6% of total calories were compared to 0% supplementation, survival was 12/22 (55%) in the 0% group, 9/22 (41%) in the 2% group, 9/22 (41%) in the 4% group, and 2/22 (9%) in the 6% group. Survival was not improved by low levels of arginine supplementation and, in fact, high levels significantly worsened mortality [59].

Since it is clear that manipulation of dietary fatty acids can affect outcome from injury and infection both negatively and positively, we conducted studies in which the guinea pigs were fed 3.5%, 14%, or 56% of total calories as either 100% Microlipid (high in linoleic acid), 100% MaxEPA, or 50% each of Microlipid and MaxEPA. Across all types of fat used, the level of fat did not affect outcome, with survival rates of 14% (6/44) at the low level of fat used, 30% (13/44) at the medium level, and 25% (11/44) at the high level ($p > 0.10$). However, fat composition significantly influenced survival across all levels of fat, with 39% (17/44) survival in the groups given equal amounts of Microlipid and MaxEPA, compared to either 20% (9/45) for the 100% Microlipid groups or 9% (4/43) for the 100% MaxEPA groups ($p < 0.05$) [121].

Future work will also focus on the optimal diet for repletion of the malnourished patient prior to elective surgery. Previous studies investigated the use of parenteral solutions prior to surgery, and divergent results have been noted [42, 87]. Restitution of the caloric deficit via the enteral route (where feasible), with careful attention to the nutrient composition of the diet, may result in reproducible beneficial effects. For example, in a study in which the animals were pair-fed for 3 weeks on diets containing 40% of total calories as fat, the fat sources safflower oil (high in omega-6 fatty acids), MaxEPA fish oil (high in omega-3 fatty acids), oleic acid (high in omega-9 fatty acids), and coconut oil (high in saturated fatty acids) were compared in a murine model of subeschar infection after thermal injury. Survival was markedly improved in the safflower oil group ($p < 0.01$), and was worst in the MaxEPA group [119]. Although omega-3 fatty acids may be important once injury has occurred or the septic state is established, saturation of cell membranes with linoleic acid prior to surgery may improve activation of the inflammatory response, especially of neutrophil function with LTB$_4$, and the high production of PGE$_2$ at the time of the injury could, at least theoretically, reduce the production of tumor necrosis factor.

Gut Function

The passage of bacteria across the intact epithelial surface of the gut is a natural process that normally does not cause disease. Disease states such as injury or infection can increase the number of viable translocated microbes cultured from the mesenteric lymph nodes by 1000-fold or more. Systemic antibiotics in these seriously ill patients may disturb intestinal microflora, exacerbating translocation. Translocation in such patients is currently thought to be a major cause of multiple-organ failure and gut origin septic states found in intensive care patients. [Editor's Note: Again, it may not be translocation of bacteria but endotoxin or other toxic bacterial products.]

In addition to simply providing continuous enteral nutrition of a properly balanced formula, there are several nutritional interventions that may decrease translocation. These include increasing the glutamine content and/or fermentable fiber content of the diets. As mentioned above, both glutamine and short-chain fatty acids (the fermentation products of carbohydrate fibers) have been found to be preferential fuel sources for enterocytes, and as such affect rates of translocation [55].

Additional nonnutritive factors may interact with the nutritive factors or have a direct effect on enterocyte growth and the preservation of the gut epithelial barrier. These include growth factors such as epidermal growth factor, urogastrone, and possibly fibroblast growth factor. Translocation can be reduced in a hemorrhagic shock model in rats by the administration of free oxygen radical scavengers [38]. Bacteremia caused by translocation from the gut was diminished from

51 to 7% following severe burn injury in rats by the administration of bombesin, a hormone that stimulates mucosal growth [32]. Thus, route and timing of administration, nutrient composition, and adjuvant hormonal or biochemical therapy can significantly affect bacterial translocation, and may play an important role in the management of critically ill patients in the future.

Autoimmunity

The impressive effects of dietary manipulation on host immune function may become important to patients with autoimmune and inflammatory diseases. New Zealand black × New Zealand white (NZB × NZW/F$_1$) mice serve as a model for systemic lupus erythematosus, since they spontaneously develop autoimmune nephritis, with circulating immune complexes and proteinuria. In these animals, both calorie restriction and enrichment of diets with fish oil have decreased circulating immune complexes, improved proteinuria, and prolonged survival [93, 128].

These experimental observations may have important clinical applications. Daily supplementation of 15 MaxEPA tablets over 14 weeks ameliorated morning fatigue and decreased the number of stiff joints in patients with rheumatoid arthritis [90]. This and other studies also found that supplementation with fish oil decreased neutrophil LTB$_4$ production, suggesting an antiinflammatory mechanism [90, 147]. Thus, dietary manipulation may prove a useful adjunct in the treatment of patients with autoimmune diseases.

Renal Function

Dietary manipulation has long been known to play a useful role in the management of patients with chronic renal failure. Restriction of protein, phosphorus, and carbohydrate has been associated with fewer renal lesions and longer life spans in experimental animals [139]. Clinical studies confirmed that a reduction in protein intake ameliorates many manifestations of the uremic syndrome. Unfortunately, anorexia frequently accompanies renal failure, leading to a state of chronic malnutrition, which may in itself compromise renal function. Therefore, there is no agreement regarding the precise stage of renal failure at which protein restriction is most likely to result in symptomatic benefit to the patient without threatening further renal damage [139].

Other avenues of dietary manipulation may hold promise. Barcelli et al. [20] showed that diets high in salmon oil (16% omega-3 fatty acids) had favorable effects on progression of renal failure in partially nephrectomized rats. TXA$_2$ generation by platelets was markedly decreased in the rats fed salmon oil, and the urinary excretion of PGE$_3$ was increased, suggesting a role for manipulation of eicosanoid synthesis in renal disease.

Pulmonary Function

Large carbohydrate intakes in patients requiring TPN result in markedly increased carbon dioxide production [10]. In the hypermetabolic patient with pulmonary failure, minute volume requirements for adequate ventilation may be increased. This has led to the recommendation that administration of nonprotein calories as lipids may be beneficial in selected patients [133]. However, high lipid loads may have adverse effects on other systems.

NUTRIENT-NUTRIENT INTERACTIONS

Vitamins E, C, and A, Superoxide Dismutase, and Catalase

Free radicals lead to a number of damaging reactions, including strand breaks in DNA, disturbance to enzyme systems, damage to proteins resulting in increased proteolysis, and destruction of cell membrane transport proteins [82, 144]. Lipid peroxidation is among the most detrimental effects of free radical damage. Free radicals are normally short-lived (the half-life of the hydroxy radical [OH·] is < 1 nanosecond) and thus their effect is limited to a radius of a few microns.

However, by reaction with polyunsaturated fatty acids in cell membranes, more stable lipid peroxides can be generated and then can exert damaging effects at a distance from the original site. In addition, lipid peroxides change membrane fluidity, increase nonspecific permeability, inactivate membrane-bound enzymes, and threaten cellular integrity [144].

There are numerous endogenous systems available for the dismutation of free radicals. The intracellular enzyme superoxide dismutase normally converts superoxide radicals into stable molecular oxygen and hydrogen peroxide. Hydrogen peroxide is further reduced by catalase (found in peroxisomes) and glutathione-peroxidase (located in mitochondria and cytosol). Many other antioxidants, including tocopherol, retinoic acid, beta carotene, ascorbic acid, cysteine, ceruloplasmin, and uric acid, are present. However, the system can be overwhelmed after intense cellular damage.

An important concept is that each of the free radical scavengers acts on specific molecules responsible for singlet oxygen production. For example, superoxide dismutase acts in soluble systems on the short-lived superoxide radicals, whereas tocopherol (vitamin E) has the important role of protection of cell membranes from lipid peroxides in a polar milieu. Fang et al. [47] demonstrated that although vitamin E given before burn injury in mice can protect against mortality from bacterial challenge, superoxide dismutase and catalase have no effect.

Since free radical generation has been implicated in several disease states, attention should be paid to increased requirements for vitamin E and other antioxidants (such as vitamin C) in the diet. Synergism among the various species of scavengers may in fact be demonstrated, leading to consideration of combinations of these agents for optimal treatment.

Mineral-Vitamin Interaction

A number of significant mineral-vitamin interactions occur and may be of potential importance in analyzing nutritional studies. Some of these are as follows: (1) High intake of vitamin C may enhance iron absorption but cause copper deficiency and elevate serum cholesterol. (2) Fat levels in the diet may influence the severity of zinc deficiency, as may dietary vitamin E. (3) Zinc deficiency may cause impaired vitamin A metabolism. (4) Riboflavin deficiency may impair iron absorption, and folate excess may impair zinc absorption.

Nutrient-Drug Interaction

This field of investigation is only now beginning to be explored. Of special importance are potential interactions between dietary lipids and immunomodulators and pharmacologic agents that influence arachidonic acid metabolism. As an example, cyclosporine and linoleic acid have synergistic effects for prolonging allogeneic graft survival. A potential mechanism for the immunosuppressive effect of linoleic acid is via PGE_2, and much of the effect of linoleic acid can be blocked, at least in part, by indomethacin. Other important interactions include arginine and immunostimulants, and glutamine or short-chain fatty acids and growth factors. Such interactions are frequently strong enough to make dietary control an almost essential component of any pharmacologic study.

CONCLUSION

During the past several years, it has become increasingly apparent that certain dietary components have pharmacologic as well as nutritional effects. Furthermore, nutrient-drug as well as nutrient-nutrient interactions strongly modulate biologic responses in addition to the considerations associated with the effects of malnutrition. Thus, the major impact that nutritional sciences will have on modern medicine in the future will be the development of nutritional pharmacology to provide both independent and auxiliary therapeutic approaches to the control of human disease. The development of the science will be both slow and difficult because of the com-

plexity of nutrient interactions as influenced by genetic background, disease, drugs, and nutritional state itself.

Acknowledgment

Supported by U.S. Public Health Service grant no. A1-12936 and the Shriners of North America.

REFERENCES

1. Alexander, J. W., Gonce, S. J., Miskell, P. W., and Peck, M. D. A new model for studying nutrition in peritonitis: The adverse effect of overfeeding. *Ann. Surg.* 209:332, 1989.
2. Alexander, J. W., and Gottschlich, M. M. Nutritional immunomodulation in burn patients. *J. Crit. Care Med.* 18(2):S149–S153, 1989.
3. Alexander, J. W., MacMillan, B. G., Stinnett, J. D., et al. Beneficial effects of aggressive protein feeding in severely burned children. *Ann. Surg.* 192:505, 1980.
4. Alexander, J. W., Saito, H., Trocki, O., and Ogle, C. K. The importance of lipid type in the diet after burn injury. *Ann. Surg.* 204:1, 1986.
5. Alverdy, J. C., Aoys, E., and Moss, G. S. Total parenteral nutrition promotes bacterial translocation from the gut. *Surgery* 104:185, 1988.
6. Anderson, R., and Lukey, P. T. A biological role for ascorbate in the selective neutralization of extracellular phagocyte-derived oxidants. *Ann. N.Y. Acad. Sci.* 498:229, 1987.
7. Anderson, R., Oosthuizen, R., Maritz, R., Theron, A., and Van Rensburg, A. J. The effects of increasing weekly doses of ascorbate on certain cellular and humoral immune functions in normal volunteers. *Am. J. Clin. Nutr.* 33:71, 1980.
8. Arita, H., Ogle, C. K., Alexander, J. W., and Warden, G. D. Induction of hypermetabolism in guinea pigs by endotoxin infused through the portal vein. *Arch. Surg.* 123:1420, 1988.
9. Arvilommi, H., Poikonen, K., Jokinen, I., et al. Selenium and immune functions in humans. *Infect. Immun.* 41:185, 1983.
10. Askanazi, J., Rosenbaum, S. H., Hyman, A., Silverberg, P. A., Milic-Emili, J., and Kinney, J. M. Respiratory changes induced by the large glucose loads of total parenteral nutrition. *J.A.M.A.* 243:1444, 1980.
11. Babayan, V. K. Medium-chain triglycerides and structured lipids. *Lipids* 22:417, 1987.
12. Baehner, R. L., Boxer, L. A., Allen, J. M.,

and Davis, J. Autooxidation as a basis for altered function by polymorphonuclear leukocytes. *Blood* 50:327, 1977.

13. Baehner, R. L., Boxer, L. A., Ingraham, L. M., Butterick, C., and Haak, R. A. The influence of vitamin E on human polymorphonuclear cell metabolism and function. *Ann. N.Y. Acad. Sci.* 383:237, 1982.

14. Bang, H. O., Dyerberg, J., and Hjorne, N. The composition of food consumed by Greenland Eskimos. *Acta Med. Scand.* 200:69, 1976.

15. Barbul, A., Sisto, D. A., Wasserkrug, H. L., and Efron, G. Arginine stimulates lymphocyte immune response in healthy human beings. *Surgery* 90:244, 1981.

16. Barbul, A., Sisto, D. A., Wasserkrug, H. L., Yoshimura, N. N., and Efron, G. Metabolic and immune effects of arginine in postinjury hyperalimentation. *J. Trauma* 21:970, 1981.

17. Barbul, A., Wasserkrug, H. L., Seifter, E., Rettura, G., Levenson, S. M., and Efron, G. Immunostimulatory effects of arginine in normal and injured rats. *J. Surg. Res.* 29:228, 1980.

18. Barbul, A., Wasserkrug, H. L., Sisto, D. A., et al. Thymic stimulatory actions of arginine. *J. Parenter. Enter. Nutr.* 4:446, 1980.

19. Barbul, A., Wasserkrug, H. L., Yoshimura, N., Tao, R., and Efron, G. High arginine levels in intravenous hyperalimentation abrogate post-traumatic immune suppression. *J. Surg. Res.* 36:620, 1984.

20. Barcelli, U. O., Miyata, J., Ito, Y., et al. Beneficial effects of polyunsaturated fatty acids in partially nephrectomized rats. *Prostaglandins* 32:211, 1986.

21. Baxter, C. R., Roberts, C., Germany, B., Heck, E., Ireton, C., and Dobke, M. Effect of Intralipid on polymorphological function. (Abstract) *Proc. Am. Burn Assoc.* 17:70, 1985.

22. Billiar, T. R., Curran, R. D., Stuehr, D. J., West, M. A., Bentz, B. G., and Simmons, R. L. An L-arginine-dependent mechanism mediates Kupffer cell inhibition of hepatocyte protein synthesis in vitro. *J. Exp. Med.* 169:1467, 1989.

23. Brennan, M. F., Cerra, F., Daly, J. M., et al. Report of a research workshop: Branched chain amino acids in stress and injury. *J. Parenter. Enter. Nutr.* 10:446, 1986.

24. Butrum, R. R., Lanza, E., and Clifford, C. K. The Diet and Cancer Branch, NCI: Current projects and future research directions. *Prog. Clin. Biol. Res.* 222:773, 1986.

25. Campbell, P. A., Cooper, H. R., Heinzerling, R. H., and Tengerdy, R. P. Vitamin E enhances in vitro immune response by normal and non-adherent spleen cells. *Proc. Soc. Exp. Biol. Med.* 146:465, 1974.

26. Cerra, F. B., Cheung, N. K., Fischer, J. E., et al. Disease-specific amino acid infusion (F080) in hepatic encephalopathy: A prospective, randomized, double-blind, controlled trial. *J. Parenter. Enter. Nutr.* 9:288, 1985.

27. Cerra, F. B., McPherson, J. P., Konstantinides, F. N., Konstantinides, N. N., and Teasley, K. M. Enteral nutrition does not prevent multiple organ failure syndrome (MOFS) after sepsis. *Surgery* 104:727, 1988.

28. Chance, W. T., Cao, L., and Fischer, J. E. Insulin and acivicin improve host nutrition and prevent tumor growth during total parenteral nutrition. *Ann. Surg.* 208:524, 1988.

29. Chance, W. T., Cao, L., and Fischer, J. E. Response of tumor and host to hyperalimentation and anti-glutamine treatments. (Abstract) *J. Parenter. Enter. Nutr.* 13(Suppl.):6, 1989.

30. Chandlee, G. C., and Fukui, G. M. The role of endotoxin induced nonspecific protection. (Abstract) *Abstr. Bacteriological Proceedings of the 65th Annual Meeting, American Society for Microbiology,* 1965, p. 45.

31. Clark, L. C. The epidemiology of selenium and cancer. *Fed. Proc.* 44:2584, 1985.

32. Coffey, J. A., Milhoan, R. A., Abdullah, A., Herndon, D. N., Townsend, C. M., and Thompson, J. C. Bombesin inhibits bacterial translocation from the gut in burned rats. *Surg. Forum* 39:109, 1988.

33. Cohen, B. E., and Cohen, I. K. Vitamin A: Adjuvant and steroid antagonist in the immune response. *J. Immunol.* 111:1376, 1973.

34. Cohen, B. E., and Elin, R. J. Vitamin A-induced nonspecific resistance to infection. *J. Infect. Dis.* 129:597, 1974.

35. Cohen, B. E., Gill, G., Cullen, P. R., and Morris, P. J. Reversal of postoperative immunosuppression in man by vitamin A. *Surg. Gynecol. Obstet.* 149:658, 1979.

36. Daly, J. M., Reynolds, J., Thom, A., et al. Immune and metabolic effects of arginine in the surgical patient. *Ann. Surg.* 208:512, 1988.

37. Dehmer, G. J., Popma, J. J., van den Berg, E. K., et al. Reduction in the rate of early restenosis after coronary angioplasty by a diet supplemented with omega-3 fatty acids. *N. Engl. J. Med.* 319:733, 1988.

38. Dietch, E. A., Bridges, W., Barker, J., et al. Hemorrhagic shock-induced bacterial translocation is reduced by xanthine oxidase inhibition or inactivation. *Surgery* 104:191, 1988.

39. Delafuente, J. C., and Panush, R. S. Modulation of certain immunologic responses by vitamin C. *Int. J. Vitam. Nutr. Res.* 50:44, 1979.

40. Delafuente, J. C., Prendergast, J. M., and Modigan, A. Immunologic modulation by vitamin C in the elderly. *Int. J. Immunopharmacol.* 8:205, 1986.

41. Demetriou, A. A., Franco, I., Bark, S., Rettura, G., Seifter, E., and Levenson, S. M. Effects of vitamin A and beta-carotene on intra-abdominal sepsis. *Arch. Surg.* 119:161, 1984.

42. Detsky, A. S., Baker, J. P., O'Rourke, K., and Goel, V. Perioperative parenteral nutrition: A meta-analysis. *Ann. Intern. Med.* 107:195, 1987.

43. Dominioni, L., Stinnett, J. D., Fang, C. H., et al. Gastrostomy feeding in normal and hypermetabolic burned guinea pigs: A model for the study of enteral diets. *J. Burn Care Rehab.* 5:100, 1984.

44. Dominioni, L., Trocki, O., Mochizuki, H., Fang, C. H., and Alexander, J. W. Prevention of severe postburn hypermetabolism and catabolism by immediate intragastric feeding. *J. Burn Care Rehab.* 5:106, 1984.

45. Dresser, D. W. Adjuvanticity of vitamin A. *Nature* 217:527, 1968.

46. Dyerberg, J., Bang, H. O., and Hjorne, N. Fatty acid composition of the plasma lipids in Greenland Eskimos. *Am. J. Clin. Nutr.* 28:958, 1975.

47. Fang, C. H., Peck, M. D., Alexander, J. W., and Babcock, G. F. The effect of free radical scavengers on outcome after infection in burned mice. *J. Trauma* 30:453–456, 1990.

48. Farrell, P. M. Vitamin E. In M. E. Shils and V. R. Young (eds.), *Modern Nutrition in Health and Disease.* Philadelphia: Lea & Febiger, 1988. P. 340.

49. Feigen, G. A., Smith, B. H., Dix, C. E., et al. Enhancement of antibody production and protection against systemic anaphylaxis by large doses of vitamin C. *Res. Commun. Chem. Pathol. Pharmacol.* 38:313, 1982.

50. Ferretti, A., Schoene, N. W., and Flanagan, V. P. Identification and quantification of prostaglandin E_3 in renal medullary tissue of three strains of rats fed fish oil. *Lipids* 16:800, 1981.

51. Fischer, J. E. Editorial: Adjuvant parenteral nutrition in the patient with cancer. *Surgery* 96:578, 1984.

52. Fischer, G. W., Hunter, K. W., Wilson, S. R., and Mease, A. D. Diminished bacterial defenses with Intralipid. *Lancet* 2:819, 1980.

53. Fischer, S., and Weber, P. C. Prostaglandin I_3 is formed in vivo in man after dietary eicosapentaenoic acid. *Nature* 307:165, 1984.

54. Forni, G., Cerutti Sola, S., Giovarelli, M., Santoni, A., Martinetto, P., and Vietti, D. Effect of prolonged administration of low doses of dietary retinoids on cell-mediated immunity and the growth of transplantable tumors in mice. *J. Natl. Cancer Inst.* 76:527, 1986.

55. Fox, A. D., Kripke, S. A., De Paula, J., Berman, J. M., Settle, R. G., and Rombeau, J. L.

Effect of a glutamine-supplemented enteral diet on methotrexate-induced enterocolitis. *J. Parenter. Enter. Nutr.* 12:325, 1988.

56. Fraker, P. J., Jardieu, P., and Cook, J. Zinc deficiency and immune function. *Arch. Dermatol.* 123:1699, 1987.

57. Frank, H. A., and Green, L. C. Successful use of a bulk laxative to control the diarrhea of tube feeding. *Scand. J. Plast. Reconstr. Surg.* 13:193, 1979.

58. Fusi, S., Kupper, T. S., Green, D. R., and Ariyan, S. Reversal of postburn immunosuppression by the administration of vitamin A. *Surgery* 96:330, 1984.

59. Gonce, S. J., Peck, M. D., Alexander, J. W., and Miskell, P. W. Arginine supplementation and its effect on established peritonitis in guinea pigs. *J. Parenter. Enter. Nutr.* 14:237–240, 1989.

60. Haberal, M., Mavi, V., and Oner, G. The stabilizing effect of vitamin E, selenium and zinc on leucocyte membrane permeability: A study in vitro. *Burns* 13:118, 1987.

61. Hamawy, K. J., Moldawer, L. L., and Gerogieff, M. The effect of lipid emulsions on reticuloendothelial system function in the injured animal. *J. Parenter. Enter. Nutr.* 9:559, 1985.

62. Hart, G. K., and Dobb, G. J. Effect of a fecal bulking agent on diarrhea during enteral feeding in the critically ill. *J. Parenter. Enter. Nutr.* 12:465, 1988.

63. Hasselgren, P. O., Pedersen, P., Sax, H. C., Warner, B. W., and Fischer, J. E. Current concepts of protein turnover and amino acid transport in liver and skeletal muscle during sepsis. *Arch. Surg.* 123:992, 1988.

64. Heinzerling, R. H., Nockels, C. F., Quarles, C. L., and Tengerdy, R. P. Protection of chicks against *E. coli* infection by dietary supplementation with vitamin E. *Proc. Soc. Exp. Biol. Med.* 146:279, 1974.

65. Heinzerling, R. H., Tengerdy, R. P., Wick, L. L., and Lueker, D. C. Vitamin E protects mice against *Diplococcus pneumoniae* Type I infection. *Infect. Immun.* 10:1292, 1974.

66. Hennekens, C. H., and Eberlein, K. Randomized trial of aspirin and beta-carotene among U.S. physicians. *Prev. Med.* 14:165, 1985.

67. Hibbs, J. B., Vavrin, Z., and Taintor, R. R. L-Arginine is required for expression of the activated macrophage effector mechanism causing selective metabolic inhibition in target cells. *J. Immunol.* 138:550, 1987.

68. Holmer, G., and Beare-Rogers, J. L. Linseed oil and marine oil as sources of omega-3 fatty acids in rat heart. *Nutr. Res.* 5:1011, 1985.

69. Hwang, D. H., and Carroll, A. E. Decreased formation of prostaglandin derived from ara-

chidonic acid by dietary linolenate in rats. *Am. J. Clin. Nutr.* 33:590, 1980.

70. Hwang, T. L., O'Dwyer, S. T., Smith, R. J., and Wilmore, D. W. Preservation of small bowel mucosa using glutamine-enriched parenteral nutrition. *Surg. Forum* 37:56, 1986.

71. Inoue, S., Epstein, M. D., Alexander, J. W., Trocki, O., and Gura, P. Prevention of yeast translocation across the gut by a single enteral feeding after burn injury. *J. Parenter. Enter. Nutr.* 13(6):565–571, 1989.

72. Inoue, S., Trocki, O., Edwards, L., and Alexander, J. W. Is glutamine beneficial in postburn nutritional support? *Curr. Surg.* 45:110, 1988.

73. Ip, C., Birt, D. F., Rogers, A. E., and Mettlin, C. (eds.). *Dietary Fat and Cancer.* New York: Alan R. Liss, 1986.

74. Ip, C., Ip, M. M., and Sylvester, P. Relevance of trans fatty acids and fish oil in animal tumorigenesis studies. In Ip, C., Birt, D. F., Rogers, A. E., and Mettlin, C. (eds.). *Dietary Fat and Cancer.* New York: Alan R. Liss, 1986. P. 283.

75. Jacobs, D., Evans, D. A., O'Dwyer, S. T., Smith, R. J., and Wilmore, D. W. Trophic effects of glutamine-enriched parenteral nutrition on colonic mucosa. (Abstract) *J. Parenter. Enter. Nutr.* 12(Suppl.):6, 1988.

76. Jarstrand, C., Berghem, L., and Lahnborg, G. Human granulocyte and reticuloendothelial system function during Intralipid infusion. *J. Parenter. Enter. Nutr.* 2:663, 1978.

77. Jeffcoat, R., Roberts, P. A., and James, A. T. The control of lipogenesis by dietary linoleic acid and its influence on the deposition of fat. *Eur. J. Biochem.* 101:447, 1979.

78. Jenkins, M., Gottschlich, M., Alexander, J. W., and Warden, G. D. A preliminary evaluation of the effect of immediate enteral feeding on the hypermetabolic response following severe burn injury. (Abstract) *Proc. Am. Burn Assoc.* 20:112, 1988.

79. Jenkins, M., Gottschlich, M., Alexander, J. W., and Warden, G. D. Effect of immediate enteral feeding on the hypermetabolic response following severe burn injury. (Abstract) *J. Parenter. Enter. Nutr.* 13(Suppl.):12, 1989.

80. Jurin, M., and Tannock, K. F. Influence of vitamin A on immunological response. *Immunology* 23:283, 1972.

81. Jurkowski, J. J., and Cave, W. T. Dietary effects of menhaden oil on the growth and membrane lipid composition of rat mammary tumors. *J. Natl. Cancer Inst.* 74:1145, 1985.

82. Kako, K. J. Free radical effects on membrane protein in myocardial ischemia/reperfusion injury. *J. Mol. Cell. Cardiol.* 19:209, 1987.

83. Karmali, R. A., Marsh, J., and Fuchs, C. Effect of omega-3 fatty acids on growth of a rat mammary tumor. *J. Natl. Cancer Inst.* 73:457, 1984.

84. Kelley, V. E., Ferretti, A., Izui, S., and Strom, T. B. A fish oil diet rich in eicosapentaenoic acid reduces cyclooxygenase metabolites and suppresses lupus in MRL-1pr mice. *J. Immunol.* 134:1914, 1985.

85. Kennes, B., Dumont, I., Brohee, D., Hubert, C., and Neve, P. Effect of vitamin C supplements on cell-mediated immunity in old people. *Gerontology* 29:305, 1983.

86. Kinsella, J. E. Effects of polyunsaturated fatty acids on factors related to cardiovascular disease. *Am. J. Cardiol.* 60:23G, 1987.

87. Klein, S., Simes, J., and Blackburn, G. L. Total parenteral nutrition and cancer clinical trials. *Cancer* 58:1378, 1986.

88. Koller, L. D., Mulhern, S. A., Frankel, N. C., Steven, M. G., and Williams, J. R. Immune dysfunction in rats fed a diet deficient in copper. *Am. J. Clin. Nutr.* 45:997, 1987.

89. Kortez, R. L. Parenteral nutrition: Is it oncologically logical? *J. Clin. Oncol.* 2:534, 1984.

90. Kremer, J. M., Jubiz, W., Michalek, A., et al. Fish-oil fatty acid supplementation in active rheumatoid arthritis: A double-blinded, controlled, crossover study. *Ann. Intern. Med.* 106:497, 1987.

91. Kripke, S. A., Fox, A. D., Berman, J. M., Settle, R. G., and Rombeau, J. L. Stimulation of mucosal growth with intracolonic butyrate infusion. *Surg. Forum* 37:47, 1987.

92. Kromann, N., and Green, A. Epidemiological studies in the Upernavik district, Greenland: Incidence of some chronic diseases 1950–1974. *Acta Med. Scand.* 208:401, 1980.

93. Kubo, C., Johnson, B. C., Day, N. K., and Good, R. A. Calorie source, calorie restriction, immunity and aging of (NZB/NZW)F_1 mice. *J. Nutr.* 114:1884, 1984.

94. Kudsk, K. A., Carpenter, G., Petersen, S., and Sheldon, G. F. Effect of enteral and parenteral feeding in malnourished rats with *E. coli* hemoglobin adjuvant peritonitis. *J. Surg. Res.* 31:105, 1981.

95. Kudsk, K. A., Stone, J. M., Carpenter, G., and Sheldon, G. F. Enteral and parenteral feeding influences mortality after hemoglobin-*E. coli* peritonitis in normal rats. *J. Trauma* 23:605, 1983.

96. Lafuze, J. E., Weisman, S. J., Alpert, L. A., and Baehner, R. L. Vitamin E attenuates the effects of FMLP on rabbit circulating granulocytes. *Pediatr. Res.* 18:536, 1984.

97. Leaf, A., and Weber, P. C. Cardiovascular effects of omega-3 fatty acids. *N. Engl. J. Med.* 318:549, 1988.

98. Likoff, R. O., Guptill, D. R., Lawrence, L. M., et al. Vitamin E and aspirin depress

prostaglandins in protection of chickens against *Escherichia coli* infection. *Am. J. Clin. Nutr.* 34:245, 1981.

99. Lim, T. S., Putt, N., Safranski, D., Chung, C., and Watson, R. R. Effect of vitamin E on cell-mediated immune responses and serum corticosterone in young and maturing mice. *Immunology* 44:289, 1981.

100. Lotan, R. Effects of vitamin A and its analogs (retinoids) on normal and neoplastic cells. *Biochem. Biophys. Acta* 605:33, 1980.

101. Madden, H. P., Breslin, R. J., Wasserkrug, H. L., Efron, G., and Barbul, A. Stimulation of T cell immunity by arginine enhances survival in peritonitis. *J. Surg. Res.* 44:658, 1988.

102. Malkovsky, M., Medawar, P. B., Thatcher, D. R., et al. Acquired immunological tolerance of foreign cells is impaired by recombinant interleukin-2 or vitamin A acetate. *Proc. Natl. Acad. Sci. USA* 82:536, 1985.

103. Marshall, L. A., Szczesniewski, A., and Johnston, P. V. Dietary alpha-linoleic acid and prostaglandin synthesis: A time course study. *Am. J. Clin. Nutr.* 38:895, 1983.

104. Mascioli, E. A., Bistrian, B. R., Babayan, V. K., and Blackburn, G. L. Medium chain triglycerides and structured lipids as unique nonglucose energy sources in hyperalimentation. *Lipids* 22:421, 1987.

105. Megadose zinc intakes impair immune responses. *Nutr. Rev.* 43:141, 1985.

106. Meydani, S. N., Meydani, M., Verdon, C. P., Shapiro, A. A., Blumberg, J. B., and Hayes, K. C. Vitamin E supplementation suppresses prostaglandin E_2 synthesis and enhances the immune response of aged mice. *Mech. Ageing Dev.* 34:191, 1986.

107. Meydani, S. N., Shapiro, A. C., Meydani, M., Macauley, J. B., and Blumberg, J. B. Effect of age and dietary fat (fish, corn and coconut oils) on tocopherol status of C57BL/6Nia mice. *Lipids* 22:345, 1987.

108. Micksche, M., Cerni, C., Kokron, O., Titscher, R., and Wrba, H. Stimulation of immune response in lung cancer patients by vitamin A therapy. *Oncology* 34:234, 1977.

109. Mochizuki, H., Trocki, O., Dominioni, L., and Alexander, J. W. Effect of a diet rich in branched chain amino acids on severely burned guinea pigs. *J. Trauma* 26:1077, 1986.

110. Mochizuki, H., Trocki, O., Dominioni, L., Ray, M. B., and Alexander, J. W. Optimal lipid content for enteral diets following thermal injury. *J. Parenter. Enter. Nutr.* 8:638, 1984.

111. Mok, K. T., Maiz, A., Yamazaki, K., et al. Structured medium-chain and long-chain triglyceride emulsions are superior to physical mixtures in sparing body protein in the burned rat. *Metabolism* 33:910, 1984.

112. Needleman, P., Raz, A., Minkes, M. S., Ferrendelli, J. A., and Sprecher, H. Triene prostaglandins: Prostacyclin and thromboxane biosynthesis and unique biological properties. *Proc. Natl. Acad. Sci. USA* 76:944, 1979.

113. Newberne, P. M., and Suphakaran, V. Preventive role of vitamin A in colon carcinogenesis in rats. *Cancer* 40:2553, 1977.

114. Newsholme, E. A., Newsholme, P., Curi, R., Challoner, E., and Ardawi, M. S. A role for muscle in the immune system and its importance in surgery, trauma, sepsis and burns. *Nutrition* 4:261, 1988.

115. Nordenstrom, J., Jarstrand, C., and Wiernik, A. Decreased chemotaxis and random migration of leukocytes during Intralipid infusion. *Am. J. Clin. Nutr.* 32:2416, 1979.

116. Oh, S. H., Lee, M. H., and Chung, C. J. Protection of phagocytic macrophages from peroxidative damage by selenium and vitamin E. *Yonsei Med. J.* 23:101, 1982.

117. Parker, C. W. Leukotrienes and prostaglandins in the immune system. *Adv. Prostaglandin Thromboxane Leukotriene Res.* 16:113, 1986.

118. Patek, P. Q., Collins, J. L., Yogeeswaran, G., and Dennert, G. Anti-tumor potential of retinoic acid: Stimulation of immune mediated effectors. *Int. J. Cancer* 24:624, 1979.

119. Peck, M. D., Ogle, C. K., Alexander, J. W., and Babcock, G. F. The effect of dietary fatty acids in response to pseudomonas infection in burned mice. *J. Trauma* 30:445–452, 1990.

120. Peck, M. D., Alexander, J. W., Gonce, S. J., and Miskell, P. W. Low protein diets improve survival from peritonitis in guinea pigs. *Ann. Surg.* 309:448, 1989.

121. Peck, M. D., Alexander, J. W., Ogle, C. K., Gonce, S. J., and Miskell, P. W. Composition of fat in enteral diets can influence outcome in experimental peritonitis. *Ann. Surg.* (In press).

122. Peck, M. D., Clouva-Molyvdas, P. M., Alexander, J. W., and Gonce, S. J. The effect of vitamin E on survival in murine models of infection. (Abstract) *J. Parenter. Enter. Nutr.* 13(Suppl.):6s, 1989.

123. Peck, M. D., Gonce, S. J., Alexander, J. W., and Miskell, P. W. Dietary iron and recovery from peritonitis in guinea pigs. *Am. J. Clin. Nutr.* 50:524, 1989.

124. Petersen, S. R., Kudsk, K. A., Carpenter, G., and Sheldon, G. F. Malnutrition and immunocompetence: Increased mortality following an infectious challenge during hyperalimentation. *J. Trauma* 21:528, 1981.

125. Popp, M. B., Enrione, E. B., Wagner, S. C., and Chance, W. T. Influence of total nitrogen, asparagine, and glutamine on MCA tumor growth in the Fischer 344 rat. *Surgery* 104:152, 1988.

126. Popp, M. B., Wagner, S. C., Enrione, E. B., and Brito, O. J. Host and tumor responses to varying rates of nitrogen infusion in the tumor-bearing rat. *Ann. Surg.* 207:80, 1988.

127. Prasad, J. S. Effect of vitamin E supplementation on leukocyte function. *Am. J. Clin. Nutr.* 33:606, 1980.

128. Prickett, J. D., Robinson, D. R., and Steinberg, A. D. Effects of dietary enrichment with eicosapentaenoic acid upon autoimmune nephritis in female NZB × NZW/F₁ mice. *Arthritis Rheum.* 26:133, 1983.

129. Rettura, G., Padawer, J., Barbul, A., Levenson, S. M., and Seifter, E. Supplemental arginine increases thymic cellularity in normal and murine sarcoma virus-inoculated mice and increases the resistance to murine sarcoma virus tumor. *J. Parenter. Enter. Nutr.* 3:409, 1979.

130. Reynolds, J. V., Daly, J. M., Zhang, S., Evantash, E., Sigal, R., and Ziegler, M. M. Immunomodulatory mechanisms of arginine. *Surgery* 104:142, 1988.

131. Ritacco, K. A., Nockels, C. F., and Ellis, R. P. The influence of supplemental vitamins A and E on ovine humoral immune response. *Proc. Soc. Exp. Biol. Med.* 182:393, 1986.

132. Robin, A. P., Askanazi, J., Cooperman, A., Carpentier, Y. A., Elwyn, D. H., and Kinney, J. M. Influence of hypercaloric glucose infusions on fuel economy in surgical patients: A review. *Crit. Care Med.* 9:680, 1981.

133. Roediger, W. E. W. Utilization of nutrients by isolated epithelial cells of the rat colon. *Gastroenterology* 83:424, 1982.

134. Rotruck, J. T., Pope, A. L., Ganther, H. E., Swanson, A. B., Hafeman, D. G., and Hoekstra, W. G. Selenium: Biochemical role as a component of glutathione peroxidase. *Science* 179:588, 1973.

135. Rundus, C., Peterson, V. M., Zapata-Sirvent, R., Hansbrough, J., and Robinson, W. A. Vitamin E improves cell-mediated immunity in the burned mouse: A preliminary study. *Burns* 11:11, 1984.

136. Saito, H., Trocki, O., Alexander, J. W., Kopcha, R., Heyd, T., and Joffe, S. N. The effect of route of nutrient administration on the nutritional state, catabolic hormone secretion, and gut mucosal integrity after burn injury. *J. Parenter. Enter. Nutr.* 11:1, 1987.

137. Saito, H., Trocki, O., Wang, S. L., Gonce, S. J., Joffe, S. N., and Alexander, J. W. Metabolic and immune effects of dietary arginine supplementation after burn. *Arch. Surg.* 122:784, 1987.

138. Sakata, T., and Englehardt, W. V. Stimulating effect of short-chain fatty acids on the epithelial cell proliferation in the rat large intestine. *Comp. Biochem. Physiol.* 74A:459, 1983.

139. Salusky, I. B., and Fine, R. N. Nutritional factors and progression of chronic renal failure. *Adv. Pediatr.* 33:149, 1986.

140. Seifter, E., Rettura, G., Barbul, A., and Levenson, S. M. Arginine: An essential amino acid for injured rats. *Surgery* 84:224, 1978.

141. Shamberger, R. C., Brennan, M. F., Goodgame, J. T., et al. A prospective randomized study of adjuvant parenteral nutrition in the treatment of sarcomas: Results of metabolic and survival studies. *Surgery* 96:1, 1984.

142. Shizgal, H. M., and Martin, M. F. Caloric requirement of the critically ill septic patient. *Crit. Care Med.* 16:312, 1988.

143. Sitren, H. S., and Fisher, H. Nitrogen retention in rats fed on diets enriched with arginine and glycine. *Br. J. Nutr.* 37:195, 1977.

144. Slater, T. F., Cheeseman, K. H., Davies, M. J., Proudfoot, K., and Xin, W. Free radical mechanisms in relation to tissue injury. *Proc. Nutr. Soc.* 46:1, 1987.

145. Sobrado, J., Moldawer, L. L., Pomposelli, J. J., et al. Lipid emulsions and reticuloendothelial system function in healthy and burned guinea pigs. *Am. J. Clin. Nutr.* 42:855, 1985.

146. Speier, C., Baker, S. S., and Neuburger, P. E. Relationships between in vitro selenium supply, glutathione peroxidase activity, and phagocytic function in the HL-60 human myeloid cell line. *J. Biol. Chem.* 260:8951, 1985.

147. Sperling, R. I., Weinblatt, M., Robin, J. L., et al. Effects of dietary supplementation with marine fish oil on leukocyte lipid mediator generation and function in rheumatoid arthritis. *Arthritis Rheum.* 30:988, 1987.

148. Spitznagel, J. K., and Allison, A. C. Mode of action of adjuvants: Retinol and other lysosome-labilizing agents as adjuvants. *J. Immunol.* 104:119, 1970.

149. Taccone-Gallucci, M., Giardini, O., Ausiello, C., et al. Vitamin E supplementation in hemodialysis patients: Effects on peripheral blood mononuclear cells lipid peroxidation and immune response. *Clin. Nephrol.* 25:81, 1986.

150. Tengerdy, R. P., Heinzerling, R. H., Brown, G. L., and Mathias, M. M. Enhancement of the humoral immune response by vitamin E. *Int. Arch. Allergy Appl. Immunol.* 44:221, 1973.

151. Tengerdy, R. P., Heinzerling, R. H., and Nockels, C. F. Effect of vitamin E on the immune response of hypoxia in normal chickens. *Infect. Immunol.* 5:987, 1972.

152. Terano, T., Salmon, J. A., Higgs, G. A., and Moncada, S. Eicosapentaenoic acid as a modulator of inflammation: Effect on prostaglandin and leukotriene synthesis. *Biochem. Pharmacol.* 35:779, 1986.

153. Thorner, R. E., Barker, C. F., and Mac-Gregor, R. R. Improvement of granulocyte adherence and in vivo granulocyte delivery by ascorbic acid in renal transplant patients. *Transplantation* 35:432, 1983.

154. Trocki, O., Mochizuki, H., Dominioni, L., and Alexander, J. W. Intact protein versus free amino acids in the nutritional support of thermally injured animals. *J. Parenter. Enter. Nutr.* 10:139, 1986.

155. Villa, S., Lorico, A., Morazzoni, G., de Gaetano, G., and Semeraro, N. Vitamin E and vitamin C inhibit arachidonate-induced aggregation of human peripheral blood leukocytes in vitro. *Agents Actions* 19:127, 1986.

156. Weinberg, E. D. Iron withholding: A defense against infection and neoplasia. *Physiol. Rev.* 64:65, 1984.

157. Windmueller, H. G., and Spaeth, A. E. Intestinal metabolism of glutamine and glutamate from the lumen as compared to glutamine from blood. *Arch. Biochem. Biophys.* 171:662, 1975.

158. Windmueller, H. G., and Spaeth, A. E. Identification of ketone bodies and glutamine as the major respiratory fuels *in vivo* for the postabsorptive rat small intestine. *J. Biol. Chem.* 253:69, 1978.

159. Yamazaki, K., Maiz, A., Moldawer, L. L., Bistrian, B. R., and Blackburn, G. L. Complications associated with the overfeeding of infected animals. *J. Surg. Res.* 40:152, 1986.

Index

Index

Parenteral nutrition—*Continued*
  educational programs, 99, 102
  vs. enteral nutrition, 433
  in fistulas, 258
  home. *See* Home parenteral nutrition
  in pediatric patients, 300–317
    Broviac catheter for, 314
    central venous access for, 314
    complications of, 315–317
    hepatobiliary dysfunction and, 315–316
    indications for, 301–304
    requirements, 304–313
      biotin, 312
      electrolytes, 312
      energy, 304–305
      fat, 306–308
      folic acid, 312
      glucose, 305–306
      minerals, 312
      pantothenic acid, 312
      protein, 308–309
      trace elements, 312–313
      vitamins, 309–312
    steatosis and, 316
    subclavian vein catheterization for, 314–315
    technique, 313–315
  peripheral, 389–401
    in burn injuries, 290–291
    clinical implications of, 400–401
    lipid emulsions and, 414
    protein-energy relationship and, 398–400
    protein-sparing effect of, 393–398
    starvation and, 389–392
    stress and, 392–393
    thrombophlebitis and, 290
  total. *See* Total parenteral nutrition
Pectin, 452
Pediatric patients. *See also* Children; Infants; Premature infants
  α_1-antitrypsin deficiency in, 317
  amino acid deficiency in, 316
  body composition, by age, 302–303
  cholestasis in, 316–317
  energy requirements, by age, 304–305
  hyperammonemia in, 51
  hyperbilirubinemia in, 316
  lipid solutions for, 306–308
  parenteral nutrition in, 299–317
    Broviac catheter for, 314
    central venous access for, 314
    complications of, 315–317
    hepatobiliary dysfunction and, 315–316

Pediatric patients—*Continued*
    indications for, 301–304
    requirements, 304–313
      biotin, 312
      electrolytes, 312
      energy, 304–305
      fat, 306–308
      folic acid, 312
      glucose, 305–306
      minerals, 312
      pantothenic acid, 312
      protein, 308–309
      trace elements, 312–313
      vitamins, 309–312
    steatosis and, 316
    subclavian vein catheterization for, 314–315
    technique, 313–315
Pellegra, 312
Penicillin G
  in parenteral nutrition solution, 81
  stability of, 85
Percutaneous endoscopic gastroscomy, 426, 427
  dressing care, 124
Pericardial tamponade, 35
Perioperative support, 9
  in cardiac disease, 204, 205
  in malnourished, 7
Peripheral parenteral nutrition. *See also* Parenteral nutrition; Total parenteral nutrition
  in burn injury, 290–291
  clinical implications of, 400–401
  lipid emulsions and, 414
  protein-energy interrelationship and, 398–400
  protein-sparing effect of, 393–398
  starvation and, 389–392
  stress and, 392–393
  thrombophlebitis and, 290
Pharmacists, educational programs for, 104
Phenylalanine
  in burn injury, 286
  deficiency, 134
  in hepatic encephalopathy, 270
Phosphate
  salts, hypocalcemia and, 48
  supplementation, 61
  ordering, 68
Phosphofructokinase, 158
Physical activity, 185–186
  energy expenditure of, total, 182
  energy requirements and, 154
Physicians
  educational programs for, 103–104

Physicians—*Continued*
  clinical rotations as, 106–107
  preceptorships, 106–107
  nutritional support, 68
Physiologic function
  assessment of, 143–144
  in nutritional assessment, 143–144
  objective evaluation of, 149
  weight loss and, 143–144
Phytohemagglutinin, 131
Phytonadione, in parenteral nutrition solutions, 78
Plasma proteins
  in body composition assessment, 143
  positive nitrogen balance and, 146
  postoperative complications and, 149
Pneumothorax, catheterization and, 33
Polymyxin B
  in parenteral nutrition solutions, 82
  stability of, 85
Polyols, lipid emulsion and, 405
Polysaccharides, fermentable, 452
Polyurethane catheter, venous thrombosis and, 36
Polyvinylchloride bags, vitamin A loss and, 77
Portal hypertension, cirrhosis and, 266
Portal-systemic encephalopathy. *See* Hepatic failure
Portal-systemic shunting, esophageal varices and, 266
Positive end expiratory pressure, 113
Postgastrectomy syndromes, 333
Potassium
  imbalance, 48
  supplementation, 61
    in burn injury, 128
    diuretics and, 208
  total body, measurement of, 327, 328
  total body exchangeable, 327
Prealbumin, 160
  protein support adequacy and, 160
  TPN response and, 224
Pregnancy
  inflammatory bowel disease in, 6
Premature infants. *See also* Infants; Pediatric patients
  body fat in, 299
  cholestasis in, 52
  copper deficiency in, 313